Allergy in Otolaryngology Practice

Cecelia Damask • Matthew Ryan
James W. Mims • Sarah K. Wise
Christine Franzese
Editors

Allergy in Otolaryngology Practice

A Comprehensive Guide

Springer

Editors
Cecelia Damask
Orlando Ear, Nose, Throat & Allergy
Orlando, FL, USA

James W. Mims
Department of Otolaryngology
Wake Forest School of Medicine
Winston-Salem, NC, USA

Christine Franzese
Department of Otolaryngology
University of Missouri
Columbia, MO, USA

Matthew Ryan
Department of Otolaryngology-Head and Neck Surgery
University of Texas Southwestern Medical Center
Dallas, TX, USA

Sarah K. Wise
Department of Otolaryngology
Emory University
Atlanta, GA, USA

ISBN 978-3-031-93454-4 ISBN 978-3-031-93455-1 (eBook)
https://doi.org/10.1007/978-3-031-93455-1

This Springer imprint is published by the registered company Springer Nature Switzerland AG
The registered company address is: Gewerbestrasse 11, 6330 Cham, Switzerland

This book is dedicated to all the allergy patients that have entrusted us with their care.

Preface

Otolaryngologists are uniquely positioned to assess for the presence of allergic disease in patients with upper aerodigestive tract symptoms. Incorporating allergy testing and immunotherapy into the otolaryngology practice allows otolaryngologists to provide comprehensive care to patients and, as an ancillary service, can help build their practice.

Allergy diagnostic testing is one of the first services that can be offered to patients. While a presumptive diagnosis of allergic disease may be made from the patient's history, allergy testing has several important roles. These include confirmation of the clinical diagnosis, identification of the patient's relevant allergen sensitivities, and selection of a safe starting dose for immunotherapy. Several different testing modalities are available. Allergen-specific IgE in the serum can be used as a marker of sensitization. An in vitro-specific IgE test may be accomplished with a simple blood draw and sent out to a reference laboratory. The most commonly employed allergy testing technique is skin testing. A simple prick test performed with an allergen extract and a plastic disposable device can identify preformed allergen-specific IgE via cutaneous mast cell degranulation and the classic "wheal and flare" reaction of the skin. Another technique is to use a small needle to inject diluted allergen into the dermis, looking for a similar reaction (intradermal test). Some practices may choose to incorporate a blended technique of both prick and intradermal tests, commonly known as "modified quantitative testing." Allergy diagnostic testing provides the clinician with important information to aid in clinical decision-making and is a cornerstone in the management of allergic disease. Most otolaryngology practices should be able to add some form of allergy diagnostic testing with minimal investment.

Most patients with allergic rhinitis (AR) are treated with allergen avoidance and pharmacotherapy. However, allergen-specific immunotherapy is the only treatment that addresses the underlying immunologic derangement in allergic disease. Successful immunotherapy decreases symptoms and improves disease-specific quality of life. Immunotherapy achieves these benefits via a variety of mechanisms. It reduces mast cell and basophil degranulation, induces the production of IgG4 "blocking antibody," upregulates tolerogenic regulatory T cell populations, and reduces allergen-specific IgE over the long term. Comprehensive allergy care thus includes allergen-specific immunotherapy.

A variety of immunotherapy options are utilized in practice. The simplest method for allergen-specific immunotherapy is sublingual immunotherapy

(SLIT) using FDA-approved sublingual tablets. These are currently available in the United States for the treatment of grass, ragweed, and dust mite allergy. Another option is SLIT utilizing a customized formulation of aqueous allergen extracts that is based upon clinical determination of a patient's relevant allergen sensitivities. The advantage of this approach is that allergens other than grass, ragweed, and dust mite can be treated.

While SLIT has many advantages, the mainstay of immunotherapy in the United States is subcutaneous injection immunotherapy (SCIT). SCIT has the longest track record of clinical use and has been demonstrated to be effective in multiple randomized placebo-controlled trials. SCIT is FDA approved and covered by most health insurance plans. While SLIT is utilized by many practices in one form or other, most allergy practices utilize SCIT for these reasons.

Otolaryngologists have a variety of reasons for incorporating comprehensive allergy care into their practices. Before initiating these services, a practice should consider its goals as well as the requirements for success.

Like any other decision involving the services offered by one's practice, incorporating allergy care should be undertaken with a business plan in mind. The business plan should include tangible metrics of success: monitoring of referral trends, financials, retention rates of patients, and analyzing patient outcomes. The primary financial investment when starting an allergy practice is the cost of supplies. These include allergen extracts, syringes, testing devices, and emergency supplies (for anaphylaxis treatment). Usually, the existing personnel in a medical office are able take on the new roles required for allergy care. These roles include performance of allergy skin tests, preparation of testing and immunotherapy vials, and administration of immunotherapy. Medical office assistants or nurses are able to perform these duties depending upon individual state regulations. Ultimately, successful allergy practices will have personnel who are completely dedicated to providing these services.

Office space for the allergy practice must also be considered. A location for preparation of allergen extracts needs to be defined as well as space for testing and administration of immunotherapy injections. Because SCIT carries with it a risk for anaphylaxis, a monitored location within the office will need to be designated for patient observation after injections are administered. When beginning an allergy practice, existing office space can be utilized. However, as the practice grows, so will requirements for space. An ideal office environment includes a dedicated check-in desk for allergy patients, a separate waiting room for observation, and an allergenic extract compounding area as well as space for testing multiple patients simultaneously and administering immunotherapy injections.

While office staff perform most of the day-to-day tasks, the physician (or advanced practice provider) is the leader of the team and should be the content expert for every aspect of the allergy practice, including the nuances of testing and immunotherapy, management of allergy emergencies, regulatory and compliance issues, proper billing and coding, and documentation. This responsibility entails considerable investment of time and energy on the part of the physician.

There is never an ideal time to get started on the journey of building an allergy practice. Fortunately, allergy services can be gradually added to what is already being offered to your patients. It's OK to start slowly. Allergy testing is a simple starting point. In vitro testing and skin prick testing are easy to introduce into practice flow. Sublingual immunotherapy tablets are a safe and effective way to begin offering immunotherapy to patients. As you and your staff learn more about allergy and are more comfortable with your knowledge and skills, you can expand to offer a full spectrum of allergy services.

Orlando, FL, USA — Cecelia Damask
Dallas, TX, USA — Matthew Ryan
Winston-Salem, NC, USA — James W. Mims
Atlanta, GA, USA — Sarah K. Wise
Columbia, MO, USA — Christine Franzese

Contents

About the Editors and Contributors[1]

About the Editors

Cecelia Damask is in private clinical practice in Orlando, Florida.

Christine Franzese is a Professor of Otolaryngology and Allergy Medical Director at the University of Missouri.

James W. Mims is a Professor of Otolaryngology at Wake Forest University School of Medicine.

Matthew Ryan is a Professor of Otolaryngology—Head & Neck Surgery at UT Southwestern Medical Center.

Sarah K. Wise is a Professor of Otolaryngology Head and Neck Surgery at Emory University School of Medicine.

Contributors

Farrukh Abbas Department of Pulmonary and Critical Care Medicine, Virginia Commonwealth University Health System, Richmond, VA, USA

Omar G. Ahmed Department of Otolaryngology-Head & Neck Surgery, University of Wisconsin School of Medicine and Public Health, Madison, WI, USA
Division of Rhinology & Skull Base Surgery, Department of Otolaryngology, Houston Methodist Hospital, Houston, TX, USA

Alicia A. Alvarez Sarasota Memorial Health Care System, FL, Sarasota, USA

Mark Arnold Department of Otolaryngology at Upstate Medical University, Syracuse, NY, USA

[1]The editors have a passion for allergy education. The editors have been teaching otolaryngologists how to incorporate allergy care into their practices for over 20 years.

Michael S. Benninger Department of Otolaryngology-Head and Neck Surgery, Cleveland Clinic Lerner College of Medicine, Head and Neck Institute, The Cleveland Clinic, Cleveland, OH, USA

J. Andrew Bird Division of Allergy and Immunology, University of Texas Southwestern Medical Center, Dallas, TX, USA

Christopher D. Brook Division of Otolaryngology, Head & Neck Surgery, Beth Israel Deaconess Medical Centre, Harvard Medical School, Boston, MA, USA

Edward G. Brooks Department of Pediatrics, Division of Immunology and Infectious Disease, The University of Texas Health Science Center at San Antonio, San Antonio, TX, USA

Mary Catherine Brown South Florida ENT Associates, Miami Lakes, FL, USA

Jeffrey M. Chambliss UT Southwestern Medical Center, Dallas, TX, USA

Sei Y. Chung, MD Department of Otolaryngology – Head and Neck Surgery, The University of Texas Southwestern Medical Center, Dallas, TX, USA

David Danis Department of Otolaryngology - Head and Neck Surgery, Boston University School of Medicine, Boston, MA, USA

John M. DelGaudio Department of Otolaryngology, Emory University, Atlanta, GA, USA

Sofia Ellen Edwards-Salmon Allergy & Immunology Fellow, PGY-5, Emory University School of Medicine, Atlanta, GA, USA

Thomas S. Edwards Department of Otolaryngology, Emory University, Atlanta, GA, USA

Ibon Eguiluz-Gracia Allergy Unit, Hospital Regional Universitario de Málaga. IBIMA-Plataforma BIONAND. RICORS Inflammatory Diseases, Málaga, Spain

Gary A. Falcetano ImmunoDiagnostics Division, U.S. Clinical Affairs Manager – Allergy, Portage, MI, USA

Amanda Gemmiti Otolaryngology-Head and Neck Surgery, SUNY Upstate Medical Center, Syracuse, NY, USA

W. Adam Gower Department of Pediatrics, Division of Pulmonary Medicine, University of North Carolina School of Medicine, Chapel Hill, NC, USA

Samuel N. Helman Department of Otolaryngology, Emory University, Atlanta, GA, USA

Jennifer L. Hsiao Department of Dermatology, University of Southern California, Los Angeles, CA, USA

Kelsey Ige Department of Pediatrics, Allergy and Asthma Medical Group of the Bay Area, Brentwood, CA, USA

Shyam Joshi Section of Allergy and Immunology, Oregon Health and Science University, Portland, OR, USA

Merin Kuruvilla (Kalangara) Division of Allergy/Immunology, Emory University School of Medicine, Atlanta, GA, USA

Rebecca J. Kamil Department of Otolaryngology-Head and Neck Surgery, Johns Hopkins University School of Medicine, Baltimore, MD, USA

Alissa Kanaan South Florida ENT Associates, Miami Lakes, FL, USA

Sandhya Khurana Pulmonary and Critical Care Medicine, University of Rochester School of Medicine, Rochester, NY, USA

Stella E. Lee, MD Division of Sinonasal Disorders and Allergy, Department of Otolaryngology-Head & Neck Surgery, Brigham and Women's Hospital, Boston, MA, USA

Joshua M. Levy Department of Otolaryngology-Head and Neck Surgery, Emory University School of Medicine, Atlanta, GA, USA

Andrea F. Lewis Department of Otolaryngology and Communicative Sciences, University of Mississippi Medical Center, Jackson, MS, USA

Sandra Y. Lin Department of Otolaryngology-Head & Neck Surgery, University of Wisconsin School of Medicine and Public Health, Madison, WI, USA

Michael Lopez Division of Internal Medicine, Scripps Clinic, San Diego, CA, USA

Ceila E. Loughlin Department of Pediatrics, Division of Pulmonary Medicine, University of North Carolina School of Medicine, Chapel Hill, NC, USA

Bradley F. Marple, MD Department of Otolaryngology – Head and Neck Surgery, The University of Texas Southwestern Medical Center, Dallas, TX, USA

Haidy Marzouk Otolaryngology-Head and Neck Surgery, SUNY Upstate Medical Center and Saint Joseph's Health, Syracuse, NY, USA

James W. Mims Department of Otolaryngology, Wake Forest School of Medicine, Winston-Salem, NC, USA

Yew Kwang Ong Department of Otolaryngology – Head and Neck Surgery, Singapore, Singapore

Michael Parker Department of Otolaryngology and Communication Sciences, State University of New York Upstate Medical University, Syracuse, NY, USA

Christopher P. Parrish Division of Allergy and Immunology, University of Texas Southwestern Medical Center, Dallas, TX, USA

Rohan Patel Otolaryngology-Head and Neck Surgery, SUNY Upstate Medical Center, Syracuse, NY, USA

Vijay A. Patel, MD Division of Pediatric Otolaryngology, Rady Children's Hospital - San Diego, San Diego, CA, USA
Department of Otolaryngology - Head and Neck Surgery, University of California San Diego, La Jolla, CA, USA

Katie M. Phillips Otolaryngology - Head & Neck Surgery, University of Cincinnati, Cincinnati, OH, USA

Michael Platt Department of Otolaryngology - Head and Neck Surgery, Boston University School of Medicine, Boston, MA, USA
Boston Medical Center, Boston, MA, USA

Murugappan Ramanathan Jr Division of Rhinology and Endoscopic Skull Base Surgery, Department of Otolaryngology-HNS, Johns Hopkins University School of Medicine, Baltimore, MD, USA

Uma S. Ramaswamy, MD Pediatric Otolaryngology-Head & Neck Surgery, Texas Children's Hospital, Houston, TX, USA

Courtney Ramos Division of Allergy, Asthma, and Immunology, Scripps Clinic, San Diego, CA, USA

Mallory J. Raymond Department of Otolaryngology-Head and Neck Surgery, Mayo Clinic, Jacksonville, FL, USA

William R. Reisacher Department of Otolaryngology – Head and Neck Surgery, Weill Cornell Medical College / NewYork-Presbyterian Hospital, New York, NY, USA

Carmen Rondón Allergy Unit, Hospital Regional Universitario de Málaga. IBIMA-Plataforma BIONAND. RICORS Inflammatory Diseases, Málaga, Spain

Matthew Ryan Department of Otolaryngology-Head and Neck Surgery, University of Texas Southwestern Medical Center, Dallas, TX, USA

Jennifer N. Shehan Department of Otolaryngology, Boston Medical Centre, Boston, MA, USA

Brandon Shepherd Mid-South Ear, Nose, Throat P.C., Jackson, MS, USA

Farrah N. Siddiqui Department of Otolaryngology, The University of Texas Medical Branch, Galveston, TX, USA

Venkataramana K. Sidhaye Division of Pulmonary Medicine, Johns Hopkins University School of Medicine, Baltimore, MD, USA

Triphoom Suwanwech Department of Otorhinolaryngology, Faculty of Medicine, Siriraj Hospital, Mahidol University, Bangkok, Thailand

Almudena Testera-Montes Allergy Unit, Hospital Regional Universitario de Málaga. IBIMA-Plataforma BIONAND. RICORS Inflammatory Diseases, Málaga, Spain

Andrew Vaughn Lake Cumberland Medical Associates ENT, Medical Clinic in Somerset, Somerset, KY, USA

Maria C. Veling UT Southwestern Medical Center, Children's Medical Center Dallas, Dallas, TX, USA

Natalie M. Villa Department of Dermatology, Dartmouth Hitchcock Medical Center, Lebanon, NH, USA

Jennifer A. Villwock Department of Otolaryngology – Head and Neck Surgery, University of Kansas Medical Center, Kansas City, KS, USA

Hannah Wangberg Division of Allergy, Asthma, and Immunology, Scripps Clinic, San Diego, CA, USA

De Yun Wang Department of Otolaryngology, Yong Loo Lin School of Medicine, National University of Singapore, Singapore, Singapore

Duncan C. Watley Department of Otolaryngology, The University of Texas Medical Branch, Galveston, TX, USA

Andrew A. White Division of Allergy, Asthma, and Immunology, Scripps Clinic, San Diego, CA, USA

Sarah K. Wise Department of Otolaryngology, Emory University, Atlanta, GA, USA

Xinni Xu Department of Otolaryngology – Head and Neck Surgery, National University Hospital, Singapore, Singapore

Part I

Introduction

Edited by Cecelia Damask

1 Allergy in Otolaryngology Practice, a Comprehensive Guide

Sei Y. Chung and Bradley F. Marple

The concept of allergy evolved through the nineteenth and early twentieth centuries as the result of clinical observation, personal experiences, and a considerable amount of loosely structured individual experimentation. It was by way of this early "experimentation" that the first in vivo demonstration of an allergic reaction was reported in 1921 [1]. Carl Prausnitz injected his own abdominal skin with serum from his colleague, Heinz Küstner. After a short period of time, Prausnitz developed a wheal and flare response at the injection site after ingestion of fish, a food to which Küstner was known to be allergic. Although we now appreciate this to represent classic "IgE-mediated Type I" hypersensitivity, the pathophysiologic mechanisms underlying this response would not be understood for several decades after Prausnitz and Küstner reported their findings. Although progress in understanding allergy and its treatment was not held to the same scientific rigor expected of today's novel medical interventions, it nevertheless advanced appreciably during the first half of the twentieth century. Antigen-specific immunotherapy was introduced in 1914 [2]. Antihistamines were first used in the 1930s [3]. Subsequently, IgE was identified in the 1960s, setting the stage for our current understanding of the allergic response [4]. While much of allergy and immunology has been attributed to other medical disciplines, the field of Otolaryngology has played a critical and sustained role in the treatment of this disease from the beginning.

As the scope of many medical specialties began to broaden during the post-World War II era, a large segment of Otolaryngology remained surgical in nature [4]. There was, however, a small group of Otolaryngologists who recognized the importance of allergy, and began incorporating it into their practice and teachings. French Hansel, who later became recognized as the father of Otolaryngic allergy, began expanding the study of this field at Washington University of St. Louis [4]. Among his numerous contributions, he observed the presence of mucosal eosinophils and plasma cells in allergic patients, as well as established the concept of dilutional titration for both allergy testing and treatment [4]. Understanding the significance of his early work, he established an allergy clinic within the department of Otolaryngology. The care provided through this clinic helped to lay the groundwork for safe antigen-specific immunotherapy that has endured to this day [4]. His work attracted many other prominent Otolaryngologists throughout the country who began to appreciate the

S. Y. Chung · B. F. Marple (✉)
Department of Otolaryngology – Head and Neck Surgery, The University of Texas Southwestern Medical Center, Dallas, TX, USA
e-mail: sei.chung@utsouthwestern.edu; bradley.marple@utsouthwestern.edu

C. Damask et al. (eds.), *Allergy in Otolaryngology Practice*,
https://doi.org/10.1007/978-3-031-93455-1_1

importance of integrating allergy into their respective practices. One such example of this was Dr. Howard House, who took interest in French Hansel's practice and recognized the potential impact of allergy upon the pathogenesis of a subset of his otologic patients [4]. In short order, Dr. Hansel's approach to allergy evaluation and treatment became a critical component in the management of patients seen at the famed House Ear Clinic in Los Angeles.

As allergy became more widely taught to Otolaryngology trainees, students of Dr. Hansel established a society of Otolaryngic Allergy in 1941, which later became known as the American Academy of Otolaryngic Allergy (AAOA) [4]. By the 1970s, the American Medical Association issued an official statement that recognized allergy as a regular part of Otolaryngic practice, and that residency training should include care of allergic patients. In 1977, the AAOA established its own fellowship examination, much of which also appeared on the American Board of Otolaryngology Examination [4]. Since then, allergy has formally remained a crucial aspect of Otolaryngology.

Today, a typical Otolaryngic practice involves caring for a large variety of inflammatory disorders of the upper airway. In many instances, the clinician is faced with recognition and management of irritative symptoms of inhalant or food allergies. However, there are several other Otolaryngic syndromes and disorders in which allergy plays a primary causative role or exists as a secondary contributing factor. Because allergic disease is so pervasive, the contemporary practice of Otolaryngology—Head and Neck Surgery requires recognition of allergy in the management of many conditions.

An allergic patient with sensitization to inhalant antigen(s) is a common scenario encountered by the Otolaryngologist. Although still far from completely understood, the pathophysiology of this allergic response is better comprehended than ever before. At a very basic level, development of a Type I Gell-Coombs reaction requires multiple steps. First, repeated exposure to an antigen is required to develop sensitization—a state in which a susceptible host begins to produce antigen-specific IgE in amounts sufficient to elicit a classic allergic response. After sensitization, subsequent exposure to the same agent will give rise to mast cell degranulation, resulting in release of pre-formed inflammatory mediators (e.g., mast cells, histamine, basophils, prostaglandins). These mediators lead to a series of end-organ responses such as increased glandular secretion, vasodilation, capillary leakage, and nerve stimulation, giving rise to characteristic symptomatology including rhinorrhea, nasal congestion, pruritus, and sneezing. The Otolaryngologist should be attuned to this mechanism that results in the hallmark signs of the early and late phase allergic response, as patients often may mistake these symptoms for respiratory infections or other inflammatory conditions.

Correct diagnosis and management of food sensitivities can be less obvious, and frequently requires careful evaluation by an experienced clinician. Food allergies or sensitivities can be acute, or delayed in nature. The former is typically identified easily by patients because they experience an immediate allergic reaction shortly after ingestion of a particular food. This patient response is typically IgE-mediated (classic Type I Gell-Coombs allergic mechanism), giving rise to its greater severity and more immediate temporal association with the food exposure.

The role that allergy may play in the development of chronic rhinosinusitis (CRS) has been a subject of great interest. Many of the inflammatory mechanisms in allergic rhinitis (AR) are recognized to also underlie endotypes of inflammatory CRS, which has historically resulted in a presumed causal link between allergy and rhinologic disorders. However, this relationship has proven to be complex. Numerous studies have demonstrated an epidemiologic coexistence of allergic diseases and inflammatory CRS, but attempts to improve inflammatory CRS through management of inhalant AR have shown little impact. For example, this has been observed in allergic fungal rhinosinusitis (AFRS) [5]. Sensitivity to fungal antigens is recognized as one of the hallmarks of AFRS. It therefore stood to reason that fungal-specific immunotherapy might play an important role in the treatment of

AFRS. Early investigations showed promise for this approach but failed to provide definitive evidence due to flaws in study design [5]. With time, at least one long-term, controlled, comparative trial demonstrated immunotherapy offered no clinical benefit in eventual outcome [6]. In the end, systematic review of the literature failed to support immunotherapy for the treatment of AFRS as anything more than an option with equal benefit to harm [7]. The example offered by our AFRS experience can generally be extrapolated to that of CRS, at present. And although there does not seem to be a consistent, causal association between allergy and CRS, this relationship continues to be explored through recently recognized phenotypes of CRS, such as such as the concept of central compartment atopic disease [8].

Symptoms of allergy may also overlap with those of other disorders impacting the larynx and esophagus, further muddling the clinical picture. Such allergy patients may present already attributing their symptoms to a laryngologic disorder, particularly if symptoms such as cough, throat clearing, post-nasal drainage, and hoarseness are most prominent. Thus, it is important to be able to recognize and discern the various influences allergy may have on these types of symptoms [9].

The impact of allergy on otologic disease is perhaps more nuanced and varied than any other Otolaryngic domain. For example, an allergic etiology of chronic otitis externa should be considered when the condition has been refractory to intensive treatment. Such patients may have allergic contact dermatitis (a Type IV Gell-Coombs hypersensitivity reaction) to metals, chemicals/cosmetics, rubber, leather, and other contact triggers [10, 11]. In some instances, the patient may be sensitized to a medication or preservative used in the topical treatment of otitis externa, such as neomycin, benzalkonium chloride, thiomersal, propylene glycol, and sorbitol [10]. Although observational studies provide low-grade evidence of e some relationship of allergy to middle ear disease as well, such as chronic otitis media, particularly the serous subtype [12, 13],high-level evidence does not support that allergy treatment is effective in resolving OME [14]. This pattern is especially observed in children. A direct causative relationship between allergy and chronic otitis media largely remains elusive [12]. In inner ear pathology, observational studies have found associations between Meniere's disease and allergy, however no data to date supports reflexive allergy testing and treatment in Meniere's disease patients without a concurrent history of allergies [14–16].

Careful review of the literature suggests that a number of disparate disease processes may serve as cofactors leading to the ultimate development of inflammatory conditions involving the structures of the head and neck. Furthermore, epidemiologic studies suggest that allergic inflammation may be associated with the development of various forms of these diseases, and its recognition and management may impact the ultimate treatment paradigms for these diseases. It is becoming increasingly apparent that the contemporary Otolaryngologist can no longer rely simply on either technical surgical skills or cognitive non-surgical skills alone to treat these patients. Instead, to be most effective, Otolaryngologists must synthesize diagnostic and treatment plans utilizing all aspects of our discipline. Whether a general Otolaryngologist or sub-specialized Otolaryngologist, a thorough knowledge of allergy will allow the clinician to understand each patient in a more comprehensive way and provide more complete care.

References

1. Cohen SG, Zelaya-Quesada M. Prausnitz and Küstner phenomenon: the PK reaction. J Allergy Clin Immunol. 2004;114(3):705–10.
2. Cooke RA. The treatment of hay fever by active immunization. Laryngoscope. 1915;25:108–12.
3. Emanuel MB. Histamine and the antiallergic antihistamines: a history of their discoveries. Clin Exp Allergy. 1999;29(Suppl 3):1–11.
4. Krouse JH, Chadwick SJ, Gordon BR, Derebery J. Allergy and immunology: an otolaryngic approach. Lippincott Williams & Wilkins; 2002.

5. Folker RJ, Marple BF, Mabry RL, Mabry CS. Treatment of allergic fungal sinusitis: a comparison trial of postoperative immunotherapy with specific fungal antigens. Laryngoscope. 1998;108:1623–7.
6. Marple B, Newcomer M, Schwade N, Mabry R. Natural history of allergic fungal rhinosinusitis: a 4- to 10-year follow-up. Otolaryngol Head Neck Surg. 2002;127:361–6.
7. Gan EC, et al. Medical management of allergic fungal rhinosinusitis following endoscopic sinus surgery: an evidence-based review and recommendations. Int Forum Allergy Rhinol. 2014;4:702–15.
8. DelGaudio JM, Loftus PA, Hamizan AW, Harvey RJ, Wise SK. Central compartment atopic disease. Am J Rhinol Allergy. 2017;31:228–34.
9. Chadwick SJ. Allergy and the contemporary laryngologist. Otolaryngol Clin N Am. 2003;36:957–88.
10. Sood S, Strachan DR, Tsikoudas A, Stables GI. Allergic otitis externa. Clin Otolaryngol Allied Sci. 2002;27:233–6.
11. Osguthorpe JD, Nielsen DR. Otitis externa: review and clinical update. S Afr Fam Pract. 2006;53(3):223–9.
12. Kreiner-Møller E, Chawes BLK, Caye-Thomasen P, Bønnelykke K, Bisgaard H. Allergic rhinitis is associated with otitis media with effusion: a birth cohort study. Clin Exp Allergy. 2012;42:1615–20.
13. Doyle WJ. The link between allergic rhinitis and otitis media. Curr Opin Allergy Clin Immunol. 2002;2:21–5.
14. Wise SK, Damask C, Roland LT, Ebert C, et al. International consensus statement on allergy and rhinology: allergic rhinitis – 2023. Int Forum Allergy Rhinol. 2023;13:293. https://doi.org/10.1002/alr.23090.
15. Derebery MJ. The role of allergy in Meniere's disease. Otolaryngol Clin N Am. 1997;30:1007–16.
16. Weinreich HM, Agrawal Y. The link between allergy and Menière's disease. Curr Opin Otolaryngol Head Neck Surg. 2014;22:227–30.

The Unified Airway

2

Hannah Wangberg, Courtney Ramos,
Michael Lopez, and Andrew A. White

Disclaimer

HW—no conflicts of interest
CR—no conflicts of interest
ML—no conflicts of interest
AW—Speakers Bureau—Regeneron/Sanofi, Astra Zeneca; Consultant—Astra-Zeneca, Regenerson, Optinose, ALK
Figure Artist: Catherine Cichon, MD, MPH
Regeneron/Sanofi – Speaker, Advisory board, Research Support
Amgen – Speaker
AstraZeneca – Speaker, Advisory Board
Blueprint – Speaker, Advisory Board
Genentech – Speaker
Elsevier – Clinical Key Editorial Board
GSK – Speaker, Advisory Board
Optinose – Speaker, Advisory Board

H. Wangberg · C. Ramos · A. A. White (✉)
Division of Allergy, Asthma, and Immunology, Scripps Clinic, San Diego, CA, USA
e-mail: Wangberg.Hannah@scrippshealth.org; Ramos.Courtney@scrippshealth.org; White.Andrew@scrippshealth.org

M. Lopez
Division of Internal Medicine, Scripps Clinic, San Diego, CA, USA
e-mail: malopez1@hs.uci.edu

Introduction

The Unified Airway

The human respiratory tract serves as a passageway for air as it shuttles critical gases such as oxygen (O_2) and carbon dioxide (CO_2) to and from the bloodstream. Conceptually, the respiratory tract has classically been subcategorized into the upper and lower airway. The upper airway consists of the paranasal sinuses, nares, oropharynx, pharynx, and larynx. The lower airway comprises the structures below the vocal cords including the trachea, bronchi, bronchioles, and alveolar structures. Despite these distinct anatomic classifications, the upper airway and lower airway do not functionally operate as separate entities. Therefore, in recent decades, the concept of the "unified airway" has gained traction—a model which highlights the interconnectedness of the human respiratory tract.

Epidemiology

Epidemiologically, there is a clear link between disorders of the upper and lower airway [1, 2]. Allergic rhinitis (AR) and nonallergic rhinitis (NAR) are both associated with a significantly increased risk of developing asthma [2–4]. Prevalence data suggests that 80% of asthmatics

C. Damask et al. (eds.), *Allergy in Otolaryngology Practice*,
https://doi.org/10.1007/978-3-031-93455-1_2

have rhinitis, a significantly increased risk relative to the general population [1, 5]. The interrelationship between these two disorders is so strong that some have coined their co-occurrence "combined allergic rhinitis and asthma syndrome" (CARAS) [6]. In patients with chronic rhinosinusitis (CRS), there is also an increased incidence of asthma relative to the general population (20% vs 5–8%, respectively) [7]. Noninfectious rhinitis was also found to be more common in a COPD population when compared with non-COPD subjects [8]. Additionally, optimized medical or surgical management of CRS has been shown to improve pulmonary outcomes [9]. Aspirin-exacerbated respiratory disease (AERD) patients present with the triad of nasal polyposis, asthma, and aspirin sensitivity. This can be found in 14.9% of severe asthmatics and 9.7% of patients with nasal polyps [10]. Cystic fibrosis (CF) is yet another disorder with an inextricable association between upper and lower airway pathology. In CF, nearly 100% of patients develop CRS which in turn contributes to the bacterial colonization and bronchiectasis of the lower airway [11, 12].

While not historically classified as part of the respiratory tract, the middle ear has been included in recent models of the unified airway [5]. The middle ear is connected to the nasopharynx (and thus, the upper airway) through the eustachian tube. One study showed that in children with persistent otitis media with effusion (OME), AR was present in 89% of these patients [13]. Patients with OME also have been found to have increased prevalence of asthma relative to healthy individuals [14]. In 15 subjects with eosinophilic otitis media and asthma, step up in asthma therapy was associated with improvement in peripheral eosinophil counts as well as inner ear symptoms [15]. These examples all support the existence of a critical relationship uniting the upper and lower airway.

Immunopathogenesis

Diseases of the upper and lower airway often share a unified immunopathogenesis. In both allergic rhinitis and allergic asthma, a type two (T2) inflammatory endotype is observed. The mucosa of both the upper and lower airways are flooded with eosinophils, mast cells, and other markers of T2 inflammation [16]. In atopic patients, allergen exposure in either the upper or lower airway broadly increases the inflammatory response in distant regions of the airway while simultaneously increasing systemic circulation of blood eosinophils and other inflammatory cell mediators such as IL-5 [16–18]. The chronic inflammation in AR, CRS, and asthma may lead to long-term remodeling of the upper and lower airway including increased mucus secretion and thickening of the basement membrane [19]. Nasal polyp development has recently been associated with fibrinolytic impairment specifically elevation in thrombin-activatable fibrinolysis inhibitor (TAFI) which is also elevated in asthma [20]. CF patients typically develop concomitant CRS and bronchiectasis (upper and lower airway disorders, respectively) which are exacerbated by identical colonies of pathologic bacteria in the upper and lower airway [21].

It is apparent that upper and lower airway disorders often share an integrated anatomy, epidemiology, and immunopathogenesis. This supports the notion of "one airway, one disease." The purpose of this chapter will be to review the impact of the unified airway model in humans.

Impact of the Upper Airway on the Lower Airway

The upper airway profoundly influences the lower airway function (Table 2.1). One means through which it does this is protecting the lower airway from various insults by warming, humidifying, and filtering inspired air [6]. Cold air is known to trigger bronchoconstriction, so heating air through the nose is imperative to avoid this adverse lower airway response [22]. The human nose provides a significant amount of heat which can raise the temperature of inspired air closer to body temperature. Therefore, nasal breathing is imperative to maintain pulmonary function [23]. Additionally, the humidification of inspired air

Table 2.1 Interactions in the unified airway

Interactions in the unified airway	
Upper airway influence on lower airway	
Upper airway process	***Lower airway response***
Warming, filtering, and humidification of air	Optimized gas exchange
Cold air in upper airway	Bronchoconstriction (possibly through activation on the TRPM8 channel)
Nasal obstruction (CRS, rhinitis, nasal polyp)	Bronchoconstriction
Upper airway allergen exposure (AR)	Inflammatory response (T2 high)
Poorly controlled rhinitis	Increased risk of asthma exacerbations
Dysbiosis of nasopharyngeal microbiome	Increased risk of wheezing in childhood
Cystic fibrosis—Bacteria "seed" lower airway	Bronchiectasis or pneumonia
Chronic inflammation from AR, NAR, CRS	Lower airway remodeling
AERD—Bulky nasal polyposis	Enhanced NSAID-triggered respiratory responses
AERD—Surgical removal of nasal polyposis	Reduced lower airway reactions during aspirin challenge and desensitization
Bitter taste receptor activation	Nitric oxide (NO) production
Lower airway influence on upper airway	
Lower airway process	***Upper airway response***
Chronic lower airway disease	Worsening SNOT-22 scores in CRS patients
Bronchial antigen exposure in patients with asthma and AR	Inflammatory response (T2 high)
Impaired mucociliary clearance (CF, primary ciliary dyskinesia, etc.)	Sinus hypoplasia
Bronchoprovocation of lower airway (with histamine, mannitol)	Laryngeal reactivity
Quorum sensing bitter taste receptor	Under investigation

occurs in the nose and the mouth as air is exposed to the moist mucous membranes of the upper airway. The point at which inspired air reaches body temperature (37 °C) and 100% relative humidity is known as the isothermic saturation boundary and typically occurs near the carina [24]. This warming and humidification of inspired air optimizes gas exchange in the alveoli. The upper airway also serves to filter potentially hazardous material from entering the lower airway and impairing gas exchange. Particles with aerodynamic equivalent diameters >15 μm are deposited in the upper respiratory tract, thus protecting the lower airway from this material [6].

The upper airway's impact on the lower airway isn't always protective. As early as the 1960s it was shown by Ogura et al. that nasal obstruction increases pulmonary resistance and bronchoconstriction [25]. Rhinitis, CRS, and nasal polyposis are disorders of nasal inflammatory obstruction, and indeed, poorly controlled rhinitis has been associated with an increased risk of asthma exacerbations [26]. Additionally, rhinitis results in increased bronchial hyperreactivity even in individuals without a former diagnosis of asthma [27, 28]. A retrospective cohort study showed that both allergic and non-allergic rhinitis were significantly associated with 30-day hospital readmission rates for asthma and COPD with hazard ratios between 2.4 and 4.4 [29]. Nasal allergen challenge increases airway responsiveness, ICAM-1 expression, induced sputum eosinophilia as well as infiltrating eosinophils in the bronchial epithelium and lamina propria [17, 30]. These findings are consistent with Oruga et al.'s initial studies and highlight the adverse influence upper airway pathology may have on the lower airways. Therefore, treatment of rhinitis, CRS, and nasal polyposis with standard medical management and/or surgical intervention likely has benefit for the lower airway function.

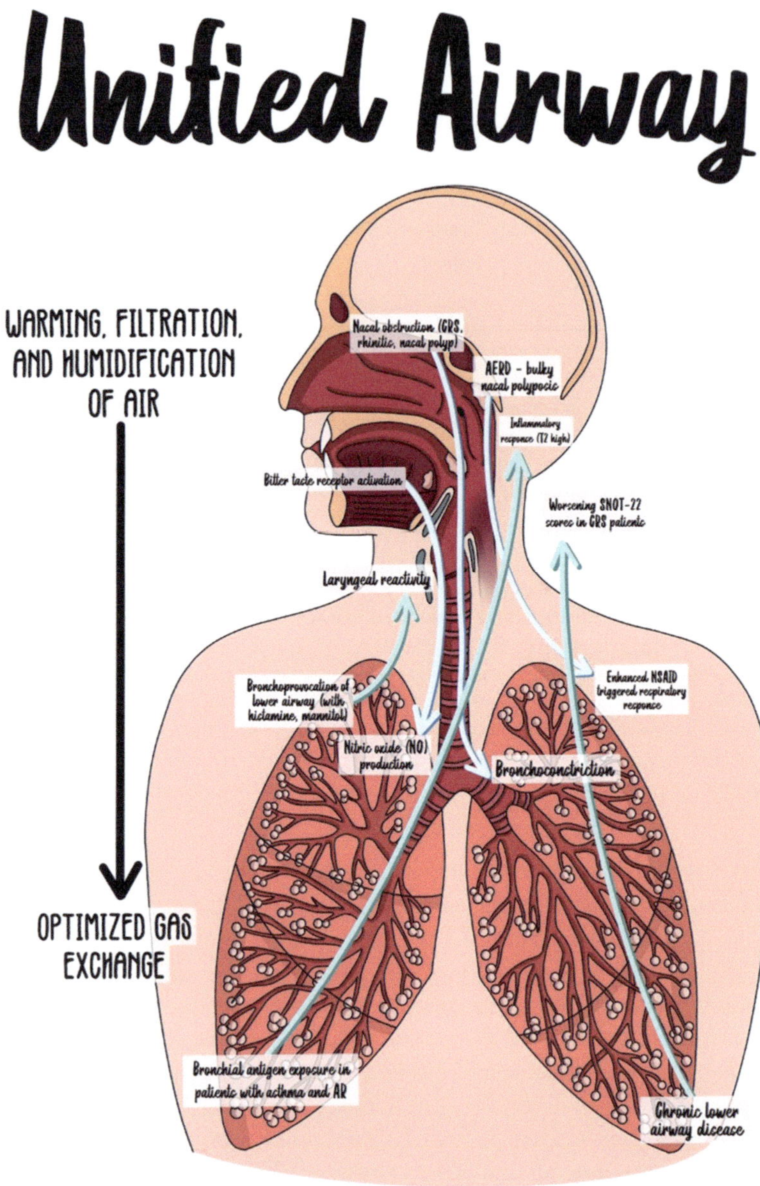

Fig. 2.1 Interactions in the unified airway. (Artwork by Catherine Cichon, MD, MPH)

Impact of the Lower Airway on the Upper Airway

The lower airway also holds significant influence on the upper airway. Among patients with CRS, it has been shown that the presence of chronic lower airway disease such as asthma or COPD led to significantly increased upper airway symptoms and SNOT-22 scores [31, 32]. In individuals with AR without a diagnosis of asthma, segmental bronchial antigen exposure led to increased mast cell and basophil numbers in the nasal mucosa [18, 27]. Impaired mucociliary clearance of the lower respiratory tract as occurs in diseases such as CF, Kartagener syndrome, and primary ciliary dyskinesia has been associated with sinus hypoplasia, though it is unclear if this relationship is causal or corollary [33]. Indeed, the lower airway has clear impact on the function of the upper airway (Fig. 2.1).

Microbiota of the Unified Airway

Microbiome

Dysbiosis refers to an abnormal microbial community associated with the disease. It is often unknown whether the dysbiosis drives the disorder or whether it occurs as a consequence of the disease. Although the microbiome of the gastrointestinal tract has garnered most attention, studies in the past decade have explored the role of the biome in the airway.

Beginning in infancy, a cycle of repeated upper respiratory viral infections can lead to alteration in the nasopharyngeal microbiome. Yet, these shifts in the biome can precede wheezing episodes, suggesting a causal role in the progression of early childhood wheezing [34]. Furthermore, specific nasopharyngeal microbiome profiles were associated with severity of respiratory illness severity regardless of specific viral pathogen [35].

In a study of severe asthmatics, bronchial brushings were significantly enriched for Actinobacteria members when compared with mild asthmatics. In matched airway epithelial gene expression microarray analysis, there were positive associations with transcriptional evidence of corticosteroid response and Th17 expression. This study also identified that in severe asthmatics, body mass index was strongly associated with Bacteroidetes and Firmicutes [36].

Microbiome and Sinusitis

Mahdavinia and colleagues examined adult CRS patients via middle meatus swabs. Corynebacterium and Peptonophilus were depleted in CRS when compared with controls. Utilizing PiCRUST, a software tool that predicts functional consequences of microbial communities, the authors identified lipopolysaccharide biosynthesis and epithelial cell invasion as two important pathways for further exploration [37].

In the unified airway, loss of microbial diversity in one anatomic location could have inflammatory consequences in a separate distant airway component. It is really only in the early childhood wheezing cohorts where nasopharyngeal diversity has been associated with lower airway outcomes. Much more work will be necessary to tie the microbiome into the unified airway model.

Taste Receptors and the Unified Airway

Intriguing work in the past decade has identified a role for taste receptors beyond that of their canonical function transmitting various gustatory sensations neurologically to the brain. A broadening role for these receptors in both the upper and lower airway is now appreciated to have effects on innate immunity and specifically in pathways activating type 2 immunity.

Bitter taste is mediated through the Taste Receptor 2 (T2R) family of approximately 25 isoforms [38]. A great deal of redundancy exists within this family of receptors, which may be activated by denatonium, strychnine, and others [39]. Among the earliest interactions with our sinonasal mucosa, pathogens and other airborne stimuli encounter mucus, ciliated respiratory epithelium, and bitter taste receptors. Bitter taste receptors sense acyl-homoserine lactones (AHLs), which are produced by many gram-negative bacteria and serve to induce biofilm formation at high enough concentrations [40]. Bitter taste receptors detect these AHLs and cause downstream nitric oxide (NO) production. NO has antimicrobial functions and may increase the ciliary beat frequency, ultimately leading to a potent innate mechanism for clearance of bacteria [41].

Bitter taste receptors are on ciliated respiratory epithelia, but also occur on a specialized cell known as a solitary chemosensory cell. These cells sense AHL and other bitter agonists, but rather than simulating NO production, acetylcholine release stimulates the trigeminal nerve and subsequent mediator release [42]. Dose-dependent inhibition of this process by glucose and sucrose has been observed. This creates a situation where bacteria consume sugars and create bitter taste agonists—a scenario which augments the antimicrobial process outlined above.

T2R38, an isoform in the T2R family, is encoded by the locus TAS2R38. A well-described polymorphism in this gene renders patients unable to taste propylthiouracil (PTU) [43]. Patients homozygous for a nonfunctional polymorphism (AVI/AVI) are unable to taste PTU, but also have a dramatically attenuated NO response to a bitter taste agonist. Those with wild type (PAV/PAV) are able to taste and have preserved function through this receptor. In patients with CRS with a "nontaster" phenotype, a correlation with worse outcomes after sinus surgery has been seen. This demonstrates the clinical relevance of this receptor specifically in patients with upper airway disease.

In separate work, the solitary chemosensory cells have been identified as a source of interleukin 25 (IL-25). In a mouse model, after allergen stimulation, airway brush cells (chemosensory cells) expand in response to cysteinyl leukotrienes, specifically through the CysLT3 receptor. Subsequent airway inflammation was dependent on IL-25. This cytokine along with TSLP and IL-33 plays a critical role in initiating an inflammatory signal through ILC2 cells among other innate cells culminating in a potent type 2 inflammatory process [44].

Similar chemosensory cells can be found in the trachea and larynx, where stimulation may influence respiratory rate and enhance airway clearance. Evidence for a "quorum sensing" bitter taste receptor in the lower airways analogous to what has been well characterized in the sinonasal cavities is developing.

These findings identify a unified system of modified taste receptors acting as sentinels of the entire respiratory tract. This system provides immediate feedback to cilia, mucociliary clearance, has an antimicrobial effect, and has the capability to initiate a more systemic and orchestrated immune response through IL-25 culminating in upregulated type 2 inflammation. Modification of these sensors through pharmacologic intervention may provide additional treatment options in many common airway diseases such as chronic rhinosinusitis and asthma.

Larynx

The larynx is not always discussed in the context of the unified airway. The larynx is a complex structure with specialized functions of phonation, coordination of swallowing, and protection of the trachea and lower airways from particulates and foreign bodies. It is in the study of cough that the role of the larynx in the unified airway may be best understood.

Common causes of cough include lower airways inflammation (asthma, infection), gastrointestinal reflux, and activation of cough receptors in the upper airways, a condition termed "upper airway cough syndrome" (discussed below). The final common pathway from any of these stimuli is the forceful explosion of air occurring immediately following an increase in intrathoracic pressure against a closed glottis. This phenomenon ties in the entire airway, where stimulation of cough receptors far from the larynx may still trigger cough.

Common triggers for asthma may also trigger laryngeal dysfunction. Methacholine, a nonspecific muscarinic receptor agonist of the parasympathetic system, is used clinically to test for bronchial hyper-reactivity—a central tenet of asthma diagnosis. An absent bronchospastic response to methacholine effectively rules out a diagnosis of asthma. Yet, the larynx may also exhibit reactivity upon exposure to methacholine. Subjects with pre-existing paradoxical vocal fold motion may selectively react with paradoxical adduction during methacholine challenge, a finding not seen in normal subjects or those with exercise induced asthma [45]. Shindoh and colleagues measured laryngeal resistance, as well as resistance above and below the larynx during methacholine and histamine challenges in 10 normal and 12 asthmatics [46]. They observed an increase in laryngeal resistance in coordination with lower airways resistance during spontaneous asthma symptoms, but not during bronchoprovocation. Guss and Mirza observed that methacholine challenge could alternatively elicit laryngeal adduction in patients with a history more consistent with PVFM and also identify lower airway hyper-reactivity in a separate group supporting a diagnosis of asthma [47]. This suggests that the airway component, either laryngeal or lower airways, may exhibit its own specific reactivity pattern with the same stimulus. Ansaranta and colleagues administered inhaled histamine to a group of patients with suspected asthma and prolonged cough [48]. Eight of 11 patients experienced voice changes, with erythema and swelling observed on videolaryngostroboscopy. This reaction was observed more in those with a history of heartburn. Mannitol is also used in bronchoprovocation tests. In 14 patients with suspected PVFM and asthma, mannitol challenge triggered vocal fold adduction in 3/7 with normal baseline laryngoscopy. Only 2 patients have bronchial hyper-responsiveness [49]. These findings of laryngeal reactivity might only be observed in those with asthma, PVFM or other airway abnormalities at baseline [50]. The finding that compounds commonly used to evaluate for bronchospasm may affect the larynx demonstrate the continuity of this response throughout the airway—consistent with a unified airway.

Aspirin-Exacerbated Respiratory Disease

Epitomizing the unified airway, both upper and lower airway inflammation occurs in aspirin-exacerbated respiratory disease (AERD). AERD is a disease consisting of asthma, CRS with nasal polyps, and sensitivity to aspirin or other nonsteroidal anti-inflammatory drugs [51, 52]. It typically presents in adulthood and is diagnosed in patients with difficult-to-control sinusitis with anosmia in conjunction with respiratory reactions in response to aspirin or other inhibitors of the cyclooxygenase-1 (COX-1) enzyme [52]. Patients with AERD tend to report symptoms within minutes to hours of ingesting the offending medication, which often was historically used without adverse sequelae. The pathophysiology of this disease is not fully known, but it does involve the downstream metabolites of the arachidonic acid (AA) pathway [53].

The AA pathway is traditionally activated by inflammatory stimuli which activates COX pathways, and in turn activates specific modulators of pain, inflammation, platelets, etc. COX-1 inhibitors such as aspirin disrupt this pathway, thereby decreasing pain and inflammation. An undesired side effect of interrupting cyclooxygenase activities in AERD patients is a significant decline in Prostaglandin 2 (PGE2) and subsequently increased production of cysteinyl leukotrienes (CysLTs) [52, 53]. In healthy airway PGE2 functions to stabilize mast cells and eosinophils while inhibiting the 5-lipoxygenase (5-LO) enzyme. When PGE2 levels decline with COX-1 inhibition, there is histamine release as well as an increase of mast cells and eosinophils in the airway by up to seven-fold compared to those without AERD [52, 53]. This results in widespread inflammation within the unified airway. CysLTs are lipid inflammatory mediators formed by 5-LO expressing cells including mast cells, eosinophils, and platelet adherent leukocytes, all of which are increased in those with AERD [53]. CysLTRs lead to airway bronchoconstriction and hyperresponsiveness, edema, increase in eosinophils and neutrophils, and this long-term inflammation may result in fibrosis of the unified airway.

AERD is a prototypical example of a unified airway disorder. Although heterogeneity within AERD exists, polyp formation is more aggressive and asthma is more severe when compared with aspirin tolerant airway disorders. In AERD, nasal polyp formation is markedly higher and sinus outcomes are far worse than in aspirin-tolerant nasal polyp sufferers [54–56]. Similarly, severe asthma is heavily enriched for severe asthmatics, and patients are more likely to be corticosteroid dependent [57, 58]. Even the NSAID-induced reactions in AERD are modifiable by debulking polypectomy, where polyp removal will lead to markedly diminished asthmatic reactions to aspirin challenge [59, 60]. In AERD, patients frequently describe asthmatic or rhinitis reactions that can occur when they ingest alcoholic beverages. The dominant part of the airway where this reaction occurs (upper vs lower) correlates with the area that is the dominant reaction during aspirin challenge [61]. In total, these findings demonstrate that both the upper and lower airway components of this disorder are inextricably combined.

Hormonal Effects on the Unified Airway

Hormones such as testosterone, estrogen, and progesterone may all impact the unified airway. Their effect is versatile and ranges from increased nasal reactivity to worsening asthma control leading to hospitalizations. Females, even those without reactive airway, can have increased nasal reactivity related to hormones, without nasal peak flow change [62]. Between 11 and 44% of women with asthma report worsening control in the weeks leading up to their menstrual cycle, and an additional subset of women (approximately 22%) report worsening asthma control during their menstrual cycle [63–66]. Women with premenstrual asthma often experience improvement in the severity of both their asthma and sinus symptoms as hormone levels change during menopause [65].

The exact mechanism of how hormones contribute to airway inflammation, mucus production, and airway hyperreactivity is unknown [65, 67]. Interestingly, Brigham and Women's AERD registry surveyed 322 women and found a strong association between those with perimenstrual asthma and aspirin-sensitive asthma, suggesting a possible pathophysiologic link between the two conditions [65]. In this cohort, women with perimenstrual asthma symptoms also simultaneously experienced worsening rhinitis and sinusitis symptoms suggesting a shared upper and lower airway hormonal sensitivity. In animal models, the withdrawal of estrogen increases bronchial contractility [63, 67]. In humans, progesterone can prevent contraction of bronchial smooth muscle, and the premenstrual withdrawal of progesterone is thought to increase constriction of the bronchial tissue [63]. In patients with premenstrual asthma, oral contraception (OCP) improves control of symptoms by regulating the withdrawal of hormones [63, 64, 67].

Upper Airway Cough Syndrome

Upper airway cough syndrome (UACS), formerly known as postnasal drip syndrome, is a common cause of subacute to chronic cough in adults. The change in nomenclature from postnasal drip syndrome to UACS conceptually reflects the unified airway concept in which cough is not unidimensionally caused by contents dripping from the nose, but rather from a broader and more nuanced effect of upper airway inflammation triggering the cough reflex. Symptoms of UACS include cough, nasal discharge, throat clearing, and the sensation of fluid dripping down the back of the throat, although cough alone may be the only symptom [68, 69].

The traditional proposed mechanism for the pathogenesis of UACS involves stimulation of cough receptors in the hypopharynx and larynx via secretions that drip downward from the nose and sinuses. However, the passage of secretions from the nose and sinuses down to the hypopharynx and larynx is often physiologic, so other mechanisms have been proposed as well. These include increased baseline sensitivity of cough receptors in the upper airways, as well as stimulation of cough receptors in the lower airways via aspiration of secretions, which would be in keeping with a unified airway model [68, 70].

UACS may be caused by several different etiologies, including allergic rhinitis, nonallergic rhinitis, vasomotor rhinitis, rhinitis medicamentosa, acute nasopharyngitis, acute sinusitis, CRS, and postinfectious rhinitis [68, 71]. The diagnosis of UACS is established by response to empiric therapy targeted toward the suspected etiology [72]. As an example, in patients with UACS that is suspected to be secondary to allergic rhinitis, intranasal glucocorticoids are recommended (in addition to avoidance of exposure to any suspected environmental aeroallergens, if possible) [68]. If a patient's cough does not improve despite 1–2 weeks of empiric upper airway cough syndrome therapy targeted toward the suspected etiology, then UACS is not likely to be the cause of the patient's cough, and other possible etiologies of chronic cough should be pursued.

Cystic Fibrosis

CF is an autosomal recessive disorder that illustrates the concept of the unified airway, as nearly all patients with CF experience dysfunction of the upper and lower airways alike [73]. Understanding why CF affects the unified airway requires an appreciation of fundamental cellular anatomy.

The luminal surface of the upper and lower airways is comprised of the same ciliated, pseudostratified, columnar, respiratory epithelial cells. CF is caused by dysfunction or deficiency of the cystic fibrosis transmembrane conductance regulator (CFTR) anion channel, which is typically present on the luminal surface of these respiratory epithelial cells [21]. Therefore, dysfunction of respiratory epithelial cells, as occurs in CF, causes disease throughout the entirety of the unified airway. This respiratory disease is classically manifested by CRS, nasal polyposis, and bronchiectasis.

More specifically, the abnormality in CTFR in CF results in impairment of transluminal chloride secretion across the respiratory epithelium [21, 73, 74]. This leads to thickening of secretions, dysfunction of the mucociliary clearance system, and chronic bacterial infections of the unified airway, ultimately resulting in bronchiectasis and respiratory failure in most patients [21, 74].

CRS has been shown to occur in nearly all CF patients, and it is suggested that in CF, exacerbations of CRS in the upper airway may lead to exacerbations of bronchiectasis in the lower airway [21]. One proposed mechanism for this involves bacterial translocation from the upper airways to the lower airways due to the impairment of mucociliary clearance in CF. In this way, it is thought that the upper airways may "seed" the lower airways with bacteria and therefore promote pulmonary infections [21]. Several studies have shown that upper airway cultures and bronchial cultures in patients with CF often yield similar pathologic bacteria [21, 75–78] although a recent study in children contradicts this notion [79].

Interestingly, there is research to suggest that aggressive management of CRS, including endoscopic sinus surgery and medical management, may improve pulmonary outcomes in patients with CF [21]. While more research is needed to confirm these findings, this demonstrates that management techniques for CF that target the unified airway as one entity hold promise.

Genetics of the Unified Airway

There is considerable variability in the heritability of disorders affecting the unified airway such as CF, asthma, CRS, and AERD. For example, CF is a monogenic disorder that is caused by mutations within the *CFTR* gene (most commonly the ΔF508 mutation, although thousands of other pathologic mutations exist) and generally follows an autosomal recessive inheritance pattern [80]. However, asthma and CRS are polygenic disorders under the influence of multiple different genes, epigenetic changes, and environmental factors, and therefore do not follow a straightforward inheritance pattern [81–84]. Moreover, AERD displays minimal heritability, and some have suggested that acquired epigenetic changes are of importance for the pathogenesis of AERD [85]. Despite these variable inheritance patterns, however, there are shared genetic factors that link disorders of the upper airway and lower airways.

Linkage analyses, candidate-gene association studies, and genome-wide association studies have identified a multitude of genetic variants that are associated with the development of CRS and asthma [84]. Notably, single nucleotide polymorphisms (SNPs) in the *IL1RL1*, *IL-4*, *IL-13*, *IL-33*, and *HLA-DQ* genes have been associated with the development of both CRS with nasal polyposis and asthma [81–84, 86]. Importantly, the type 2 inflammatory pathway serves as a key therapeutic target for both CRS with nasal polyposis and asthma. Additionally, polymorphisms of bitter taste receptors have been linked to the development of both asthma and CRS [86–89].

While CF is caused by mutations of the *CFTR* gene and nearly all patients with CF develop CRS (with or without nasal polyposis), there are some mutations of the *CFTR* gene that have been associated with the development of CRS in the absence of other clinical features of CF [84]. This suggests that dysfunction of the CFTR protein is an important factor in the pathogenesis of some types of CRS, and it is conceivable that the CFTR protein or the downstream effects of CFTR dysfunction could be targeted for the treatment of CRS in the future.

The AA pathway is well known to contribute to AERD, but it is hypothesized that the AA pathway may play a role in the pathophysiology of CRS with nasal polyposis outside of the context of AERD as well. Some studies have shown that genetic polymorphisms involving AA metabolism may result in CRS with nasal polyposis, but these findings have not been consistently replicated [84]. Rather than genetic polymorphisms, however, epigenetic factors involving the AA pathway may be at play in the development of nasal polyposis. One study suggested that epigenetic regulation of prostaglandin E2-mediated fibroblast proliferation may contribute to the nasal polyposis seen in AERD [85], yet it remains to be seen whether this specific epigenetic pathway is implicated in CRS with nasal polyposis outside of the context of AERD.

There is considerable heterogeneity in the presentation, severity, and heritability of the disorders of the unified airway, but there are common genetic variants that link upper and lower airway pathology. Gene expression studies, which evaluate for differential expression of implicated genes as a result of inherited, environmental, and epigenetic factors, have helped elucidate the molecular mechanisms that contribute to various asthma phenotypes [90, 91], and future gene expression studies will undoubtedly further our understanding of the unified airway as a whole.

Treatments Targeting the Unified Airway

Optimal treatment of the unified airway varies widely depending upon the disease being managed. In atopic disorders, treatment generally has three broad categories for consideration: allergen avoidance, immunotherapy, and pharmacotherapy. As avoidance of allergens is not always a feasible option, immunotherapy has been utilized for the past century to gradually desensitize an individual's inflammatory response to environmental aeroallergens. Immunotherapy is available both sublingually (SLIT) and subcutaneously (SCIT). There are multiple options available for the medical management of AR and allergic asthma. Topical corticosteroids (intranasal and inhaled) have been utilized for several decades as a first-line therapeutic modality to reduce airway inflammation. Well known to improve upper airway symptoms, nasal corticosteroids have also been shown to improve lower airway symptoms in individuals with mild asthma [92]. NAR symptoms also improve with nasal corticosteroids [4]. H_1-receptor antagonists (antihistamines) work well in AR but there is less benefit in allergic asthma [5]. Leukotriene modifiers are useful adjuvants for atopic disorders of both the upper and lower airways [5].

The available treatments targeting the unified airway of atopic patients is rapidly expanding with the increased availability of biologic therapies. The shared T2 inflammatory pathways in AR and allergic asthma make biologic therapies that target inflammatory cell mediators such as IL-5. IL-4/IL-13, and IgE ideal for treating the unified airway. Dupilumab has benefit on both nasal polyposis and asthma, demonstrating the importance of the IL-4/IL-13 axis in these conditions [93, 94]. Omalizumab has also recently been shown to be effective in nasal polyposis in addition to its improvement in asthma and allergic rhinitis [95]. Mepolizumab, reslizumab, and benralizumab have demonstrated efficacy for asthma management, but the effect of these biologics on the upper airway remains to be seen.

In AERD, high-dose aspirin therapy (650–1300 mg daily) following induced aspirin tolerance is considered the first-line medical management in conjunction with standard medical management for rhinitis and asthma. While aspirin has been shown to improve upper airway symptoms in AERD, it has demonstrated less benefit for lower airway disease [52]. Additionally, there are risks of long-term high-dose aspirin such as bleeding and gastrointestinal upset [96]. Therefore, the above biologic therapies have emerged as promising new therapeutic modality uniquely positioned to target the unified airway in AERD [97–100]. Leukotriene modifiers such as zileuton have been shown to improve upper and lower airway symptoms in AERD [101]. In addition to the above medical therapies, surgical debulking of nasal polyposis is typically necessary in the treatment of AERD, and improves upper and lower airway symptom severity during aspirin challenges and desensitization [60, 102].

When managing the unified airway in CF, particular consideration must be placed on infection control. Interventions should be implemented to reduce the spread of pathogens among individuals with CF. Antimicrobial therapy targeting *Pseudomonas aeruginosa, Staphylococcus aureus*, and fungal pathogens such as *Aspergillus fumigatus* is another critical aspect of CF respiratory management [103, 104]. Treatments targeting optimized mucociliary clearance and CFTR modulators are also integral in the management of this disorder [103, 104].

Conclusion

The upper and lower airway demonstrate an interconnectedness with regard to anatomy, function, immunopathogenesis, microbial diversity, genetics, and more. It has been shown that numerous diseases of the lower airway have significant impact on the upper airway, and vice versa (Table 2.1). Many upper and lower airway diseases are linked by a shared immunology driving these conditions (such as type 2 inflammation observed in AR and asthma). Inflammatory events in one region may trigger an inflammatory cascade that impacts distant regions of the airway. As such, treatment targeting a localized region of the airway (such as minimizing bulky nasal polyposis) often has beneficial implications for the airway as a whole.

Specialists in airway diseases must therefore keep in mind that their organ system does not exist in isolation. A disease in one segment of the airway is likely to influence pathology in another area. This concept requires integration in the treatment of complex disorders, and may require input from head and neck surgeons, pulmonologists, and allergists to gain control of severe airway disease. The identification of novel bitter taste receptors throughout the airway demonstrates how even a seemingly insignificant cell type can influence the entire airway. Indeed, an understanding of the integrated relationship between all aspects of the respiratory tract is critical when providing treatment for any facet of the unified airway.

References

1. Corren J. Allergic rhinitis and asthma: how important is the link? J Allergy Clin Immunol. 1997;99(2):S781–6.
2. Guerra S, et al. Rhinitis as an independent risk factor for adult-onset asthma. J Allergy Clin Immunol. 2002;109(3):419–25.
3. European Community Respiratory Health Survey, I.I.S.C. The European Community respiratory health survey II. Eur Respir J. 2002;20(5):1071–9.
4. Lieberman P, Pattanaik D. Nonallergic rhinitis. Curr Allergy Asthma Rep. 2014;14(6):439.
5. Marple BF. Allergic rhinitis and inflammatory airway disease: interactions within the unified airspace. Am J Rhinol Allergy. 2010;24(4):249–54.
6. Paiva Ferreira LKD, et al. Combined allergic rhinitis and asthma syndrome (CARAS). Int Immunopharmacol. 2019;74:105718.
7. Hamilos DL. Chronic sinusitis. J Allergy Clin Immunol. 2000;106(2):213–27.
8. Bergqvist J, et al. New evidence of increased risk of rhinitis in subjects with COPD: a longitudinal population study. Int J Chron Obstruct Pulmon Dis. 2016;11:2617–23.
9. Batra PS, et al. Outcome analysis of endoscopic sinus surgery in patients with nasal polyps and asthma. Laryngoscope. 2003;113(10):1703–6.

10. Rajan JP, et al. Prevalence of aspirin-exacerbated respiratory disease among asthmatic patients: a meta-analysis of the literature. J Allergy Clin Immunol. 2015;135(3):676–81 e1.
11. Chang EH. New insights into the pathogenesis of cystic fibrosis sinusitis. Int Forum Allergy Rhinol. 2014;4(2):132–7.
12. Gentile VG, Isaacson G. Patterns of sinusitis in cystic fibrosis. Laryngoscope. 1996;106(8):1005–9.
13. Alles R, et al. The prevalence of atopic disorders in children with chronic otitis media with effusion. Pediatr Allergy Immunol. 2001;12(2):102–6.
14. Nguyen LH, et al. Similar allergic inflammation in the middle ear and the upper airway: evidence linking otitis media with effusion to the united airways concept. J Allergy Clin Immunol. 2004;114(5):1110–5.
15. Seo Y, et al. Optimal control of asthma improved eosinophilic otitis media. Asia Pac Allergy. 2018;8(1):e5.
16. Braunstahl GJ, Hellings PW. Nasobronchial interaction mechanisms in allergic airways disease. Curr Opin Otolaryngol Head Neck Surg. 2006;14(3):176–82.
17. Braunstahl GJ, et al. Nasal allergen provocation induces adhesion molecule expression and tissue eosinophilia in upper and lower airways. J Allergy Clin Immunol. 2001;107(3):469–76.
18. Braunstahl GJ, et al. Segmental bronchial provocation induces nasal inflammation in allergic rhinitis patients. Am J Respir Crit Care Med. 2000;161(6):2051–7.
19. Bachert C, et al. Allergic rhinitis, rhinosinusitis, and asthma: one airway disease. Immunol Allergy Clin N Am. 2004;24(1):19–43.
20. Imoto Y, et al. Increased thrombin-activatable fibrinolysis inhibitor levels in patients with chronic rhinosinusitis with nasal polyps. J Allergy Clin Immunol. 2019;144(6):1566–1574 e6.
21. Illing EA, Woodworth BA. Management of the upper airway in cystic fibrosis. Curr Opin Pulm Med. 2014;20(6):623–31.
22. McLane ML, et al. Integrated response of the upper and lower respiratory tract of asthmatic subjects to frigid air. J Appl Physiol (1985). 2000;88(3):1043–50.
23. Krouse JH. The unified airway. Facial Plast Surg Clin North Am. 2012;20(1):55–60.
24. Shelly MP. The humidification and filtration functions of the airways. Respir Care Clin N Am. 2006;12(2):139–48.
25. Ogura JH, Harvey JE. Nasopulmonary mechanics-experimental evidence of the influence of the upper airway upon the lower. Acta Otolaryngol. 1971;71(2):123–32.
26. Brozek JL, et al. Allergic rhinitis and its impact on asthma (ARIA) guidelines-2016 revision. J Allergy Clin Immunol. 2017;140(4):950–8.
27. Stachler RJ. Comorbidities of asthma and the unified airway. Int Forum Allergy Rhinol. 2015;5(Suppl 1):S17–22.
28. Jones CA, Holt PG. Immunopathology of allergy and asthma in childhood. Am J Respir Crit Care Med. 2000;162(2 Pt 2):S36–9.
29. Singh U, Wangia-Anderson V, Bernstein JA. Chronic rhinitis is a high-risk comorbidity for 30-day hospital readmission of patients with asthma and chronic obstructive pulmonary disease. J Allergy Clin Immunol Pract. 2019;7(1):279–285 e6.
30. Bonay M, et al. Changes in airway inflammation following nasal allergic challenge in patients with seasonal rhinitis. Allergy. 2006;61(1):111–8.
31. Luu K, et al. The impact of chronic airway disease on symptom severity and global suffering in Canadian rhinosinusitis patients. J Otolaryngol Head Neck Surg. 2018;47(1):40.
32. Hens G, et al. Sinonasal pathology in nonallergic asthma and COPD: 'united airway disease' beyond the scope of allergy. Allergy. 2008;63(3):261–7.
33. Marino MJ, et al. The unified airway: does asthma influence paranasal sinus Pneumatization? Ear Nose Throat J. 2020;99(2):89–93.
34. Teo SM, et al. Airway microbiota dynamics uncover a critical window for interplay of pathogenic bacteria and allergy in childhood respiratory disease. Cell Host Microbe. 2018;24(3):341–352 e5.
35. Teo SM, et al. The infant nasopharyngeal microbiome impacts severity of lower respiratory infection and risk of asthma development. Cell Host Microbe. 2015;17(5):704–15.
36. Huang YJ, et al. The airway microbiome in patients with severe asthma: associations with disease features and severity. J Allergy Clin Immunol. 2015;136(4):874–84.
37. Mahdavinia M, et al. The nasal microbiome in patients with chronic rhinosinusitis: analyzing the effects of atopy and bacterial functional pathways in 111 patients. J Allergy Clin Immunol. 2018;142(1):287–290 e4.
38. Roudnitzky N, et al. Receptor polymorphism and genomic structure interact to shape bitter taste perception. PLoS Genet. 2015;11(9):e1005530.
39. Patel NN, Workman AD, Cohen NA. Role of taste receptors as sentinels of innate immunity in the upper airway. J Pathog. 2018;2018:9541987.
40. Li Z, Nair SK. Quorum sensing: how bacteria can coordinate activity and synchronize their response to external signals? Protein Sci. 2012;21(10):1403–17.
41. Salathe M. Regulation of mammalian ciliary beating. Annu Rev Physiol. 2007;69:401–22.
42. Saunders CJ, et al. Cholinergic neurotransmission links solitary chemosensory cells to nasal inflammation. Proc Natl Acad Sci USA. 2014;111(16):6075–80.
43. Bufe B, et al. The molecular basis of individual differences in phenylthiocarbamide and propylthiouracil bitterness perception. Curr Biol. 2005;15(4):322–7.
44. Bankova LG, et al. The cysteinyl leukotriene 3 receptor regulates expansion of IL-25-producing airway brush cells leading to type 2 inflammation. Sci Immunol. 2018;3(28)

45. Perkins PJ, Morris MJ. Vocal cord dysfunction induced by methacholine challenge testing. Chest. 2002;122(6):1988–93.
46. Shindoh C, et al. Upper airway response during bronchoprovocation and asthma attack. Am Rev Respir Dis. 1985;132(3):671–8.
47. Guss J, Mirza N. Methacholine challenge testing in the diagnosis of paradoxical vocal fold motion. Laryngoscope. 2006;116(9):1558–61.
48. Ansaranta M, et al. Laryngeal mucosal reaction during bronchial histamine challenge test visualized by Videolaryngostroboscopy. J Voice. 2017;31(4):470–5.
49. Tay TR, et al. Inhaled mannitol as a laryngeal and bronchial provocation test. J Voice. 2017;31(2):247 e19–23.
50. England SJ, Ho V, Zamel N. Laryngeal constriction in normal humans during experimentally induced bronchoconstriction. J Appl Physiol. 1985;58(2):352–6.
51. Babu KS, Salvi SS. Aspirin and asthma. Chest. 2000;118(5):1470–6.
52. White AA, Stevenson DD. Aspirin-exacerbated respiratory disease. N Engl J Med. 2018;379(11):1060–70.
53. Laidlaw TM, Boyce JA. Aspirin-exacerbated respiratory disease--new prime suspects. N Engl J Med. 2016;374(5):484–8.
54. Mascia K, et al. Chronic hyperplastic eosinophilic sinusitis as a predictor of aspirin-exacerbated respiratory disease. Ann Allergy Asthma Immunol. 2005;94(6):652–7.
55. Kim JE, Kountakis SE. The prevalence of Samter's triad in patients undergoing functional endoscopic sinus surgery. Ear Nose Throat J. 2007;86(7):396–9.
56. Cho KS, et al. Long-term sinonasal outcomes of aspirin desensitization in aspirin exacerbated respiratory disease. Otolaryngol Head Neck Surg. 2014;151(4):575–81.
57. Stevens WW, et al. Clinical characteristics of patients with chronic Rhinosinusitis with nasal polyps, asthma, and aspirin-exacerbated respiratory disease. J Allergy Clin Immunol Pract. 2017;5(4):1061–1070 e3.
58. Mascia K, et al. Aspirin sensitivity and severity of asthma: evidence for irreversible airway obstruction in patients with severe or difficult-to-treat asthma. J Allergy Clin Immunol. 2005;116(5):970–5.
59. Jerschow E, et al. Sinus surgery is associated with a decrease in aspirin-induced reaction severity in patients with aspirin exacerbated respiratory disease. J Allergy Clin Immunol Pract. 2019;7(5):1580–8.
60. Huang GX, et al. Sinus surgery improves lower respiratory tract reactivity during aspirin desensitization for AERD. J Allergy Clin Immunol Pract. 2019;7(5):1647–9.
61. Cardet JC, et al. Alcohol-induced respiratory symptoms are common in patients with aspirin exacerbated respiratory disease. J Allergy Clin Immunol Pract. 2014;2(2):208–13.
62. Paulsson B, et al. Nasal mucosal congestion during the menstrual cycle. J Laryngol Otol. 1997;111(4):337–9.
63. Haggerty CL, et al. The impact of estrogen and progesterone on asthma. Ann Allergy Asthma Immunol. 2003;90(3):284–91; quiz 291–3, 347.
64. van den Berge M, et al. The role of female sex hormones in the development and severity of allergic and non-allergic asthma. Clin Exp Allergy. 2009;39(10):1477–81.
65. Eid RC, Palumbo ML, Cahill KN. Perimenstrual asthma in aspirin-exacerbated respiratory disease. J Allergy Clin Immunol Pract. 2020;8(2):573–578 e4.
66. Sanchez-Ramos JL, et al. Risk factors for premenstrual asthma: a systematic review and meta-analysis. Expert Rev Respir Med. 2017;11(1):57–72.
67. Yung JA, Fuseini H, Newcomb DC. Hormones, sex, and asthma. Ann Allergy Asthma Immunol. 2018;120(5):488–94.
68. Patrick H, Patrick F. Chronic cough. Med Clin North Am. 1995;79(2):361–72.
69. Pratter MR, et al. An algorithmic approach to chronic cough. Ann Intern Med. 1993;119(10):977–83.
70. Yu L, et al. Advances in upper airway cough syndrome. Kaohsiung J Med Sci. 2015;31(5):223–8.
71. Pratter MR. Chronic upper airway cough syndrome secondary to rhinosinus diseases (previously referred to as postnasal drip syndrome): ACCP evidence-based clinical practice guidelines. Chest. 2006;129(1 Suppl):63S–71S.
72. Irwin RS, et al. Diagnosis and management of cough executive summary: ACCP evidence-based clinical practice guidelines. Chest. 2006;129(1 Suppl):1S–23S.
73. Davies JC, Alton EW, Bush A. Cystic fibrosis. BMJ. 2007;335(7632):1255–9.
74. Reis FJ, Damaceno N. Cystic fibrosis. J Pediatr. 1998;74(Suppl 1):S76–94.
75. Aanaes K, et al. The effect of sinus surgery with intensive follow-up on pathogenic sinus bacteria in patients with cystic fibrosis. Am J Rhinol Allergy. 2013;27(1):e1–4.
76. Koch C. Early infection and progression of cystic fibrosis lung disease. Pediatr Pulmonol. 2002;34(3):232–6.
77. Munck A, et al. Genotypic characterization of Pseudomonas aeruginosa strains recovered from patients with cystic fibrosis after initial and subsequent colonization. Pediatr Pulmonol. 2001;32(4):288–92.
78. Johansen HK, et al. Colonisation and infection of the paranasal sinuses in cystic fibrosis patients is accompanied by a reduced PMN response. J Cyst Fibros. 2012;11(6):525–31.
79. Kirst ME, et al. Upper versus lower airway microbiome and metagenome in children with cystic fibrosis and their correlation with lung inflammation. PLoS One. 2019;14(9):e0222323.
80. Gallati S. Disease-modifying genes and monogenic disorders: experience in cystic fibrosis. Appl Clin Genet. 2014;7:133–46.

81. Thomsen SF. Genetics of asthma: an introduction for the clinician. Eur Clin Respir J. 2015;2:2.
82. Willis-Owen SAG, Cookson WOC, Moffatt MF. The genetics and genomics of asthma. Annu Rev Genomics Hum Genet. 2018;19:223–46.
83. Hernandez-Pacheco N, Pino-Yanes M, Flores C. Genomic predictors of asthma phenotypes and treatment response. Front Pediatr. 2019;7:6.
84. Hsu J, et al. Genetics of chronic rhinosinusitis: state of the field and directions forward. J Allergy Clin Immunol. 2013;131(4):977–93, 993 e1–5.
85. Cahill KN, et al. Impaired E Prostanoid2 expression and resistance to prostaglandin E2 in nasal polyp fibroblasts from subjects with aspirin-exacerbated respiratory disease. Am J Respir Cell Mol Biol. 2016;54(1):34–40.
86. Workman AD, Kohanski MA, Cohen NA. Biomarkers in chronic Rhinosinusitis with nasal polyps. Immunol Allergy Clin N Am. 2018;38(4):679–92.
87. Nayak AP, et al. Bitter taste receptors for asthma therapeutics. Front Physiol. 2019;10:884.
88. Yoon SY, et al. Association between polymorphisms in bitter taste receptor genes and clinical features in Korean asthmatics. Respiration. 2016;91(2):141–50.
89. Adappa ND, et al. Genetics of the taste receptor T2R38 correlates with chronic rhinosinusitis necessitating surgical intervention. Int Forum Allergy Rhinol. 2013;3(3):184–7.
90. Modena BD, et al. Gene expression in relation to exhaled nitric oxide identifies novel asthma phenotypes with unique biomolecular pathways. Am J Respir Crit Care Med. 2014;190(12):1363–72.
91. Modena BD, et al. Gene expression correlated with severe asthma characteristics reveals heterogeneous mechanisms of severe disease. Am J Respir Crit Care Med. 2017;195(11):1449–63.
92. Scichilone N, et al. The effect of intranasal corticosteroids on asthma control and quality of life in allergic rhinitis with mild asthma. J Asthma. 2011;48(1):41–7.
93. Rabe KF, et al. Efficacy and safety of Dupilumab in glucocorticoid-dependent severe asthma. N Engl J Med. 2018;378(26):2475–85.
94. Bachert C, et al. Efficacy and safety of dupilumab in patients with severe chronic rhinosinusitis with nasal polyps (LIBERTY NP SINUS-24 and LIBERTY NP SINUS-52): results from two multicentre, randomised, double-blind, placebo-controlled, parallel-group phase 3 trials. Lancet. 2019;394(10209):1638–50.
95. Gevaert P, et al. Omalizumab is effective in allergic and nonallergic patients with nasal polyps and asthma. J Allergy Clin Immunol. 2013;131(1):110–6 e1.
96. Walters KM, et al. Long-term clinical outcomes of aspirin desensitization with continuous daily aspirin therapy in aspirin-exacerbated respiratory disease. Am J Rhinol Allergy. 2018;32(4):280–6.
97. Laidlaw TM, et al. Dupilumab improves nasal polyp burden and asthma control in patients with CRSwNP and AERD. J Allergy Clin Immunol Pract. 2019;7(7):2462–2465 e1.
98. Lang DM, et al. Omalizumab can inhibit respiratory reaction during aspirin desensitization. Ann Allergy Asthma Immunol. 2018;121(1):98–104.
99. Mahdavinia M, Batra PS, Codispoti C. Mepolizumab utility in successful aspirin desensitization in aspirin-exacerbated respiratory disease in a refractory case. Ann Allergy Asthma Immunol. 2019;123(3):311–2.
100. Weinstein SF, et al. Effects of Reslizumab on asthma outcomes in a subgroup of eosinophilic asthma patients with self-reported chronic Rhinosinusitis with nasal polyps. J Allergy Clin Immunol Pract. 2019;7(2):589–596 e3.
101. Laidlaw TF, DJ, Want Y. Efficacy of Zileuton in patients with asthma and history o faspirin sensitivity: a retrospective analysis of dat from two phase 3 studies. J Allergy Clin Immunol. 2017;139(1):AB384.
102. White AA, Doherty TA. Role of group 2 innate lymphocytes in aspirin-exacerbated respiratory disease pathogenesis. Am J Rhinol Allergy. 2018;32(1):7–11.
103. Savant AP, McColley SA. Cystic fibrosis year in review 2018, part 1. Pediatr Pulmonol. 2019;54(8):1117–28.
104. Savant AP, McColley SA. Cystic fibrosis year in review 2018, part 2. Pediatr Pulmonol. 2019;54(8):1129–40.

Immunology in Allergy

3

Xinni Xu, Yew Kwang Ong, and De Yun Wang

Introduction

An allergy is an exaggerated immune response to a specific innocuous substance (an allergen), which is reproducible on re-exposure. Allergic rhinitis, allergic conjunctivitis, allergic asthma, atopic dermatitis (eczema), and food allergy are among the most common immune-mediated ailments. An allergic reaction causes undesirable reactions, such as rhinorrhoea, wheezing, and itch. In severe circumstances, it can result in life-threatening anaphylaxis.

An allergic reaction is mediated by the immune system. Whilst immune (patho)physiology is perhaps not the most exciting subject to most clinicians, knowing how it works is important in the appropriate selection of investigations and treatments, which has implications on patient care.

This chapter is written with the practicing otolaryngologist in mind. It is not intended to be an exhaustive description on all the inflammatory mediators of immune system or the latest research on new immune mechanisms, for it is a continually evolving field (and there is always Pubmed). We have chosen instead to provide an overview of the immune system, the pathophysiology of an allergic response and concepts on the development of allergy. Each segment is correlated with clinical applications as far as possible in the hope that readers will find relevance to their clinical practice.

The Immune System

The immune system is crucial in defending the body against foreign entities whilst recognizing and avoiding attack on self-components. It is described in terms of the innate and adaptive systems (Table 3.1). Both have roles in the pathophysiology of allergy.

(i) **Innate Immune System**

The innate immune is the first line of defence against pathogens. Its response is immediate and non-specific in nature. It consists of physical barriers, antimicrobial compounds, and immune

The authors have no conflict of interests to declare.

X. Xu · Y. K. Ong
Department of Otolaryngology – Head and Neck Surgery, National University Hospital, Singapore, Singapore
e-mail: xinni_xu@nuhs.edu.sg; entoyk@nus.edu.sg

D. Y. Wang (✉)
Department of Otolaryngology, Yong Loo Lin School of Medicine, National University of Singapore, Singapore, Singapore
e-mail: entwdy@nus.edu.sg

C. Damask et al. (eds.), *Allergy in Otolaryngology Practice*,
https://doi.org/10.1007/978-3-031-93455-1_3

Table 3.1 Innate versus adaptive immunity

	Innate immunity	Adaptive immunity
Response	Fast: Within minutes to hours	Days
Specificity	Non-specific. Recognizes pathogen-associated molecular patterns (PAMPs)—Highly conserved DNA sequences—in pathogens	Highly specific. Recognizes pathogens via specific antigens.
Key components	Cellular: Phagocytes (e.g., neutrophils, eosinophils, macrophages, dendritic cells, monocytes, mast cells, basophils), innate lymphoid cells Non-cellular: Epithelial barrier, complement system, and other antimicrobial peptides	T and B lymphocytes
Effectors	Antimicrobial peptides, cytokines	Antibodies (immunoglobulins)
Immunologic memory	None	Present
Diversity	Limited.	Highly diverse. Receptors can undergo genetic rearrangement to recognize an array of antigens.
Ability to discriminate self	High integrity	Errors can occur here, which result in autoimmune conditions

cells. In the nose, tight junctions across ciliated columnar epithelium hinder the passage of pathogens across the epithelial barrier. The overlying mucous blanket traps pathogens and is eliminated by mucociliary clearance. Antimicrobial peptides (e.g., lacteroferrin, lysozyme, defensins) within the secretions of upper and lower airway have microbicidal and bacteriostatic properties. The complement system opsonizes foreign particles, activates phagocytes and induces lysis of target cells.

The cellular component of the innate immune system comprises of activated phagocytes (e.g., neutrophils, monocytes, macrophages, eosinophils, mast cells) and innate lymphoid cells (ILCs). Phagocytes have pattern recognition receptors (a well-known example is the Toll-like receptor) on their surface or intracellularly. These receptors recognize highly conserved sequences or molecules on cell wall components that are shared by many microorganisms, which triggers the inflammatory response. ILCs belong to the lymphoid lineage, like B and T lymphocytes. However, ILCs do not express antigen receptors or undergo clonal expansion. They are activated by alarmins from damaged tissue and not antigens, unlike B and T lymphocytes. There are three subsets of ILCs—ILC1, ILC2, and ILC3 – which closely mirror the function of T helper 1 (Th1), T helper 2 (Th2) and T helper 17 (Th17) cells respectively and hence are considered the innate counterparts to these lymphoid cells. ILC1s produce Th1 cytokines interferon-gamma (IFNγ) and tumour necrosis factor-alpha (TNF-α), which target viruses and intracellular pathogens. ILC1s also include natural killer (NK) cells, which were first recognized for their ability to kill tumour cells without prior priming or activation. ILC2s produce Th2 cytokines interleukin (IL)-4, IL-5 and IL-13 in response to helminths and protozoa. They play an important role in allergy as they are additional sources of Th2 cytokines that amplify the allergic, type 2 immune response and induce IgE production. ILC3s produce IL-17A and IL-22 in response to extracellular microorganisms.

In allergic rhinitis, the innate immune system is primed to favour a Th2 response. Some allergens, such as Der p 1 in the house dust mite *Dermatophagoides pteronyssinus*, have protease activity that can penetrate the epithelial barrier. Others, such as Der p 2, activate pattern recognition receptors on phagocytes. Upon contact, allergens trigger the epithelium to release alarmins, which are immune-activating molecules released in response to tissue damage. Some well-known examples are IL-1, IL-25, IL-33, and thymic stromal lymphopoietin (TSLP). These epithelial cytokines promote development of pro-allergic dendritic cells and preferential Th2 cell differentiation [1]. They also amplify and maintain ILC2-driven inflammation, thus perpetuating Th2 cytokine-mediated inflammation [2].

(ii) **Adaptive Immune System**

The adaptive immune system is activated if the innate immune system is unable to remove the offending invader. A key characteristic of the adaptive immune system is its highly specific nature and capability for memory.

The adaptive immune system is composed of T and B lymphocytes. They are derived from pluripotent hematopoietic stem cells in the bone marrow (Fig. 3.1). B cells mature in the bone marrow and aggregate in follicles within lymphoid organs. Naive B cells express membrane-bound antibodies on their surfaces. When a naive B cell encounters an antigen specific to its B cell receptor, the antigen-antibody binding triggers the B cell to differentiate into memory B cells and plasma cells. Memory B cells express the same membrane-bound antibody as the naive B cell. Plasma cells secrete antibodies (immunoglobulins) which are free-floating in the serum and are not bound to membrane. There are five classes of immunoglobulins: IgE, IgM, IgG, IgA, and IgD. They coordinate antibody-mediated immunity. This is also known as the humoral response, so named because it involves immunoglobulins free-floating in extracellular fluids (or "humours", a term often credited to Hippocrates). In the context of infections, the humoral response acts against bacteria or bacterial products. Of the five immunoglobulins, IgE is involved in allergy and its production is stimulated mainly by IL-4 and IL-13. IgE binds with very high affinity to mast cells and basophils. It also binds to macrophages, neutrophils, eosinophils, and dendritic cells, albeit with much lower affinity [3, 4].

Once formed, T progenitor cells travel from bone marrow to the thymus, where they mature and ultimately develop T cell receptors (TCR) with either CD4 or CD8 receptors. TCRs undergo

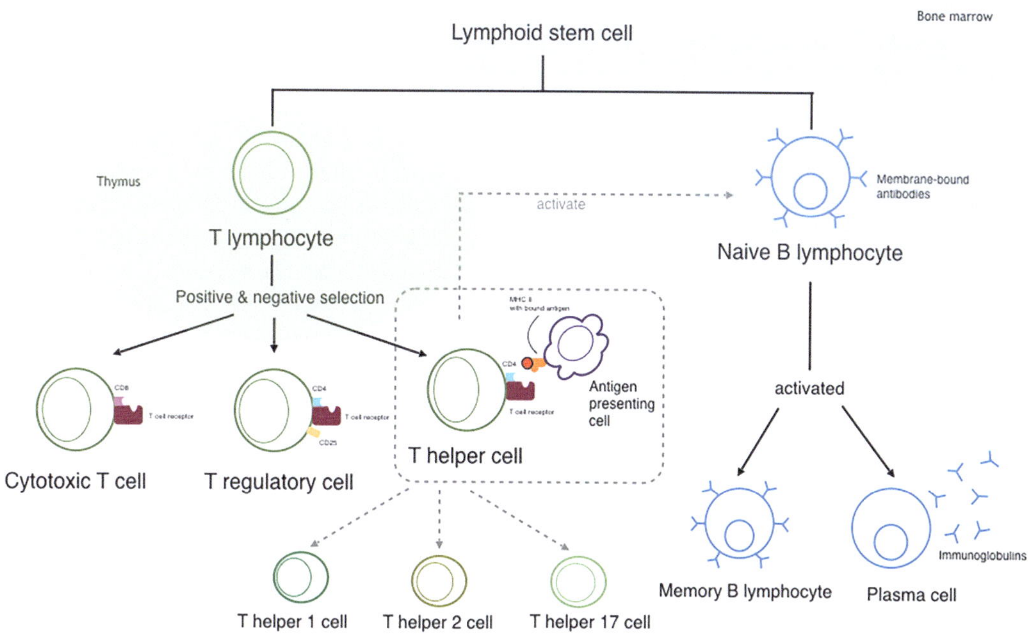

Fig. 3.1 Cells of the adaptive immune system

gene segment rearrangements, which result in multiple genetic recombinations that result in immense antigen-binding diversity. Within the thymus, T cells undergo two selection processes: positive and negative selection. T cells that express both CD4 and CD8 undergo positive selection, in which these T cells survive only if they can recognize self-antigens. The T cells then drop either CD4 to become C8+ T cells (cytotoxic T cells), or drop CD8 to become CD4+ T cells (T helper cells). T cells also undergo negative selection, in which T cells that bind strongly to self-antigens undergo apoptosis and are eliminated. These two selection processes allow for self-tolerance. Errors in these processes can lead to autoimmune conditions.

After positive and negative selection, there are three main types of mature T cells: cytotoxic T (Tc) cells, T helper (Th) cells, and T regulatory (Treg) cells. Mature T cells congregate mainly at the paracortical lymph nodes and spleen. T cells participate in cellular-mediated immunity, which act primarily against viral and fungal infections. They interact with major histocompatibility complex (MHC) molecules, which are glycoproteins found on the surface of all nucleated cells on the body. They function primarily to present antigens to T cells. There are two main classes of MHC: MHC I and MHC II. MHC I are found on all nucleated cells in the body and platelets. They can present both self- and non-self-antigens. MHC I bound to self-antigens are recognized by immune cells and are left alone. However, if a cell is infected, it processes and binds pathogenic antigens to the cell's MHC I, which signals the cell for destruction. MHC II are found on antigen-presenting cells, which are macrophages, dendritic cells, Langerhans cells, and B cells. MHC IIs present non-self-antigens.

Th cells (CD4+ T cells) interact with MHC II-antigen complex on antigen-presenting cells. These naive CD4+ T cell then differentiates into a specialized subtype, depending on cues from innate immune cells. For a long time, the better-known subtypes are Th1 and Th2 cells [5]. Th1 cells secrete IL-2, IFN-γ, TNF-α, and TNF-β, which eliminate intracellular pathogens. Th2 cells secrete IL-4, IL-5, and IL-13, which eliminate extracellular organisms. IL-4, IL-13, and CD40L from Th2 cells also induce B cell immunoglobulin class switching in the nasal mucosa and promote IgE synthesis [6]. More recently, a new Th cell subset, Th17, was identified [7]. Th17 cells secrete IL-17A, as well as other cytokines IL-17F, IL-21, and IL-22. Th17 cells stimulate epithelial cells, endothelial cells, and fibroblasts to produce inflammatory cytokines that recruit neutrophils against extracellular pathogens. Aberrant Th17 activation has also been linked to the pathogenesis of various autoimmune diseases [8].

Tc cells (CD8+ T cells) interact with MHC I bound to pathogenic antigens. Tc cells then secrete Th1 cytokines to destroy the infected host cell.

Treg cells are characterized by surface expression of CD4 and CD25 and the intracellular presence of transcription factor Foxp3. They are immunomodulators that regulate the Th1-Th2 balance and promote tolerance. There are two major subsets of Treg cells: natural Treg (nTreg) and induced Treg (iTreg) cells. nTreg cells develop in the thymus, directly from CD4+ T cell precursors [9]. iTreg cells differentiate in the periphery from conventional naive T cells and are responsible for peripheral tolerance to self-antigens. Two types of iTreg cells have been described. Inducible regulatory T class 1 cells (Tr1 cells) produce IL-10 and low to moderate transforming growth factor beta (TGF-β), whereas Th3 cells preferentially secrete TGF-β. iTreg cells downregulate allergen-specific Th1 and Th2 responses [10]. Dysfunctional Tregs have been implicated in a variety of autoimmune conditions, including type 1 diabetes mellitus [11], multiple sclerosis [12], and inflammatory bowel disease [13].

The Allergic Response

Broadly speaking, allergic reactions can be considered as IgE- or non-IgE-mediated allergy. IgE-mediated allergy is the archetypal allergic response. Under the Gel and Coombs classification, it is a Type I hypersensitivity reaction, which is immediate and involves IgE-mediated release of inflammatory mediators, including cytokines, histamine, bradykinin, prostaglandins, and leukotrienes. This response includes allergic rhinitis and anaphylaxis, and also plays a protective role against parasites. The diagnosis of IgE-mediated allergy is dependent on investigations that measure the IgE response.

Atopy is not the same as allergy. Atopy refers to the genetic tendency to develop IgE-mediated allergic diseases, such as allergic rhinitis, asthma, atopic dermatitis (eczema), and food allergy [14]. Atopic individuals have a family history of the aforementioned conditions. They are predisposed to heightened immune responses to common allergens, such as inhaled allergens and food allergens. They may or may not have symptoms of allergy. Atopic individuals who do not have symptoms of allergy can be sensitized to certain allergens, but are not considered allergic. Therefore, for a diagnosis of an allergic disease, *both* a suggestive history and a positive test that proves the IgE-mediated allergic reaction are necessary.

Non-IgE immune responses include Types II, III, and IV hypersensitivity reactions, which are mediated by other antibody classes, immune cell complexes, or T cells respectively. Non-IgE-mediated food allergies do not fall into any of the above classes of hypersensitivity. They are a heterogenous group, amongst which the more commonly known conditions are food protein-induced enterocolitis syndrome (FPIES), celiac disease and eosinophilic esophagitis. Their immune pathophysiology is not very well known, but is thought to be mediated by T cells in some conditions [15]. Adverse reactions to foods that do not involve an immune response are considered food intolerances and not allergies. Some common food intolerances include lactose intolerance, irritable bowel syndrome, sensitivity to sulphites in preserved foods and red wine.

Compared to IgE-mediated allergy, the symptoms of non-IgE-mediated allergy generally appear more slowly, sometimes several hours after exposure. However, this is not the rule of thumb. In aspirin-exacerbated respiratory disease (AERD), inherent dysregulation of the arachidonic acid metabolic pathway leads to overproduction of pro-inflammatory cysteinyl leukotrienes and underproduction of anti-inflammatory prostaglandin-E2 [16]. Following ingestion of cyclooxygenase-1 (COX-1) inhibitors, such as aspirin and non-steroidal anti-inflammatory drugs, prostaglandin-E2 is quickly depleted, resulting in uninhibited, massive leukotriene production and mast cell histamine release. Clinically, AERD patients experience symptoms as early as within 30 min of exposure to COX-1 inhibitors, especially in those with unstable asthma [17]. These symptoms typically involve the upper airway first (rhinorrhoea, sneezing, congestion), followed by the lower airway (wheezing, coughing, laryngospasm). Less commonly, cutaneous (flushing, urticaria) and gastrointestinal (abdominal pain, vomiting) symptoms are also seen.

Pathophysiology of IgE-Mediated Allergy

The development of IgE-mediated allergy first requires sensitization of host. Upon subsequent antigen exposure, mast cells and basophils degranulate, releasing inflammatory mediators which result in early-phase (immediate) symptoms. In some patients, a late-phase response is seen hours after initial antigen exposure as a result of influx of immune cells and their inflammatory mediators. Allergic rhinitis was chosen as an example to illustrate the mechanism of IgE-mediated allergy, although it is applicable to other IgE-mediated allergic conditions.

(i) **Sensitization**

The first contact with an allergen can occur via inhalation, orally or through altered skin such as in atopic dermatitis. When an atopic person encounters an allergen for the first time, the antigen-presenting cell at body surfaces (e.g., Langerhans cells in the epidermis or dendritic cells in nasal mucosa) internalizes the antigen,

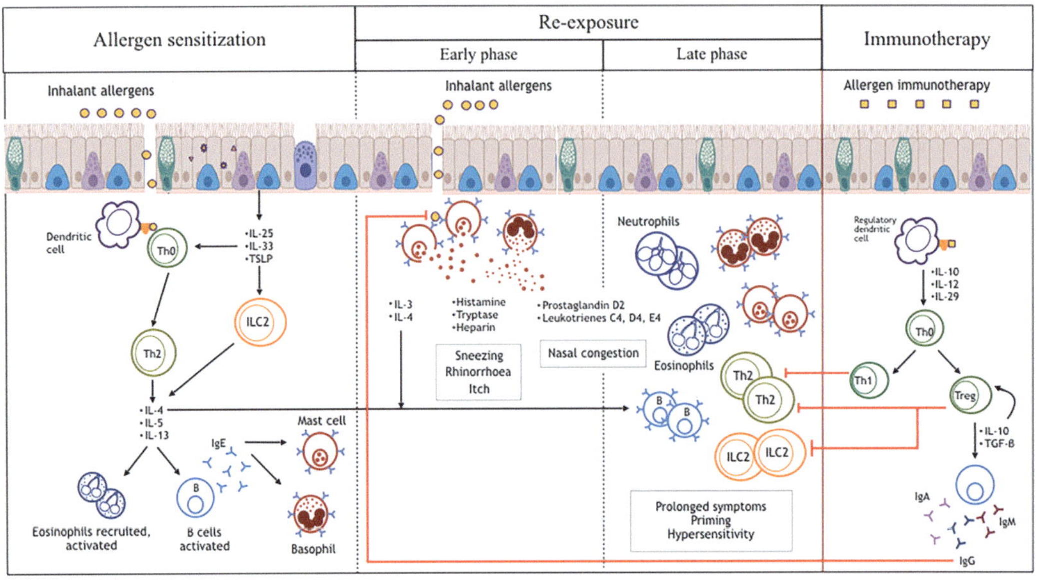

Fig. 3.2 Immune mechanism of allergic rhinitis and allergen immunotherapy. **Sensitization:** When an allergen is encountered for the first time, the dendritic cell processes it and presents it to the naive CD4+ T cell. This activates the T cell, which differentiates to form an antigen-specific Th2 cell. The Th2 cell secretes IL-4, IL-5, and IL-13, recruiting eosinophils and activating B cells to produce IgE. IgEs bind to their receptors on mast cells and basophils. **Early phase:** Upon re-exposure to the specific allergen, the allergen crosslinks cell-bound IgE. This causes mast cell and basophil degranulation. This results in the symptoms of rhinorrhoea, sneezing, and itch. **Late phase:** Chemotactic factors and cytokines produced by Th2 cells and mast cells recruit multiple inflammatory cells, which in turn become activated and perpetuate the inflammatory response. This typically leads to nasal congestion, prolongation of the allergic symptoms, priming and hypersensitivity. **Allergen immunotherapy:** Immunotherapy promotes the development of regulatory dendritic cells, which produce IL-10, IL-12, and IL-27 that preferentially skew the immune response toward a Th1 response. The production of Treg cells also increases, which suppresses Th2 cell production and induces B cells to generate allergen-specific IgG, IgA, and IgM. IgG4 competes with IgE for allergen and blocks cross-linkage of IgE on mast cells and basophils. IgA and IgM may boost barrier function against antigen penetration at mucosal surfaces. *TSLP* thymic stromal lymphopoietin, *Th0* naive T cell, *Th1*, *T* helper 1 cell, *Th2* T helper 2 cell, *Treg* T regulatory cell, *ILC2* innate lymphoid cell 2

processes it, and re-presents it on the cell surface as a MHC II-antigen complex (Fig. 3.2). The antigen-presenting cell then migrate to lymph nodes, where the antigen is presented to naive CD4+ T cell. The T cell is then activated and differentiates to form an antigen-specific Th2 cell. The Th2 cell secretes IL-4, IL-5, and IL-13. IL-5 recruits and activates eosinophils, whilst IL-4 and IL-13 activate B cells and promote immunoglobulin heavy chain class-switching to IgE. Once released into the blood, IgE binds to the numerous high-affinity IgE receptors on mast cells or basophils. The patient remains asymptomatic and may not be aware of the potential allergy.

(ii) **Re-exposure: Early Phase**

Upon subsequent antigen re-exposure in a sensitized host, symptoms and signs of allergy manifest, which have an early and late phase. As its name suggests, the early response occurs within minutes of antigen exposure. Mast cells are the dominant effectors here. Antigens bind to their specific IgEs on mast cells and basophils, resulting in cross-linkage of adjacent surface IgEs. Mast cells rapidly degranulate and release their secretory granules, which contain preformed inflammatory mediators such as histamine, heparin, tryptase, and other enzymes. Histamine is responsible for itch, sneezing, and mucus secretion. Mast cells also release newly synthesized (not pre-formed) inflammatory mediators derived from arachidonic acid within membrane phospholipids, such as prostaglandin D2 and leukotrienes (LTC4, LTD4 and LTE4), which promotes vascular permeability and the resultant mucosal oedema. The nasal-ocular reflex, in which stimulation of the nasal mucosa produces nasal and ocular symptoms, is the reason why allergic rhinitis is associated with ocular itch and watering [18]. Correspondingly, intranasal corticosteroids and antihistamines can improve both nasal and ocular symptoms of allergic rhinitis even without systemic absorption.

(iii) **Late Phase**

The late phase occurs hours after antigen exposure and lasts up to 24 h. Clinically, affected individuals remain symptomatic for prolonged periods after initial allergen exposure and removal from the allergen source. The chief symptom is nasal congestion, although rhinorrhoea and sneezing may persist. IL-4 released by mast cells and Th cells induce vascular endothelial cells to express vascular cell adhesion molecule 1 (VCAM-1) and E-selectin. These chemotactic factors then attract many other inflammatory cells to the site, including eosinophils, neutrophils, Th2 cells, and ILC2s. These cells, in turn, become activated and release additional inflammatory mediators, thus sustaining the allergic response. For example, neutrophils produce reactive oxygen species and the enzymes elastase, metallopeptidase 9 and myeloperoxidase that damage the epithelial barrier and promote recruitment of more immune cells [19]. Eosinophils generate major basic protein, eosinophil cationic protein, and leukotrienes that can penetrate the epithelial barrier. Eosinophils, Th2 cells, and mast cells release IL-5, which promotes eosinophil activation and survival [20]. In spite of tissue eosinophilia, airway remodelling is not a feature of allergic rhinitis, even in severe cases [21]. This is in contrast to eosinophilic chronic rhinosinusitis, in which airway remodelling is a characteristic feature [22].

The influx of inflammatory cells and their cumulative inflammatory processes result in a phenomenon called priming, in which the amount of allergen required to produce the allergic response decreases with repeated allergen exposure [23]. Another effect of this immune cell surge is hypersensitivity, in which the nasal mucosa becomes hyperresponsive even to non-specific stimuli, such as changes in environmental temperature or humidity [24]. This may be related to eosinophil-mediated epithelial damage and exposure of underlying nerve fibres [25]. This is associated with a stimulated parasympathetic state, which releases acetylcholine that acts on muscarinic receptors in nasal mucous glands, resulting in rhinorrhoea and mucous [26].

In some patients, allergen-specific IgE is produced locally by B cells in the nasal mucosa rather than systemically. This phenotype is known as local allergic rhinitis. The concept of IgE-mediated reaction localized to the nasal mucosa is called entopy, as opposed to systemic atopy. Hence, patient symptoms are similar to that of allergic rhinitis; however, systemic allergy tests are negative. The diagnosis is made through a positive nasal allergen challenge and/or identification of specific IgE in nasal secretions [23]. It appears to be a distinct phenotype independent of allergic rhinitis and does not evolve to systemic allergy even after many years [24, 25].

Clearly, the pathophysiology of the allergic reaction is as sophisticated as it is complex. It should come as no surprise that a single drug, usually acting only on a particular pathway, is often not sufficient to contain the inflammatory storm caused by an allergen. Nor is a single drug often able to treat adequately treat all the symptoms of an allergy. For example, intranasal corticosteroids are effective in broadly suppressing the inflammation of an allergic reaction, but its onset of action is slower as it works mainly by inactivating transcription factors that regulate expression of inflammatory proteins, which perpetuate the inflammatory response and recruit additional effector immune cells [27]. In an acute allergic reaction, anti-histamines have a quick onset of action and are effective in relieving histamine-activated symptoms of sneezing, itch, and rhinorrhoea but have little effect on nasal congestion. Nasal decongestants have no effect on histamine-activated symptoms, because they work by activating postsynaptic α1- and α2-adrenergic receptors on smooth muscles lining nasal capacitance vessels. This causes vasoconstriction and reduces fluid leakage into nasal tissue, which relieves oedema and nasal congestion. Intranasal anticholinergics inhibit acetylcholine-induced mucous production, but do not affect sneezing, itch, or nasal congestion. Biologics are monoclonal antibodies that target specific components of the allergic pathway. Whilst not used in allergic rhinitis, omalizumab (anti-IgE) is indicated in severe allergic asthma and dupilumab (anti-IL-4) is used in moderate to severe atopic dermatitis. These examples of pharmacologic treatment for allergy are not exhaustive, but they illustrate why combination therapy achieves superior clinical relief by acting on different pathways of the allergic response compared to monotherapy.

Implications on Allergy Testing

A sound understanding on the pathophysiology of allergy helps physicians select the most appropriate investigation for their patients with suspected allergy. It is also important to understand the mechanism that the chosen test is designed to uncover in order to interpret the results correctly. For example, in AERD, the mechanism of hypersensitivity is not mediated by IgE, hence ordering a skin prick test or serum IgE is not going to be relevant or useful.

Allergy tests are most useful when guided by the patient's clinical history. Atopy is far more common than allergy. Hence doing a smorgasbord of allergy tests in individuals without a convincing history of allergy can produce positive results which are difficult to interpret. This is not clinically meaningful. For example, if food allergy tests are performed for vague symptoms such as fatigue or headache, positive results may lead to unhelpful recommendations on restrictive diets. Allergy testing should only be done when there is reasonable clinical suspicion of sensitivity to a particular allergen.

(i) **Skin Prick Test**

The skin prick test works by detecting antigen-specific IgE bound to mast cells in the skin. The IgE response in a positive skin prick test is the classic wheal and flare, which is an early phase response in an allergic reaction. When the skin is pricked with a lancet, antigen is introduced to its specific IgE bound to mast cells in the epidermis, leading to IgE cross-linkage, mast cell degranulation and the inflammatory cascade as described earlier. Within 10 to 20 min, this manifests as itching, redness, and whealing on the skin of an allergic patient. This makes the skin prick test a quick, simple, and sensitive method of detecting specific IgE. Drugs with anti-histamine activity should be avoided for a few days or more before a skin prick test, as they result in a negative skin response. In some patients, a late phase reaction develops, seen as diffuse redness, warmth, or swelling 2 to 3 h after the initial prick test, peaking at 6 to 12 h and disappearing within 12 to 24 h [28].

When performed correctly, the skin prick test has high sensitivity and good specificity for diagnosing IgE-mediated allergy. False negatives are extremely unusual, and a negative skin prick test makes the presence of IgE-mediated allergic reactivity very unlikely.

Prick testing is not the same as a patch test. A patch test detects antigen-specific T cells and not IgE. The main indication of a patch test is to detect antigens responsible for conditions involved in Type IV delayed hypersensitivity, such as contact dermatitis, rather than atopic conditions.

(ii) **Intradermal Skin Test**

An intradermal skin test is performed by injecting a small volume (0.01 to 0.05 ml) of allergen extract into the dermis to create a bleb. It is used to demonstrate IgE-dependent response (early reading, similar to a skin prick test) or T cell-dependent, type IV hypersensitivity response (delayed reading). An example of intradermal testing for delayed-type hypersensitivity is the Mantoux test, which detects exposure to tuberculosis by reading the extent of skin induration at 48 to 72 h after inoculation.

The intradermal test is far more sensitive (100- to 1000-fold higher) than the skin prick test. This is also associated with a higher rate of false positive results (i.e., lower specificity). This confers some benefits in certain situations, such as in the testing of suspected hymenoptera venom or drug allergies in patients with negative skin prick tests, as failure to identify these allergies may have life-threatening consequences. On the other hand, routine intradermal testing for inhalant allergens in the context of negative skin prick tests is not routinely performed as a positive result has not been shown to correlate well with clinical allergy [29, 30]. Intradermal testing carries a higher risk of anaphylaxis compared skin prick test, and is not carried out for food or latex allergy in the United States.

(iii) **In-vitro Immunoassays**

In-vitro immunoassays test for allergen-specific IgE that are free-floating in the serum and not cell-bound IgE. Traditionally, these tests were radioallergosorbent (RAST) tests, which used radioactively labelled antigens. This term has prevailed, even though these have mostly been replaced with the enzyme-linked immunosorbent assay (ELISA). The test serum is incubated with antigen that is bound to a solid support, usually a filter paper disc. Following this, the presence of serum IgE is detected by adding labelled antibodies that are specific for human IgE. The result is quantitatively given as the concentration of serum IgE detected. It is also semi-quantitatively designated into 5 or 6 classes, which broadly classify serum IgE from the lowest to the highest concentration.

In-vitro immunoassays are generally thought to be slightly less sensitive than the skin prick test. The accuracy of immunoassays varies with the system being used and the quality of the allergen produced by the laboratory, which can differ amongst laboratories [31]. Most IgE is cell-bound, with only a small proportion of IgE that is free in the serum [32]. Antigen-specific IgG is also produced in allergy, and its levels are significantly more abundant than IgE (75% versus 0.004% of total serum immunoglobulins), which can lead to competition for available allergen binding sites [33]. Free serum IgE has a short half-life of approximately 2 days, compared to mast cell-bound IgE which persists for 2 months [34]. Therefore IgE can only be detected in serum if it is being produced during the time of testing. Tests that use batches of related allergens, such as food or inhalant allergen mix, are even less sensitive than individual allergen testing. In allergen mixes, the amount of each individual allergen is limited, leading to binding of only a small amount of specific IgE which can give a negative result.

Causes of Allergy

The development of allergy is a complex process. It is likely due to a combination of genetic predisposition, environmental factors, and timing of exposure to environmental triggers.

(i) **Genetic Factors**

A family history of atopic diseases is a risk factor for the development of allergic rhinitis, asthma, and atopic dermatitis. A child without allergic parents may have up to a 20% risk of developing allergy. However, the risk increases to 40–50% with one allergic parent, and as high as 90% when both parents are allergic [35].

The development of atopic eczema early in life, especially severe types, appears to facilitate penetration of food allergens through the disrupted skin barrier to induce allergic sensitization [36]. The major genetic risk factors for atopic dermatitis are genetic variants that cause impaired skin barrier function. Loss-of-function mutations in the gene encoding for filaggrin, a filament-binding protein in the stratum corneum, is associated with a significant increase in the risk of peanut allergy [37].

(ii) **Environmental Factors: "Hygiene Hypothesis" Versus "Old Friends Hypothesis"**

Hygiene Hypothesis

The incidence of allergic conditions is on the rise over the last two decades, especially in industrialized and rapidly developing nations [38, 39]. At around the same time, the incidence of infectious diseases such as mumps and tuberculosis has drastically fallen due to improvement in hygiene, living conditions, and vaccines. Is there a link between the two?.

The "hygiene hypothesis" was introduced in 1989, when it was observed that children with older siblings were less likely to develop allergic rhinitis, possibly because of exposure to germs from their siblings [40]. This led to the theory that early, repeated exposure to various pathogens in childhood promotes the development of both Th1 and Th2 immune responses, which are kept balanced by Tregs and reduce the risk of developing allergic and autoimmune conditions. Excess hygiene is postulated to remove the pathogen burden, thus favouring the Th2 immune response which is heightened in atopic individuals. This may explain why children in developed countries who are relatively protected from infectious diseases appear to be at increased risk of developing allergy.

This concept is supported by several epidemiologic studies. In a well-known cross-sectional study of rural areas in Austria, Germany, and Switzerland, early life exposure before 1 year of age and long-term exposure until 5 years of age to stables and farm milk was protective against asthma, allergic rhinitis and atopic sensitization [41]. This was thought to be because exposure to farm animals increased exposure to endotoxins, which stimulated the Th1 immune response and reduced Th2-dependent antibody isotype switching on exposure to inhalant allergens. Amongst urban populations, daycare attendance before 3 to 24 months of age was associated with decreased risk of asthma [42], atopy [43], and decreased total IgE levels in later childhood [44]. Hence, infections during infancy may actually downregulate IgE production and protect against subsequent development of allergic rhinitis [45, 46].

Nonetheless, there are flaws with this theory. Parasitic infections trigger the Th2 immune response and these infections are common in developing countries; however, allergic disorders are unusual occurrences in these regions [47]. Treatment of children with intestinal helminths in endemic, rural areas was not associated with increase in prevalence of atopy or clinical allergy [48]. A large-scale epidemiological study on the Danish national birth cohort found that measles and many respiratory diseases did not protect against allergic disease [49].

Old Friends Hypothesis

In 2003, Rook et al. proposed the alternative "old friends" hypothesis. It suggests that it is not exposure to childhood infectious diseases, but rather early and regular exposure to harmless symbiotic microbiome (or "old friends"), such as helminths, saprophytic mycobacteria, and lactobacilli that are important in immune regulation [50]. These beneficial microbes induce Tregs and regulate the immune system to react appropriately to pathogens whilst remaining neutral toward non-pathogenic foreign. Modern lifestyle changes may have impacted on the exposure to and composition of these microbiomes. Altered maternal diet [51] and antibiotic use in the first year of life [52, 53] may alter the composition and amount of microbiome, whilst increase in Caesarean section births, smaller family sizes, and less time outdoors have been implicated in reduced exposure to friendly microbes, and therefore increased incidence of allergies over the years.

Atopic March

The atopic march refers to the natural history of allergic disease manifestation from infancy to childhood [54]. The classic concept of this "march" starts with atopic dermatitis and advances toward IgE-mediated food allergy, asthma, and allergic rhinitis [55]. Each atopic condition has a different peak age of onset, which supports this theory of sequential disease progression. An accepted, looser definition of the atopic march is the early onset of atopic dermatitis followed by increased risk of developing one or more allergic disorders characterized by the Th2 immune response [56].

Atopic dermatitis is the first manifestation of allergic disease. The resultant skin inflammation, barrier defect, and alteration in skin microbiome sets the stage for sensitization and development of subsequent allergic disorders. Even so, this is not the only factor that leads to allergies. Several large-scale, longitudinal cohort studies examining children from birth or infancy to childhood observe that nearly 50% of children with atopic dermatitis do not develop other allergic conditions [57–61]. In fact, less than 5% of children in the general population "complete" the course of the atopic march [58, 62]. Certain risk factors are required to increase the risk of progression to other allergic disorders. These included early-onset, severe and/or persistent atopic dermatitis, parental atopy, polysensitization, and filaggrin mutation [57–61, 63].

The association between early-onset or severe subtypes of atopic dermatitis and food allergy is well recognized. A study from the Avon Longitudinal Study of Parents and Children found that application of peanut oil to eczematous skin in children is associated with sensitization to peanut [64]. The seminal Learning Early About Peanut Allergy (LEAP) study identified 640 infants with severe eczema and/or egg allergy, considered high-risk for peanut allergy, and randomly assigned them to consume or avoid peanuts until 60 months old [65]. The study found that early introduction of peanuts significantly decreased the incidence of peanut allergy by about 80%. However, a follow-up study by the same group found that early introduction of peanut did not hasten resolution of atopic dermatitis, prevent development of other allergic diseases, or prevent sensitization to other food allergens [66]. In other words, the protective effect of early consumption of peanuts in this group of infants is allergen-specific.

Progression from atopic dermatitis to food allergy, especially peanut allergy is associated with sensitization to multiple allergens and development of asthma [62]. Food allergy at 1 year of age is associated with increased risk of asthma at 4 years old, regardless of whether the food allergy resolves [67]. Sensitization to inhalant allergens, particularly cat and dust mites, are risk factors for wheeze and asthma in children [68–70]. In the Finnish Twin Cohort Study, which followed up over 11,000 patients over 15 years, subjects with allergic rhinitis had a fourfold increase in asthma compared to normal subjects [71].

Prevention of Allergy?

In terms of primary prevention of food allergy, studies have examined the impact of modifying maternal and infantile diet. Maternal avoidance of cow's milk, eggs, or peanuts during pregnancy or lactation has no effect on the development of allergic diseases in offspring [72]. Peanut-specific IgE has not been detected in cord blood despite peanut consumption during pregnancy, suggesting that peanut sensitization does not occur in-utero [64]. Conversely, a maternal diet rich in fruit, vegetables, fish, vitamin D, and Mediterranean diet appears to lower risk of allergic disease in their offspring [73].

The extent to which breastfeeding prevents atopy is controversial. Exclusive breastfeeding for 3 to 4 months appears to decrease the cumulative incidence of eczema in the first 2 years of life [74]. However, beyond 3 to 4 months, there were no short- or long-term advantages for prevention of atopic disease by exclusive breastfeeding [75]. There is no evidence on breastfeeding in preventing or delaying the onset of food allergies [14]. Although there is no specific association between exclusive breastfeeding and prevention of atopic disease or any specific food allergy, it is nonetheless universally recommended for all mothers due to other substantial benefits of breastfeeding.

The use of hydrolysed formulas, in which cow's milk proteins have been broken down to smaller peptides, has been considered in reducing the risk of atopic disease in high-risk, non-exclusively breastfed children. A large randomized prospective study, the German Infant Nutritional Intervention Study, seemed to suggest that extensively and partially hydrolysed formulas reduced the incidence of atopic dermatitis in infancy compared to standard infant formulas [76]. However, the 15-year follow-up of this study found that whilst extensively hydrolysed formula significantly reduced the prevalence of atopic dermatitis at 7 to 10 years of age, it did not prevent the development of asthma or allergic rhinitis [77]. A meta-analysis of 37 studies concluded there was no consistent evidence that partially or extensively hydrolysed formulas reduce the risk of allergic disease, even in high-risk infants [78].

The timing in which allergenic complementary foods are introduced into the diet is well studied.

The Enquiring About Tolerance (EAT) study found that early introduction of six allergenic foods—milk, peanut, sesame, fish, egg, wheat—into the infant weaning diet at 3 months of age reduced their risk of developing allergies to these foods [79]. A meta-analysis of the LEAP and the EAT studies found that early peanut introduction at 4 to 11 months of age was associated with a reduced risk of peanut allergy [80]. Conversely, there was no evidence of benefit in delaying the introduction of allergenic foods beyond 4 to 6 months to prevent atopic disease [14].

With regard to atopic dermatitis, two large prevention trials have found no evidence that daily emollient use in a population-based or high-risk cohort of newborns prevented the development of atopic dermatitis [81, 82]. A Cochrane meta-analysis similarly found that skin care interventions are probably not effective in preventing atopic dermatitis and may increase the risk of skin infection [83]. The same meta-analysis also found that it wasn't clear whether skin care interventions during infancy change the risk of IgE-mediated food allergy or sensitization to food allergen by one to two years of age, due to very low-certainty evidence for these outcomes [83].

There is some evidence that immunotherapy in children with allergic rhinitis may prevent the onset of asthma. In a large study of children with grass-induced allergic rhinitis and no evidence of pre-existing asthma, development of summer- and winter-time asthma was significantly reduced in the group that underwent treatment with Timothy SLIT tablets for three years compared to those who had received placebo treatment [84]. A meta-analysis on immunotherapy in preventing allergic disease found that immunotherapy reduced the short-term risk of developing asthma in individuals with allergy rhinitis, although there was insufficient evidence for the long-term maintenance of this benefit [85].

Immunotherapy

Allergen immunotherapy goes beyond symptomatic treatment of allergy. It is the only treatment that modulates the immune system and can potentially modify the course of allergy. Immunotherapy is administered over at least 3 years, because immune modulation and building sustainable tolerance takes time. Its action is specific to the allergen of interest and can be administered via the subcutaneous or sublingual route. Its mechanisms of action are still not completely understood, although several immunologic changes have been described following immunotherapy (Fig. 3.2).

On initiating immunotherapy, an early increase in allergen-specific serum IgE is seen [86, 87]. This is followed by a gradual decrease to pre-treatment levels during maintenance. In grass pollen allergy, seasonal bursts of serum IgE are blunted during maintenance immunotherapy. A gradual decrease in serum IgE occurs over the next few years, which may contribute to long-term allergen tolerance, although the concentration of IgE does not necessarily correlate with clinical response [88]. Even with successful immunotherapy, serum IgE may not consistently reduce or become undetectable, signifying that reversal of the sensitization process is not required to develop allergen tolerance [89]. In fact, the development of tolerance is more likely to be related to the development of Tregs [90].

Allergen-specific IgG (especially IgG4) and IgA also increase soon after immunotherapy.

IgG4 competes with IgE for allergen and blocks cross-linkage of IgE on mast cells and basophils [91]. Within a year of completing immunotherapy, IgG1 and IgG4 levels reduce to near pre-immunotherapy levels; however, the inhibitory bioactivity of allergen-specific IgG antibodies appears to persist and is accompanied by long-term clinical tolerance [92, 93].

Desensitization to the inflammatory mediators released by mast cells and basophils in the event of antigen exposure is also seen in patients soon after undergoing very fast bee venom immunotherapy [94]. This early desensitization may be related to reduced granule content in mast cells and basophils or increase in threshold for their activation.

As the allergen dose is increased, a tolerant state is induced in peripheral T cells. This is characterized by a change in the distribution of T cell subsets. Allergen-specific Treg cells are generated [95, 96]. Tr1 cells produce IL-10 and TGF-β, which further induce production of Treg cells and maintain peripheral tolerance. This is associated with induction of Th1 cells and suppression of Th2 cells. Decrease in nasal Th2 cells and their corresponding IL-4, IL-5, and IL-13 cytokines is associated with clinical improvement with two years of immunotherapy [93]. One year following discontinuation of immunotherapy, a rebound in Th2 cells and cytokines was associated with seasonal symptom flares, which may suggest that two years of immunotherapy is insufficient to induce lasting tolerance, which is seen in the re-emergence of Th2 immunity. In sublingual immunotherapy, an increase in serum regulatory dendritic cells (DCreg) was seen [97]. These DCregs produce IL-10, IL-12, and IL-27, which further promote the immune deviation from Th2 to Th1 response [98].

In the late response, IgG4 blocking antibodies prevent IgE-mediated presentation of antigen to T cells [99]. IL-10 induces B lymphocytes to switch immunoglobulin production from IgE to IgA and IgM production, which theoretically boosts barrier function against antigen penetration at mucosal surfaces [100].

Conclusion

Good clinical practice in allergy goes hand-in-hand with a sound understanding of the basic principles in immunology. Whilst providing symptomatic relief of the patient's allergic reaction is usually the immediate aim, application of these principles will ensure appropriate selection of investigations and therapies. It is hoped this would translate to improved long-term disease control and better overall patient care.

References

1. Gueguen C, et al. Changes in markers associated with dendritic cells driving the differentiation of either TH2 cells or regulatory T cells correlate with clinical benefit during allergen immunotherapy. J Allergy Clin Immunol. 2016;137(2):545–58.
2. Xue L, et al. Prostaglandin D2 activates group 2 innate lymphoid cells through chemoattractant receptor-homologous molecule expressed on TH2 cells. J Allergy Clin Immunol. 2014;133(4):1184–94.
3. Gounni AS, et al. Human neutrophils express the high-affinity receptor for immunoglobulin E (fc epsilon RI): role in asthma. FASEB J. 2001;15(6):940–9.
4. Kayaba H, et al. Human eosinophils and human high affinity IgE receptor transgenic mouse eosinophils express low levels of high affinity IgE receptor, but release IL-10 upon receptor activation. J Immunol. 2001;167(2):995–1003.
5. Mosmann TR, et al. Two types of murine helper T cell clone. I. Definition according to profiles of lymphokine activities and secreted proteins. J Immunol. 1986;136(7):2348–57.
6. Punnonen J, Yssel H, de Vries JE. The relative contribution of IL-4 and IL-13 to human IgE synthesis induced by activated CD4+ or CD8+ T cells. J Allergy Clin Immunol. 1997;100(6 Pt 1):792–801.
7. Harrington LE, et al. Interleukin 17-producing CD4+ effector T cells develop via a lineage distinct from the T helper type 1 and 2 lineages. Nat Immunol. 2005;6(11):1123–32.
8. Maddur MS, et al. Th17 cells: biology, pathogenesis of autoimmune and inflammatory diseases, and therapeutic strategies. Am J Pathol. 2012;181(1):8–18.
9. Ling EM, et al. Relation of CD4+CD25+ regulatory T-cell suppression of allergen-driven T-cell activation to atopic status and expression of allergic disease. Lancet. 2004;363(9409):608–15.
10. Akdis M, et al. Immune responses in healthy and allergic individuals are characterized by a fine balance between allergen-specific T regulatory 1 and T helper 2 cells. J Exp Med. 2004;199(11):1567–75.

11. McClymont SA, et al. Plasticity of human regulatory T cells in healthy subjects and patients with type 1 diabetes. J Immunol. 2011;186(7):3918–26.
12. Kitz A, et al. AKT isoforms modulate Th1-like Treg generation and function in human autoimmune disease. EMBO Rep. 2016;17(8):1169–83.
13. Cao AT, et al. TLR4 regulates IFN-gamma and IL-17 production by both thymic and induced Foxp3+ Tregs during intestinal inflammation. J Leukoc Biol. 2014;96(5):895–905.
14. Greer FR, et al. The effects of early nutritional interventions on the development of atopic disease in infants and children: the role of maternal dietary restriction, breastfeeding, hydrolyzed formulas, and timing of introduction of allergenic complementary foods. Pediatrics. 2019;143(4):e20190281.
15. Cianferoni A. Non-IgE mediated food allergy. Curr Pediatr Rev. 2020;16(2):95–105.
16. Cahill KN, Boyce JA. Aspirin-exacerbated respiratory disease: mediators and mechanisms of a clinical disease. J Allergy Clin Immunol. 2017;139(3):764–6.
17. Kowalski ML, et al. Diagnosis and management of NSAID-exacerbated respiratory disease (N-ERD)-a EAACI position paper. Allergy. 2019;74(1):28–39.
18. Baroody FM, et al. Nasal ocular reflexes and eye symptoms in patients with allergic rhinitis. Ann Allergy Asthma Immunol. 2008;100(3):194–9.
19. Arebro J, et al. A possible role for neutrophils in allergic rhinitis revealed after cellular subclassification. Sci Rep. 2017;7:43568.
20. Yamaguchi Y, et al. Analysis of the survival of mature human eosinophils: interleukin-5 prevents apoptosis in mature human eosinophils. Blood. 1991;78(10):2542–7.
21. Eifan AO, et al. Severe persistent allergic Rhinitis. Inflammation but no histologic features of structural upper airway remodeling. Am J Respir Crit Care Med. 2015;192(12):1431–9.
22. Tsuda T, et al. Eosinophil-derived neurotoxin enhances airway remodeling in eosinophilic chronic rhinosinusitis and correlates with disease severity. Int Immunol. 2019;31(1):33–40.
23. Connell JT. Quantitative intranasal pollen challenges. 3. The priming effect in allergic rhinitis. J Allergy. 1969;43(1):33–44.
24. Gerth van Wijk RG, de Graaf-in't Veld C, Garrelds IM. Nasal hyperreactivity. Rhinology. 1999;37(2):50–5.
25. Ayars GH, et al. Injurious effect of the eosinophil peroxide-hydrogen peroxide-halide system and major basic protein on human nasal epithelium in vitro. Am Rev Respir Dis. 1989;140(1):125–31.
26. Undem BJ, Taylor-Clark T. Mechanisms underlying the neuronal-based symptoms of allergy. J Allergy Clin Immunol. 2014;133(6):1521–34.
27. Coutinho AE, Chapman KE. The anti-inflammatory and immunosuppressive effects of glucocorticoids, recent developments and mechanistic insights. Mol Cell Endocrinol. 2011;335(1):2–13.
28. Skin tests used in type I allergy testing position paper. Sub-committee on skin tests of the European academy of Allergology and clinical immunology. Allergy. 1989;44(s10):11–59.
29. Nelson HS, et al. An assessment of the role of intradermal skin testing in the diagnosis of clinically relevant allergy to timothy grass. J Allergy Clin Immunol. 1996;97(6):1193–201.
30. Wood RA, et al. A comparison of skin prick tests, intradermal skin tests, and RASTs in the diagnosis of cat allergy. J Allergy Clin Immunol. 1999;103(5 Pt 1):773–9.
31. Cox L, et al. Pearls and pitfalls of allergy diagnostic testing: report from the American College of Allergy, asthma and immunology/American Academy of allergy, asthma and immunology specific IgE test task force. Ann Allergy Asthma Immunol. 2008;101(6):580–92.
32. Laffer S, et al. A high-affinity monoclonal anti-IgE antibody for depletion of IgE and IgE-bearing cells. Allergy. 2008;63(6):695–702.
33. Wachholz PA, Dearman RJ, Kimber I. Detection of allergen-specific IgE antibody responses. J Immunotoxicol. 2005;1(3):189–99.
34. Stone KD, Prussin C, Metcalfe DD. IgE, mast cells, basophils, and eosinophils. J Allergy Clin Immunol. 2010;125(2 Suppl 2):S73–80.
35. Van Bever HP, Samuel ST, Lee BW. Halting the allergic march. World Allergy Organ J. 2008;1(4):57–62.
36. Bartnikas LM, et al. Epicutaneous sensitization results in IgE-dependent intestinal mast cell expansion and food-induced anaphylaxis. J Allergy Clin Immunol. 2013;131(2):451–60 e1–6.
37. Asai Y, et al. Filaggrin gene mutation associations with peanut allergy persist despite variations in peanut allergy diagnostic criteria or asthma status. J Allergy Clin Immunol. 2013;132(1):239–42.
38. Worldwide variation in prevalence of symptoms of asthma, allergic rhinoconjunctivitis, and atopic eczema: ISAAC. The International Study of Asthma and Allergies in Childhood (ISAAC) Steering Committee. Lancet. 1998;351(9111):1225–32.
39. Asher MI, et al. Worldwide time trends in the prevalence of symptoms of asthma, allergic rhinoconjunctivitis, and eczema in childhood: ISAAC phases one and three repeat multicountry cross-sectional surveys. Lancet. 2006;368(9537):733–43.
40. Strachan DP. Hay fever, hygiene, and household size. BMJ. 1989;299(6710):1259–60.
41. Riedler J, et al. Exposure to farming in early life and development of asthma and allergy: a cross-sectional survey. Lancet. 2001;358(9288):1129–33.
42. Celedon JC, et al. Day care attendance in early life, maternal history of asthma, and asthma at the age of 6 years. Am J Respir Crit Care Med. 2003;167(9):1239–43.
43. Haby MM, et al. Daycare attendance before the age of two protects against atopy in preschool age children. Pediatr Pulmonol. 2000;30(5):377–84.

44. Rothers J, et al. Influence of early day-care exposure on total IgE levels through age 3 years. J Allergy Clin Immunol. 2007;120(5):1201–7.
45. Martinez FD, et al. Association of non-wheezing lower respiratory tract illnesses in early life with persistently diminished serum IgE levels. Group Health Med Assoc Thorax. 1995;50(10):1067–72.
46. Holt PG, Sly PD, Bjorksten B. Atopic versus infectious diseases in childhood: a question of balance? Pediatr Allergy Immunol. 1997;8(2):53–8.
47. Yazdanbakhsh M, Kremsner PG, van Ree R. Allergy, parasites, and the hygiene hypothesis. Science. 2002;296(5567):490–4.
48. Cooper PJ, et al. Effect of albendazole treatments on the prevalence of atopy in children living in communities endemic for geohelminth parasites: a cluster-randomised trial. Lancet. 2006;367(9522):1598–603.
49. Benn CS, et al. Cohort study of sibling effect, infectious diseases, and risk of atopic dermatitis during first 18 months of life. BMJ. 2004;328(7450):1223.
50. Rook GA, Martinelli R, Brunet LR. Innate immune responses to mycobacteria and the downregulation of atopic responses. Curr Opin Allergy Clin Immunol. 2003;3(5):337–42.
51. Dunstan JA, et al. Fish oil supplementation in pregnancy modifies neonatal allergen-specific immune responses and clinical outcomes in infants at high risk of atopy: a randomized, controlled trial. J Allergy Clin Immunol. 2003;112(6):1178–84.
52. Wickens K, et al. Antibiotic use in early childhood and the development of asthma. Clin Exp Allergy. 1999;29(6):766–71.
53. Ni J, et al. Early antibiotic exposure and development of asthma and allergic rhinitis in childhood. BMC Pediatr. 2019;19(1):225.
54. Cohen S, Dworetzky M, Frick OL. Coca and Cooke on the classification of hypersensitiveness. J Allergy Clin Immunol. 2003;111(1):205–10.
55. Hill DA, et al. The epidemiologic characteristics of healthcare provider-diagnosed eczema, asthma, allergic rhinitis, and food allergy in children: a retrospective cohort study. BMC Pediatr. 2016;16:133.
56. Paller AS, et al. The atopic march and atopic multimorbidity: many trajectories, many pathways. J Allergy Clin Immunol. 2019;143(1):46–55.
57. Illi S, et al. The natural course of atopic dermatitis from birth to age 7 years and the association with asthma. J Allergy Clin Immunol. 2004;113(5):925–31.
58. Belgrave DC, et al. Developmental profiles of eczema, wheeze, and rhinitis: two population-based birth cohort studies. PLoS Med. 2014;11(10):e1001748.
59. Roduit C, et al. Phenotypes of atopic dermatitis depending on the timing of onset and progression in childhood. JAMA Pediatr. 2017;171(7):655–62.
60. Abo-Zaid G, et al. Association of Infant Eczema with childhood and adult asthma: analysis of data from the 1958 birth cohort study. Int J Environ Res Public Health. 2018;15(7)
61. Tran MM, et al. Predicting the atopic march: results from the Canadian healthy infant longitudinal development study. J Allergy Clin Immunol. 2018;141(2):601–607 e8.
62. Davidson WF, et al. Report from the National Institute of Allergy and Infectious Diseases workshop on "atopic dermatitis and the atopic march: mechanisms and interventions". J Allergy Clin Immunol. 2019;143(3):894–913.
63. Ziyab AH, et al. Epistasis between FLG and IL4R genes on the risk of allergic sensitization: results from two population-based birth cohort studies. Sci Rep. 2018;8(1):3221.
64. Lack G, et al. Factors associated with the development of peanut allergy in childhood. N Engl J Med. 2003;348(11):977–85.
65. Du Toit G, et al. Randomized trial of peanut consumption in infants at risk for peanut allergy. N Engl J Med. 2015;372(9):803–13.
66. du Toit G, et al. Allergen specificity of early Peanut consumption and effect on development of allergic disease in the learning early about Peanut allergy study cohort. J Allergy Clin Immunol. 2018;141(4):1343–53.
67. Vermeulen EM, et al. Food allergy is an important risk factor for childhood asthma, irrespective of whether it resolves. J Allergy Clin Immunol Pract. 2018;6(4):1336–1341 e3.
68. Erwin EA, et al. Contribution of dust mite and cat specific IgE to total IgE: relevance to asthma prevalence. J Allergy Clin Immunol. 2007;119(2):359–65.
69. Platts-Mills TA, et al. Pro: the evidence for a causal role of dust mites in asthma. Am J Respir Crit Care Med. 2009;180(2):109–13; discussion 120–1.
70. Wisniewski JA, et al. Sensitization to food and inhalant allergens in relation to age and wheeze among children with atopic dermatitis. Clin Exp Allergy. 2013;43(10):1160–70.
71. Huovinen E, et al. Incidence and prevalence of asthma among adult Finnish men and women of the Finnish twin cohort from 1975 to 1990, and their relation to hay fever and chronic bronchitis. Chest. 1999;115(4):928–36.
72. Kramer MS, Kakuma R. Maternal dietary antigen avoidance during pregnancy or lactation, or both, for preventing or treating atopic disease in the child. Evid Based Child Health. 2014;9(2):447–83.
73. Netting MJ, Middleton PF, Makrides M. Does maternal diet during pregnancy and lactation affect outcomes in offspring? A systematic review of food-based approaches. Nutrition. 2014;30(11–12):1225–41.
74. Lodge CJ, et al. Breastfeeding and asthma and allergies: a systematic review and meta-analysis. Acta Paediatr. 2015;104(467):38–53.
75. Kramer MS, Kakuma R. Optimal duration of exclusive breastfeeding. Cochrane Database Syst Rev. 2012;8:CD003517.

76. von Berg A, et al. The effect of hydrolyzed cow's milk formula for allergy prevention in the first year of life: the German infant nutritional intervention study, a randomized double-blind trial. J Allergy Clin Immunol. 2003;111(3):533–40.
77. von Berg A, et al. Allergic manifestation 15 years after early intervention with hydrolyzed formulas–the GINI Study. Allergy. 2016;71(2):210–9.
78. Boyle RJ, et al. Hydrolysed formula and risk of allergic or autoimmune disease: systematic review and meta-analysis. BMJ. 2016;352:i974.
79. Perkin MR, et al. Randomized trial of introduction of allergenic foods in breast-fed infants. N Engl J Med. 2016;374(18):1733–43.
80. Ierodiakonou D, et al. Timing of allergenic food introduction to the infant diet and risk of allergic or autoimmune disease: a systematic review and meta-analysis. JAMA. 2016;316(11):1181–92.
81. Chalmers JR, et al. Daily emollient during infancy for prevention of eczema: the BEEP randomised controlled trial. Lancet. 2020;395(10228):962–72.
82. Skjerven HO, et al. Skin emollient and early complementary feeding to prevent infant atopic dermatitis (PreventADALL): a factorial, multicentre, cluster-randomised trial. Lancet. 2020;395(10228):951–61.
83. Kelleher MM, et al. Skin care interventions in infants for preventing eczema and food allergy. Cochrane Database Syst Rev. 2021;2:CD013534.
84. Valovirta E, et al. Results from the 5-year SQ grass sublingual immunotherapy tablet asthma prevention (GAP) trial in children with grass pollen allergy. J Allergy Clin Immunol. 2018;141(2):529–538 e13.
85. Kristiansen M, et al. Allergen immunotherapy for the prevention of allergy: a systematic review and meta-analysis. Pediatr Allergy Immunol. 2017;28(1):18–29.
86. Muller U, Helbling A, Bischof M. Predictive value of venom-specific IgE, IgG and IgG subclass antibodies in patients on immunotherapy with honey bee venom. Allergy. 1989;44(6):412–8.
87. Dahl R, et al. Sublingual grass allergen tablet immunotherapy provides sustained clinical benefit with progressive immunologic changes over 2 years. J Allergy Clin Immunol. 2008;121(2):512–518 e2.
88. Gleich GJ, et al. Effect of immunotherapy on immunoglobulin E and immunoglobulin G antibodies to ragweed antigens: a six-year prospective study. J Allergy Clin Immunol. 1982;70(4):261–71.
89. Hedlin G, et al. Comparison of the in-vivo and in-vitro response to ragweed immunotherapy in children and adults with ragweed-induced rhinitis. Clin Exp Allergy. 1990;20(5):491–500.
90. Akdis CA, Akdis M. Mechanisms of allergen-specific immunotherapy. J Allergy Clin Immunol. 2011;127(1):18–27; quiz 28–9.
91. Rispens T, et al. Mechanism of immunoglobulin G4 fab-arm exchange. J Am Chem Soc. 2011;133(26):10302–11.
92. James, L.K., et al., Long-term tolerance after allergen immunotherapy is accompanied by selective persistence of blocking antibodies. J Allergy Clin Immunol, 2011. 127(2): p. 509–516 e1–5.
93. Renand A, et al. Synchronous immune alterations mirror clinical response during allergen immunotherapy. J Allergy Clin Immunol. 2018;141(5):1750–1760 e1.
94. Jutel M, et al. Influence of bee venom immunotherapy on degranulation and leukotriene generation in human blood basophils. Clin Exp Allergy. 1996;26(10):1112–8.
95. Jutel M, et al. IL-10 and TGF-beta cooperate in the regulatory T cell response to mucosal allergens in normal immunity and specific immunotherapy. Eur J Immunol. 2003;33(5):1205–14.
96. Suarez-Fueyo A, et al. Grass tablet sublingual immunotherapy downregulates the TH2 cytokine response followed by regulatory T-cell generation. J Allergy Clin Immunol. 2014;133(1):130–8 e1–2.
97. Zimmer A, et al. A regulatory dendritic cell signature correlates with the clinical efficacy of allergen-specific sublingual immunotherapy. J Allergy Clin Immunol. 2012;129(4):1020–30.
98. Angelini F, et al. Dendritic cells modification during sublingual immunotherapy in children with allergic symptoms to house dust mites. World J Pediatr. 2011;7(1):24–30.
99. Kuehr J, et al. Efficacy of combination treatment with anti-IgE plus specific immunotherapy in polysensitized children and adolescents with seasonal allergic rhinitis. J Allergy Clin Immunol. 2002;109(2):274–80.
100. Wachholz PA, et al. Inhibition of allergen-IgE binding to B cells by IgG antibodies after grass pollen immunotherapy. J Allergy Clin Immunol. 2003;112(5):915–22.

Part II

Allergic and Non-Allergic Rhinitis

Edited by Whit Mims

4 Allergic Rhinitis: Epidemiology and Evaluation

James W. Mims

Introduction and Definition

At first glance, allergic rhinitis (AR) appears to have annoying, but harmless, symptoms brought about by known allergic triggers which can be easily diagnosed and reliably confirmed with testing. However, a closer examination reveals a more heterogeneous disease which often deceives providers and patients.

With allergy testing that has a high false positive rate in the general population and symptoms that overlap with non-allergic nasal conditions, AR is a common chronic condition that can be difficult to distinguish from other causes of nasal inflammation. Additionally, moderate/severe AR has a substantial negative impact on sleep efficiency, school performance, and work productivity.

There are multiple definitions of AR in the medical literature. Most definitions agree that AR is nasal inflammation caused by IgE-mediated allergy. A highly referenced definition comes from the 2008 ARIA (Allergic Rhinitis Impact on Asthma) Guidelines developed through the World Health Organization which states, "Allergic rhinitis is clinically defined as a symptomatic disorder of the nose induced after allergen exposure by an IgE–mediated inflammation." [1].

Symptoms and Evaluation

Primary Symptoms

There are four primary symptoms of allergic rhinitis: nasal obstruction, rhinorrhea, nasal itching, and sneezing. Of these, nasal obstruction has the greatest negative effect on quality of life and sleep [2, 3]. Interestingly, one of the most common therapies for allergic rhinitis are oral antihistamines, which have very limited effect on nasal obstruction. Nasal obstruction is thought to be the predominant symptom in those with "year-round", or perennial, allergic rhinitis [4]. Table 4.1 shows the symptoms and percentage of allergic rhinitis patients that report having each.

There has been some contention that allergic rhinitis and allergic conjunctivitis are so frequently found together that allergic rhinoconjunctivitis is a better description of the natural disease state [4]. In this chapter, allergic conjunctivitis is discussed later in "Associated Conditions".

J. W. Mims (✉)
Department of Otolaryngology, Wake Forest School of Medicine, Winston-Salem, NC, USA
e-mail: wmims@wakehealth.edu

C. Damask et al. (eds.), *Allergy in Otolaryngology Practice*, https://doi.org/10.1007/978-3-031-93455-1_4

Table 4.1 Symptoms of allergic rhinitis [5]

Symptoms	Percentage
Sneezing	84
Rhinorrhea	77
Nasal obstruction	71
Nasal itching	57

Classification

Traditionally, allergic rhinitis was divided into "Seasonal" and "Perennial". In the 2001 ARIA guideline it was recommended that "Intermittent Allergic Rhinitis" (IAR) and "Persistent Allergic Rhinitis" (PER) were more appropriate as one might be intermittently exposed to an allergic source (e.g. a cat) irrespective of season [6]. PER was defined by having symptoms 4 or more consecutive days a week and for more than 4 consecutive weeks, but most classified as PER have daily symptoms throughout the year and seasonal variations [1, 6].

Severity

One of the confounders to guiding the epidemiology and treatment recommendations for AR is the variability in severity. ARIA Guidelines have divided allergic rhinitis into two categories by severity, "Mild" and "Moderate/Severe". The criteria for "Moderate/Severe" is listed in Box 4.1, while the absence of all the "Moderate/Severe" criteria qualifies as "Mild". The classification of AR "severity" is almost entirely subjective and quantified allergy test results (wheal size or sIgE level) do not correlate with symptom severity [7, 8].

Box 4.1 ARIA Criteria for "Moderate/Severe" AR

Sleep disturbance
Impairment of daily activities, leisure, and/or sport
Impairment of work or school
Troublesome symptoms

If one or more of the criteria are present, AR is classified as "moderate/severe" [1, 6].

Physical Findings

The physical findings of AR are non-specific and little is known about the sensitivity, specificity, or inter-observer reliability of physical exam. Classically, turbinate hypertrophy, nasal secretions, supra-nasal tip crease, infra-orbital skin edema and discoloration, pharyngeal mucosal thickening, and pharyngeal drainage have been physical signs attributed to AR [9]. As nasal and ocular itching can be present, nasal or eye rubbing can be observed.

Imaging/Endoscopy

On nasal endoscopy, polypoid changes limited to the head of the middle turbinate are associated with allergic rhinitis [10–12]. Also, CT scans demonstrating enlarged inferior and middle turbinates with clear (or minimal) sinus disease, referred to as sino-nasal "Central Compartment" inflammation, is also associated with AR [13].

AR guidelines generally do not recommend imaging or nasal endoscopy for the diagnosis of AR alone, [14] but in 2020 there is some discordance between the newer endoscopic and imaging literature and the guidelines. As some of the symptoms of chronic sinusitis and AR overlap, recognizing signs specific for AR on CT scans and nasal endoscopy is helpful for the practicing otolaryngologist.

Burdon of Disease

There is evidence that AR has a substantial impact on quality of life (QOL), sleep, ambulatory health care utilization, pharmaceutical expense, work productivity, and school performance.

Quality of Life

The 2018 International Consensus Statement on Allergic Rhinitis found two systematic reviews on AR and QOL [15]. Both found evidence of measurable decrease in quality of life from AR [16, 17]. The effect on QOL was similar to other chronic diseases including epilepsy, liver disease, and migraines [16]. In Spain, one study found the decrease in health-related QOL was 25% for AR compared to controls using the Short Form 12 [18]. Perennial AR has been found to have a greater impact on QOL than Seasonal AR [16].

Sleep

Contributing to AR's negative impact on well-being, AR has been found to disturb sleep. A large 2020 meta-analysis of AR and sleep was reported on 240 million cumulative subjects. Impaired sleep latency, higher sleep disturbance scores, lower sleep efficiency, increased insomnia, increased restless sleep, increased nocturnal enuresis, increased sleep disorder breathing, increased obstructive sleep apnea, and increased snoring were found more frequently in AR patients compared to controls [2]. Subjects with AR also reported daytime dysfunction associated with poor sleep including morning headaches, sleepiness, and use of sleeping pills [2].

Costs

The direct costs and indirect costs of AR have been estimated but vary between countries and studies. Many of these studies predate non-sedating antihistamines and may not be applicable to the current environment where better pharmacologic options are available over the counter. Generally, indirect costs are probably higher than direct costs [16].

Work Productivity

Work productivity has been shown to be negatively affected by AR. AR is associated with "presenteeism" which refers to workers' decreased productivity without absence. In one study, 36% of workers with AR reported decreased workplace performance due to AR [19]. In the United States, the annual loss associated with presenteeism from AR was estimated for 1995 at $600 million [20]. In 2003, indirect costs from AR calculations ranged a hundred-fold from $100 million to $9.7 billion US$ [21, 22].

School Performance

As the incidence of AR peaks in the teenage and young adult age groups, the impact of AR on school performance has been evaluated in several studies. Grass pollen allergy has been shown to lower summer college entrance exam scores for allergic students compared to controls as matched against winter pre-test scores [23]. Sedating antihistamines confound the issue by also impairing school performance [23, 24].

Epidemiology

Self-Reported/Parent-Reported AR: Survey Data

One method to assess the prevalence of AR is to survey populations and ask about AR symptoms, self-diagnosis, or health care provider (HCP) diagnosis. The results of these surveys have varied with region, age, and how the question is worded. Some surveys use the term "Hay Fever" to be consistent with historical surveys (even though "Hay Fever" is not recommended terminology in current guidelines).

Questionnaire data on 54,178 children (8–12 years of age) varied markedly between different sites in the International Study of Asthma and Allergies in Childhood (ISAAC) phase II study. Rhinoconjunctivitis symptoms in the absence of URI varied from 1.5% in Ecuador to 24.5% in Spain [25]. The ISAAC phase I study reported on questionnaires across the world in 463,801 children aged 13–14 and 257,800 aged 6–7 years old. The 50%tile (range per testing center) for "rhinitis within the past year with itchy watery eyes" was 5.9% (0.8–14.9) in 6–7-year olds and 13.6% (1.4–39.7) for 13–14-year olds. The 50%tile for ever having "hay fever" was 7.2% (0.0–39.4) in 6–7-year olds and 16.4% (0.0–54.4) for 13–14-year olds [26].

In the United States, a national screening of 35,757 households by phone was conducted to assess nasal allergies in children aged 4–17 years old in 2006. The survey asked if they had been diagnosed with AR, "hay fever", or nasal allergies by an HCP. They reported "13% of children had an HCP-confirmed diagnosis of AR and were symptomatic during the year before the survey." [3] Approximately 50% of those with HCP-confirmed AR reported prior allergy testing. The authors compared this to an estimated 14% of adults citing an unpublished survey [3]. In a separate study of adults, a survey was mailed to weighted sample of the US population in 2004. Of 19,678 adults in the surveyed households, 30.2% reported nasal symptoms attributed to allergies >6 days in the last 12 months and 15.7% > 29 days. The subjects that reported HCP-confirmed AR and symptoms was 22% independent of allergy testing [27].

Population Allergy Testing

Population testing surveys of inhalant allergen sensitivity, independent of symptoms, have been done using skin prick testing or sIgE testing of common allergens. These studies typically show a much higher rate of positive allergen tests (allergic sensitivity) than the prevalnece of surveyed symptoms. The CDC has conducted surveys of a representative sample of the US population finding positive allergy tests in 54.3% (by Skin Prick Test 1988–94) [28] and 43.7% (by sIgE in 2005–6) of participants [29].

In 31,759 international school-aged children, the ISAAC Phase II study found large variations in Skin Prick Tests (SPT) to 6 common aero-allergens. For perennial allergens, positive SPT ranged from 1.4% in Ghana to 45.2% in Hong Kong [25]. For seasonal allergens, positive SPT ranged from 0.1% in Ghana to 25.8% in Norway [25].

There are substantially more people with positive allergy tests than report bothersome rhinitis symptoms. There is a potential for clinicians to over-diagnose AR if too reliant on testing alone.

AR Diagnosed by History and Positive Allergy Testing

Epidemiologic studies that assess allergy history and allergy testing have also been performed. This shows a smaller percentage with AR than either history or testing alone (Table 4.2).

Cohort studies also provide some insight. The Multicenter Allergy Study (MAS) in Germany followed 1314 children from birth to age 20 years. Thirty-eight percent were selected as a high-risk group skewing the cohort toward more allergic than the general population. They found a cumulative incidence of AR between ages 4 and 20 years of age to be 290/1314 (22%) [32].

Family History of Allergy

Taking a family history can be helpful in assessing for AR. In the MAS cohort, 14% of 20-year olds with one allergic parent were diagnosed with AR (history + sIgE testing) compared to 7% with no allergic parents [32, 33]. However, in the 30,000 children in the ISAAC II studies, parental allergies did not influence their results and were omitted [25]. Discrepancies between high-risk cohorts and the general population are common in allergy epidemiology.

Table 4.2 Percentage of population with positive allergic history and positive allergy testing [30]

Study	Age in years	Size	Allergic history and testing (%)
SAPALDIA [31]	18–60	$N = 8329$	12
NHANES 2005–2006 [29, 30]	≥6	$N = 7398$	13.6

Allergic Rhinitis and Age

Allergic rhinitis generally begins to present in school-aged children, increases till the late teens or early 20s, and then decreases [34]. For example, the MAS cohort showed steadily rising incidence to the ages of 15 and 20 years of age [32].

The ISAAC studies of children were notable for profound variability across countries but the mean prevalence of rhinoconjunctivitis by questionnaire was higher in the 13–15 years of age cohort than the 6–7 years of age cohort [35]. Testing sensitivity and symptoms may change discordantly with age. A Swedish study in 2009 compared a cohort's SPTs at ages 7–8 years old and again 10 years later and found an increase from 20.6% to 29.9% ($p < 0.001$) in those with at least one positive SPT. However, the prevalence of rhinitis symptoms in the same subjects only changed from 14.5% to 15.1% [36].

Assessing AR in the preschool age group is clinically difficult due to the ubiquity of viral rhinitis. Assessing allergic rhinitis in older adults is complicated by the increased prevalence of chronic non-allergic rhinitis. Generally, burdensome AR is uncommon in the elderly (allergic senescence), but there is some debate on this issue as inhalant allergy testing can remain positive despite clinical tolerance (which is also observed in other settings such as allergy immunotherapy).

Allergic Rhinitis and Gender

AR was more common in school-aged boys than school-aged girls in the MAS cohort [32]. However, allergic asthma is known to change from being common in boys before puberty but more common in females after puberty. Similarly, the male-to-female ratio in AR narrowed after puberty [32]. However, in the ISAAC Phase II international survey of AR in school-aged children, gender did not influence the models and was omitted [25]. This is another example of discordances between high-risk and general populations in allergy epidemiology.

Allergic Rhinitis and Socioeconomics

Several cohorts have looked at socio-economic status and the prevalence of AR. The results have been contradictory. The 2018 International Consensus on Allergic Rhinitis concluded that pediatric cohorts in developed nations showed more AR in higher socio-economic groups, but after 1990, lower socio-economic status appeared to be a risk factor for AR [15]. Air quality, industrialization, and early childhood infections are commonly researched variables.

Allergic Rhinitis: Risk and Protective Factors

Risk factors vary between studies, but a list of commonly investigated risk factors is provided in Table 4.3 and protective factors in Table 4.4. The controversies and nuances of the conflicting studies are beyond the scope of this chapter, but it is important to remember that AR is a heterogeneous disease that appears to be influenced by a multitude of genetic and environmental factors.

Table 4.3 Potential risk factors for AR [15]

Risk factor	Evidence
Genetics	Supported by genealogy and genetic studies, but genetic underpinnings of AR unclear
Early mite exposure	Studies conflict
Early pollen exposure	Studies conflict
Early dander exposure	Studies conflict
Maternal diet	No association with AR
Food allergy when >2 y.o.	Risk factor for AR
Air pollution	Unclear
Tobacco smoke	Associated with non-allergic rhinitis
High socioeconomic status	Inconsistent risk factor

Table 4.4 Potential protective factors [15]

Protective factor	Evidence
Breastfeeding	Unclear, less rhinitis (viral?) under age 5 y.o.
Childhood pet exposure	Dog exposure in non-allergic families probably protective. Results vary between high-risk AR (harmful) and non-allergic populations (helpful)
Siblings	More siblings associated with less AR
Early-life farm living	Protective, especially animal farms
Microbial flora diversity	Probably protective

Allergic Rhinitis: Associated Conditions

The conditions associated with AR tend to be other allergic conditions such as allergic asthma, allergic conjunctivitis, food allergy, and atopic dermatitis. In several cohorts, childhood allergic asthma (AA) may precede AR with an odds ratio ranging from 3.4 to 4.8 compared to non-asthmatic children [37]. Classically, the Atopic March is considered the progression from atopic dermatitis and food allergy in infancy to AR and AA in childhood or later. It has been observed that only 3.1% of children follow this model, [38] and the search for reproducible endotypes of atopic disease is an area of current interest and research [37].

Many with AR also have allergic conjunctivitis. A survey of rhinitis symptoms, eye symptoms, and SPT was performed in 2120 Swiss children. Of children who reported rhinitis without a cold, 59.6% reported itchy-watery eyes. Adding itchy-watery eyes to rhinitis symptoms increased the specificity (83–92.8%) of having a positive allergy test but the sensitivity decreased and was low (37.5–25.7%) [39].

There is not a clear causal relationship between AR and chronic sinusitis (CRS) with or without polyps, although having both AR and CRS appears have a negative effect on QOL and recidivism of CRS [15].

Conclusion

Allergic rhinitis is primarily diagnosed by history and symptoms that may include variable combinations of intermittent rhinorrhea, nasal congestion, nasal/ocular itching, and sneezing. In persistent allergic rhinitis, the most common symptom is nasal congestion. While exam is often non-specific, most persons with moderate/severe AR have physical findings. If isolated polypoid changes to the head of the middle turbinate are seen on nasal endoscopy, AR is highly correlated (specific, but not sensitive).

There are complex genetic and environmental contributions to AR resulting in varied epidemiology across different populations. In the United States approximately 50% will have a positive allergy test, 30% report some nasal allergies with half to a fourth being more severe. Both positive testing and symptoms are seen in roughly 15%. Having an allergic parent or other allergic conditions is associated with higher prevalence of AR. AR is associated with allergic asthma and allergic conjunctivitis.

AR is most accurately diagnosed by history and corresponding allergic testing, but testing should be reserved for when it is useful in clinical management. While not life-threatening, AR can have a substantial impact on quality of life, sleep, and school/work productivity.

Familiarity with the presentation and epidemiology of AR is clinically useful in otolaryngology to provide more accurate assessment which can lead to a better quality of life for our patients.

References

1. Bousquet J, Khaltaev N, Cruz AA, Denburg J, Fokkens WJ, Togias A, et al. Allergic rhinitis and its impact on asthma (ARIA) 2008 update (in collaboration with the World Health Organization, GA(2)LEN and AllerGen). Allergy. 2008;63(Suppl 86):8–160. https://doi.org/10.1111/j.1398-9995.2007.01620.x.
2. Liu J, Zhang X, Zhao Y, Wang Y. The association between allergic rhinitis and sleep: a systematic review and meta-analysis of observational studies. PLoS One. 2020;15(2):e0228533. https://doi.org/10.1371/journal.pone.0228533.

3. Meltzer EO, Blaiss MS, Derebery MJ, Mahr TA, Gordon BR, Sheth KK, et al. Burden of allergic rhinitis: results from the pediatric allergies in America survey. J Allergy Clin Immunol. 2009;124(3 Suppl):S43–70. https://doi.org/10.1016/j.jaci.2009.05.013.
4. Dykewicz MS, Fineman S, Skoner DP, Nicklas R, Lee R, Blessing-Moore J, et al. Diagnosis and management of rhinitis: complete guidelines of the joint task force on practice parameters in allergy, asthma and immunology. American Academy of allergy, asthma, and immunology. Ann Allergy Asthma Immunol. 1998;81(5 Pt 2):478–518. https://doi.org/10.1016/s1081-1206(10)63155-9.
5. Marple BF, Fornadley JA, Patel AA, Fineman SM, Fromer L, Krouse JH, et al. Keys to successful management of patients with allergic rhinitis: focus on patient confidence, compliance, and satisfaction. Otolaryngol Head Neck Surg. 2007;136(6 Suppl):S107–24. https://doi.org/10.1016/j.otohns.2007.02.031.
6. Bousquet J, et al. Allergic rhinitis and its impact on asthma. J Allergy Clin Immunol. 2001;108(5 Suppl):S147–334. https://doi.org/10.1067/mai.2001.118891.
7. Graif Y, Goldberg A, Tamir R, Vigiser D, Melamed S. Skin test results and self-reported symptom severity in allergic rhinitis: the role of psychological factors. Clin Exp Allergy. 2006;36(12):1532–7. https://doi.org/10.1111/j.1365-2222.2006.02589.x.
8. Pastorello EA, Incorvaia C, Ortolani C, Bonini S, Canonica GW, Romagnani S, et al. Studies on the relationship between the level of specific IgE antibodies and the clinical expression of allergy: I. Definition of levels distinguishing patients with symptomatic from patients with asymptomatic allergy to common aeroallergens. J Allergy Clin Immunol. 1995;96(5 Pt 1):580–7. https://doi.org/10.1016/s0091-6749(95)70255-5.
9. Franzese CB. AAOA allergy primer: history and physical examination. Int Forum Allergy Rhinol. 2014;4(Suppl 2):S28–31. https://doi.org/10.1002/alr.21390.
10. White LJ, Rotella MR, DelGaudio JM. Polypoid changes of the middle turbinate as an indicator of atopic disease. Int Forum Allergy Rhinol. 2014;4(5):376–80. https://doi.org/10.1002/alr.21290.
11. Hamizan AW, Christensen JM, Ebenzer J, Oakley G, Tattersall J, Sacks R, et al. Middle turbinate edema as a diagnostic marker of inhalant allergy. Int Forum Allergy Rhinol. 2017;7(1):37–42. https://doi.org/10.1002/alr.21835.
12. Brunner JP, Jawad BA, McCoul ED. Polypoid change of the middle turbinate and paranasal sinus polyposis are distinct entities. Otolaryngol Head Neck Surg. 2017;157(3):519–23. https://doi.org/10.1177/0194599817711887.
13. DelGaudio JM, Loftus PA, Hamizan AW, Harvey RJ, Wise SK. Central compartment atopic disease. Am J Rhinol Allergy. 2017;31(4):228–34. https://doi.org/10.2500/ajra.2017.31.4443.
14. Seidman MD, Gurgel RK, Lin SY, Schwartz SR, Baroody FM, Bonner JR, et al. Clinical practice guideline: allergic rhinitis. Otolaryngol Head Neck Surg. 2015;152(1 Suppl):S1–43. https://doi.org/10.1177/0194599814561600.
15. Wise SK, Lin SY, Toskala E, Orlandi RR, Akdis CA, Alt JA, et al. International consensus statement on allergy and rhinology: allergic rhinitis. Int Forum Allergy Rhinol. 2018;8(2):108–352. https://doi.org/10.1002/alr.22073.
16. Linneberg A, Dam Petersen K, Hahn-Pedersen J, Hammerby E, Serup-Hansen N, Boxall N. Burden of allergic respiratory disease: a systematic review. Clin Mol Allergy. 2016;14:12. https://doi.org/10.1186/s12948-016-0049-9.
17. Hahn-Pedersen J, Boxall N, Maier W, Linneberg A, Serup-Hansen N. Systematic literature review assessing data on the burden of allergic rhinitis from a cost and quality of life perspective. Value Health. 2014;17(7):A602. https://doi.org/10.1016/j.jval.2014.08.2087.
18. Navarro A, Colas C, Anton E, Conde J, Davila I, Dordal MT, et al. Epidemiology of allergic rhinitis in allergy consultations in Spain: Alergologica-2005. J Investig Allergol Clin Immunol. 2009;19(Suppl 2):7–13.
19. Blanc PD, Trupin L, Eisner M, Earnest G, Katz PP, Israel L, et al. The work impact of asthma and rhinitis: findings from a population-based survey. J Clin Epidemiol. 2001;54(6):610–8. https://doi.org/10.1016/s0895-4356(00)00349-8.
20. Settipane RA, Schwindt C. Chapter 15: allergic rhinitis. Am J Rhinol Allergy. 2013;27(Suppl 1):S52–5. https://doi.org/10.2500/ajra.2013.27.3928.
21. Simoens S, Laekeman G. Pharmacotherapy of allergic rhinitis: a pharmaco-economic approach. Allergy. 2009;64(1):85–95. https://doi.org/10.1111/j.1398-9995.2008.01909.x.
22. Reed SD, Lee TA, McCrory DC. The economic burden of allergic rhinitis: a critical evaluation of the literature. PharmacoEconomics. 2004;22(6):345–61. https://doi.org/10.2165/00019053-200422060-00002.
23. Walker S, Khan-Wasti S, Fletcher M, Cullinan P, Harris J, Sheikh A. Seasonal allergic rhinitis is associated with a detrimental effect on examination performance in United Kingdom teenagers: case-control study. J Allergy Clin Immunol. 2007;120(2):381–7. https://doi.org/10.1016/j.jaci.2007.03.034.
24. Jauregui I, Mullol J, Davila I, Ferrer M, Bartra J, del Cuvillo A, et al. Allergic rhinitis and school performance. J Investig Allergol Clin Immunol. 2009;19(Suppl 1):32–9.
25. Weinmayr G, Forastiere F, Weiland SK, Rzehak P, Abramidze T, Annesi-Maesano I, et al. International variation in prevalence of rhinitis and its relationship with sensitisation to perennial and seasonal allergens. Eur Respir J. 2008;32(5):1250–61. https://doi.org/10.1183/09031936.00157807.

26. Strachan D, Sibbald B, Weiland S, Ait-Khaled N, Anabwani G, Anderson HR, et al. Worldwide variations in prevalence of symptoms of allergic rhinoconjunctivitis in children: the international study of asthma and allergies in childhood (ISAAC). Pediatr Allergy Immunol. 1997;8(4):161–76. https://doi.org/10.1111/j.1399-3038.1997.tb00156.x.
27. Nathan RA, Meltzer EO, Derebery J, Campbell UB, Stang PE, Corrao MA, et al. The prevalence of nasal symptoms attributed to allergies in the United States: findings from the burden of rhinitis in an America survey. Allergy Asthma Proc. 2008;29(6):600–8. https://doi.org/10.2500/aap.2008.29.3179.
28. Arbes SJ Jr, Gergen PJ, Elliott L, Zeldin DC. Prevalences of positive skin test responses to 10 common allergens in the US population: results from the third National Health and nutrition examination survey. J Allergy Clin Immunol. 2005;116(2):377–83. https://doi.org/10.1016/j.jaci.2005.05.017.
29. Salo PM, Calatroni A, Gergen PJ, Hoppin JA, Sever ML, Jaramillo R, et al. Allergy-related outcomes in relation to serum IgE: results from the National Health and nutrition examination survey 2005-2006. J Allergy Clin Immunol. 2011;127(5):1226–35 e7. https://doi.org/10.1016/j.jaci.2010.12.1106.
30. Mims JW. Epidemiology of allergic rhinitis. Int Forum Allergy Rhinol. 2014;4(Suppl 2):S18–20. https://doi.org/10.1002/alr.21385.
31. Tschopp JM, Sistek D, Schindler C, Leuenberger P, Perruchoud AP, Wuthrich B, et al. Current allergic asthma and rhinitis: diagnostic efficiency of three commonly used atopic markers (IgE, skin prick tests, and Phadiatop). Results from 8329 randomized adults from the SAPALDIA study. Swiss study on air pollution and lung diseases in adults. Allergy. 1998;53(6):608–13. https://doi.org/10.1111/j.1398-9995.1998.tb03937.x.
32. Lau S, Matricardi PM, Wahn U, Lee YA, Keil T. Allergy and atopy from infancy to adulthood: messages from the German birth cohort MAS. Ann Allergy Asthma Immunol. 2019;122(1):25–32. https://doi.org/10.1016/j.anai.2018.05.012.
33. Gough H, Grabenhenrich L, Reich A, Eckers N, Nitsche O, Schramm D, et al. Allergic multimorbidity of asthma, rhinitis and eczema over 20 years in the German birth cohort MAS. Pediatr Allergy Immunol. 2015;26(5):431–7. https://doi.org/10.1111/pai.12410.
34. Ghouri N, Hippisley-Cox J, Newton J, Sheikh A. Trends in the epidemiology and prescribing of medication for allergic rhinitis in England. J R Soc Med. 2008;101(9):466–72. https://doi.org/10.1258/jrsm.2008.080096.
35. Asher MI, Montefort S, Bjorksten B, Lai CK, Strachan DP, Weiland SK, et al. Worldwide time trends in the prevalence of symptoms of asthma, allergic rhinoconjunctivitis, and eczema in childhood: ISAAC phases one and three repeat multicountry cross-sectional surveys. Lancet. 2006;368(9537):733–43. https://doi.org/10.1016/S0140-6736(06)69283-0.
36. Ronmark E, Bjerg A, Perzanowski M, Platts-Mills T, Lundback B. Major increase in allergic sensitization in schoolchildren from 1996 to 2006 in northern Sweden. J Allergy Clin Immunol. 2009;124(2):357–63. https://doi.org/10.1016/j.jaci.2009.05.011.
37. Aw M, Penn J, Gauvreau GM, Lima H, Sehmi R. Atopic march: collegium Internationale Allergologicum update 2020. Int Arch Allergy Immunol. 2020;181(1):1–10. https://doi.org/10.1159/000502958.
38. Belgrave DC, Simpson A, Buchan IE, Custovic A. Atopic dermatitis and respiratory allergy: what is the link. Curr Dermatol Rep. 2015;4(4):221–7. https://doi.org/10.1007/s13671-015-0121-6.
39. Braun-Fahrlander C, Wuthrich B, Gassner M, Grize L, Sennhauser FH, Varonier HS, et al. Validation of a rhinitis symptom questionnaire (ISAAC core questions) in a population of Swiss school children visiting the school health services. SCARPOL-team. Swiss study on childhood allergy and respiratory symptom with respect to air pollution and climate. International study of asthma and allergies in childhood. Pediatr Allergy Immunol. 1997;8(2):75–82. https://doi.org/10.1111/j.1399-3038.1997.tb00147.x.

5 Pathophysiology of Allergic Rhinitis

William R. Reisacher

The European Academy of Allergy and Clinical Immunology (ECAAI) has defined "atopy" as, "*A personal or familial tendency to produce IgE antibodies in response to low doses of allergens, usually proteins, and to develop typical symptoms such as asthma, rhinoconjunctivitis, or eczema/dermatitis*" [1]. While many asymptomatic individuals may be able to produce IgE specific to allergens in our environment, the term "allergy" is reserved for those individuals who have a high enough level of sensitization to an allergen, combined with sufficient exposure, to produce symptoms which are bothersome when they are exposed to that allergen. In the nose, this phenomenon is called allergic rhinitis (AR).

Allergic Rhinitis

AR is one of the most common chronic diseases in humans. The condition decreases the quality of life for up to 30% of children and adults, particularly in industrialized countries, and is quickly becoming more prevalent in the urban regions of developing countries [2, 3]. The symptoms produced by AR, such as nasal congestion, rhinorrhea, sneezing, and pruritis, are mediated by immunoglobulin E (IgE), which also plays a role in other Type I inflammatory conditions, such as asthma, eczema, and anaphylaxis [4, 5]. Through the early history of humans, this type of inflammation was very beneficial for fighting parasitic infections, a common cause for infant mortality, which may help explain why AR has persisted in the modern world [6].

W. R. Reisacher (✉)
Department of Otolaryngology – Head and Neck Surgery, Weill Cornell Medical College / NewYork-Presbyterian Hospital, New York, NY, USA
e-mail: Wir2011@med.cornell.edu

The Nasal Cavity

The nasal cavity, which is strategically positioned at the entry point of the respiratory tract, is designed to detect stimuli that are presented to it from the environment. The range of stimuli is quite large, including infectious microbes, small chemical molecules, or allergen proteins to other factors related to air quality, such as particle density, temperature, and humidity. The nasal cavity must decide whether or not what has been detected is dangerous to the body, and then take the necessary steps to either mount a defense against it or tolerate it. To perform this function, the nasal cavity possesses an elaborate system of both innate and adaptive immune mechanisms. The innate immune system is the first line of defense, and uses both specific as well as non-specific mechanisms, while the adaptive immune system, as seen with AR, demonstrates both

C. Damask et al. (eds.), *Allergy in Otolaryngology Practice*,
https://doi.org/10.1007/978-3-031-93455-1_5

specificity and memory through the clonal proliferation of T and B lymphocytes [5].

The vestibule of the nasal cavity is lined with keratinized, stratified squamous epithelium, which is contiguous with the skin of the external nose. This squamous epithelium transitions to non-ciliated cuboidal or columnar epithelium at the *limen nasi* before becoming the true respiratory epithelium which lines the remainder of the nasal cavity and paranasal sinuses. This respiratory mucosa is a pseudostratified, ciliated, columnar epithelium comprised of three types of cells: ciliated cells, goblet cells, and basal cells. Ciliated cells are the most prevalent cell, each containing over 200 cilia which beat at 10–20 cycles per second to power mucociliary clearance. Goblet cells rest on the basement membrane, producing mucus that is expelled from the apical surface. The third cell type is the basal cell, which sits on the basement membrane and serves as a source of regenerating ciliated and goblet cells [7]. Other cell types which can be found in the nasal cavity include melanocytes, intraepithelial lymphocytes, plasma cells, mast cells, and eosinophils.

Mucus, which is primarily composed of high-molecular-weight, heavily glycosylated macromolecules, sits on a less dense layer of serous fluid produced from seromucinous glands in the underlying lamina propria. The viscous mucinous layer traps inhaled particulate matter, such as protein allergens, while the serous layer allows the underlying cilia to beat freely and direct mucous-trapped foreign matter toward the nasopharynx to prevent damage to the respiratory tract. The efficiency of this system is regulated by the physical properties of mucus as well as the ciliary beat frequency [8].

IgA is the most prevalent immunoglobulin in the nasal cavity. It exists in monomeric and dimeric forms, but the vast majority of IgA in the nasal cavity and paranasal sinuses is in the dimeric form of secretory IgA (SIgA). SIgA is a 390 kDa dimer linked by a J chain and containing a secretory component which allows for active passage across the nasal epithelium. This secretory IgA found in nasal mucus coats bacterial and other antigenic material and prohibits it from breaching the nasal mucosa [9].

Cells of the Adaptive Immune System

Antigen-presenting cells (APC) include macrophages and dendritic cells which engulf allergens and internalize them. This function is enhanced by opsonization, which involves coating allergenic particles with either antibodies or complement. Opsonization also attracts and activates other inflammatory cells in the lamina propria, such as lymphocytes, neutrophils, eosinophils, basophils, mast cells, and plasma cells. While this is largely a non-specific process, certain opsonins can be specific as well [10]. Serum amyloid A, an opsonin secreted by respiratory epithelial cells, has the ability to bind and agglutinate specific allergens, as well as bacteria, fungi, and inorganic particles [11, 12].

The mucosal lymphocyte population within the nasal cavity is composed predominately of T cells. This likely explains the finding that the majority of lymphomas of the nasal cavity are natural killer (NK) cell/T cell lymphomas. In contrast, lymphomas of the paranasal sinuses tend to originate from B cells [13]. T cells originate in the thymus, where they mature and undergo differentiation. After leaving the thymus, these cells move to other lymphoid organs under the control of cellular signals. T cells differentiate into one of two lineages: T helper cells which are positive for CD4 and cytotoxic T cells which are positive for CD8. CD4+ T helper cells further differentiate into either Th1 or Th2 cells based on their different cytokine profiles and functionality [14].

Th1 cells produce IL-2 and IFN-γ, which are involved in cytotoxic inflammatory reactions in response to intracellular pathogens, such as viruses or bacteria. They also participate in delayed-type hypersensitivity reactions, acting primarily through cell-mediated interactions and cytokine communication channels. Th2 cells, on the other hand, produce IL-1, IL-4, IL-5, IL-9, and IL-10, which favor IgE-mediated allergic inflammation and eosinophil production. Cytokines produced by each cell type, Th1 and Th2, inhibit the activation of the other cell type, thus preventing the activation of conflicting inflammatory pathways [14].

Differential activation of Th1 and Th2 pathways within the nasal cavity also promotes differential expression of rhinologic disease. In individuals with chronic rhinosinusitis with nasal polyps (CRSwNP), the local inflammatory environment exhibits a predominance of Th2 cells and the Th2-related cytokines, IL-4 and IL-5. This is significantly different from chronic rhinosinusitis without nasal polyps (CRSsNP), which is generally a Th1-driven process. Activation of the Th2 cytokine profile is associated with the influx of eosinophils, which compose 60–90% of the cell population in nasal polyps. The inflammatory products of eosinophils have the capacity to inflict local tissue damage which has been proposed to account for the inflammatory reactions that occur in nasal polyposis. The predominance of Th2 and eosinophilia-mediated reactions also account for the association of nasal polyps in individuals with AR and asthma, also Th2-driven processes [15].

B cells, the second class of lymphocytes that make up the adaptive immune system, originate in the bone marrow and are initially coated with IgM and IgD on their surfaces. After leaving the bone marrow, they migrate to secondary lymphoid organs and proliferate in response to antigen-stimulation and T cell interactions. When activated, B cells mature into plasma cells which secrete a monoclonal population of immunoglobulins specific to the activating allergen, including classes IgA, IgG, and IgE, each of which has a specific role in immune defense. This process is referred to as class-switching or isotype-switching [14].

Allergen Sensitization

When a sensitizing protein or carbohydrate allergen on the mucosal surface of the nose is detected by the surface receptors of an APC in a susceptible individual, it is taken up by that cell and transported to naïve CD4+ T cells either in the mucosa itself or in the locoregional lymph tissue. When that allergen is encountered on the major histocompatibility complex (MHC) of the APC, that T cell becomes activated and undergoes clonal expansion as a T helper type 2 (Th2) cells with specificity to that allergen [16].

Under the influence of cytokines, particularly IL-4, the activated Th2 cell stimulates a naïve B cell to undergo class-switching and begin producing IgE specific to the allergen. IgE is the main immunoglobulin involved in the allergic response and is very important in the pathophysiology of allergic rhinitis. The activation of B cells also produces proliferation of eosinophils, mast cells, and neutrophils [17]. The IgE which has been produced then binds to mast cells, basophils, lymphocytes, and other APCs through the high-affinity IgE receptor, FcεRI.

For many years, it was believed that class-switching occurred primarily in the large lymphoid structures of the body, such as the spleen or mesenteric lymph nodes, and that IgE was transported to the mucosa of the upper aerodigestive tract via the serum [18]. The idea that specific IgE could be produced in local nasal tissue began around 1947, two decades before the actual identification of IgE, when Sampter reported that nasal secretions from individuals with ragweed allergy could passively transfer symptoms to non-allergic individuals [19]. Then, in 1975, Huggins and Brostoff observed that specific IgE to dust mites was present in nasal secretions after nasal challenge, but not on skin prick testing (SPT) [20]. The following year, it was demonstrated that 78% of individuals with clinical AR, but no evidence of specific IgE in the serum, had specific IgE to airborne allergens on nasal lavage [21].

While it was known that the nasal mucosa contained all the cells (APCs, B cells, T cells) and cytokines (IL-4 and IL-13) required for class-switching, the actual production of specific IgE from functional nasal B cells cultured in a CD40-stimulating environment was finally demonstrated in 1996 [22, 23]. Four years later, KleinJan and colleagues used immunohistochemical analysis to demonstrate that specific IgE is produced in the nasal mucosa of individuals with seasonal and perennial AR, but not in healthy controls without AR [24].

Specific Allergic Inflammation

When a previously sensitized individual is exposed to a particular allergen again, the immune system reacts in two distinct reaction phases: early and late. Initiating the early phase, the allergen binds to IgE molecules present on the surface of mast cells and basophils. This cross-linking of IgE molecules causes the cell surface to become unstable and degranulate, releasing chemicals such as histamine, tryptase, prostaglandins, leukotrienes, cytokines, and platelet-activating factor, producing the common symptoms of sneezing, itching, rhinorrhea, and edema. Increased cytokine production results in the recruitment of additional inflammatory cells along with further amplification of the immune response [5]. This initial phase of the allergic reaction occurs within minutes of exposure and can last minutes to hours depending on the level of exposure of the individual to that allergen [25].

The late phase of allergic inflammation typically begins approximately 6 h after initial exposure, producing nasal congestion which subsides very slowly. The mechanism of this phase involves eosinophil chemotaxis promoted by the mediators released in the early phase. This cellular influx into the nasal mucosa, which also includes additional lymphocytes and mast cells, causes the breakdown and eventual remodeling of tissue [26].

Non-specific Hyperresponsiveness

Damage to the nasal mucosa caused by eosinophilic inflammation and other mediators can lead to exposure of sensory nerve C fibers, causing them to be more sensitive to normal and allergic stimuli. These excited fibers stimulate afferent as well as efferent fibers, causing them to secrete neuropeptides such as substance P and neurokinin A, producing what is known as neurogenic inflammation [27]. Substance P can also interact with receptors on mast cell membranes, leading to further degranulation. Smooth muscle contraction, goblet cell mucus secretion, and plasma exudate from capillaries produce the classic symptoms of congestion, sneezing, itching, and rhinorrhea [28]. This condition can be even more severe for individuals diagnosed with multiple chemical sensitivity.

Non-allergic rhinitis (NAR) is a clinical condition that resembles AR, characterized by inflammation of the sinonasal mucosa, congestion, rhinorrhea, sneezing, pruritus, and postnasal drainage, but results from non-allergen stimuli [29, 30]. NAR can exist along with AR (referred to as mixed rhinitis), and typical causes include rhinitis medicamentosa (through prolonged use of medications such as topical decongestants), gustatory rhinitis, weather-induced rhinitis, hormone-induced rhinitis, infectious rhinitis, NARES (non-allergic rhinitis eosinophilia syndrome), occupational rhinitis, senile rhinitis, atrophic rhinitis, and vasomotor rhinitis. After a complete evaluation, approximately 25% of individuals with clinical AR will receive the diagnosis of idiopathic NAR, based on the absence of antigen-specific IgE on skin or serum testing [31].

It has been reported that local sensitization can be demonstrated on nasal prevocational testing (NPT) in approximately 47% to 63% of individuals with perennial and seasonal AR who were previously diagnosed with idiopathic NAR [32–35]. These individuals are often described as having local allergic rhinitis, or LAR. Ohashi and colleagues detected antigen-specific IgE from homogenized nasal mucosa in 100% of individuals previously diagnosed with NAR based on negative skin and serum IgE testing [36]. Reisacher and colleagues also reported that 100% of individuals with idiopathic NAR had detectable antigen-specific IgE to at least one of nine airborne antigens on nasal mucosal brush biopsy (MBB) of the inferior turbinates, with 90% of the inner-city study participants sensitized to cockroach [37]. For a Type 1 inflammatory reaction to occur in the nose, however, there must be locally present IgE, whether it was produced in the mucosa or not, though the reasons systemic evidence of sensitization are often absent remain elusive.

References

1. Johansson SGO, Hourihane JOB, Bousquet J, et al. A revised nomenclature for allergy: an EAACI position statement from the EAACI nomenclature task force. Allergy. 2001;56:813–24.
2. Mallol J, Crane J, von Mutius E, et al. The international study of asthma and allergies in childhood (ISAAC) phase three: a global synthesis. Allergol Immunopathol (Madr). 2013;41:73.
3. Solé D, Cassol VE, Silva AR, et al. Prevalence of symptoms of asthma, rhinitis, and atopic eczema among adolescents living in urban and rural areas in different regions of Brazil. Allergol Immunopathol (Madr). 2007;35:248.
4. Mattos JL, Woodard CR, Payne SC. Trends in common rhinologic illnesses: analysis of U.S. healthcare surveys 1995–2007. Int Forum Allergy Rhinol. 2011;1:3–12.
5. Min YG. The pathophysiology, diagnosis and treatment of allergic rhinitis. Allergy Asthma Immunol Res. 2010;2(2):65–76.
6. Santiago HDC, Ribeiro-Gomes FL, Bennuru S, Nutman TB. Helminth infection alters IgE responses to allergens structurally related to parasite proteins. J Immunol. 2015;194:93–100.
7. Avery JK, Steele PF, Avery N. In: Avery JK, editor. Oral development and histology. 3rd ed. Thieme New York; 2002. p. 343–4.
8. Knowles MR, Boucher RC. Mucus clearance as a primary innate defense mechanism for mammalian airways. J Clin Invest. 2002;109:571–7.
9. Brandtzaeg P. Immunocompetent cells of the upper airway: functions in normal and diseased mucosa. Eur Arch Otorrinolaringol. 1995;252(Suppl 1):S8–21.
10. Ramanathan M, Lane AP. Innate immunity of the sinonasal cavity and its role in chronic rhinosinusitis. Otolaryngol Head Neck Surg. 2007;136:348–56.
11. Lane AP, Truong-Tran QA, Myers A, et al. Serum amyloid a, properdin, complement 3, and toll-like receptors are expressed locally in human sinonasal tissue. Am J Rhinol. 2006;20:117–23.
12. Madan T, Kishore U, Shah A, et al. Lung surfactant proteins a and D can inhibit specific IgE binding to the allergens of aspergillus fumigatus and block allergen-induced histamine release from human basophils. Clin Exp Immunol. 1997;110:241–9.
13. Balogh K, Pantanowitz L. Mouth, nose, and paranasal sinuses. In: Mills SE, editor. Histology for pathologists. 3rd ed. Philadelphia PA: Lippincott Williams & Wilkins; 2007. p. 403–30.
14. Kircher S, Marquardt D. Introduction to the immune system. In: Adelman DC, Casale TB, Corren J, editors. Manual of allergy and immunology. 4th ed. Philadelphia PA: Lippincott Williams & Wilkins; 2002. p. 1–23.
15. DeMarcantonio MA, Han JK. Nasal polyps: pathogenesis and treatment implications. Otolaryngol Clin N Am. 2011;44(3):685–95.
16. Chaplin DD. 1. Overview 1111 of the human immune response. J Allergy Clin Immunol. 2006;117:S430–5.
17. Broide DH. The pathophysiology of allergic rhinoconjunctivitis. Allergy Asthma Proc. 2007;28:398–403.
18. He JS, Narayanan S, Subramaniam S, et al. Biology of IgE production: IgE cell differentiation and the memory of IgE responses. Curr Top Microbiol Immunol. 2015;388:1–19.
19. Samter M. Ragweed reagins in nasal secretion. Proc Soc Exp Biol Med. 1947;65(1):140–1.
20. Huggins KG, Brostoff J. Local production of specific IgE antibodies in allergic rhinitis patients with negative skin tests. Lancet. 1975;2:148–50.
21. Merrett TG. Measurement of specific IgE antibodies in nasal secretion--evidence for local production. Clin Allergy. 1976;6:69–73.
22. Bradding P, Feather IJ, Wilson S, et al. Immunolocalization of cytokines in the nasal mucosa of normal and perennial rhinitis subjects. The mast cell as a source of IL-4, IL-5 and IL-6 in human allergic mucosal inflammation. J Immunol. 1993;151:3853–65.
23. Zurcher AW, Derer T, Lang AB, Stadler BM. Culture and IgE synthesis of nasal B cells. Int Arch Allergy Immunol. 1996;111:77–82.
24. KleinJan A, Vinke JG, Severijnen LWFM, Fokkens WJ. Local production and detection of (specific) IgE in nasal B-cells and plasma cells of allergic rhinitis patients. Eur Respir J. 2000;15:491–7.
25. Prussin C, Metcalfe DD. IgE, mast cells, basophils, and eosinophils. J Allergy Clin Immunol. 2006;117:S450–6.
26. Kay AB. Allergy and allergic diseases. Second of two parts. N Engl J Med. 2001;344:109–13.
27. Togias A. Unique mechanistic features of allergic rhinitis. J Allergy Clin Immunol. 2000;105:S599–604.
28. Gerth van Wijk RG, de Graaf-int' veld C, Garrelds IM. Nasal hyperreactivity. Rhinology. 1999;37:50–5.
29. Settipane RA, Charnock DR. Epidemiology of rhinitis: allergic and nonallergic. Clin Allergy Immunol. 2007;19:23–34.
30. Forester JP, Calabria CW. Local production of IgE in the respiratory mucosa and the concept of entopy: does allergy exist in nonallergic rhinitis? Ann Allergy Asthma Immunol. 2010;105:249–56.
31. Settipane RA. Other causes of rhinitis: mixed rhinitis, rhinitis medicamentosa, hormonal rhinitis, rhinitis of the elderly, and gustatory rhinitis. Immunol Allergy Clin N Am. 2011;31:457–67.
32. Carney AS, Powe DG, Huskisson RS, et al. Atypical nasal challenges in patients with idiopathic rhinitis: more evidence for the existence of allergy in the absence of atopy? Clin Exp Allergy. 2002;32:1436–40.
33. Rodon C, Romero JJ, Lopez S, et al. Local IgE production and positive nasal provocation test in patients with persistent nonallergic rhinitis. J Allergy Clin Immunol. 2007;119:899–905.
34. Rodon C, Dona I, Lopez S, et al. Seasonal idiopathic rhinitis with local inflammatory response and spe-

cific IgE in absence of systemic response. Allergy. 2008;63:1352–8.

35. Wedback A, Enbom H, Ericksson NE, et al. Seasonal non-allergic rhinitis (SNAR)—a new disease entity? A clinical and immunological comparison between SNAR, seasonal allergic rhinitis and persistent non-allergic rhinitis. Rhinology. 2005;43:86–92.
36. Ohashi Y, Nakai Y, Kuroki K, et al. Topical immunology of nasal allergy and mucosal IgE antibodies. Arch Otorhinolaryngol. 1985;241:169–74.
37. Reisacher WR, Bremberg MG. Prevalence of antigen-specific immunoglobulin E on mucosal brush biopsy of the inferior turbinates in patients with nonallergic rhinitis. Int Forum Allergy Rhinol. 2014;4(4):292–7.

Allergic Rhinitis Therapy: Environmental, Pharmacotherapy, and Immunotherapy

6

Maria C. Veling

Environmental Controls—Allergen Avoidance

After identifying the offending indoor allergens, allergic patients should minimize exposure to them as much as possible. This strategy is frequently discussed with patients as part of their treatment plan, so it's important to understand the available evidence regarding the effectiveness of this approach. Reducing exposure to the more common allergens of house dust mite, cockroach and pet dander have been studied in depth. Although there are successful strategies for minimizing allergen load and exposure, the clinical response to these difficult and expensive measures has had mixed results. The literature contains many studies that assessed a single intervention, which often fail to demonstrate efficacy [1]. Studies looking at multimodality approaches to environmental controls suggest a more robust response [2].

The following is a synopsis of the available data as it relates to these allergens.

M. C. Veling (✉)
UT Southwestern Medical Center, Children's Medical Center Dallas, Dallas, TX, USA
e-mail: Maria.Veling@UTSouthwestern.edu

House Dust Mite (HDM)

Techniques for house dust mite control have been studied extensively in the management of allergic rhinitis. Measures include physical barriers such as specialized covers for bedding and upholstered furniture, vacuuming, and air filtration [4]. Other strategies that minimize dust mite count include chemical treatment using acaricides [5], keeping the relative humidity below 50 percent in the home, and decreasing areas that can harbor the mite antigen such as carpets, drapes, upholstered furniture, etc.

While multiple studies have demonstrated reduced measurable allergen with these strategies [4, 5], improvement of symptoms has not been reliably demonstrated using isolated interventions [4]. A 2010 Cochrane review found acaricides to be the most effective as a single measure or in combination with other measures to decrease HDM levels and improve AR symptoms [6].

Cockroach

Interventions for the management of roach infestations include educating patients, minimizing cockroach access by sealing cracks and crevices, and using pesticides or bait traps [7]. Though more expensive, the most effective treatment for eliminating infestation and reducing allergen

C. Damask et al. (eds.), *Allergy in Otolaryngology Practice*,
https://doi.org/10.1007/978-3-031-93455-1_6

load is professional pest control [8]. Of note, Sever et al. [9] found that placement of insecticide bait traps was more effective than insecticide applications over a 12-month period,. With appropriate intervention, studies have shown reduction of cockroach allergen load in the home [10], but unfortunately, there is a scarcity of information regarding its effects on allergic rhinitis symptoms.

Pet Dander

When patients are allergic to their pets, as confirmed by testing and clinically significant symptomatology, avoidance is usually recommended. Pet removal is a difficult subject and one that is not likely to be welcomed with a reported low compliance rate [11]. A more tolerable approach is that of decreasing exposure, such as by removing the pet from the bedroom, pet washing, etc. However, demonstration of clinical improvement has been mixed [12].

Pharmacotherapy

Most patients with allergic rhinitis will require medical management for control of their symptoms. There are many pharmacologic options, and therapy is aimed at managing the particular symptoms for each patient. Patient's age, preference, comorbidities, chronicity of symptoms, and previous treatment are among the variables considered when choosing among pharmacologic agents.

Antihistamines

Histamine is a prominent mediator of the allergic response. It causes mucus secretion and vascular permeability resulting in the symptoms of rhinorrhea, sneezing, and pruritis. Over the years, different generations of oral antihistamines have been developed. An antihistamine works as a histamine receptor antagonist that decreases the inflammatory response and results in a reduction of allergic symptoms such as itching, sneezing, and rhinorrhea [13].

Oral H_1 Antihistamines

First-generation antihistamines, including brompheniramine, chlorpheniramine, hydroxyzine, and diphenhydramine, have the disadvantage of being lipophilic and therefore able to cross the brain-blood barrier. Unwanted side effects of these medications include sedation, fatigue, and impaired coordination, making first-generation antihistamines difficult and dangerous to use. In addition, their effect on the CYP2D6 enzyme pathway can interfere with the metabolism of other medications using the same hepatic enzymes. For these reasons, the use of first-generation antihistamines is no longer recommended as a first-line treatment option in allergic rhinitis [13].

Second- and third-generation antihistamines were developed to improve the adverse effect profile. These lipophobic agents have similar efficacy and fewer central nervous system effects. Their onset of action is usually within one hour, dosing is every 12 to 24 hours, and they appear to be similarly efficacious to each other [14]. Their metabolism by the cytochrome P450 CYP3A4 system has the potential to interfere with other medications, which can result in increased drug concentrations and toxicity. Second- and third-generation antihistamines include cetirizine, loratadine, fexofenadine, desloratadine, and levocetirizine.

The use of oral antihistamines has been studied in depth and in general has been shown to be effective in relieving the histamine-mediated symptoms of allergic rhinitis. In its latest clinical practice guidelines on allergic rhinitis, the American Academy of Otolaryngology - Head and Neck Surgery recommended the use of newer generation antihistamines in allergic rhinitis patients [15].

Intranasal Antihistamines (INAH)

Azelastine hydrochloride and olopatadine hydrochloride are available in the United States and appear to be similarly effective [16]. Azelastine is available in two strengths, 0.1% or 0.15%. The lower strength preparation can be used in patients 5 years old and older. Olopatadine is indicated for patients starting at age 6 years old.

INAH have a rapid onset of action (within 15 minutes) and appear to have some anti-inflammatory effect that can improve nasal congestion [17]. They are generally well tolerated with unpleasant taste being the most commonly reported adverse reaction. When comparing intranasal antihistamines, one study reported a better taste profile for olopatadine [18]. Other side effects reported include epistaxis, nasal irritation, sedation, and headache [15].

The efficacy of intranasal compared to oral antihistamines has been examined. There are studies which support improved clinical response to INAH treatment [17] while others show equivalency of response when compared to oral antihistamines [19–21]. Choice between the oral or intranasal antihistamine options are usually determined by patient age, preference, and experience with previous treatment.

Studies have also compared the use of INAH and INCS. The results have been mixed, with some favoring the use of INAH alone [22, 23], others the use of INCS [24, 25], and still others show no significant difference between the two [26–29]. Most guidelines recommend the use of INCS over INAH, but in clinical practice patient demographics, history, and findings of physical exam need to be considered when choosing a specific treatment option.

Corticosteroids

The anti-inflammatory effect of corticosteroids has been well documented and its long-standing use in the treatment of allergic rhinitis has evolved over time. The different steroid preparations in the treatment of allergic rhinitis include oral, parenteral, and intranasal delivery options.

Systemic Corticosteroids

Although short courses of oral steroids usually effectively reduce the symptoms of allergic rhinitis, their safety profile and the availability of the intranasal preparation, make it a less desirable treatment option [3]. The adverse effects of steroids are of particular concern when using the parenteral and oral preparations due to their bioavailability, unpredictable absorption, and the inability to dose adjust if side effects occur.

The major adverse effects seen with systemic steroid therapy are dose and duration dependent and include suppression of the hypothalamic-pituitary-adrenal axis which can reduce growth. Other systems negatively impacted by systemic steroids are immune, musculoskeletal system, ophthalmologic, psychiatric, endocrine, and gastrointestinal systems [30, 31]. Because of these possible systemic effects, the use of oral or parenteral steroids in the treatment of allergic rhinitis has been largely replaced by intranasal preparations.

Intranasal Corticosteroids (INCSs)

Intranasal corticosteroid sprays are the most effective therapy for allergic rhinitis with a good safety profile at recommended doses [3, 15, 32]. The rationale for using INCS in the treatment of AR is that effective drug concentrations can be achieved locally with minimal risk of systemic adverse effects. Their anti-inflammatory action is effective in the reduction of nasal symptoms including congestion, sneezing, pruritis, and rhinorrhea [33], as well as ocular symptoms such as itching, tearing, redness, and puffiness [34]. INCS therapy has also been shown to improve QOL [35] and sleep [36, 37] in affected individuals.

INCS are usually well tolerated. The most common side effects are usually mild and are due to local mucosal irritation. Patients may complain of mucosal dryness, burning, and stinging and some may experience epistaxis, which can be more frequent with prolonged use [38, 39]. Septal perforation is another rare complication of nasal sprays [3]. The more concerning systemic effects of adrenal suppression are slowed growth in children, cataract formation, and decrease in bone density. However, the occurrence of systemic steroid adverse effects is rare with the use of INCS. Multiple studies in both adults and children have failed to demonstrate that these are common or clinically relevant [3]. However, because adverse effects are possible, growth in children using INCS should be monitored and dosages of INCS should be tapered to the lowest effective dose in all patients.

Multiple agents are available including fluticasone, mometasone, flunisolide, ciclesonide, triamcinolone, and budesonide, with most being available without a prescription. Comparative studies have not demonstrated a significant difference in efficacy between INCS preparations [40].

Combination Steroid-Antihistamine Spray

A combination spray of INCS and INAH may be helpful in patients who do not obtain sufficient relief with one agent [16]. In the United States, the only available combination spray contains azelastine hydrochloride and fluticasone propionate and is indicated down to 6 years of age. Studies comparing the use of INCS/INAH combination with INCS, INAH, or placebo treatment have shown that improved patient-reported symptom control and QOL improvement is seen with the use of combination therapy [3]. Advantages include a more rapid onset of action and better response in the relief of multiple symptoms. However, due to the increased financial cost and need for prescription, it is usually recommended as a second-line treatment option when monotherapy with either INCS or antihistamine does not provide adequate symptom control [3].

Decongestants

Oral Decongestants

Decongestants act on adrenergic receptors with resultant vasoconstriction and improvement of nasal congestion in patients with allergic rhinitis. In the United States, pseudoephedrine has been limited to behind-the-counter pharmacies due to its potential for abuse, both as a stimulant and more importantly due to its use in the illegal production of methamphetamine. Phenylephrine has been substituted in OTC decongestant products but may not provide improvement in nasal congestion when compared with placebo [41].

Decongestants have a variety of side effects including insomnia, increased blood pressure, irritability, nervousness, tremors, urinary retention, and palpitations [15]. They should be used with caution in patients at risk for hypertension and those with hyperthyroidism, closed angle glaucoma, cardiovascular or cerebrovascular disease, and are contraindicated in patients receiving monoamine oxidase inhibitor therapy.

For the pediatric population (>2 years old to 6 years old), its use and possible benefits, should be weighted against the potential for CNS stimulatory effects which may result in psychosis, hallucinations, and ataxia in this age group [42, 43].

Intranasal Decongestants

Nasal decongestant sprays are highly effective in the treatment of nasal congestion. Available preparations include phenylephrine, xylometazoline, and oxymetazoline. Direct application to the nasal mucosa results in immediate vasoconstriction and reduction of nasal mucosal edema. Intranasal decongestants are not recommended for prolonged treatment of nasal congestion due to the potential to cause rhinitis medicamentosa.

The downregulation of alpha-adrenergic receptors results in rebound nasal congestion [15]. Studies have shown variable definitions of "continued use" with some suggesting the development of rhinitis medicamentosa within 3 days of continued use [44], while others have shown that use of up to 8 weeks does not produce rebound nasal congestion [45]. Its use is commonly limited to no more than 3 days in an effort to avoid potential complications.

Leukotriene Receptor Antagonists (LTRAs)

Montelukast, a leukotriene receptor antagonist, has been used and studied in the treatment of asthma and allergic rhinitis. For the symptoms of allergic rhinitis, montelukast monotherapy has been shown to be more effective than placebo, but less effective than INCS [46–48]. In the latest CPG on AR published by the AAO-HNS, montelukast is not recommended as first-line therapy [15]. More recently (2020), due to its potential for neuropsychiatric effects, a boxed warning was added to the product, with the US Food and Drug Administration (FDA) recommendation against its use in patients with allergic rhinitis or mild asthma in favor of other treatment options.

Cromolyn

Cromolyn sodium is a mast cell stabilizer. It inhibits mast cell release of histamine and other inflammatory mediators. Its mechanism of action is through its influence in chloride channel pathways, which results in preventing mast cell degranulation [49, 50]. It also inhibits other pro-allergic inflammatory cells such as eosinophils, macrophages, monocytes, and platelets [51]. It is most effective when used as a preventive measure prior to exposure to the triggering allergens. Cromolyn is available as a nasal spray, in inhaled form to treat mild asthma, as an eye drop for allergic conjunctivitis, and as an oral preparation, which has been used in the treatment of allergic reactions to foods. Cromolyn nasal spray is available OTC and can be used in children as young as 2 years old. Because of its short half-life, dosing may be needed 3–6 times daily. Side effects are few with most being due to local irritation [52].

Although studies comparing its effectiveness against placebo have shown it to be superior in the treatment of seasonal allergic rhinitis [53], when compared with intranasal steroids or oral antihistamines it is less effective [54, 55].

Cromolyn is a safe treatment option for patients with predictable, episodic allergic rhinitis symptoms, limited by its need for frequent dosing and lower efficacy relative to other treatment options.

Ipratropium Bromide

Ipratropium bromide nasal spray can be useful in decreasing rhinorrhea. It can be used in adults and children, though it is not a first-line therapy in allergic rhinitis. It has a quick onset of action but a short half-life requiring administration up to 6 times per day. At therapeutic dosing, it has a low side-effect profile consisting mostly of symptoms related to local irrigation including epistaxis and burning [56].

The combined use with INCS has shown it to be more effective than either agent alone in the treatment of chronic rhinitis [56].

Nasal Saline

Nasal saline is another option in the treatment of allergic rhinitis. How saline irrigation works is not fully understood, but it is believed to be, at least in part, due to its ability to thin out and remove mucus and some of the pertinent allergens causing allergic symptoms. Studies have also shown improved mucociliary clearance function with the use of isotonic saline irrigations [57]. There are wide varieties of choices that can be used to deliver a variety of saline volumes to the nasal cavity.

Nasal irrigation carries little risk if properly performed and studies suggest improvement of symptoms and QOL scores over no treatment [58]. In a 2018 Cochrane review, which included 14 studies with 747 adult and pediatric participants, it was concluded that saline irrigation may improve patient-reported disease severity, in adults and children, compared to no saline. The evidence was considered low quality due to the inconsistent reporting of outcome measures between studies. They were unable to conclude if there was a significant difference in patient-reported disease severity between nasal saline and INCS, or nasal saline vs. no saline with adjuvant use of INCS or oral antihistamines [59].

Since saline irrigation is safe, cheap, and appears effective in some patients, it can be considered as an adjunct treatment for allergic rhinitis.

Combination Therapy

Oral Antihistamine and Oral Decongestant

The combination of an oral non-sedating antihistamine and oral decongestant has been shown to provide better symptom relief in patients with allergic rhinitis than placebo [60, 61] or than either agent alone [62]. In addition to the previously mentioned unfavorable systemic side effects, oral decongestants are not recommended in children under 4 years of age [63]. A combination of oral antihistamine and oral decongestant preparations should be prescribed with caution in patients with cardiovascular or urologic comorbidities.

Oral Antihistamine and Intranasal Corticosteroid (INCS)

INCS have been shown to be more effective than oral antihistamines in controlling nasal symptoms in the treatment of allergic rhinitis [64, 65]. However, a combination of an oral antihistamine and INCS is often used in clinical practice. Several large RCTs have examined the efficacy of combining the two classes of drugs to achieve greater symptom control but failed to demonstrate an added benefit of combination therapy [66, 67]. In contrast, a meta-analysis by Feng et al. concluded that combination therapy was superior in the improvement of allergic rhinitis symptom scores when compared to an antihistamine alone, but no improvement was noted if the antihistamine was added to an effective INCS [68].

Unless patient preference limits their use, INCS should be first-line therapy in the treatment of nasal symptoms in allergic rhinitis.

Allergen Immunotherapy (AIT)

Allergen immunotherapy is usually considered when other treatments, such as allergen avoidance and pharmacotherapy, have not resulted in effective management of the patient's allergic rhinitis symptoms. Indications for AIT include having documented specific IgE to an inhalant antigen, which must correlate with allergic symptoms when exposed to that allergen. In addition to unsatisfactory response to conservative management, AIT is an option for those patients who have experienced unacceptable adverse effects to the medications and those wishing to obtain a lasting response by modifying the immunologic process [69].

The safety of allergen immunotherapy in certain patient groups warrants special consideration. Absolute contraindications to AIT include patients with uncontrolled or poorly controlled asthma, active autoimmune disorders, and malignancy [70]. Relative contraindications of AIT are patients with cardiovascular disease, those on beta-blocker therapy, and patients with partially controlled asthma [69]. AIT should not be initiated during pregnancy, but may be continued in those patients at maintenance dosing prior to the pregnancy [69].

Clinical studies do not support the use of inhalant immunotherapy in the treatment of food hypersensitivity [71], pollen-food allergy syndrome [72], chronic urticaria, angioedema, or latex allergy [73].

Once a decision is made to proceed with immunotherapy, there are several considerations to be addressed. These include allergen extracts, vial preparation options including the number of allergens to be included, mode of delivery, optimal dosing, and length of treatment, among others.

Allergen Extract Units, Potency, and Standardization

Variation in the composition of available allergen extracts used in immunotherapy has historically been a problem. Because the allergen extract is made up of, not only the desired allergenic protein, but also non-allergic proteins, glycoproteins, polysaccharides, proteases, and micromolecules, there is potential for significant variation in the antigenicity and composition of each [74, 75]. For this reason, an effort to standardize aeroallergens, a process that insures composition and potency, has been undertaken with the result of multiple inhalant allergens now available in their standardized form.

In the United States, the US Food and Drug Administration (FDA) and the Center for Biologics Evaluation and Research (CBER) regulate the manufacturing of allergen extracts.

Several units of measure are in use and they do not necessarily reflect potency. These units can be grouped into standardized, nonstandardized, or proprietary. Examples of units that are used in non-standardized allergens and do not reflect potency include protein nitrogen units (PNU), which measures the total protein content, but does not distinguish between allergenic and non-allergenic proteins [76], and weight by volume (w/v), a measure of raw material per volume of extract solvent [76]. Currently, most allergen extracts available are non-standardized, and can vary widely in their potency, especially when produced by different manufacturers.

Standardization of allergen extracts offers a more consistent composition and potency. In the United States, standardized allergen extracts have a unit of potency assigned, and each lot is tested for conformance to a specified reference range. This allows the clinician relative certainty that a known amount of the pertinent allergen is being delivered with each dose, and decreases the risk of inducing a systemic reaction when different lots or manufacturers are used during treatment [3].

Allergy Units (AU) or Bioequivalent Allergy Units (BAU) are commonly used in standardized allergen extracts. The method for assigning BAU involves intradermal skin tests with serial threefold dilutions of a reference extract in highly allergic subjects. Potency is measured by how many dilutions are needed to obtain a certain flare reaction [77]. The dilution that produces an area of erythema with the sum of the longest diameter and midpoint (orthogonal) diameter equaling 50 mm is the D50 (ID50 EAL). The result is used to calculate the potency based on a D50 of 14 threefold dilutions, designated as 100,000 BAU/mL [77].

Standardized inhalant allergens available in the United States include cat, *Dermatophagoides pteronyssinus*, *Dermatophagoides farinae*, short ragweed, and multiple grass species [77].

In Europe, the potency is based on the dose of allergen extract that produces a wheal comparable in size to one produced by a given concentration of histamine. This unit is termed the biologic unit (BU). However, each manufacturer uses company-specific units based on in-house reference standards, making it difficult to compare potency of allergen extracts from different manufacturers.

Modification of Allergen Extracts

Recombinant-derived allergens, synthetic peptides, allergoids, and adjuvants are undergoing clinical development in an effort to improve safety, consistency, and availability of allergen extracts [78]. Extract modification can be accomplished by chemical, physical, or a combination of both processes, which may enhance an immunologic response while decreasing the risk of adverse reactions. Studies looking at the effectiveness of multiple recombinant allergens suggest equivalent or improved clinical outcomes when compared to their native counterparts [79].

The coupling of adjuvants to the native allergen has been popularized by European manufacturers, using such adjuvants as aluminum hydroxide, calcium phosphate, or L-tyrosine. This physical modification has shown a more pronounced immune response [80]. However, the adjuvant can induce an initial IgE immune response, which limits its therapeutic application [81]. There is limited availability of alum-precipitated extracts approved in the United States.

There are multiple immunotherapeutic options being investigated, with the goal of safer delivery and long-term lasting therapeutic efficacy. Long-term data is needed to allow for further recommendations.

Subcutaneous (SCIT) and Sublingual (SLIT) Immunotherapy

Allergy immunotherapy involves the sequential administration of allergen in the treatment of IgE-mediated sensitivity, for the purpose of modulating the untoward immune response and alleviating allergic symptoms. Immunotherapy is the only treatment that alters the abnormal immune response underlying allergic disease [82]. Response to immunotherapy is usually measured by the degree of symptom improvement and the ability to decrease or stop allergy medication use.

Other benefits that have been identified in patients undergoing allergen immunotherapy include a decrease in the development of asthma and in new allergen sensitizations. A 2017 meta-analysis evaluating the preventive effects of allergen immunotherapy (both SCIT and SLIT) found evidence of a reduction in the risk of developing asthma in patients with allergic rhinitis, as well as the ability to prevent sensitization to new allergens [83].

Subcutaneous Immunotherapy (SCIT)

Subcutaneous immunotherapy is the best-established form of AIT, having been practiced for over 100 years using aqueous or glycerinated extracts of naturally occurring allergens [84]. Its efficacy is supported by an extensive body of evidence, which supports its use in the management of allergic rhinitis, allergic asthma, and hymenoptera allergy [3].

The dose of allergen administered in AIT is an important variable. Studies have repeatedly shown that clinical response is dependent on an effective dose range for most allergens and efficacy may be compromised with low or underdose treatment. Effective doses for standardized and non-standardized allergens can be found in the Immunotherapy Practice Parameters third update [69].

Another important consideration in the administration of SCIT is the use of single or multiple allergens in polysensitized patients. In the United States, it is common practice to include in the treatment vial(s) the multiple allergens to which the patient is sensitized producing concomitant symptoms [85]. In contrast, European guidelines recommend treating with one or two allergens that appear to cause the most troublesome allergic symptoms [86]. Though some studies support the use of multiple allergens when treating these patients [87, 88], its effectiveness has not been extensively analyzed and further well-designed, well-powered clinical trials are needed [89].

When preparing treatment vials with multiple allergens for SCIT, proteolytic activity of the allergen must be taken into account, so that those with strong proteolytic activity (i.e., mold and cockroach) are not mixed with those susceptible to it (i.e., pollens, dust mite, and animal dander). Cross-reactivity among treatment allergens, the type of diluent, and the use of preservatives are also important considerations [90]. Diluent options in the United States include glycerin, phenolated saline, and human serum albumin [91].

There is significant variation in the way SCIT is administered throughout the world. Conventional immunotherapy usually consists of weekly injections, which deliver progressive allergen amounts to the desired final dose, followed by a maintenance phase with a total treatment time of 3–5 years [3]. There are more aggressive build-up schedules where maintenance dosing and clinical response can be more quickly achieved. However, research supports that rush regimens, where many injections are administered per day on consecutive days, reaching maintenance in 1–3 days, have an increased rate of systemic reactions compared to conventional dosing [92].

Though rare, SCIT can induce anaphylaxis necessitating prompt and appropriate response [93]. For this reason, current guidelines recommend that allergy injections be given only in a medical facility where prompt recognition and treatment are immediately available [69].

SCIT is recommended for 3–5 years and desensitization persists after discontinuation. The cost-effectiveness of SCIT in patients with allergic rhinitis surpasses that of long-term pharmacotherapy [94].

Sublingual Immunotherapy (SLIT)

An alternate approach of administering allergens is via sublingually (SLIT). This can be accomplished by either administering a dissolvable tablet or as a liquid extract. Oral immunotherapy was proposed as a method of treatment for allergic rhinitis over 100 years ago [95] and was recognized as a treatment option by the World Health Organization (WHO) in 1998 [96].

There are several advantages of sublingual immunotherapy over subcutaneous immunotherapy. First, studies show that SLIT has a better safety profile than SCIT with a much lower risk of anaphylaxis [97]. Also, SLIT is self-administered by the patient or caretaker at home, decreasing the expense and time associated with SCIT with its need to miss school, work, and transportation to the medical facility.

Delivery options for SLIT include rapidly dissolving sublingual immunotherapy tablets (SLIT tablets) and sublingual aqueous or glycerinated preparations (SLIT drops). Currently, in the United States, there are grass tablets, short ragweed, and house dust mite SLIT-tablets available. SLIT has been shown to be effective and safe in the treatment of allergic rhinitis in both children and adults [98–100]. In adults, most of the available research shows a low to moderate efficacy of SLIT over placebo with a trend for greater improvement with treatments longer than one year [101].

Compared to pharmacotherapy, HDM SLIT-tablets are superior to any pharmacologic therapies for perennial allergic rhinitis [102]. For seasonal allergic rhinitis due to pollens, the efficacy of grass and ragweed tablets appears to be similar to that of intranasal steroid sprays, and more effective than antihistamines and montelukast [102].

Due to a lack of heterogeneity between studies, the compared efficacy of SLIT and SCIT has been difficult to determine. Most meta-analyses are based on indirect comparisons, and though considered weak evidence, studies show a greater overall benefit of SCIT over SLIT [103].

The incidence of systemic adverse events, such as anaphylaxis, is rare with SLIT compared with SCIT [97]. The most common adverse effects of SLIT are oral mucosal pruritis and edema, which is usually self-limited to early treatment [104]. A possible association has been reported between eosinophilic esophagitis and sublingual immunotherapy [105]. Discontinuation of SLIT and consideration of eosinophilic esophagitis is recommended in patients who develop persistent gastroesophageal symptoms [105].

There is data supporting the preventive effects of SLIT on the development of asthma, especially in children, and the development of new allergy sensitizations in treated patients [106].

Contraindications to SLIT therapy include a history of eosinophilic esophagitis, any severe systemic reaction or severe local reaction after taking SLIT, or hypersensitivity to any of the inactive ingredients. SLIT-tablets are labeled as contraindicated in patients with severe, unstable, or uncontrolled asthma [107–109].

There are other options in allergen immunotherapy under investigation, including transcutaneous/epicutaneous, and intralymphatic immunotherapy. At this time, there are no specific recommendations regarding their use.

References

1. Leas BF, D'Anci KE, Apter AJ, et al. Effectiveness of indoor allergen reduction in asthma management: a systematic review. J Allergy Clin Immunol. 2018;141:1854.
2. Wood RA, Johnson EF, Van Natta ML, Chen PH, Eggleston PA. A placebo-controlled trial of a HEPA air cleaner in the treatment of cat allergy. Am J Respir Crit Care Med. 1998;158:115–20.
3. Wise SK, Lin SY, Toskala E, et al. International consensus statement on allergy and rhinology: allergic rhinitis. Int Forum Allergy Rhinol. 2018;8:108–352.
4. Terreehorst I, Hak E, Oosting AJ, et al. Evaluation of impermeable covers for bedding in patients with allergic rhinitis. N Engl J Med. 2003;349:237–46.
5. Geller-Bernstein C, Pibourdin JM, Dornelas A, Fondarai J. Efficacy of the acaricide: acardust for the prevention of asthma and rhinitis due to dust mite allergy, in children. Allerg Immunol (Paris). 1995;27:147–54.
6. Sheikh A, Hurwitz B, Nurmatov U, van Schayck CP. House dust mite avoidance measures for perennial allergic rhinitis. Cochrane Database Syst Rev. 2010;7:CD001563.
7. Le Cann P, Paulus H, Glorennec P, Le Bot B, Frain S, Gangneux JP. Home environmental interventions for the prevention or control of allergic and respiratory diseases: what really works. J Allergy Clin Immunol Pract. 2017;5:66–79.
8. Arbes SJ Jr, Sever M, Mehta J, et al. Abatement of cockroach allergens (Bla g 1 and Bla g 2) in low income, urban housing: month 12 continuation results. J Allergy Clin Immunol. 2004;113:109–14.
9. Sever ML, Arbes SJ Jr, Gore JC, et al. Cockroach allergen reduction by cockroach control alone in low income urban homes: a randomized control trial. J Allergy Clin Immunol. 2007;120:849–55.
10. McConnell R, Jones C, Milam J, et al. Cockroach counts and house dust allergen concentrations after professional cockroach control and cleaning. Ann Allergy Asthma Immunol. 2003;91:546–52.
11. Sanchez J, Dıez S, Cardona R. Pet avoidance in allergy cases: is it possible to implement it? Biomedica. 2015;35:357–62.
12. Bjornsdottir US, Jakobinudottir S, Runarsdottir V, Juliusson S. The effect of reducing levels of cat allergen (Fel d 1) on clinical symptoms in patients with cat allergy. Ann Allergy Asthma Immunol. 2003;91:189–94.
13. Seidman MD, Gurgel RK, Lin SY, et al. Clinical practice guideline: allergic rhinitis executive summary. Otolaryngol Head Neck Surg. 2015;152:197–206.
14. Stübner P, Zieglmayer R, Horak F. A direct comparison of the efficacy of antihistamines in SAR and PAR: randomised, placebo-controlled studies with levocetirizine and loratadine using an environmental exposure unit - the Vienna challenge chamber (VCC). Curr Med Res Opin. 2004;20:891.
15. Seidman MD, Gurgel RK, Lin SY, et al. Clinical practice guideline: allergic rhinitis. Otolaryngol Head Neck Surg. 2015;152:S1–S43.
16. Berger WE, Meltzer EO. Intranasal spray medications for maintenance therapy of allergic rhinitis. Am J Rhinol Allergy. 2015;29:273.
17. Berger W, Hampel F Jr, Bernstein J, Shah S, Sacks H, Meltzer EO. Impact of azelastine nasal spray on symptoms and quality of life compared with cetirizine oral tablets in patients with seasonal allergic rhinitis. Ann Allergy Asthma Immunol. 2006;97:375–81.
18. Meltzer EO, Garadi R, Laforce C, et al. Comparative study of sensory attributes of two antihistamine nasal sprays: olopatadine 0.6% and azelastine 0.1%. Allergy Asthma Proc. 2008;29:659–68.
19. Berger WE, White MV, Rhinitis Study Group. Efficacy of azelastine nasal spray in patients with an unsatisfactory response to loratadine. Ann Allergy Asthma Immunol. 2003;91:205–11.
20. Meltzer EO, Weiler JM, Dockhorn RJ, Widlitz MD, Freitag JJ. Azelastine nasal spray in the management of seasonal allergic rhinitis. Ann Allergy. 1994;72:354–9.
21. Gambardella R. A comparison of the efficacy of azelastine nasal spray and loratidine tablets in the treatment of seasonal allergic rhinitis. J Int Med Res. 1993;21:268–75.
22. Patel P, D'Andrea C, Sacks HJ. Onset of action of azelastine nasal spray compared with mometasone nasal spray and placebo in subjects with seasonal allergic rhinitis evaluated in an environmental exposure chamber. Am J Rhinol. 2007;21:499–503.
23. Patel D, Garadi R, Brubaker M, et al. Onset and duration of action of nasal sprays in seasonal allergic rhinitis patients: olopatadine hydrochloride versus mometasone furoate monohydrate. Allergy Asthma Proc. 2007;28:592–9.
24. Stern MA, Wade AG, Ridout SM, Cambell LM. Nasal budesonide offers superior symptom relief in perennial allergic rhinitis in comparison to nasal azelastine. Ann Allergy Asthma Immunol. 1998;81:354–8.
25. Newson-Smith G, Powell M, Baehre M, Garnham SP, MacMahon MT. A placebo controlled study comparing the efficacy of intranasal azelastine and beclomethasone in the treatment of seasonal allergic rhinitis. Eur Arch Otorrinolaringol. 1997;254:236–41.

26. Carr WW, Ratner P, Munzel U, et al. Comparison of intranasal azelastine to intranasal fluticasone propionate for symptom control in moderate to severe seasonal allergic rhinitis. Allergy Asthma Proc. 2012;33:450–8.
27. Kaliner MA, Storms W, Tilles S, et al. Comparison of olopatadine 0.6% nasal spray versus fluticasone propionate 50 microg in the treatment of seasonal allergic rhinitis. Allergy Asthma Proc. 2009;30:255–62.
28. Davies RJ, Lund VJ, Harten-Ash VJ. The effect of intranasal azelastine and beclomethasone on the symptoms and signs of nasal allergy in patients with perennial allergic rhinitis. Rhinology. 1993;31:159–64.
29. Gastpar H, Aurich R, Petzold U, et al. Intranasal treatment of perennial allergic rhinitis. Comparison of azelastine nasal spray and budesonide nasal aerosol. Arzneimittelforschung. 1993;43:475–9.
30. Huscher D, Thiele K, Gromnica-Ihle E, et al. Dose-related patterns of glucocorticoid-induced side effects. Ann Rheum Dis. 2009;68:1119.
31. Bousquet J, Khaltaev N, Cruz AA, et al. Allergic rhinitis and its impact on asthma (ARIA) 2008 update (in collaboration with the World Health Organization, GA(2)LEN and AllerGen). Allergy. 2008;63(Suppl 86):8–160.
32. Dykewicz MS, Wallace DV, Baroody F, et al. Treatment of seasonal allergic rhinitis: an evidence-based focused 2017 guideline update. Ann Allergy Asthma Immunol. 2017;119:489.
33. Wallace DV, Dykewicz MS, Bernstein DI, et al. The diagnosis and management of rhinitis: an updated practice parameter. J Allergy Clin Immunol. 2008;122:S1–S84.
34. Ratner P, Van Bavel J, Mohar D, et al. Efficacy of daily intranasal fluticasone propionate on ocular symptoms associated with seasonal allergic rhinitis. Ann Allergy Asthma Immunol. 2015;114:141–7.
35. Rodrigo GJ, Neffen H. Efficacy of fluticasone furoate nasal spray vs. placebo for the treatment of ocular and nasal symptoms of allergic rhinitis: a systematic review. Clin Exp Allergy. 2011;41:160–70.
36. Craig TJ, Mende C, Hughes K, Kakumanu S, Lehman EB, Chinchilli V. The effect of topical nasal fluticasone on objective sleep testing and the symptoms of rhinitis, sleep, and daytime somnolence in perennial allergic rhinitis. Allergy Asthma Proc. 2003;24:53–8.
37. Meltzer EO, Munafo DA, Chung W, Gopalan G, Varghese ST. Intranasal mometasone furoate therapy for allergic rhinitis symptoms and rhinitis disturbed sleep. Ann Allergy Asthma Immunol. 2010;105:65–74.
38. Rosenblut A, Bardin PG, Muller B, et al. Long-term safety of fluticasone furoate nasal spray in adults and adolescents with perennial allergic rhinitis. Allergy. 2007;62:1071–7.
39. Ratner PH, Meltzer EO, Teper A. Mometasone furoate nasal spray is safe and effective for 1-year treatment of children with perennial allergic rhinitis. Int J Pediatr Otorhinolaryngol. 2009;73:651–7.
40. Herman H. Once-daily administration of intranasal corticosteroids for allergic rhinitis: a comparative review of efficacy, safety, patient preference, and cost. Am J Rhinol. 2007;21:70–9.
41. Meltzer EO, Ratner PH, McGraw T. Oral phenylephrine HCl for nasal congestion in seasonal allergic rhinitis: a randomized, open-label, placebo controlled study. J Allergy Clin Immunol Pract. 2015;3:702–8.
42. Roberge RJ, Hirani KH, Rowland PL 3rd, Berkeley R, Krenzelok EP. Dextromethorphan- and pseudoephedrine-induced agitated psychosis and ataxia: case report. J Emerg Med. 1999;17:285–8.
43. Sauder KL, Brady WJ Jr, Hennes H. Visual hallucinations in a toddler: accidental ingestion of a sympathomimetic over-the-counter nasal decongestant. Am J Emerg Med. 1997;15:521–6.
44. Morris S, Eccles R, Martez SJ, Riker DK, Witek TJ. An evaluation of nasal response following different treatment regimes of oxymetazoline with reference to rebound congestion. Am J Rhinol. 1997;11:109–15.
45. Watanabe H, Foo TH, Djazaeri B, Duncombe P, Mackay IS, Durham SR. Oxymetazoline nasal spray three times daily for four weeks in normal subjects is not associated with rebound congestion or tachyphylaxis. Rhinology. 2003;41:167–74.
46. Grainger J, Drake-Lee A. Montelukast in allergic rhinitis: a systematic review and meta-analysis. Clin Otolaryngol. 2006;31:360–7.
47. Rodrigo GJ, Yanez A. The role of antileukotriene therapy in seasonal allergic rhinitis: a systematic review of randomized trials. Ann Allergy Asthma Immunol. 2006;96:779–86.
48. Ratner PH, Howland WC 3rd, Arastu R, et al. Fluticasone propionate aqueous nasal spray provided significantly greater improvement in daytime and nighttime nasal symptoms of seasonal allergic rhinitis compared with montelukast. Ann Allergy Asthma Immunol. 2003;90:536–42.
49. Altounyan RE. Review of clinical activity and mode of action of sodium cromoglycate. Clin Allergy. 1980;10(Suppl):481–9.
50. Kay AB, Walsh GM, Moqbel R, et al. Disodium cromoglycate inhibits activation of human inflammatory cells in vitro. J Allergy Clin Immunol. 1987;80:1–8.
51. Holgate ST. Reflections on the mechanism(s) of action of sodium cromoglycate (Intal) and the role of mast cells in asthma. Respir Med. 1989;83 (SupplA):25–31:25.
52. NasalCrom. Cromolyn nasal. Drug monograph. Dosing Epocrates, Inc; 2017. http://online.epocrates.com/drugs/otcs/211701/NasalCrom/Dosing. Accessed 19 Dec 2017.
53. Lejeune M, Lefebvre PP, Delvenne P, El-Shazly AE. Nasal sodium cromoglycate (Lomusol) modulates the early phase reaction of mild to moderate persistent allergic rhinitis in patients

mono-sensitized to house dust mite: a preliminary study. Int Immunopharmacol. 2015;26:272–6.
54. Pitsios C, Papadopoulos D, Kompoti E, et al. Efficacy and safety of mometasone furoate vs nedocromil sodium as prophylactic treatment for moderate/severe seasonal allergic rhinitis. Ann Allergy Asthma Immunol. 2006;96:673.
55. Lange B, Lukat KF, Rettig K, Holtappels G, Bachert C. Efficacy, cost-effectiveness, and tolerability of mometasone furoate, levocabastine, and disodium cromoglycate nasal sprays in the treatment of seasonal allergic rhinitis. Ann Allergy Asthma Immunol. 2005;95:272–82.
56. Dockhorn R, Aaronson D, Bronsky E, et al. Ipratropium bromide nasal spray 0.03% and beclomethasone nasal spray alone and in combination for the treatment of rhinorrhea in perennial rhinitis. Ann Allergy Asthma Immunol. 1999;82:349–59.
57. Ural A, Oktemer TK, Kizil Y, Ileri F, Uslu S. Impact of isotonic and hypertonic saline solutions on mucociliary activity in various nasal pathologies: clinical study. J Laryngol Otol. 2009;123:517–21.
58. Rogkakou A, Guerra L, Massacane P, et al. Effects on symptoms and quality of life of hypertonic saline nasal spray added to antihistamine in persistent allergic rhinitis—a randomized controlled study. Eur Ann Allergy Clin Immunol. 2005;37:353–6.
59. Head K, Snidvongs K, Glew S, Scadding G, Schilder AGM, Philpott C, Hopkins C. Saline irrigation for allergic rhinitis. Cochrane Database Syst Rev 2018, Issue 6. Art. No.: CD012597. DOI: https://doi.org/10.1002/14651858.CD012597.pub2, CD012597.
60. Badorrek P, Dick M, Schauerte A, et al. A combination of cetirizine and pseudoephedrine has therapeutic benefits when compared to single drug treatment in allergic rhinitis. Int J Clin Pharmacol Ther. 2009;47:71–7.
61. Brozek JL, Bousquet J, Baena-Cagnani CE, et al. Allergic rhinitis and its impact on asthma (ARIA) guidelines: 2010 revision. J Allergy Clin Immunol. 2010;126:466–76.
62. Pleskow W, Grubbe R, Weiss S, Lutsky B. Efficacy and safety of an extended-release formulation of desloratadine and pseudoephedrine vs the individual components in the treatment of seasonal allergic rhinitis. Ann Allergy Asthma Immunol. 2005;94:348–54.
63. Yau WP, Mitchell AA, Lin KJ, Werler MM, Hernandez-Diaz S. Use of decongestants during pregnancy and the risk of birth defects. Am J Epidemiol. 2013;178:198–208.
64. Weiner JM, Abramson MJ, Puy RM. Intranasal corticosteroids versus oral H1 receptor antagonists in allergic rhinitis: systematic review of randomized controlled trials. BMJ. 1998;317:1624–9.
65. Benninger M, Farrar JR, Blaiss M, et al. Evaluating approved medications to treat allergic rhinitis in the United States: an evidence-based review of efficacy for nasal symptoms by class. Ann Allergy Asthma Immunol. 2010;104:13–29.
66. Barnes ML, Ward JH, Fardon TC, Lipworth BJ. Effects of levocetirizine as add-on therapy to fluticasone n seasonal allergic rhinitis. Clin Exp Allergy. 2006;36:676–84.
67. Di Lorenzo G, Pacor ML, Pellitteri ME, et al. Randomized placebo-controlled trial comparing fluticasone aqueous nasal spray in mono-therapy, fluticasone plus cetirizine, fluticasone plus montelukast and cetirizine plus montelukast for seasonal allergic rhinitis. Clin Exp Allergy. 2004;34:259–67.
68. Feng S, Fan Y, Liang Z, Ma R, Cao W. Concomitant corticosteroid nasal spray plus antihistamine (oral or local spray) for the symptomatic management of allergic rhinitis. Eur Arch Otorrinolaringol. 2016;273:3477–86.
69. Cox L, Nelson H, Lockey R, et al. Allergen immunotherapy: a practice parameter third update. J Allergy Clin Immunol. 2011;127:S1–S55.
70. Pitsios C, Demoly P, Bilo MB, et al. Clinical contraindications to allergen immunotherapy: an EAACI position paper. Allergy. 2015;70:897–909.
71. Nelson HS, Lahr J, Rule R, et al. Treatment of anaphylactic sensitivity to peanuts by immunotherapy with injections of aqueous peanut extract. J Allergy Clin Immunol. 1997;99:744.
72. Sampson HA, Aceves S, Bock SA, et al. Food allergy: a practice parameter update—2014. J Allergy Clin Immunol. 2014;134:1016–1025.e43.
73. Leynadier F, Herman D, Vervloet D, Andre C. Specific immunotherapy with a standardized latex extract versus placebo in allergic healthcare workers. J Allergy Clin Immunol. 2000;106:585.
74. Zimmer J, Vieths S, Kaul S. Standardization and regulation of allergen products in the European Union. Curr Allergy Asthma Rep. 2016;16:21.
75. Carnes J, Iraola V, Gallego M, Leonor JR. Control process for manufacturing and standardization of allergenic molecules. Curr Allergy Asthma Rep. 2015;15:37.
76. Mason WW, Ward WA. Standardized extracts. Otolaryngol Clin N Am. 1992;25:101–17.
77. Jutel M, Agache I, Bonini S, et al. International consensus on allergen immunotherapy II: mechanisms, standardization, and pharmacoeconomics. J Allergy Clin Immunol. 2016;137:358–68.
78. Creticos PS. Allergen immunotherapy: vaccine modification. Immunol Allergy Clin N Am. 2016;36:103–24.
79. Nony E, Bouley J, Le Mignon M, et al. Development and evaluation of a sublingual tablet based on recombinant bet v 1 in birch pollen-allergic patients. Allergy. 2015;70:795–804.
80. Mellerup MT, Hahn GW, Poulsen LK, Malling H, Safety of allergen-specific immunotherapy. Relation between dosage regimen, allergen extract, disease and systemic side-effects during induction treatment. Clin Exp Allergy. 2000;30:1423.

81. Francis JN, Durham SR. Adjuvants for allergen immunotherapy: experimental results and clinical perspectives. Curr Opin Allergy Clin Immunol. 2004;4:543–8.
82. Jutel M, Akdis M, Budak F, et al. IL-10 and TGF beta cooperate in the regulatory T cell response to mucosal allergens in normal immunity and specific immunotherapy. Eur J Immunol. 2003;33:1205–14.
83. Kristiansen M, Dhami S, Netuveli G, et al. Allergen immunotherapy for the prevention of allergy: a systematic review and meta-analysis. Pediatr Allergy Immunol. 2017;28:18.
84. Passalacqua G, Canonica GW. Allergen immunotherapy: history and future developments. Immunol Allergy Clin N Am. 2016;36:1–12.
85. Blume SW, Yeomans K, Allen-Ramey F, et al. Administration and burden of subcutaneous immunotherapy for allergic rhinitis in U.S. and Canadian clinical practice. J Manag Care Spec Pharm. 2015;21:982–90.
86. Van Cauwenberge P, Bachert C, Passalacqua G, et al. Consensus statement on the treatment of allergic rhinitis. European academy of Allergology and clinical immunology. Allergy. 2000;55:116–34.
87. Franklin W, Lowell FC. Comparison of two dosages of ragweed extract in the treatment of pollenosis. JAMA. 1967;201:915–7.
88. Lowell FC, Franklin W. A double-blind study of the effectiveness and specificity of injection therapy in ragweed hay fever. NEngl J Med. 1965;273:675–9.
89. Calderon MA, Cox L, Casale TB, Moingeon P, Demoly P. Multiple-allergen and single-allergen immunotherapy strategies in polysensitized patients: looking at the published evidence. J Allergy Clin Immunol. 2012;129:929–34.
90. Nelson HS. Subcutaneous injection immunotherapy for optimal effectiveness. Immunol Allergy Clin N Am. 2011;31:211–26. viii
91. Plunkett G. Update: stability of allergen extracts to establish expiration dating. Curr Opin Otolaryngol Head Neck Surg. 2016;24:261–9.
92. Calabria CW, Cox L. Accelerated immunotherapy schedules and premedication. Immunol Allergy Clin N Am. 2011;31(251–263):ix.
93. Bernstein DI, Wanner M, Borish L, Liss GM. American Academy of Allergy Asthma and Immunology immunotherapy committee, immunology. Twelve year survey of fatal reactions to allergen injections and skin testing: 1990–2001. J Allergy Clin Immunol. 2004;113:1129–36.
94. Hankin CS, Cox L, Bronstone A, Wang Z. Allergy immunotherapy: reduced health care costs in adults and children with allergic rhinitis. J Allergy Clin Immunol. 2013;131:1084–91.
95. Noon L. Prophylactic inoculation against hayfever. Lancet. 1911;1:1572–3.
96. Bousquet J, Lockey R, Malling HJ. Allergen immunotherapy: therapeutic vaccines for allergic diseases. A WHO position paper. J Allergy Clin Immunol. 1998;102:558–62.
97. Creticos PS, Bernstein DI, Casale TB, Lockey RF, Maloney J, Nolte H. Coseasonal initiation of allergen immunotherapy: a systematic review. J Allergy Clin Immunol Pract. 2016;4:1194–1204.e4.
98. Lin SY, Erekosima N, Kim JM, et al. Sublingual immunotherapy for the treatment of allergic rhinoconjunctivitis and asthma: a systematic review. JAMA. 2013;309:1278–88.
99. Radulovic S, Wilson D, Calderon M, Durham S. Systematic reviews of sublingual immunotherapy (SLIT). Allergy. 2011;66:740–52.
100. Di Bona D, Plaia A, Scafidi V, Leto-Barone MS, Di Lorenzo G. Efficacy of sublingual immunotherapy with grass allergens for seasonal allergic rhinitis: a systematic review and meta-analysis. J Allergy Clin Immunol. 2010;126:558–66.
101. Radulovic S, Calderon MA, Wilson D, Durham S. Sublingual immunotherapy for allergic rhinitis. Cochrane Database Syst Rev. 2010;(12):CD002893.
102. Durham SR, Creticos PS, Nelson HS, et al. Treatment effect of sublingual immunotherapy tablets and pharmacotherapies for seasonal and perennial allergic rhinitis: pooled analyses. J Allergy Clin Immunol. 2016;138:1081–1088.e4.
103. Di Bona D, Plaia A, Leto-Barone MS, La Piana S, LorenzoG D. Efficacy of subcutaneous and sublingual immunotherapy with grass allergens for seasonal allergic rhinitis: a meta-analysis-based comparison. J Allergy Clin Immunol. 2012;130:1097–1107.e2.
104. Bernstein DI, Kleine-Tebbe J, Nelson HS, et al. SQ house dust mite sublingual immunotherapy tablet subgroup efficacy and local application site reaction duration. Ann Allergy Asthma Immunol. 2018;121:105.
105. Miehlke S, Alpan O, Schröder S, Straumann A. Induction of eosinophilic esophagitis by sublingual pollen immunotherapy. Case Rep Gastroenterol. 2013;7:363.
106. Marogna M, Tomassetti D, Bernasconi A, et al. Preventive effects of sublingual immunotherapy in childhood: an open randomized controlled study. Ann Allergy Asthma Immunol. 2008;101:206–11.
107. Prescribing information for Oralair is available at http://www.fda.gov/downloads/BiologicsBloodVaccines/Allergenics/UCM391580.pdf. Accessed 24 Nov 2014.
108. Prescribing information for Grastek. http://www.merck.com/product/usa/pi_circulars/g/grastek/grastek_pi.pdf. Accessed on 15 April 2014.
109. Prescribing information for Ragwitek is available at http://www.merck.com/product/usa/pi_circulars/r/ragwitek/ragwitek_pi.pdf. Accessed on 24 April 2021.

Non-allergic Rhinitis: Evaluation and Epidemiology

7

James W. Mims

Introduction

Non-allergic rhinitis (NAR) is a collection of different entities often characterized as NAR subtypes. NAR could be defined a group of conditions causing nasal symptoms in the absence of allergies, chronic sinusitis, foreign body, neoplasm, or infection. While "rhinitis", etymologically, implies inflammation, some subtypes of non-allergic rhinitis may not be inflammatory, for example, rhinitis medicamentosa. Additionally, rhinitis with negative allergy skin tests or sIgE blood tests is generally characterized as NAR, but some of these individuals have inhalant-specific IgE detectable in their nasal secretions raising the possibility that they are "locally allergic." Local nasal reactivity was present in 26.5% of NAR patients (defined by negative skin or sera allergy testing) in one review [1]. This chapter will discuss the evaluation and epidemiology of NAR.

J. W. Mims (✉)
Department of Otolaryngology, Wake Forest School of Medicine, Winston-Salem, NC, USA
e-mail: wmims@wakehealth.edu

Evaluation of Non-allergic Rhinitis by Subtype

The diversity among subtypes of NAR makes broad descriptions difficult. History and physical exam are important. NAR subjects are reported to be older and have less self-reported asthma than patients with AR [2]. A study comparing patient questionnaires to an allergy-immunology physician's diagnosis of vasomotor rhinitis found that "no outdoor symptoms in spring", "no parental history of allergy", "no symptoms around cats", "presence of symptoms around perfumes and fragrances", and "older age" were predictive of NAR compared to AR [3]. Exposure history can be helpful in diagnosing NAR such as exposure to topical decongestants (such as oxymetazoline), illicit nasal drug use, vapors, chemicals, smoke, or other irritants. Reviewing the medication list for possible nasal side effects should be part of the evaluation. Medications that cause dry mouth also commonly effect the nasal mucosa too.

History and physical exam can distinguish nasal inflammation (congestion and rhinorrhea) from dry and widely patent nasal cavity (empty nose, age-related changes). Triggering events may differ between AR and NAR. AR is triggered by allergens, while irritants or autonomic stimuli, such as gustation, more likely trigger NAR. However, patient with AR may also be

C. Damask et al. (eds.), *Allergy in Otolaryngology Practice*,
https://doi.org/10.1007/978-3-031-93455-1_7

more sensitive to non-allergic irritants. Clear thin "watery" secretions that can drip out the anterior nose are more commonly encountered in vasomotor rhinitis than AR. Unilateral clear rhinorrhea should prompt concern for a possible cerebral spinal fluid leak. In school-aged children with rhinitis, the absence of eye itching is associated with negative allergy testing [4].

The diagnosis of NAR is clinical with no confirmatory testing indicated. Allergy provocation and allergy testing is not recommended when NAR is suspected and the high false positivity does not accurately exclude AR. Microbiological assays fail to differentiate between colonization and infection. Nasal cytology is not diagnostic of NAR. Cerebral spinal fluid tests should be limited to skull base defects, unilateral rhinorrhea, or idiopathic intracranial hypertension. Computerized tomography is not appropriate to diagnose NAR [5].

What constitutes a subtype of non-allergic rhinitis (a diagnosis of exclusion) compared to what is included on the differential diagnosis of nasal symptoms is not uniformly agreed upon, but a distinction can be offered between primary and secondary NAR. Primary NAR subtypes tend to be non-allergic, non-infectious conditions that primarily affect the nose, while secondary NAR includes multi-system conditions that also cause nasal symptoms. Some conditions such as "autoimmune rhinitis" could be classified either way. Subtypes of non-allergic rhinitis are listed in Table 7.1 and a brief differential diagnosis of secondary non-allergic rhinitis in Table 7.2. In practice, there is likely overlap between AR and NAR and among different NAR subtypes with many patients having "mixed rhinitis" [5]. For example, a patient could have chronic sinusitis and vasomotor rhinitis.

Table 7.1 Primary subtypes of non-allergic rhinitis (NAR)

NAR subtype	Description
"Recreational" drug-induced rhinitis	Intranasal illicit drug use
Rhinitis medicamentosa	Chronic use of intranasal decongestants
Pharmacologically induced rhinitis	Dry mouth (and dry nose) are common side effects of common medications including many psychiatric and antihypertensive medications
Occupational/chemical rhinitis	Chemical vapors may irritate nasal mucosa
Tobacco smoke-induced rhinitis	Smoke may irritate nasal mucosa
Hormonal rhinitis	Endocrine disorders or pregnancy may cause nasal symptoms
Food induced rhinitis	Food ingredients such as triptans can cause nasal symptoms
Alcohol-induced rhinitis	Ingestion of EtOH can cause nasal congestion and rhinorrhea
Vasomotor (idiopathic) rhinitis	Cholinergic-mediated autonomic dysfunction
Empty nose syndrome	Loss of nasal structures can be associated with nasal drying
Atrophic rhinitis	Mucosal atrophy
Radiation/chemotherapy-induced rhinitis	Therapies targeting cell mitosis adversely affect nasal mucosa
Age-related rhinitis	Ciliary function and mucus production change with age
Autoimmune rhinitis	Sarcoid, granulomatous diseases, Sjogrens, etc. effect the nasal mucosa
Non-allergic rhinitis with eosinophilia syndrome (NARES)	NAR classified by nasal cytology noted an eosinophilic sub-type

Table 7.2 Secondary NAR and differential diagnosis

Differential diagnosis	Description
Allergic rhinitis	Nasal inflammation from IgE-mediated allergies
Chronic sinusitis	Inflammation of the paranasal sinuses and nasal passage for >3 months
Infectious rhinitis	Viral, bacterial, fungal, or parasitic infections of the nasal passages
Cerebral spinal fluid leak	Clear nasal drainage can be mistaken for rhinitis
Nasal foreign bodies	Often cause unilateral symptoms
Neoplasms	Can cause rhinorrhea and obstruction
Ciliary dyskinesia	Primary ciliary dyskinesia and cystic fibrosis cause nasal inflammation

Subtypes of NAR

"Recreational" Intranasal Drug Use

"Recreational" or illicit intranasal drug use is a well-known cause of damage to the nasal mucosa most commonly seen with cocaine and opioid medications but not limited to those. Mucosal dryness, tissue necrosis, septal perforation, drug residue, loss of smell, epistaxis, and nasal-oral fistulas have been described. It is estimated that 0.6% of the US population uses cocaine illicitly [6].

Rhinitis Medicamentosa (RM)

RM has been diagnosed in 1–9% of rhinitis clinic patients in otolaryngology and allergy-immunology offices. Characterized by use of a topical nasal decongestant for more than 3 days with "rebound" congestion causing primarily nasal obstruction. The pathophysiology for RM is not known and there are discrepancies in the literature of the dose and time needed to illicit RM. Large turbinates, thickened nasal mucosa, and poor nasal decongestion are commonly cited physical findings [7].

Rhinitis as a Medication Side Effect

A variety of prescription medications have nasal side effects that tend to be drying and thickening of mucus drainage. Alpha antagonists, presynaptic alpha-2 agonists, beta-antagonists, phosphodiesterase inhibitors, angiotensin-converting enzyme inhibitors, psychotropic medications, immunomodulators (cyclosporine), hormones, and other antihypertensives have been implicated. Although poorly studied, it is logical that polypharmacy of these classes may have an increased effect [8].

Occupational/Chemical Rhinitis

A variety of chemicals and irritants can be associated with rhinitis. Exposure to chemical fumes (e.g., cleaning products and hair products), wood dust, and industrial irritants such as processing metals among others have been associated with rhinitis symptoms. History of exposure to fumes or chemicals is important in assessing rhinitis patients [9].

Tobacco Smoke-Induced Rhinitis

Second-hand smoke has been associated with more prevalent rhinitis in children and tobacco smokers also have more rhinitis symptoms. History is the primary means of evaluation. Poor ciliary clearance has been reported in active smokers [10].

Hormonal Rhinitis

The archetype is Rhinitis of Pregnancy affecting 22% of pregnancies and most severe in the second trimester. It has been suggested and refuted that oral birth control pills are associated with nasal congestion. Menopause and estrogen replacement may also have some influence on nasal symptoms. Hormonal rhinitis in males is less discussed. Hypothyroidism has been associated with nasal congestion and drainage [8].

Food-Induced Rhinitis

Food allergy has only rarely been associated with isolated rhinitis. Some foods that are "spicy" may cause rhinorrhea, which is thought to be neurologically mediated along with gustatory rhinitis (see vasomotor rhinitis). Science on other types of food-induced rhinitis is lacking but evaluation would rely mostly on history and possibly challenge testing [8].

Alcohol-Induced Rhinitis

Alcohol-induced rhinitis is part of alcohol-induced upper airway symptoms and seen in the general population (14%) but is higher in asthmatics and aspirin-exacerbated respiratory disease patients. Symptoms are rhinorrhea and nasal congestion secondary to vasodilation. Evaluation is primarily by history [11].

Vasomotor (Idiopathic) Rhinitis

Vasomotor rhinitis has been assessed to comprise 71% of the NAR population. Classically, elderly patients present with clear rhinorrhea that is often gustatory. This presentation is thought to be cholinergically mediated from autonomic dysfunction. However, there is also a population of patients described presenting to allergy-immunology clinics with nasal congestion who are allergy-test negative and are also classified as having vasomotor rhinitis. The lack of distinction between "local allergy", vasomotor dysfunction, gustatory rhinitis, and age-related rhinitis in the literature creates a lack of clarity [8, 11, 12].

Empty Nose Syndrome (ENS)

ENS and atrophic rhinitis are sometimes used interchangeably but there are efforts to characterize ENS as resulting from nasal surgery (generally from turbinate resection) and atrophic being non-surgical. With loss of nasal tissue, the nasal neurosensory functions, humidification, and temperature regulation can be disrupted. This can be associated with nasal dryness, crusting, discomfort, and the sensation of nasal obstruction despite objective nasal patency. In some patients, this condition can be profoundly bothersome [13].

Atrophic Rhinitis

Atrophic rhinitis refers to atrophic nasal mucosa with complains of dryness and sometimes paradoxical subjective nasal obstruction. When not associated with prior surgery, nutritional disorders (e.g., vitamin deficiency), Klebsiella infection, and chronic inflammation are possible causes. Assessment is primarily history and examination [13].

Radiation/Chemotherapy-Induced Rhinitis

Radiation and chemotherapy preferentially affect the nasal mucosa due to a higher rate of cellular mitosis. Mucus gland metaplasia, neutrophilia, and decreased smell thresholds have been reported during and at the end of radiation therapy with improvement at 3 months after radiation. Long-term nasal assessments are lacking [14].

Age-Related Rhinitis

There are multiple age-related changes in the nose including increased clear rhinorrhea, decreased mucociliary clearance, increased dryness, and disruption of the nasal cycle. While symptoms of post-nasal drip, clear rhinorrhea, and nasal obstruction are similar to AR, the exam and mechanisms appear to be different in the elderly population [8].

Non-allergic Rhinitis with Eosinophilia Syndrome (NARES)

NARES is chronic nasal inflammation that displays eosinophilia on biopsy or nasal cytology while allergy tests are negative. There is probably a spectrum of nasal eosinophilic disorders spanning from NARES to Eosinophilic Rhinosinusitis with Polyps to Aspirin-Exacerbated Respiratory Disease. All of these can be non-allergic and may be associated with other eosinophilic diseases such as asthma. Assessment of chronic nasal inflammation should include consideration of chronic diseases of the upper and lower respiratory tracts [8].

Burden of Disease

The economic costs of outpatient visits, medications, and lost work productivity have not been widely studied for NAR. However, NAR does have a negative impact on quality of life.

Quality of Life (QOL)

Segboer et al. demonstrated impairment in QOL in NAR subjects. Using the mini-RQLQ (Rhinitis Quality of Life Questionnaire), they found QOL was equally or more impaired in NAR than in AR patients, and they reported that more than 50% of NAR subjects were "unsatisfied" with treatment. Compared to healthy controls, NAR patients were impaired over all domains of the mini-RQLQ. Compared to AR controls, NAR showed significantly greater impairment of "nasal symptoms" and "other symptoms." [15].

Epidemiology

The prevalence of NAR is not well known. The European Position Paper on Chronic Sinusitis in 2020 cited that 10–19% of the population report NAR symptoms [16–18].

Studies examining the prevalence of NAR in children have shown a wide range of values suggesting regional differences and variance with age. The prevalence of NAR in eight-year-olds in Sweden was 6.3% [19] compared to 24.9% in Singapore [20]. In Singapore, the prevalence of NAR decreased to 10–15% in older children [20].

The International Study of Asthma and Allergies (ISAAC) phase II studies evaluated NAR, defined as rhinitis symptoms with negative allergy SPT, indirectly when assessing children for AR. They uniformly asked questions about rhinitis (without a cold) and rhinoconjuctivitis (without a cold) and allergy tested (SPT) 31,000 children (age 8–12 years) across the globe. The variation of rhinitis without conjunctivitis (which was generally associated with negative allergy testing) varied from 1.4% to 45.2% across 22 countries [4]. The overall Population Attributable Fraction (PAF) of allergy (determined by skin testing) for rhinitis symptoms with and without eye itching was 33%, meaning 66% of those with rhinitis had negative skin testing (or non-allergic rhinitis) [4]. Tables 7.3 and 7.4 show the PAF of children with rhinitis (with and without conjunctivitis) with positive allergy testing (the remainder could be classified as NAR). Interestingly, there was no association of rhinitis without eye itching and seasonal allergy testing. The overall PAF of AR for those with rhinoconjuctivitis was 56%, thus we can infer 44% of rhinoconjuctivitis could be labeled as NAR. However, the regional variability was marked [4].

In conclusion, this data found that 66% of 8–12 year olds with rhinitis tested negative for allergies suggesting that internationally most school-aged rhinitis is NAR. Also, rhinitis with an absence of eye symptoms is a strong predictor of negative allergy testing in this population.

Table 7.3 Population attributed fraction (PAF) of allergy sensitization for those with rhinoconjunctivitis symptoms ISAAC Phase II [4]

	Seasonal	Perennial	All
Affluent countries	35.9% (23.6–46.2%)	25% (18.1–31.4)	Not provided
Non-affluent countries	1.3% (0–2.8%)	12.6% (2.7–21.6)	Not provided
All	Not provided	Not provided	56%

Table 7.4 Population attributed fraction (PAF) of allergy sensitization for those with rhinitis without conjunctivitis symptoms ISAAC Phase II [4]

	Seasonal	Perennial
Affluent countries	2.1% (−0.3 to +4.5)	8.0% (5.5–10.5)
Non-affluent countries	0.6% (−0.5 to +1.6)	4.0% (1.2–6.6)

Conclusion

NAR is a heterogeneous condition composed of several different subtypes. NAR negatively affects QOL and may be at least as common as AR. Evaluation is primarily by history and physical exam with particular attention to watery rhinorrhea, medication use, patient age, eye symptoms, and triggers. Familiarity with the different subtypes allows better clinician recognition of NAR and may direct therapy and patient expectations.

References

1. Hamizan AW, Rimmer J, Alvarado R, Sewell WA, Kalish L, Sacks R, et al. Positive allergen reaction in allergic and nonallergic rhinitis: a systematic review. Int Forum Allergy Rhinol. 2017;7(9):868–77. https://doi.org/10.1002/alr.21988.
2. Hamizan AW, Azer M, Alvarado R, Earls P, Barham HP, Tattersall J, et al. The distinguishing clinical features of nonallergic rhinitis patients. Am J Rhinol Allergy. 2019;33(5):524–30. https://doi.org/10.1177/1945892419850750.
3. Brandt D, Bernstein JA. Questionnaire evaluation and risk factor identification for nonallergic vasomotor rhinitis. Ann Allergy Asthma Immunol. 2006;96(4):526–32. https://doi.org/10.1016/S1081-1206(10)63546-6.
4. Weinmayr G, Forastiere F, Weiland SK, Rzehak P, Abramidze T, Annesi-Maesano I, et al. International variation in prevalence of rhinitis and its relationship with sensitisation to perennial and seasonal allergens. Eur Respir J. 2008;32(5):1250–61. https://doi.org/10.1183/09031936.00157807.
5. Hellings PW, Klimek L, Cingi C, Agache I, Akdis C, Bachert C, et al. Non-allergic rhinitis: position paper of the European academy of allergy and clinical immunology. Allergy. 2017;72(11):1657–65. https://doi.org/10.1111/all.13200.
6. Moreno-Artero E, Querol-Cisneros E, Rodriguez-Garijo N, Tomas-Velazquez A, Antonanzas J, Secundino F, et al. Mucocutaneous manifestations of cocaine abuse: a review. J Eur Acad Dermatol Venereol. 2018;32(9):1420–6. https://doi.org/10.1111/jdv.14912.
7. Ramey JT, Bailen E, Lockey RF. Rhinitis medicamentosa. J Investig Allergol Clin Immunol. 2006;16(3):148–55.
8. Wise SK, Lin SY, Toskala E, Orlandi RR, Akdis CA, Alt JA, et al. International consensus statement on allergy and rhinology: allergic rhinitis. Int Forum Allergy Rhinol. 2018;8(2):108–352. https://doi.org/10.1002/alr.22073.
9. Shao Z, Bernstein JA. Occupational rhinitis: classification, diagnosis, and therapeutics. Curr Allergy Asthma Rep. 2019;19(12):54. https://doi.org/10.1007/s11882-019-0892-0.
10. Shargorodsky J. Secondhand smoke and rhinitis. Curr Opin Otolaryngol Head Neck Surg. 2016;24(3):241–4. https://doi.org/10.1097/MOO.0000000000000250.
11. Dykewicz MS, Wallace DV, Amrol DJ, Baroody FM, Bernstein JA, Craig TJ, et al. Rhinitis 2020: a practice parameter update. J Allergy Clin Immunol. 2020;146(4):721–67. https://doi.org/10.1016/j.jaci.2020.07.007.
12. Pattanaik D, Lieberman P. Vasomotor rhinitis. Curr Allergy Asthma Rep. 2010;10(2):84–91. https://doi.org/10.1007/s11882-010-0089-z.
13. Kuan EC, Suh JD, Wang MB. Empty nose syndrome. Curr Allergy Asthma Rep. 2015;15(1):493. https://doi.org/10.1007/s11882-014-0493-x.
14. Riva G, Franco P, Provenzano E, Arcadipane F, Bartoli C, Lava P, et al. Radiation-induced rhinitis: cytological and olfactory changes. Am J Rhinol Allergy. 2019;33(2):153–61. https://doi.org/10.1177/1945892418822448.
15. Segboer CL, Terreehorst I, Gevorgyan A, Hellings PW, van Drunen CM, Fokkens WJ. Quality of life is significantly impaired in nonallergic rhinitis patients. Allergy. 2018;73(5):1094–100. https://doi.org/10.1111/all.13356.
16. Fokkens WJ, Lund VJ, Hopkins C, Hellings PW, Kern R, Reitsma S, et al. European position paper on Rhinosinusitis and nasal polyps 2020. Rhinology. 2020;58(Suppl S29):1–464. https://doi.org/10.4193/Rhin20.600.
17. Cazzoletti L, Ferrari M, Olivieri M, Verlato G, Antonicelli L, Bono R, et al. The gender, age and risk factor distribution differs in self-reported allergic and non-allergic rhinitis: a cross-sectional population-based study. Allergy Asthma Clin Immunol. 2015;11:36. https://doi.org/10.1186/s13223-015-0101-1.
18. Olsson P, Berglind N, Bellander T, Stjarne P. Prevalence of self-reported allergic and non-allergic rhinitis symptoms in Stockholm: relation to age, gender, olfactory sense and smoking. Acta Otolaryngol. 2003;123(1):75–80. https://doi.org/10.1080/0036554021000028071.
19. Westman M, Stjarne P, Asarnoj A, Kull I, van Hage M, Wickman M, et al. Natural course and comorbidities of allergic and nonallergic rhinitis in children. J Allergy Clin Immunol. 2012;129(2):403–8. https://doi.org/10.1016/j.jaci.2011.09.036.
20. Chiang WC, Chen YM, Tan HK, Balakrishnan A, Liew WK, Lim HH, et al. Allergic rhinitis and non-allergic rhinitis in children in the tropics: prevalence and risk associations. Pediatr Pulmonol. 2012;47(10):1026–33. https://doi.org/10.1002/ppul.22554.

Non-allergic Rhinitis Pathophysiology

8

Vijay A. Patel, Uma S. Ramaswamy, and Stella E. Lee

Introduction

Non-allergic rhinitis (NAR) describes a set of symptoms that traditionally indicates a state of inflammation, including nasal rhinorrhea, obstruction, and/or congestion, without objective evidence of an IgE-mediated process by either skin or in vitro testing. The diagnosis of NAR is often challenging as it is one of exclusion; once diagnosed, it can be difficult to treat, as the mechanism of this disease process is not well-defined. As there are several subsets of rhinopathy, it is important to understand the potential underlying mechanisms and effective management principles of NAR. There is an extensive differential for patients who have NAR, including the most common, non-allergic rhinopathy, termed "vasomotor rhinitis" or "idiopathic rhinitis," as well as inflammation related to medications, environmental triggers, hormonal changes, infections, or autoimmune, vasculitic, and granulomatous processes. At this time, research suggests that the pathophysiology of NAR may be partly explained by entopy, neural dysregulation, and/or chemoreceptor activation.

Clinical Features

Patients who present with NAR have symptoms that are often non-distinguishable from allergic rhinitis including rhinorrhea, congestion, nasal obstruction, sneezing, and nasal irritation. The differential diagnosis is broad and patients may have elements of both conditions. Types of rhinitis may be attributed to "vasomotor", or non-allergic rhinopathy, medications as well as a myriad of other possible etiologies: occupational exposures, chemical sensitivities, pregnancy or hormonal changes, food- and/or alcohol-induced, nonallergic rhinitis with eosinophilia syndrome (NARES), vasculitides, granulomatous, or autoimmune conditions [1]. History is the most important factor in the diagnosis of NAR, and in combination with a complete nasal exam, can direct further work-up. Further detailed discussion regarding the epidemiology, evaluation, and treatment of NAR can be found in Chaps. 7, 8 and 9.

V. A. Patel (✉)
Division of Pediatric Otolaryngology, Rady Children's Hospital - San Diego, San Diego, CA, USA

Department of Otolaryngology - Head and Neck Surgery, University of California San Diego, La Jolla, CA, USA
e-mail: vpatel2@rchsd.org

U. S. Ramaswamy
Pediatric Otolaryngology-Head & Neck Surgery, Texas Children's Hospital, Houston, TX, USA
e-mail: usramaw@texaschildrens.org

S. E. Lee
Division of Sinonasal Disorders and Allergy, Department of Otolaryngology-Head & Neck Surgery, Brigham and Women's Hospital, Boston, MA, USA
e-mail: lees6@upmc.edu

C. Damask et al. (eds.), *Allergy in Otolaryngology Practice*,
https://doi.org/10.1007/978-3-031-93455-1_8

Classic Inflammatory Pathway

Entopy (local atopy) refers to localized allergy in the nasal cavity without positive skin prick testing, elevated serum IgE, or serum allergen-specific IgE [2]. Support for this theory in the pathogenesis of NAR is directly related to the influx of type 2 inflammatory cells and associated immune effectors within nasal mucosal tissue. A preliminary study of 17 non-allergic rhinopathy patients who underwent inferior turbinate sampling followed by immunohistochemical analysis detected a six-fold mean increase in mean mast cell population ($P < 0.03$), increased epithelial and superficial mucosal IgE^{+} cell population ($P < 0.05$), and elevated eosinophil levels ($P < 0.05$) relative to normal nasal mucosa [3]. A follow-up study of 22 nonatopic rhinitis patients who underwent inferior turbinate sampling followed by immunohistochemical analysis found a significant proportion of $CD8^{+}$ lymphocytes ($P = 0.02$) in superficial submucosa and fewer HLA-DR α^{+} cells ($P = 0.007$) compared to healthy subjects [4]. Further investigation of 50 perennial NAR patients who underwent nasal lavage mucosal sampling revealed a higher density of albumin ($P < 0.05$), $CD3^{+}$ T cells ($P < 0.001$), eosinophils ($P < 0.05$), and eosinophil catatonic protein ($P < 0.05$) on flow cytometry compared to healthy participants [5]. However, it appears the inflammatory profile in NAR may have cell types other than eosinophils in different patient populations, which may have a direct influence on disease severity. A cross-sectional study of 519 adults with NAR who underwent nasal cytology identified four inflammatory groups: NAR with neutrophilia ($n = 171$, 32.95%), NAR with eosinophilia ($n = 81$, 15.61%), NAR with mast cells ($n = 19$, 3.66%), and NAR with mast cells and eosinophils ($n = 17$, 3.28%) [6]. Similarly, in a series of 114 children with NAR who underwent nasal cytology, eosinophils were the predominant cell type in 53 patients (46.5%) followed by neutrophils which were the predominant cell type present in 46 patients (40.4%) [7]. By extension, it appears cytokine expression also differs in NAR; a study comparing 45 NAR and 45 allergic rhinitis patients notes significantly elevated interleukin-16 and interleukin-17 levels compared to healthy controls. Naturally, these findings have led researchers to question if the localized inflammatory response in NAR may lead to the development of systemic atopy with IgE antibody production. A prospective cohort study of 176 localized allergic rhinitis patients and 115 controls determined skin prick tests and/or serum-specific IgE became positive in 6.81% of patients with local allergic rhinitis compared to 4.5% of controls over a 5-year period [8]. Multiple studies have also challenged the validity of the classic inflammatory pathway given negative mucosal biopsies [9, 10] and negative allergen challenges [11, 12]. Future research efforts are necessary to better elucidate the exact role of entopy as a pathogenic mechanism in NAR.

Neural Deregulation Pathway

Role of the Trigeminal Nerve

The fifth cranial nerve predominantly relays sensory innervation to the nose. The ophthalmic (V1) and maxillary (V2) divisions of the trigeminal nerve innervate the anterior nasal floor, inferior meatus, lateral nasal wall, septum, and vestibule and provide the sensation of nasal airflow, pain, pruritus, temperature, and touch. These sensory nerves, which supply deep venous sinusoids and submucosal glands consist of both fast-conducting, myelinated-type Aδ fibers and slow-conducting, nonmyelinated C-type fibers. Rapidly transmitted sensations perceived at the cortical level via Aδ fibers include heat, burning pain (first pain), and cold [13]. Conversely, C-type fibers convey the slower onset sensations of discomfort, mechanical stretch, paresthesia, and gentle touch, as they are the most relevant type of sensory nerves in NAR [14, 15].

An important characteristic of C-type fibers is that their dendrites can be antidromically stimulated by action potentials that originate at different terminals of the same neuron [16]. This mechanism, referred to as the axon reflex, mediates inflammatory neuropeptide release from peripheral neurosecretory varicosities, producing vasodilatation and increased vascular permeability collectively termed as neurogenic inflammation [17]. These C-type fibers contain neuropeptides including calcitonin G-related peptide, gastrin-releasing peptide, tachykinins (substance P and neurokinin A), and urocortin [18]. Immunohistochemical analysis has confirmed that these neuropeptide-containing fibers colocalize with their respective receptors at sphenopalatine ganglion cells, regional microvasculature, and nasal epithelium [19, 20]. Additional neuropeptide effects include glandular activation, leukocyte recruitment, and differentiation as well as activation of inflammatory cells (lymphocytes, eosinophils, mast cells, and macrophages) [17]. It is thought that stimulation of C-fibers innervating nasal mucosal endothelial and epithelial cells increases vascular permeability and glandular secretion, resulting in secretory rhinorrhea observed in NAR [21]. Finally, solitary chemoreceptor cells that are scattered throughout the nasal cavity and synapse with trigeminal nerve fibers may play a role in NAR by reacting to chemical stimuli and nasal irritants through the canonical taste transduction cascade [22]. The trigeminal system appears to constitute a major component in the pathophysiology of NAR, additional scientific attention is necessary to explore this important phenomenon.

Autonomic System Dysfunction

Since 1959, the etiology of NAR has been linked to an imbalance of the autonomic nervous system, with either excessive autonomic activity or reduced sympathetic activity. Serving as the efferent arc of the nasal reflex, postganglionic parasympathetic fibers primarily innervate seromucous and serous nasal glands. The cholinergic component of parasympathetic reflexes is the predominant stimulus for mucus secretion; parasympathetics not only release neurotransmitters such as acetylcholine but also neuropeptides such as vasoactive intestinal peptide and peptide histidine isoleucine. There are five different subtypes of muscarinic receptors that are distributed on glands, arteries, veins, and epithelial cells. The M3 subtype is the most abundant, with a predominant effect of stimulating glandular secretion through the action of physiologically released acetylcholine [18]. Sympathetic nerves reach the nasal mucosa via the superior cervical ganglion and are distributed to nasal blood vessels by the vidian and trigeminal nerves. Sympathetic nerves contain the primary neurotransmitter of norepinephrine as well as neuropeptides (neuropeptide Y). Norepinephrine carries a predominant vasoconstrictive action via α-adrenergic receptors as well as vasodilation of resistance vessels through β1- and β2- adrenergic receptors, this results in an increase in blood flow as well as a direct influence on nasal glandular activity [23]. Neuropeptide Y and its receptor are present in the walls of arterioles, arteriovenous anastomoses, and other vessels within the nasal mucosa, suggestive of the relevance of neuropeptide Y as a regulator of vascular tone as a vasoconstrictor peptide [24]. The potential link between autonomic dysfunction and NAR has been evaluated by performing autonomic nervous system testing in 19 vasomotor rhinitis patients, where marked abnormalities in sudomotor, cardiovagal, and adrenergic subscores were appreciated, with a composite autonomic scale score that was significantly impaired ($P < 0.005$) compared to controls [25]. Further characterization of autonomic dysfunction in NAR was measured by calculating heart rate variability parameters in 26 vasomotor rhinitis patients. A decrease in root mean square of adjacent differences in N-N intervals ($P < 0.001$) and standard deviations of all N-N intervals for all 5 min segments of the entire recording ($P < 0.001$) were found, suggesting a hyperactive parasympathetic nervous system when compared to control patients [26]. A prospective study of 78 idiopathic perennial rhinitis patients revealed either a hypervagal response (59%) or mixed response (41%) when compared to healthy controls ($P < 0.05$) and that the hypervagal response correlated with rhinorrhea severity ($r = 0.52$, $P < 0.05$) [27]. Finally, a small study of 19 intrinsic rhinitis patients revealed an abnormal nasal response to isometric exercise with a moderate rise in nasal resistance compared to controls ($P < 0.05$). Despite this body of evidence, it remains to be seen whether dysautonomia can be a predictor of therapeutic response in NAR.

Environmental Triggers

Increased sensitivity to environmental factors (chemical fumes, climate change, floral fragrances, occupational exposures, pollution, strong odors, tobacco smoke, and perfumes) triggers symptoms in NAR [28]. Sudden temperature changes (e.g., leaving or entering an air-conditioned room), humidity, or barometric pressure, as well as ingestion of some foods (hot, spicy) or alcohol, also serve as inciting factors for many NAR patients.

Nitric Oxide

Nitric oxide (NO) is a diffusible free radical generated from the amino acid L-arginine by the action of nitric oxide synthase, which requires the co-factor nicotinamide adenine dinucleotide phosphate (NADPH). NO has been proposed as a mediator of important nasal functions, including relaxation of vascular smooth muscle cells as well as modulation of glandular secretion and ciliary beat frequency. In an ultrastructural localization analysis of 7 vasomotor rhinitis patients who underwent inferior turbinate sampling, strong NADPH-diaphorase activity was appreciated in vascular smooth muscle cells of the cavernous sinuses, a venous erectile tissue of the nasal respiratory mucosa [29]. Additional histopathological study of 10 partial inferior turbinectomy specimens from NAR patients revealed both damaged epithelial and basal cells were found to have strong NADPH-diaphorase activity relative to healthy subjects. These findings were also accompanied by basement membrane disruption, complete ciliary loss, absence of tight junctions, and widening of intercellular spaces in NAR patients [30]. Interestingly, postganglionic nerve bodies (pterygopalatine ganglion) have also been shown to contain nitric oxide synthase, which is responsible for NO production [31]. Through neurally generated nitric oxide and potential contribution of various neuropeptides, noradrenergic noncholinergic neural control of nasal blood vessels may exist. Additional support for NO in the pathogenesis of NAR can be found in a time series model of 16 non-allergic noninfectious perennial rhinitis patients, where environmental NO correlated with symptom scores ($r = 0.32$) as well as visual analog scores for secretions ($r = 0.53$) and sneezing ($r = 0.46$) [32]. Although promising, the clinical significance of NO levels in NAR requires further exploration.

Transient Receptor Potential Receptors

Of increasing importance is the recognition that a superfamily of 28 nociceptors facilitate the nasal response. Specifically, the transient receptor potential (TRP) receptor is a calcium ion channel involved in transducing external stimuli to sensory neurons [33]. These channels mediate neurovascular reflexes and detect as well as react to noxious chemical, mechanical, and osmotic stimuli. TRP ankyrin 1 (TRPA1) mediates the effects of noxious stimuli, such as allicin (garlic and onion), cold temperatures, dietary isothiocyanates (mustard, wasabi, horseradish), environmental irritants (chlorite, formalin, isothiocyanates, ozone, toluene), and smoke (acrolein, crotonaldehyde, methacrolein) [34]. TRPA1 channels are expressed on sensory neurons, particularly C-fibers, innervating nasal mucosa and acting as oxidant sensors. When stimulated, these channels initiate neuronal excitation followed by a physiological response through neuropeptide release [35]. Significant overexpression and activity of TRPA1 in small-diameter nociceptive neurons has been demonstrated in NAR and results in an exaggerated sensation to noxious stimuli leading to marked neurogenic inflammation [36]. TRP vanilloid-1 (TRPV1), which is co-expressed with TRPA1, is activated by capsaicin, ethanol, H^+, local anesthetics, and warm temperatures (>42 °C). A double-blind, placebo-controlled randomized trial of 33 idiopathic rhinitis patients revealed baseline mRNA expression of TRPV1 was significantly higher ($P = 0.031$) compared to controls and that an increased threshold to allyl isothiocyanate at 4 weeks ($P = 0.0406$) and 12 weeks ($P = 0.0325$) was appreciated following capsaicin treatment compared to placebo with accompanying changes in visual analog scale major symptom ($P = 0.0004$) and total symptom ($P = 0.0018$) scores. Extreme temperatures (>52 °C) activate TRP vanilloid-2 (TRPV2), which results in Aδ nerve fiber depolarization. TRP vanilloid-4 (TRPV4) channels respond to osmotic stress, mechanical stimuli, and temperature changes. These channels regulate intracellular volume and physiologic responses to osmotic stress and mucus homeostasis [37]. Extremely cool temperatures (<22 °C) result in the activation of TRP melastatin member 4 (TRPM4) and TRP melastatin member-8 (TRPM8). TRPM4 is primarily a chemoreceptor activated by mint and TRPM8 serves as a menthol receptor. TRPM8 channels are expressed extensively on sensory nerve fibers branching to nasal mucosa subepithelium and regional microvasculature [22]. TRPM8 Aδ nerve fibers are critical for assessing breath-to-breath evaporation of water from superficial nasal mucosa (cooling). Greater cooling implies faster airflow, increased evaporation, and low airflow resistance, suggesting nasal patency. TRPM8 input to the brainstem also helps determine the muscular force necessary for air inhalation, dysfunction of this system may contribute to dyspnea [14].

Conclusion

Current literature suggests that there are multiple mechanisms that mediate non-allergic rhinitis, suggesting several key pathways and potential targets for therapy. The underlying physiology of NAR may be multifactorial, as certain subsets could be a result of a combination of pathologic processes. Efforts to further analyze and understand these differences are key to determining targeted therapies that can better manage this unique condition.

References

1. Wise SK, Lin SY, Toskala E, Orlandi RR, Akdis CA, Alt JA, et al. International consensus statement on allergy and rhinology: allergic rhinitis. Int Forum Allergy Rhinol. 2018;8(2):108–352.
2. Powe DG, Jagger C, Kleinjan A, Carney AS, Jenkins D, Jones NS. 'Entopy': localized mucosal allergic disease in the absence of systemic responses for atopy. Clin Exp Allergy. 2003;33(10):1374–9.
3. Powe DG, Huskisson RS, Carney AS, Jenkins D, Jones NS. Evidence for an inflammatory pathophysiology in idiopathic rhinitis. Clin Exp Allergy. 2001;31(6):864–72.
4. Powe DG, Huskisson RS, Carney AS, Jenkins D, McEuen AR, Walls AF, et al. Mucosal T-cell phenotypes in persistent atopic and nonatopic rhinitis show an association with mast cells. Allergy. 2004;59(2):204–12.
5. Rondon C, Romero JJ, Lopez S, Antunez C, Martin-Casanez E, Torres MJ, et al. Local IgE production and positive nasal provocation test in patients with persistent nonallergic rhinitis. J Allergy Clin Immunol. 2007;119(4):899–905.
6. de Corso E, Battista M, Pandolfini M, Liberati L, Baroni S, Romanello M, et al. Role of inflammation in non-allergic rhinitis. Rhinology. 2014;52(2):142–9.
7. Maselli Del Giudice A, Barbara M, Russo GM, Fiocca Matthews E, Cassano M. Cell-mediated non-allergic rhinitis in children. Int J Pediatr Otorhinolaryngol. 2012;76(12):1741–5.
8. Rondon C, Campo P, Zambonino MA, Blanca-Lopez N, Torres MJ, Melendez L, et al. Follow-up study in local allergic rhinitis shows a consistent entity not evolving to systemic allergic rhinitis. J Allergy Clin Immunol. 2014;133(4):1026–31.
9. Blom HM, Godthelp T, Fokkens WJ, Klein Jan A, Holm AF, Vroom TM, et al. Mast cells, eosinophils and IgE-positive cells in the nasal mucosa of patients with vasomotor rhinitis. An immunohistochemical study. Eur Arch Otorrinolaringol. 1995;252(Suppl 1):S33–9.
10. van Rijswijk JB, Blom HM, KleinJan A, Mulder PG, Rijntjes E, Fokkens WJ. Inflammatory cells seem not to be involved in idiopathic rhinitis. Rhinology. 2003;41(1):25–30.
11. Khan DA. Allergic rhinitis with negative skin tests: does it exist? Allergy Asthma Proc. 2009;30(5):465–9.
12. Wierzbicki DA, Majmundar AR, Schull DE, Khan DA. Multiallergen nasal challenges in non-allergic rhinitis. Ann Allergy Asthma Immunol. 2008;100(6):533–7.
13. Dray A, Urban L, Dickenson A. Pharmacology of chronic pain. Trends Pharmacol Sci. 1994;15(6):190–7.
14. Baraniuk JN. Pathogenic mechanisms of idiopathic nonallergic rhinitis. World Allergy Organ J. 2009;2(6):106–14.

15. Belmonte C, Viana F. Molecular and cellular limits to somatosensory specificity. Mol Pain. 2008;4:14.
16. Kenins P. Identification of the unmyelinated sensory nerves which evoke plasma extravasation in response to antidromic stimulation. Neurosci Lett. 1981;25(2):137–41.
17. Sarin S, Undem B, Sanico A, Togias A. The role of the nervous system in rhinitis. J Allergy Clin Immunol. 2006;118(5):999–1016.
18. Salib RJ, Harries PG, Nair SB, Howarth PH. Mechanisms and mediators of nasal symptoms in non-allergic rhinitis. Clin Exp Allergy. 2008;38(3):393–404.
19. Baraniuk JN, Lundgren JD, Goff J, Mullol J, Castellino S, Merida M, et al. Calcitonin gene-related peptide in human nasal mucosa. Am J Phys. 1990;258(2 Pt 1):L81–8.
20. Baraniuk JN, Lundgren JD, Okayama M, Goff J, Mullol J, Merida M, et al. Substance P and neurokinin a in human nasal mucosa. Am J Respir Cell Mol Biol. 1991;4(3):228–36.
21. Evans MJ, Plopper CG. The role of basal cells in adhesion of columnar epithelium to airway basement membrane. Am Rev Respir Dis. 1988;138(2):481–3.
22. Bernstein JA, Singh U. Neural abnormalities in nonallergic rhinitis. Curr Allergy Asthma Rep. 2015;15(4):18.
23. Hall LJ, Jackson RT. Effects of alpha and beta adrenergic agonists on nasal blood flow. Ann Otol Rhinol Laryngol. 1968;77(6):1120–30.
24. Cervin A, Onnerfalt J, Edvinsson L, Grundemar L. Functional effects of neuropeptide Y receptors on blood flow and nitric oxide levels in the human nose. Am J Respir Crit Care Med. 1999;160(5 Pt 1):1724–8.
25. Jaradeh SS, Smith TL, Torrico L, Prieto TE, Loehrl TA, Darling RJ, et al. Autonomic nervous system evaluation of patients with vasomotor rhinitis. Laryngoscope. 2000;110(11):1828–31.
26. Vayisoglu Y, Ozcan C, Pekdemir H, Gorur K, Pata YS, Camsari A. Autonomic nervous system evaluation using heart rate variability parameters in vasomotor rhinitis patients. J Otolaryngol. 2006;35(5):338–42.
27. Elsheikh MN, Badran HM. Dysautonomia rhinitis: associated otolaryngologic manifestations and characterization based on autonomic function tests. Acta Otolaryngol. 2006;126(11):1206–12.
28. Pattanaik D, Lieberman P. Vasomotor rhinitis. Curr Allergy Asthma Rep. 2010;10(2):84–91.
29. Ruffoli R, Fattori B, Giambelluca MA, Soldani P, Giannessi F. Ultracytochemical localization of the NADPH-d activity in the human nasal respiratory mucosa in vasomotor rhinitis. Laryngoscope. 2000;110(8):1361–5.
30. Giannessi F, Fattori B, Ursino F, Giambelluca MA, Soldani P, Scavuzzo MC, et al. Ultrastructural and ultracytochemical study of the human nasal respiratory epithelium in vasomotor rhinitis. Acta Otolaryngol. 2003;123(8):943–9.
31. Hanazawa T, Tanaka K, Chiba T, Konno A. Distribution and origin of nitric oxide synthase-containing nerve fibers in human nasal mucosa. Acta Otolaryngol. 1997;117(5):735–7.
32. Braat JP, Mulder PG, Duivenvoorden HJ, Gerth Van Wijk R, Rijntjes E, Fokkens WJ. Pollutional and meteorological factors are closely related to complaints of non-allergic, non-infectious perennial rhinitis patients: a time series model. Clin Exp Allergy. 2002;32(5):690–7.
33. Eijkelkamp N, Quick K, Wood JN. Transient receptor potential channels and mechanosensation. Annu Rev Neurosci. 2013;36:519–46.
34. Lieberman PL, Smith P. Nonallergic rhinitis: treatment. Immunol Allergy Clin N Am. 2016;36(2):305–19.
35. Wang YY, Chang RB, Waters HN, McKemy DD, Liman ER. The nociceptor ion channel TRPA1 is potentiated and inactivated by permeating calcium ions. J Biol Chem. 2008;283(47):32691–703.
36. Van Gerven L, Alpizar YA, Wouters MM, Hox V, Hauben E, Jorissen M, et al. Capsaicin treatment reduces nasal hyperreactivity and transient receptor potential cation channel subfamily V, receptor 1 (TRPV1) overexpression in patients with idiopathic rhinitis. J Allergy Clin Immunol. 2014;133(5):1332–9.
37. Guilak F, Leddy HA, Liedtke W. Transient receptor potential vanilloid 4: the sixth sense of the musculoskeletal system? Ann N Y Acad Sci. 2010;1192:404–9.

Nonallergic Rhinitis Therapy

9

Omar G. Ahmed and Sandra Y. Lin

Introduction

Rhinitis is a broad clinical entity defined by symptomatic inflammation of the nasal mucosal lining. It can be broken into three broad categories which include allergic, nonallergic, and infectious rhinitis. By definition, a diagnosis of nonallergic rhinitis (NAR) can be made by the presence of at least 2 nasal symptoms such as nasal obstruction, rhinorrhea, sneezing, and nasal or ocular itching, without clinical evidence of infection or signs of sensitization to inhalant allergens [1]. Chronic nonallergic rhinitis is a heterogenous syndrome with multiple underlying etiologies. The pathophysiology is not completely understood and a lack of universally accepted diagnostic criteria makes it difficult to estimate the true incidence and prevalence. Some studies estimate the prevalence to be at least 200 million worldwide, while others predict the prevalence to be 30–40% in industrialized nations [2]. The economic impact from nonallergic rhinitis can be deduced from allergic rhinitis data given the similarities in symptoms and often overlap of the disease. In fact, 34% of chronic rhinitis patients presenting to otolaryngology clinics have a mixed allergic and nonallergic rhinitis diagnosis. This economic burden including costs to the health care system and lost productivity could approach 3.8 billion dollars [3]. This has a significant impact to society and thus a better understanding of the pathophysiology of the different subtypes of the disease and appropriate medical treatments is needed.

Subtypes of Nonallergic Rhinitis

Nonallergic rhinitis is divided into various subtypes as defined by the World Allergy Organization which include idiopathic nonallergic rhinitis (formerly vasomotor rhinitis), nonallergic rhinitis with eosinophilia (NARE), atrophic rhinitis, senile rhinitis, hormonal rhinitis (rhinitis of pregnancy), drug-induced rhinitis or rhinitis medicamentosa, gustatory rhinitis, and cerebrospinal fluid (CSF) leak [3]. CSF leak however is a completely different entity which is beyond the scope of this chapter. Although these are listed as separate subtypes of NAR, there is frequent overlap. The primary goal of treatment is to decrease

O. G. Ahmed
Department of Otolaryngology-Head & Neck Surgery, University of Wisconsin School of Medicine and Public Health, Madison, WI, USA

Division of Rhinology & Skull Base Surgery, Department of Otolaryngology, Houston Methodist Hospital, Houston, TX, USA

S. Y. Lin (✉)
Department of Otolaryngology-Head & Neck Surgery, University of Wisconsin School of Medicine and Public Health, Madison, WI, USA
e-mail: slin362@wisc.edu

C. Damask et al. (eds.), *Allergy in Otolaryngology Practice*,
https://doi.org/10.1007/978-3-031-93455-1_9

symptom burden. There is no specific treatment that can modify the underlying the disease course other than avoidance of specific irritants or triggers. Allergy immunotherapy does not play a role in the treatment of NAR. Before diving into specific treatments for NAR, an understanding of the potential underlying mechanisms is needed. In general terms, NAR can be divided into two broad categories, inflammatory and non-inflammatory.

Pathophysiology: Role of Inflammation

Evidence regarding the role of inflammation in the pathogenesis of NAR has been somewhat contradictory. Initially, a study by van Rijswijk et al. in 2003 concluded that inflammation likely did not play a big role in the pathogenesis of NAR [4]. They examined nasal biopsies taken from 65 NAR patients with significant nasal complaints and compared them to 20 healthy control patients and found no difference in inflammatory cells including lymphocytes, macrophages, antigen-presenting cells, eosinophils, monocytes, mast cells, and other IgE-positive cells. NAR patients treated with intranasal corticosteroids resulted in a reduction of inflammatory cells but no associated improvement in symptoms. However, other studies such as Powe et al. demonstrated an increase in nasal mucosal inflammation in NAR [5]. They compared the nasal mucosa of 11 patients with perennial allergic rhinitis (PAR), 17 patients with NAR, and 9 control subjects who were undergoing partial turbinectomies and found that there was an increased number of mast cells, IgE cells, eosinophils, and plasma cells in the PAR and NAR group compared to control subjects. The same group also studied the T-lymphocyte differences between PAR, NAR, and control subjects and found a significant overlap in T-lymphocytes and mast cells in the PAR and NAR groups [6].

Increased inflammation in NAR patients is also supported in the pediatric literature. Maselli et al. examined nasal cytology of 114 children with NAR and found there were different predominantly inflammatory cells in these patients, where neutrophils were present in 40.4%, eosinophils in 46%, mast cells in 10.5%, and eosinophils and mast cells in 2.6% of children. These histological findings may be associated with different clinical manifestations. For example, nasal obstruction was more common in children with a predominantly mast cell and eosinophil infiltrate, whereas rhinorrhea and sneezing were more common in patients with predominantly eosinophils. Nasal itching was more common in patients with primary mast cell infiltrates [7].

The predominate cellular infiltrate and symptoms profile can have potential therapeutic implications, as patients with a predominantly eosinophilic infiltrate may respond better to corticosteroids. A more recent study in the adult literature also demonstrated similar findings in regard to symptoms and inflammatory cells. De Corso et al. looked at nasal cytology from 519 NAR patients enrolled from a rhinology tertiary clinic and were able to distinguish several NAR phenotypes based on symptoms and inflammation pattern [8]. They found about 55% of NAR patients had a predominantly inflammatory phenotype, compared to 45% of patients who did not. Of the inflammatory phenotype, 33% had predominantly neutrophilia, 16% had eosinophilia, 4% had mast cells, and 3% had increased mast cells and eosinophils. Patients with the neutrophil predominant subtype had milder symptoms, similar to patients with NAR without inflammation.

In summary, after a thorough review of the literature, it is likely that inflammation does play a role in certain subtypes of NAR. Studies which demonstrated that inflammation did not play a significant role likely evaluated a subset of NAR patients with a different pathogenic cause.

Pathophysiology: Role of Neurogenic Mechanisms

Imbalances in the autonomic nervous system and neurogenic innervation of the nasal mucosa are a leading underlying cause of non-inflammatory NAR. The parasympathetic and sympathetic components of the autonomic nervous system maintain a fine balance between vasoconstriction and vasodilation of the nasal vasculature and secretion of the nasal mucosal glands in the healthy state. Patients with non-inflammatory causes of NAR will often have an imbalance of this, leading to symptoms such as excess nasal secretion and congestion [9]. Several recent studies have also implicated important neuropeptides which may be involved in the pathogenesis of non-inflammatory NAR [10–12]. Neuropeptides such as substance P, vasoactive intestinal peptide, and calcitonin gene-related peptide can be secreted by unmyelinated nociceptive C fibers and parasympathetic and sympathetic nerve endings and their respective receptors found in veins, arteries, and glands of the nasal mucosa. These neuropeptides can activate their respective receptors and produce symptoms seen in NAR. Functional MRI studies provide additional evidence that NAR can be caused by a neurogenic mechanism. Bernstein et al. looked at 12 subjects diagnosed with NAR and evaluated blood flow to odor-sensitive regions of the brain in response to pleasant and unpleasant odors and saw an increased response using functional MRI. The increased response was associated with increased nasal symptoms seen in NAR [10]. Gustatory rhinitis, a subtype of NAR, likely has a predominantly non-inflammatory, cholinergic-mediated mechanism. Pre-treatment of patients with atropine significantly decreased food-induced rhinorrhea in 12 patients [10]. The transient receptor potential (TRP) family of calcium ion channels involved in transducing external stimuli to sensory neurons provides additional proof of the neurogenic role in the pathogenesis of NAR. Specifically TRP vanilloid-1 (TRPV1), sensitive to capsaicin and TRP ankyrin 1 (TRPA1) mediate the effects of noxious stimuli such as cold temperatures, pungent compounds, and environmental irritants and are likely involved in the pathophysiology of certain subtypes of NAR [13].

Treatment Overview

Nonallergic rhinitis is a heterogenous group of diseases lumped into one broad category. Treatment can be challenging and is usually less effective compared to allergic rhinitis. Immunotherapy, typically used as a treatment option for severe AR by sensitizing a patient's immune system, has no role in NAR. By taking a thorough history and physical, a clinician should try to distinguish the subtype of NAR. Treatment should be guided based on the subtype of NAR and target the underlying pathophysiology. If a predominantly inflammatory-mediated NAR is suspected, treatment with topical corticosteroids and antihistamines should be used to help decrease the inflammatory response. If a neurogenic mechanism is suspected, treatments such as ipratropium bromide or topical capsaicin can be considered. If an occupational irritant or medication is suspected to be the main culprit, an emphasis on avoidance of the trigger should be practiced. The remainder of this chapter will discuss the different classes of medications and the evidence for their use in NAR and their application (Table 9.1).

Table 9.1 Summary of treatments

	Commonly prescribed	Mechanism of action	What symptoms does it reduce?
Intranasal corticosteroids (INCS)	Fluticasone propionate Fluticasone furoate Mometasone Budesonide Triamcinolone Dexamethasone Beclomethasone Flunisolide	Decreases neutrophil and eosinophil chemotaxis Reduces mast cell and basophil mediator release Decreases edema and inflammation	Nasal congestion Rhinorrhea Nasal obstruction Post-nasal drip

(continued)

Table 9.1 (continued)

	Commonly prescribed	Mechanism of action	What symptoms does it reduce?
Topical antihistamines (TA)	Azelastine Olopatadine	Local H1 inhibitor Decreases eosinophil activation, adhesion molecule expression and suppresses generation of inflammatory cytokines Potential inhibition of nasal neurogenic excitation	Nasal congestion Rhinorrhea Nasal obstruction Post-nasal drip
Combination (INCS+TA)	fluticasone propionate+ azelastine	Anti-inflammatory	Nasal congestion Rhinorrhea Nasal obstruction Post-nasal drip
Topical anticholinergic	Ipratropium bromide	Blocks parasympathetic input of the nasal mucosal glands	Rhinorrhea
Topical capsaicin	Intranasal capsaicin spray (formulations can be mixed with eucalyptus to decrease burning sensation)	Agonist of TRPV1 Chronic activation of this receptor causes a decrease in conduction of nociceptive C-fibers in the trigeminal nerve and diminishes neurogenic response to irritant	Rhinorrhea, overall decreases nasal response to irritant
Decongestants	Oral pseudoephedrine Intranasal oxymetazoline Intranasal phenylephrine	Alpha-adrenergic agonist causing vasoconstriction of the blood vessels of the nasal mucosa	Nasal congestion

Topical Intranasal Corticosteroids (INCS)

Topical intranasal corticosteroids are one of the main treatments for NAR. They penetrate the nasal mucosa with the result of decreased neutrophil chemotaxis, decreased eosinophil chemotaxis, reduced mast cell mediator release, and reduced basophil mediator release [14]. Fluticasone and beclomethasone are the only two topical intranasal corticosteroids approved by the Food and Drug Administration (FDA) for NAR. In general, this class of medications is well tolerated with minimal systemic side effects. These medications are likely more beneficial in inflammatory-mediated forms of NAR such as NARE compared to non-inflammatory forms. There have been multiple randomized placebo-controlled trials which demonstrate the effectiveness of various forms of INCS for NAR symptoms [15–17]. One studied looked at pooled data from 3 RCTs of 983 patients and evaluated the effect of fluticasone propionate at 200 micrograms, 400 micrograms, and placebo in NAR patients both with and without eosinophilia for 4 weeks. They found both treatment groups had a significant improvement in total nasal symptom score compared to placebo. This was true in both the NARES and non-NARES groups. However, there are other studies which show INCS is likely not beneficial for all subtypes of NAR patients. For example, Jacobs et al. examined pooled data from two RTCs (*n*=699) and found that fluticasone treatment for four weeks compared to placebo showed no improvement in total nasal symptom score in vasomotor rhinitis patients [18]. This subset of vasomotor rhinitis patients had mainly weather-related onset of symptoms and were refractory to INCS.

Antihistamines

H1 antihistamines come in both a topical intranasal spray and an oral form. The traditional oral antihistamines have a limited role in the treatment of NAR. First-generation H1 antihistamines (chlorpheniramine or diphenhydramine) are more potent and have anticholinergic effects which may be helpful in NAR patients with persistent post-nasal drip and anterior rhinorrhea despite first-line treatments [19]. These medications cross the blood-brain barrier and are limited in use due to potential central nervous system effects such as sedation, drowsiness, and cognitive impairment. Second-generation antihistamines (loratadine, desloratadine, cetirizine, levocetirizine, and fexofenadine) are less sedating and can be beneficial in NAR patients who have sneezing and itching as part of their symptoms [20].

Intranasal H1 antihistamine sprays such as azelastine and olopatadine have been studied, and play an important role in the treatment of NAR. Azelastine is available in 0.1% and 0.15% formulations and is thought to improve symptoms because of its anti-inflammatory properties. This medication has been shown to diminish eosinophil activation, adhesion molecule expression and suppress the generation of inflammatory cytokines [21, 22]. Azelastine may also reduce neurogenic excitation from olfactory stimuli. In vitro studies show that azelastine can activate TRPV1 receptors and with continuous exposure, desensitize these receptors, similar to capsaicin [23]. Functional brain MRI has shown NAR patients exposed to both pleasant and unpleasant odors have increased blood flow to certain odor-sensitive regions of the brain relevant to olfactory sensation and sensory processing. This increased blood flow response was blunted with the use of azelastine, thus suggesting this medication may decrease neurogenic activation by olfactory stimuli [24]. Two multicenter, randomized, double-blind, placebo-controlled, parallel-group clinical trials (n=200) showed azelastine was an effective treatment for NAR patients after 3 weeks of treatment [25]. All symptoms measured including total vasomotor rhinitis symptoms score improved in the azelastine treatment group compared to placebo. Bitter taste, a common side effect of the medication, was seen in 19% of patients.

Olopatadine, another topical H1 antihistamine, is not FDA approved for the treatment of NAR. However, there is evidence for its effectiveness in the treatment of this disease. Liberman et al. look at 129 patients with NAR in a randomized, double-blind, multi-centered study and compared olopatadine to azelastine. They found both medications were equally as effective in reducing symptoms of nasal congestion, rhinorrhea, postnasal drip, and sneezing after 14 days of treatment [26]. Both medications had a similar efficacy and safety profile.

Combination of Intranasal Corticosteroids and Topical Antihistamines

The combined use of INCS and intranasal topical antihistamines is considered to be an effective treatment for nonallergic rhinitis [27]. It is more effective than either medication alone. The combination of the two medications can be given separately or through a combined spray with azelastine (137 mcg) and fluticasone propionate (50 mcg) called Dymista. Price et al. evaluated 612 chronic rhinitis patients (424 perennial allergic rhinitis and 188 NAR) who were treated with either Dymista for fluticasone propionate nasal spray for 52 weeks in a randomized, open-label, parallel-group study [28]. They found that total nasal symptom score (nasal congestion, pruritis, rhinorrhea, sneezing) was reduced to a greater degree in the Dymista group compared to the fluticasone propionate group starting at day 1 of treatment, up to 28 weeks of treatment. This benefit in nasal symptoms persisted for the 52-week duration of the study in both the NAR and perennial allergic rhinitis patients. Thus, combination treatment should be used in NAR patients if symptoms are not adequately controlled with either medication alone.

Anticholinergics

Anticholinergic medications take effect by blocking the action of the neurotransmitter acetylcholine at the synapses of the nervous system. Anticholinergics are useful for the symptom of rhinorrhea in NAR patients. The oral forms of the medication have significant systemic side effects including blurred vision, dry eyes and mouth, thickened secretions, and are not well tolerated. Therefore, oral anticholinergics are not indicated for the treatment of NAR. The only topical intranasal form that is FDA approved for NAR is ipratropium bromide which acts locally by blocking the parasympathetic input of the nasal mucosal glands. Ipratropium is available in two strengths, 0.03% and 0.06%; however only the 0.03% dosed three times daily is approved for NAR. Grossman et al. looked at 285 patients with NAR and treated them with 0.03% of ipratropium bromide in an open-label trial over 1 year and found the treatment effective for NAR symptoms with minimal side effects. There was demonstrated improvement in patient quality of life and a reduction in the need for other medications [29]. Bronsky evaluated 283 patients in an 8-week, double-blind parallel comparison trial of ipratropium bromide and placebo saline sprays for the treatment of NAR and found a 30% reduction in rhinorrhea [30]. However, there was no significant difference in other symptoms such as postnasal drip, sneezing, and congestion.

Overall, ipratropium bromide is an effective treatment for the symptom rhinorrhea in NAR with good tolerability. This medication is especially helpful in gustatory rhinitis and vasomotor rhinitis where there is a specific trigger for the onset of rhinorrhea. Patients can take this medication prophylactically prior to exposure of the known trigger or irritant to help control symptoms.

Decongestants

Decongestants are available in systemic or topical forms and can be used as an adjunct for the treatment of NAR. These medications work by causing vasoconstriction in the nasal mucosa leading to decreased edema. Oral decongestants including pseudoephedrine and phenylephrine can cause systemic side effects such as irritability, tachycardia, and hypertension and should be used with caution for patients with a cardiac history. Topical decongestants including oxymetazoline and phenylephrine are effective in temporarily improving nasal congestion, but there is concern that prolonged use greater than 3–14 days can lead to rebound congestion. However, a pilot study by Rael et al. demonstrated that combined treatment with intranasal corticosteroid and intranasal oxymetazoline for 20 days did not cause any rebound nasal congestion in both NAR and AR patients [31]. They also found the combination treatment had significantly improved quality of life measures including sleep compared to INCS treatment alone.

Although there are specific studies of NAR patients, decongestants can be used to help with the symptoms of nasal congestion in otherwise medically refractory NAR patients. Topical decongestants should be used in combination with INCS when prescribed for greater than 3–14 days in order to prevent rebound congestion. Caution should be used if patients do examine rebound effects from topical decongestants and then patients will need to be counseled appropriately so as not to develop rhinitis medicamentosa.

Topical Capsaicin

Capsaicin is an active compound found in chili peppers and has been used as treatment for various pathologies including NAR. Capsaicin is a selective agonist of TRPV1. Chronic activation of TROV1 is thought to cause a decrease in conduction of nociceptive C-fibers in the trigeminal nerve and diminish a neurogenic response to inhaled irritants. A Cochrane review attempted to perform a meta-analysis of 4 studies to evaluate the effectiveness of topical capsaicin for NAR, but found heterogeneity too great between these studies to pool the studies. They also found a high risk of bias in 2 of the studies and overall low to moderate quality of evidence. The authors concluded that capsaicin may be an option for treatment for NAR, and benefits of improved nasal symptoms may be seen up to 36 weeks after treatment based on a few small studies with low-quality evidence [32]. A more recent study by Bernstein et al. evaluated the treatment of a formulation of capsaicin spray mixed with eucalyptol in order to decrease burning for NAR [33]. They studied 42 NAR patients in a randomized double-blinded parallel trial treated with either topical capsaicin mixed with eucalyptol twice daily for 2 weeks compared to placebo and found significant improvement in total nasal symptom score and good tolerability in the treatment arm. Although this study has promising results, future larger RCTs are required in order to make a strong scientific recommendation regarding the use of topical capsaicin for NAR.

Nasal Saline Irrigation

There is no strong evidence pertaining to the use of nasal irrigations or nasal saline sprays for the treatment of NAR. A recent Cochrane review of 14 pooled studies (n=747) evaluated the use of nasal irrigations for allergic rhinitis [34]. The authors concluded that saline irrigation may reduce patient-reported disease severity compared to no saline irrigation at up to 3 months of treatment. The overall quality of evidence was considered low or very low. Based on the literature, the role of nasal saline rinses in NAR is undefined, and further studies are needed to investigate this.

References

1. Hellings PW, Klimek L, Cingi C, et al. Non-allergic rhinitis: position paper of the european academy of allergy and clinical immunology. Allergy. 2017;72:1657–65. https://doi.org/10.1111/all.13200.
2. Bousquet J, Fokkens W, Burney P, et al. Important research questions in allergy and related diseases: nonallergic rhinitis: a GA2LEN paper. Allergy. 2008;63:842–53. https://doi.org/10.1111/j.1398-9995.2008.01715.x.
3. Schoenwetter WF, Dupclay L, Appajosyula S, et al. Economic impact and quality-of-life burden of allergic rhinitis. Curr Med Res Opin. 2004;20:305–17. https://doi.org/10.1185/030079903125003053.
4. van Rijswijk JB, Blom HM, KleinJan A, et al. Inflammatory cells seem not to be involved in idiopathic rhinitis. Rhinology. 2003;41:25–30.
5. Powe DG, Huskisson RS, Carney AS, et al. Evidence for an inflammatory pathophysiology in idiopathic rhinitis. Clin Exp Allergy. 2001;31:864–72. https://doi.org/10.1046/j.1365-2222.2001.01106.x.
6. Powe DG, Huskisson RS, Carney AS, et al. Mucosal T-cell phenotypes in persistent atopic and nonatopic rhinitis show an association with mast cells. Allergy. 2004;59:204–12. https://doi.org/10.1046/j.1398-9995.2003.00315.
7. Maselli Del Giudice A, Barbara M, Russo GM, et al. Cell-mediated non-allergic rhinitis in children. Int J Pediatr Otorhinolaryngol. 2012;76:1741–5. https://doi.org/10.1016/j.ijporl.2012.08.013.
8. de Corso E, Battista M, Pandolfini M, et al. Role of inflammation in non-allergic rhinitis. Rhinology. 2014;52:142–9. https://doi.org/10.4193/Rhin.
9. Baroody FM. Nonallergic rhinitis: mechanism of action. Immunol Allergy Clin. 2016;36:279–87. https://doi.org/10.1016/j.iac.2015.12.005.
10. Baraniuk JN, Lundgren JD, Goff J, et al. Calcitonin gene-related peptide in human nasal mucosa. Am J Phys Lung Cell Mol Phys. 1990;258:L81–8. https://doi.org/10.1152/ajplung.1990.258.2.L81.
11. Lung MA, Widdicombe JG. Lung reflexes and nasal vascular resistance in the anaesthetized dog. J Physiol. 1987;386:465–74. https://doi.org/10.1113/jphysiol.1987.sp016545.
12. de Mendonça JC, Dolci JEL. Neuropeptide immunofluorescence in human nasal mucosa: assessment of the technique for vasoactive intestinal peptide (VIP). Rev Bras Otorrinolaringol. 2005;71:123–31. https://doi.org/10.1016/s1808-8694(15)31299-4.
13. Raphael G, Raphael MH, Kaliner M. Gustatory rhinitis: a syndrome of food-induced rhinorrhea. J Allergy Clin Immunol. 1989;83:110–5. https://doi.org/10.1016/0091-6749(89)90484-3.
14. Pipkorn U, Proud D, Lichtenstein LM, et al. Inhibition of mediator release in allergic rhinitis by pretreatment with topical glucocorticosteroids. N Engl J Med. 1987;316:1506–10. https://doi.org/10.1056/NEJM198706113162403.
15. Scadding GK, Lund VJ, Jacques LA, Richards DH. A placebo-controlled study of fluticasone propionate aqueous nasal spray and beclomethasone dipropionate in perennial rhinitis: efficacy in allergic and non-allergic perennial rhinitis. Clin Exp Allergy. 1995;25:737–43. https://doi.org/10.1111/j.1365-2222.1995.tb00011.
16. Small P, Black M, Frenkiel S. Effects of treatment with beclomethasone dipropionate in subpopulations of perennial rhinitis patients. J Allergy Clin Immunol. 1982;70:178–82. https://doi.org/10.1016/0091-6749(82)90039-2.
17. Wight RG, Jones AS, Beckingham E, et al. A double blind comparison of intranasal budesonide 400 micrograms and 800 micrograms in perennial rhinitis. Clin Otolaryngol Allied Sci. 1992;17:354–8. https://doi.org/10.1111/j.1365-2273.1992.tb01012.
18. Jacobs R, Lieberman P, Kent E, et al. Weather/temperature-sensitive vasomotor rhinitis may be refractory to intranasal corticosteroid treatment. Allergy Asthma Proc. 2009;30:120–7. https://doi.org/10.2500/aap.2009.30.3206.
19. Meltzer EO. An overview of current pharmacotherapy in perennial rhinitis. J Allergy Clin Immunol. 1995;95:1097–110. https://doi.org/10.1016/s0091-6749(95)70213.

20. Purello-D'Ambrosio F, Isola S, Ricciardi L, et al. A controlled study on the effectiveness of loratadine in combination with flunisolide in the treatment of nonallergic rhinitis with eosinophilia (NARES). Clin Exp Allergy. 1999;29:1143–7. https://doi.org/10.1046/j.1365-2222.1999.00598.
21. Ciprandi G, Pronzato C, Passalacqua G, et al. Topical azelastine reduces eosinophil activation and intercellular adhesion molecule-1 expression on nasal epithelial cells: an antiallergic activity. J Allergy Clin Immunol. 1996;98:1088–96. https://doi.org/10.1016/s0091-6749(96)80196-5.
22. Yoneda K, Yamamoto T, Ueta E, Osaki T. Suppression by azelastine hydrochloride of NF-kappa B activation involved in generation of cytokines and nitric oxide. Jpn J Pharmacol. 1997;73:145–53. https://doi.org/10.1254/jjp.73.145.
23. Singh U, Bernstein JA, Haar L, et al. Azelastine desensitization of transient receptor potential vanilloid 1: a potential mechanism explaining its therapeutic effect in nonallergic rhinitis. Am J Rhinol Allergy. 2014;28:215–24. https://doi.org/10.2500/ajra.2014.28.4059.
24. Bernstein JA, Hastings L, Boespflug EL, et al. Alteration of brain activation patterns in nonallergic rhinitis patients using functional magnetic resonance imaging before and after treatment with intranasal azelastine. Ann Allergy Asthma Immunol. 2011;106:527–32. https://doi.org/10.1016/j.anai.2011.02.014.
25. Banov CH, Lieberman P. Efficacy of azelastine nasal spray in the treatment of vasomotor (perennial nonallergic) rhinitis. Ann Allergy Asthma Immunol. 2001;86:28–35. https://doi.org/10.1016/S1081-1206(10)62352-6.
26. Lieberman P, Meltzer EO, LaForce CF, et al. Two-week comparison study of olopatadine hydrochloride nasal spray 0.6% versus azelastine hydrochloride nasal spray 0.1% in patients with vasomotor rhinitis. Allergy Asthma Proc. 2011;32:151–8. https://doi.org/10.2500/aap.2011.32.3439.
27. Meltzer EO, LaForce C, Ratner P, et al. MP29-02 (a novel intranasal formulation of azelastine hydrochloride and fluticasone propionate) in the treatment of seasonal allergic rhinitis: a randomized, double-blind, placebo-controlled trial of efficacy and safety. Allergy Asthma Proc. 2012;33:324–32. https://doi.org/10.2500/aap.2012.33.3587.
28. Price D, Shah S, Bhatia S, et al. A new therapy (MP29-02) is effective for the long-term treatment of chronic rhinitis. J Investig Allergol Clin Immunol. 2013;23:495–503.
29. Grossman J, Banov C, Boggs P, et al. Use of ipratropium bromide nasal spray in chronic treatment of nonallergic perennial rhinitis, alone and in combination with other perennial rhinitis medications. J Allergy Clin Immunol. 1995;95:1123–7. https://doi.org/10.1016/s0091-6749(95)70216-4.
30. Bronsky EA, Druce H, Findlay SR, et al. A clinical trial of ipratropium bromide nasal spray in patients with perennial nonallergic rhinitis. J Allergy Clin Immunol. 1995;95:1117–22. https://doi.org/10.1016/s0091-6749(95)70215-6.
31. Rael EL, Ramey J, Lockey RF. Oxymetazoline hydrochloride combined with mometasone nasal spray for persistent nasal congestion (pilot study). World Allergy Organ J. 2011;4:65–7. https://doi.org/10.1097/WOX.0b013e31820f8fae.
32. Gevorgyan A, Segboer C, Gorissen R, et al. Capsaicin for non-allergic rhinitis. Cochrane Database Systemat Rev. 2015:CD010591. https://doi.org/10.1002/14651858.CD010591.pub2.
33. Bernstein JA, Davis BP, Picard JK, et al. A randomized, double-blind, parallel trial comparing capsaicin nasal spray with placebo in subjects with a significant component of nonallergic rhinitis. Ann Allergy Asthma Immunol. 2011;107:171–8. https://doi.org/10.1016/j.anai.2011.05.016.
34. Head K, Snidvongs K, Glew S, et al. Saline irrigation for allergic rhinitis. Cochrane Database Syst Rev. 2018;6:CD012597. https://doi.org/10.1002/14651858.CD012597.pub2.

Part III

Allergy Testing

Edited by Matthew Ryan

10 Indications and Interpretation of Allergy Testing

Triphoom Suwanwech

The prevalence of allergic diseases has steadily increased in Western industrialized countries and is at present estimated to be between 30% and 40% [1]. Every fifth child and every second to third adult are affected [2]. The hygiene hypothesis, infant feeding factors, and other lifestyle factors may have a differential effect depending on the genetic status of the individual, which favors allergic status.

IgE-mediated respiratory allergic diseases are caused by exposure to allergens. The clinical steps that explain the development of allergic diseases are as follows: First, a switch to the production of allergen-specific IgE detectable in serum leads to the sensitization of a patient. Next, mast cells, basophils activation, and various mediators are released and subsequently develop further chronic tissue inflammation of the primary organ reflecting its atopic status. The diagnosis of allergic diseases is based on the correlation between a typical history of allergic symptoms and diagnostic tests. Thus, *in vivo* and *in vitro* tests used in the diagnosis of allergic diseases are directed toward the detection of free or cell-bound IgE in blood and specific organs (Table 10.1). Confirmation of allergy and identification of causative allergens are crucial to correctly manage allergic diseases.

T. Suwanwech (✉)
Department of Otorhinolaryngology, Faculty of Medicine, Siriraj Hospital, Mahidol University, Bangkok, Thailand
e-mail: triphoom.suw@mahidol.ac.th

C. Damask et al. (eds.), *Allergy in Otolaryngology Practice*,
https://doi.org/10.1007/978-3-031-93455-1_10

Table 10.1 Method and indications for the diagnosis of allergic diseases

In vivo	Method	Indication
Skin testing	Skin prick test Intradermal test Patch test	Inhalant, food allergy Venom, drug allergy Contact hypersensitivity
Organ challenge tests	Nasal allergen challenge Bronchial challenge Conjunctival challenge Oral challenge	Inhalant, occupational allergy Asthma Ocular allergy Food, drug allergy
Cellular testing	Basophil activation	Drug, venom, food, pollen allergy
Mediators detection	Histamine, leukotriene, eosinophil cationic protein Tryptase	Inhalant, drug allergy Anaphylaxis
IgE detection	Total IgE Serum-specific IgE	Atopic disposition Inhalant, food allergy

In Vivo Test

Skin Testing

Skin tests are the most accurate diagnostic tool for demonstrating that a specific allergen has induced an IgE antibody response that is used for the identification of causative allergens and selection of therapy, including environmental control and immunotherapy. These tests were introduced in 1865 by Blackley [3], some years later, in 1908 intradermal test was proposed by Mantoux [4]. The procedures were subsequently refined, and further standardized technique. Furthermore, the diagnosis of respiratory allergy has also been improved by allergen standardization providing satisfactory extracts for most inhalant allergens as well as by recombinant allergens.

Skin test methods are convenient, simple, biologically relevant, reproducible, easy, and rapid to perform, with low cost. They require a degree of training and experience to interpret the results and correlate them with the history and physical findings. Attention should be given to the selection of allergens to be tested according to the pattern of allergens in the environment, as derived from epidemiological studies, and taking into account the stability and concentration of the extracts [5]. The allergens that are tested for should be relevant to the patient's clinical condition and exposure. In general, the smallest number of allergens required to establish a diagnosis and adequately manage the patient should be used. There are no strict age limits for performance of skin tests. However, skin test reactivity may be diminished in infants and in the elderly [6]. Tests must be performed in clinics with emergency equipment available for the treatment of anaphylaxis.

Epicutaneous Skin Test

Epicutaneous skin test or skin prick/puncture test is widely practiced providing high sensitivity and specificity for the presence of allergen-specific IgE, and in some cases, is more sensitive than in vitro testing for specific IgE in serum [7, 8]. The discomfort is small and the risk of systemic reactions is minimal although not negligible.

Indications for Epicutaneous Skin Test [5, 6]

1. Rhinitis/rhinoconjunctivitis/allergic conjunctivitis.
2. Allergic asthma.
3. Food reactions such as those manifested by anaphylaxis, immediate acute urticaria, or acute flare of eczema.
4. Latex allergy.
5. Rarer disorders such as allergic bronchopulmonary aspergillosis.

Contraindications for Epicutaneous Skin Test

1. Diffuse or active dermatological conditions (e.g., urticarial, eczema).
2. Severe dermatographism.
3. Poor subject cooperation.
4. Persistent severe or unstable asthma.
5. Pregnancy because of the l risk of anaphylaxis with hypotension and uterine contractions.
6. Patient on beta-blockers (*relative contraindication*).

Conditions Not Routinely Indicated

- Nonspecific rash without allergic/atopic characteristics.
- Chronic urticaria in the absence of allergic features on history.
- Food intolerance without allergic features (e.g., irritable bowel syndrome).
- Assessment of the effectiveness of allergen immunotherapy.
- Reactions to respiratory irritants (smoke, fumes, perfumes, etc.).

Performance of the epicutaneous skin test involves placing a drop of allergen, often in glycerinated saline, onto the normal skin surface of the upper back or volar forearm. A variety of single-, dual-, and multiple-point standardized test devices are currently available to gently create a small break of the skin thus introducing the allergen into the epidermis [9, 10]. Separate test sites need to be spaced sufficiently and the distance should be at least 2 cm apart from each other to prevent overlap of any erythema. Excess allergen is then removed with gauze or tissue paper, and any immediate reaction (wheal and erythema) is read at 15–20 min as it reaches a maximum diameter.

False-positive results can occur as a result of bleeding or direct skin irritation by some extracts that might contain naturally occurring histamine. Dermographism which is a constitutional wheal-ing tendency, in which firm stroking of the skin can cause capillary and arteriolar dilatation and transudation of fluid causing edema, can also lead to a false-positive wheal and erythema and invalidation of the skin test result. False-negative results can occur as improper technique (no or weak puncture) and a result of prior consumption of antihistamines, high-potency topical corticosteroids, tricyclic antidepressants, and some tranquilizers [5, 11, 12]. Some herbal supplements such as *Curcumae rhizome, Adhota vasica, Glycyrrhiza glabra, Cyperus rotundus, Mentha piperita, Ocemium tenoflorium,* and *Nigella sativa* can suppress epicutaneous test results [13] (Table 10.2). A positive control comprising of histamine (1.8 or 10 mg/mL) and a negative control of saline and/or 50% glycerin must be applied in parallel with the test allergen extracts to document validity and control for confounding problems associated with antihistamine premedication and dermographism [12] (Table 10.3).

Skin prick tests are highly reproducible when carried out by trained individuals and results will depend on the devices, potency and stability of the extracts, the depth of the needle puncture and force, angle of the application device, and duration between testing and reading.

Interpretation of Epicutaneous Skin Test

In general, epicutaneous skin test with a response of at least 3 mm wheal diameter more than diluent control done at the same time is interpreted as a positive result demonstrating the presence of cutaneous allergen-specific IgE. Suggested proficiency testing and quality assurance technique for prick skin testing include [11]:

- Using desired skin test device, performing skin testing with positive (histamine) and negative controls (saline and/or 50% glycerin).
- Record histamine results at 10 minutes.
- Record negative control results at 20 minutes.
- All negative controls should be <3 mm wheals

Table 10.2 Suppressant effects of medications on immediate skin tests [11]

Generic names	Mean days suppressed	Maximum days suppressed	Dose
First-generation antihistamines			
Chlorpheniramine	2–3	6	4 mg 4 times daily
Clemastine	5	10	1 mg twice daily
Cyproheptadine	9	11	8 mg/d
Diphenhydramaine	2	5	50 mg 4 times daily
Hydroxyzine	5	8	25 mg 4 times daily
Promethazine	3	5	25 mg 4 times daily
Tripelennamine	3	7	50 mg 4 times daily
Second-generation antihistamines			
Azelastine nasal	2		1% twice daily
Cetirizine	3		10 mg/d
Fexofenadine	2		60 mg twice daily
Loratadine	7		10 mg/d
Levocabastine nasal	0		50 micro/sp. twice daily
Levocabastine Opth	0		0.05% twice daily
Tricyclic antidepressants and tranquilizers			
Desipramine	2		25 mg single dose
Imipramine	>10		
Doxepin	6		25 mg single dose
Doxepin topical	11		
Histamine$_2$ antihistamines			
Ranitidine	<1		
Cysteinyl leukotriene antagonists			
Montelukast	0		
Zafirlukast	0		
Corticosteroid			
Short-term systemic therapy	0		30 mg prednisone daily for 1 week
High-potency topical therapy	Suppress skin response over apply areas		
Local anesthetic			
EMLA cream	0 effect on wheal, 150–100% inhibit flare response		5 g over volar surface of arm 1 h before test

Table 10.3 Factors that cause false skin test results

Factors	False positive	False negative
Biological factors	Dermographism Intracutaneous bleeding	Age, area of the body Local production IgE
External factors	Cross-reactivity Extract irritation	Medication, herbal supplement Extract quality Incorrect technique

Intradermal Skin Test

Intradermal (intracutaneous) skin tests are relevant to both immediate IgE-mediated allergy and delayed-type hypersensitivity. These tests are useful for evaluation of anaphylaxis, particularly drug (e.g., penicillin) and *Hymenoptera* venom anaphylaxis [6, 11, 14, 15]. Generally used when increased sensitivity is the main goal of testing followed negative prick/puncture test results despite very convincing history of exposure. They permit identification of a larger number of clinically reactive patients, especially those with lower skin test sensitivity. In addition, skin sensitivity to low-potency allergenic extracts may best be evaluated by this method [11]. The use of positive intradermal tests after negative epicutaneous tests may not be an appropriate basis for selecting patients for immunotherapy because of lack of specificity. However, an intradermal test is used for the vial test before starting immunotherapy.

Indications for Intradermal Skin Test

1. Insect venom hypersensitivity.
2. Immediate drug allergy.
3. Immediate hypersensitivity to some vaccines.

Intradermal testing is performed on skin of the volar forearm rather than the back to allow the placement of a tourniquet above the injection site in case of a systemic reaction. Because epicutaneous tests are less likely to result in systemic reaction, they are often performed on the back. Technical administration of allergen (0.01–0.05 mL) can be accomplished by using a tuberculin syringe with a 26- to 27-gauge needle. The skin test is then read at 10 min, when the wheal and erythema are considered maximal. The intradermal skin test requires approximately 1000-fold lower concentrations of antigen than the epicutaneous skin test to produce a same-sized skin reaction [16]. In clinical practice with an extract concentration of 1:500 or 1:1000 for intradermal versus 1:20 wt/vol for epicutaneous skin testing, is a bigger dose by approximately 100- to 1000-fold because of the differential volumes and concentrations [11, 12, 17]. Therefore, the intradermal skin tests are more sensitive partially explained by the larger volumes of test solutions administered by the intracutaneous route that induce the predefined wheal or erythema diameter. On the other hand, the epicutaneous skin tests are more specific because the increased sensitivity at a fixed high concentration may be responsible for a small but reproducible number of false positive reactions, presumably because of an irritant effect [11].

Interpretation of Intradermal Skin Test

Reading results should occur after 10 min if immediate reactions are analyzed. Any reaction larger than the negative control may indicate the presence of specific IgE antibody. There are no evidence-based studies on standardized intradermal test grading [15]. However, several qualitative scoring systems are available and used in different centers [12, 17, 18].

Both epicutaneous and intracutaneous tests are safe for immediate hypersensitivity cutaneous reaction. However, possible severe immediate reactions can occur.

Organ Challenge Tests

Provocation challenge tests with inhalant allergens have been used to clarify the role of allergens in specific organs. They may occasionally facilitate or confirm the diagnosis of clinical sensitivity when the history is suggestive but skin and/or specific IgE test results are negative [19–24]. These tests should be performed by trained allergists who can do them properly; who know how to interpret and analyze the results, and who have experience in treating adverse reactions. Challenges may be conducted by conjunctival, nasal, bronchial, skin, and oral routes depending on the clinical history. Occupational exposures may occur via fluids, aerosols, vapors, or dust [25–27]. Provocation tests are often the tools of research protocols that require an objective gold standard for establishing clinical sensitivity.

Nasal Provocation Test

Principle of nasal challenge is the observation of intensity of nasal symptoms such as itching, sneezing, rhinorrhea, nasal obstruction as well as ocular and bronchial symptoms after nasal challenge with allergen extracts or other non-specific stimuli agents. It is important to differentiate AR from non-allergic rhinitis since management may be different. The mechanism of nasonasal reflex involves ipsilateral activation of afferent sensory nerves, resulting in bilateral parasympathetic efferent responses which cause nasal obstruction and rhinorrhea on both sides. The most important outcome parameter is nasal obstruction which can be assessed by various objective methods such as peak nasal inspiratory flow (PNIF), rhinomanometry (RMM) or acoustic rhinometry (ARM) [25, 28–30]. Moreover, sampling of mediators, cells, and secretion from respiratory mucosa has been used in the investigations of allergen-induced immediate- and late-phase responses, and the dose-dependent nature of such reactions [29, 31, 32].

Nasal provocation test should be performed at least 2–4 weeks after any acute allergic episode or respiratory tract infections. Nasal reactivity is also decreased for 4–8 weeks after nasal or sinus surgery, since atypical reactions may be induced [25, 33]. The pathologies affecting nasal patency should be excluded such as choanal atresia, chronic rhinosinusitis with nasal polyps, septal perforation, severe septal deviation, atrophic rhinitis, and adenoids obstructing nasal ventilation.

Indications for Nasal Provocation Test [25, 29]

1. Local allergic rhinitis; to assess the role of allergens implicated by a patient's history when allergy skin test and/or RAST are negative, or when the reactions of the nasal mucosa to an allergen are more pronounced than those of skin.
2. To confirm the clinical relevance of a specific allergen in patients with multiple positive allergy skin tests.
3. To identify a role of an individual, nonstandardized, novel, or unique specific allergen in the nasal target organ using allergen preparations.
4. Occupational rhinitis; to confirm the role of a special occupational agent.
5. To confirm nasal reactivity prior to starting local nasal immunotherapy.
6. For allergy research such as the identification of new allergens or in the process of evaluating new treatments for allergic conditions.

Contraindications for Nasal Provocation Test

1. Previous anaphylactic reaction to the allergen.
2. During an acute inflammation of the nose or paranasal sinuses.
3. Severe comorbidities (e.g., cardiopulmonary diseases, impairment of lung capacity FEV1 < 70% of predicted).
4. Extremely high grade of sensitization (e.g., severe and uncontrolled bronchial asthma or chronic obstructive pulmonary disease).
5. Other severe systemic diseases (e.g., malignant tumors, autoimmune diseases).
6. During pregnancy.
7. Infants under the age of 5 (*relative contraindication*).
8. Unstandardized allergen extracts due to a lack of comparability and reproducibility (*relative contraindication*).

Allergen challenge should preferably be performed in the morning. Patients should avoid any irritant effects (e.g., tobacco, smoke, spicy food) to minimize false results. In addition, physical or mental stress may have an influence in the test performance. Room condition and environmental variations should be avoided. There are different manufacturers of allergen provocation solutions or freeze-dried lyophilisate on the market. Numerous concentration units (SQ-U/mL, SBU/mL, AU/mL, or w/v %) unfortunately make it impossible to compare the allergen concentration of the different allergen solutions. Several methods for allergen application have been used, i.e., pump-aerosol nasal spray, paper disc place on the turbinate, pipettes or dropper into the nasal mucosa. Pump-aerosol nasal spray has been claimed to be the easiest and most reliable device available. The instructions are to take a deep breath before, hold breath during, and exhale profoundly after application of the allergen [25, 26, 33]. This technique prevents aerosol penetration of the lower respiratory tract via the nasopharynx, which is one possible adverse event. The procedure can be divided into 3 steps of measurements, containing a baseline measurement, a control challenge, and the allergen challenge, subjectively and objectively assessing nasal ventilation at each step. Testing continues with increasing concentrations of the allergen challenge and measurement at regular every 10–15 min intervals.

There are some medications which are advised to withdraw before nasal provocation test as follows [29, 33, 34]:

- Antihistamines (48 h to 1 week).
- Astemizole (4–12 weeks).
- Ketotifen (2 weeks).
- Nasal corticosteroids (6 h to 2, or 3–6 weeks).
- Sodium cromoglycate (1 or 3 weeks).
- Nasal alpha-adrenergic agonist (0 or 1 day).
- Oral corticosteroids, more than 10 mg (2–4 weeks).
- Nonsteroidal analgesics (1 week).
- Central nervous antihypertensives such as resperine, clonidine (3 weeks).
- Imipramines and related tricyclic drugs (2–3 weeks).

Interpretation of Nasal Provocation Test

Both subjective and objective assessments of the nasal airways should be performed before and after nasal provocation test. Symptom score is commonly used as a subjective parameter, for example, Likert scale of organ-related symptom (0 = none, 1 = mild, 2 = moderate, or 3 = severe) [35], Total Nasal Symptom Score (TNSS) which is a 12-point scale derived by summing scores for 4 symptoms (rhinorrhea, nasal obstruction, sneezing, and nasal itching) or visual analog scales (VAS) [36, 37] reporting the severity of symptoms on a 0- to 100-mm horizontal scale (mild: 0–30 mm; moderate: 31–70 mm; and severe: 71–100 mm) [26]. The task force members concurred that the ideal subjective scale would contain the following 5 symptoms: sneezing, nasal pruritus, rhinorrhea, nasal obstruction, and ocular symptoms. These key symptoms are also included in Linder and Lebel scores [27, 38, 39]. The objective assessment has been used to identify change of nasal patency by the following methods: PNIF, ARM, ARM, and 4-phase rhinomanometry.

There are various valid ways to interpret the reaction nasal provocation test, which are summarized [25] (Table 10.4). However, in clinical practice, nasal provocation test is still much underused because of the time-consuming procedure and many factors that may affect the clinical outcomes (Table 10.5).

Table 10.4 Positive criteria after nasal provocation test

Method	Clearly positive	Moderately positive
Subjective measures		
Visual analog scale	Symptoms ≥55 mm	Symptoms ≥23 mm
Lebel score	Increase of ≥5 points	Increase of ≥3 points
Linder score	Increase of ≥5 points	Increase of ≥3 points
Total nasal symptom score	Increase of ≥5 points	Increase of ≥3 points
Objective measures		
Peak nasal inspiratory flow	Flow decrease of ≥40%	Flow decrease of ≥20%
Acoustic rhinometry	CSA-2 decrease of ≥40%	Decrease in the sum of 2–6 cm^3 ≥ 27% bilaterally
Active anterior rhinomanometry	Flow decrease of ≥40% at 150 pa	Flow decrease in ≥20% at 150 pa
4-phase rhinomanometry	≥ 40% increase in logarithmic (lg) effective resistance	≥ 20% increase in lg effective resistance

Table 10.5 Possible causes lead to false positive and negative outcomes after nasal provocation test

Factors	False positive	False negative
Biological factors	Changes in the nasal cycle Recent allergen exposure Lack of adaptation to room climate	Post exercise Lack of adaptation to room climate After specific immunotherapy
External factors	Medication Temperature and humidity pH (< 5 or > 8) or hypo−/hyperosmolality of extracts Preservatives in extracts Faulty delivery of test solution	Medication Lack of standardized some extracts Expired test extracts Faulty delivery of test solution

In Vivo Test

Cellular Testing

Basophil Activation Test

Basophils and mast cells both express the high-affinity receptor for IgE on the cell surface. The basophil activation test (BAT) documents type I sensitization to an allergen, as fraction of blood basophils activated by soluble allergen that comes closest to the results of challenge testing. BAT is used when the patient history and specific IgE or skin tests are discordant, when there is no reliable specific IgE or skin test, or if the patient history indicates that skin tests may elicit a systemic response. Determination of basophil sensitivity with serial dilutions of allergen can be used to measure the point of inflection or half maximal allergen concentration as measure of allergic response [14].

Indications for Basophil Activation Test

1. Diagnosis of allergy drug, i.e., insect venom, food, and some pollen allergy.
2. Diagnosis of chronic spontaneous urticaria.
3. Monitoring allergic diseases, i.e., resolution of food allergy, allergen immunotherapy, anti-IgE treatment.

BAT reflects a functional response as basophil activation can be induced by cross-linking of FcƐRI, which requires more than binding of sIgE to allergen [40]. The technique involves flow cytometry to identify basophils in fresh serum (within 3 h of collection), stimulating such with interleukin 3 (IL-3), and then adding the allergen in question. If sIgE to that allergen is bound to the basophils it crosslinks, the cells degranulate and expression of cluster of differentiation 63 (CD63), sometimes also CD203c, greatly increases, evidence of clinical sensitivity [41, 42]. Basophil activation is measured as either histamine release or as upregulation of granule proteins to the cell surface in response.

IgE Detection

The first assay for allergen -specific IgE was reported in 1967 and was termed the radioallergosorbent test (RAST) based on degree of radioactivity [43]. Next-generation technology has been made from enzyme labels immunoassay which substitutes radioactive labels method. Improvements of this method include better characterized allergen solid phases, monoclonal antibodies, automation, decreased assay time, and less expensive instrumentation. In addition, they can calibrate strategy among assay methods, permit a uniform system of reporting IgE antibody, and result in quantitative kU/L units traceable to a common IgE standard.

There is general agreement that, for most allergens, allergen-specific immunoassays detect IgE antibody in the serum of most but not all patients who are clinically allergic. The precise sensitivity of these immunoassays compared with prick/puncture skin tests has been reported to range from less than 50% to greater than 90%, with the average being approximately 70–75% for most studies [23, 44–53]. More recently, novel diagnostic tests based on allergen microarrays have been introduced both in research and clinical practice. Multiplex-based in vitro tools for allergy diagnosis allow a component resolved diagnostics of the atopy status of a patient in a cost-effective way.

Total Serum IgE Assays

Total serum IgE has traditionally demonstrated atopic disposition. It does not identify specific allergens thereby low total IgE indicates less atopic risk. However, approximately half of allergic patients have a total IgE within the normal range. There is great overlap between normal and allergic subjects, thus the utility of total IgE in diagnosing these common conditions is limited [11, 12]. An elevated IgE should stimulate further investigations for specific IgE sensitivity. False positive may occur in subjects with high total IgE without allergic disorders. Other conditions that are associated with increased serum IgE include helminthic infestations, allergic bronchopulmonary aspergillosis, Buckley's syndrome (hyper IgE, eosinophilia, and recurrent infections), other primary immunodeficiencies, and IgE myeloma.

Interpretation of Total Serum IgE

The serum total IgE level in healthy individuals increases during childhood from <1 kU/L at birth to a peak at the age of about 10–15 years. The geometric mean of total IgE in healthy adults is about 10 kU/L and the mean + 2SD is slightly above 100 kU/L [54]. It is recommended that allergy investigation is done in children with levels higher than the mean for the age + 1SD, and in adults if the level is higher than 100 kU/L [55]. The validity of the original adult reference values, mean = 13.2 kU/L, mean + 2SD = 114 kU/L [56] was confirmed with UniCAP, testing in 63 healthy without known allergy.

Allergen-Specific IgE Assays

Assays of specific IgE are modified as manufacturers improve allergens or change reagents to optimize test performance, and enhance accuracy and sensitivity. Allergen-specific IgE in serum is a marker for sensitization and a prerequisite for the development of an IgE-mediated allergy, but is not sufficient for the induction of symptoms. The results of serum-specific IgE and epicutaneous tests are usually concordant. Its high negative predictive value is useful to rule out the presence of sensitization in an individual whose clinical history does not suggest IgE-mediated allergic disease.

Advantages of Serum-Specific IgE Testing [6]

- Widely available in any medical setting.
- No risk to patient; may be first line with certain high-risk allergens.
- Can be done where there is extensive skin disease.
- Can be done where the patient has taken antihistamines or is unable to stop certain medications which might interfere with skin test.
- Little patient effort or cooperation required.
- Many allergens available, including some which are not available for skin test.
- Laboratory test, subject to quality control and standardization.

Disadvantages of Serum-Specific IgE Testing

- Results may take days or weeks.
- Results are not directly meaningful to patients.
- Minor pain or anxiety-provoking particularly in children.
- Some allergens particularly foods may show low sensitivity in certain clinical situations.
- False positives possible with high total IgE levels, i.e., hyperimmunoglobulin E syndrome.

Indications for Allergen-Specific IgE

1. Allergic (IgE-mediated) diseases.
2. Life-threatening allergy (e.g., anaphylaxis).
3. Impossibility of skin tests (skin lesions, unstable medical underlying, medication, extract irritation).

Interpretation of Allergen-Specific IgE

Testing result only gives information about sensitization (the presence of IgE directed to a certain allergen) but not possible clinical consequences. Furthermore, the sensitivity and specificity of both tests depend on the cut-off of the serum IgE level [57] (Table 10.6). For exam-

Table 10.6 Interpretation of serum -specific IgE and management options

Class	Specific IgE (kU/L)	Level	Clinical correlation	Management options
0	<0.35	Undetectable	Consider non-allergic causes	Consider causes other than allergic disease
I	0.35–0.69	Low	Uncertain clinical relevance; weak IgE antibody response may be a risk factor for future sensitization	Allergen avoidance Trial of pharmacotherapy
II	0.70–3.49	Moderate	Probably a contributing factor to total allergic load	Allergen avoidance Trial of pharmacotherapy
III	3.50–17.49	High	Clinically relevant	Allergen avoidance Trial of pharmacotherapy
IV	17.50–49.99	Very high	High clinically relevant	Same as II/III if not controlled consider referral to an allergist
V	50.00–100.0	Very high	High clinically relevant	
VI	>100	Very high	High clinically relevant	

ple, if the result is markedly positive (e.g., a class III, VI), the history suggests a past reaction to the allergen, and the allergen is well-characterized, then the diagnosis of an allergy can usually be made without further evaluation. If weakly positive (e.g., a class I), then further evaluation is usually needed. Skin testing and possible challenge may be indicated, based upon the patient's clinical history.

Negative immunoassay result with the strongly suggestive history does not exclude allergy. In this situation, a skin test should be considered (if not contraindicated).

In vitro tests are occasionally indicated to confirm negative skin tests. As an example, a patient who experienced a systemic reaction following a Hymenoptera sting and had a negative skin test should have in vitro IgE testing done as well to assure that the skin test was not false negative, as this allergy is potentially life-threatening.

The presence of allergen-specific IgE is correctly interpreted as that patient is sensitized to that allergen and may react upon exposure. The likelihood of clinical reactivity is influenced by the degree of positivity, the allergen in question, and the patient's clinical history [11].

Conclusion

Allergy test results (blood or skin) should always be interpreted with the patient's clinical presentation and relevant allergen exposures. Particularly, positive test results only indicate sensitization, not always clinical allergy. Allergy testing should be done in standard laboratory tests by trained individuals to make sure that results are reliable. Finally, the treatment of allergic patients should be based on the appropriate diagnosis and the identification of causative allergens.

References

1. Wüthrich B. Epidemiology of the allergic diseases: are they really on the increase? Int Arch Allergy Immunol. 1989;90(Suppl. 1):3–10.
2. Smits WL, Letz KL, Evans TS, Giese JK. Evaluating the response of patients undergoing both allergy skin testing and in vitro allergy testing with the ImmunoCAP technology system. J Am Acad Nurse Pract. 2003;15(9):415–23.
3. Blackley C. Hay fever: its causes, treatment and effective prevention. Experimental researches. 2nd ed. Bailliere: Tindal & Cox; 1880.
4. Mantoux C. Intradermoréaction de la tuberculose. CR Acad Sci. 1908;147:355.

5. Pawankar R, Walter C, Holgate ST, Lockey RF. WAO, white book on allergy. Milwaukee, WI: World Allergy Organ. 2012;52:55–8.
6. Australasian Society of Clinical Immunology and Allergy. Skin prick testing guide for diagnosis of allergic disease. 2020.
7. van der Zee JS, de Groot H, van Swieten P, Jansen HM, Aalberse RC. Discrepancies between the skin test and IgE antibody assays: study of histamine release, complement activation in vitro, and occurrence of allergen-specific IgG. J Allergy Clin Immunol. 1988;82(2):270–81.
8. Wood RA, Phipatanakul W, Hamilton RG, Eggleston PA. A comparison of skin prick tests, intradermal skin tests, and RASTs in the diagnosis of cat allergy. J Allergy Clin Immunol. 1999;103(5 Pt 1):773–9.
9. Nelson HS, Lahr J, Buchmeier A, McCormick D. Evaluation of devices for skin prick testing. J Allergy Clin Immunol. 1998;101(2 Pt 1):153–6.
10. van der Veen MJ, Mulder M, Witteman AM, van Ree R, Aalberse RC, Jansen HM, et al. False-positive skin prick test responses to commercially available dog dander extracts caused by contamination with house dust mite (Dermatophagoides pteronyssinus) allergens. J Allergy Clin Immunol. 1996;98(6 Pt 1):1028–34.
11. Bernstein IL, Li JT, Bernstein DI, Hamilton R, Spector SL, Tan R, et al. Allergy diagnostic testing: an updated practice parameter. Ann Allergy Asthma Immunol. 2008;100(3 Suppl 3):S1–148.
12. Hamilton RG, Adkinson NF Jr. Clinical laboratory assessment of IgE-dependent hypersensitivity. J Allergy Clin Immunol. 2003;111(2 Suppl):S687–701.
13. Qureshi TA, Qadri Q, Shafi T, Shah ZA, Kundangar A, Rasool R. Pre skin prick testing: a curfew required on herbals too. J Cell Immunother. 2018;4(2):83–6.
14. Braunstahl G-J. Global atlas of allergy. European Academy of Allergy and Clinical Immunology; 2014. p. 153–5.
15. Kränke B, Aberer W. Skin testing for IgE-mediated drug allergy. Immunol Allergy Clin N Am. 2009;29(3):503–16.
16. Turkeltaub PC, Rastogi SC, Baer H, Anderson MC, Norman PS. A standardized quantitative skin-test assay of allergen potency and stability: studies on the allergen dose-response curve and effect of wheal, erythema, and patient selection on assay results. J Allergy Clin Immunol. 1982;70(5):343–52.
17. Demoly P, Pipet A, Bousquet J. Skin testing in diagnosis and management of respiratory allergic diseases. Allergy Allergic Dis. 2009;2:1335–45.
18. Norman P. In: Middleton E, Ellis EF, Reed C, editors. Allergy: principles and practice. 2nd ed. St Louis: Mosby; 1982.
19. Gould HJ, Takhar P, Harries HE, Durham SR, Corrigan CJ. Germinal-Centre reactions in allergic inflammation. Trends Immunol. 2006;27(10):446–52.
20. Gurgenidze GV, Baraban EI, Gamkrelidze AG. Local humoral immunity in patients with pollen allergy. Allergol Immunopathol (Madr). 1990;18(6):315–9.
21. Kontou-Fili K. Patients with negative skin tests. Curr Opin Allergy Clin Immunol. 2002;2(4):353–7.
22. Leonardi A, Battista MC, Gismondi M, Fregona IA, Secchi AG. Antigen sensitivity evaluated by tear-specific and serum-specific IgE, skin tests, and conjunctival and nasal provocation tests in patients with ocular allergic disease. Eye (Lond). 1993;7(Pt 3):461–4.
23. Miadonna A, Leggieri E, Tedeschi A, Zanussi C. Clinical significance of specific IgE determination on nasal secretion. Clin Allergy. 1983;13(2):155–64.
24. Tamura G, Satoh K, Chao CL, Inoue H, Takishima T. Do diagnostic procedures other than inhalation challenge predict immediate bronchial responses to inhaled allergen? Clin Exp Allergy. 1991;21(4):497–502.
25. Auge J, Vent J, Agache I, Airaksinen L, Campo Mozo P, Chaker A, et al. EAACI position paper on the standardization of nasal allergen challenges. Allergy. 2018;73(8):1597–608.
26. Bachert C, editor. Nasal provocation test: critical evaluation. New trends in allergy IV. Berlin, Heidelberg: Springer; 1997.
27. Hohlfeld JM, Holland-Letz T, Larbig M, Lavae-Mokhtari M, Wierenga E, Kapsenberg M, et al. Diagnostic value of outcome measures following allergen exposure in an environmental challenge chamber compared with natural conditions. Clin Exp Allergy. 2010;40(7):998–1006.
28. Fokkens W, Lund V, Mullol J. European position paper on rhinosinusitis and nasal polyps 2007. Rhinol Suppl. 2007;20:1–136.
29. Litvyakova LI, Baraniuk JN. Human nasal allergen provocation for determination of true allergic rhinitis: methods for clinicians. Curr Allergy Asthma Rep. 2002;2(3):194–202.
30. Tantilipikorn P, Vichyanond P, Lacroix JS. Nasal provocation test: how to maximize its clinical use? Asian Pac J Allergy Immunol. 2010;28(4):225–31.
31. Horak F, Toth J, Hirschwehr R, Marks B, Stubner UP, Jager S, et al. Effect of continuous allergen challenge on clinical symptoms and mediator release in dust-mite-allergic patients. Allergy. 1998;53(1):68–72.
32. Pelikan Z. Late and delayed responses of the nasal mucosa to allergen challenge. Ann Allergy. 1978;41(1):37–47.
33. Andersson M, Greiff L, Svensson C, Persson C. Various methods for testing nasal responses in vivo: a critical review. Acta Otolaryngol. 1995;115(6):705–13.
34. Demoly P, Campbell A, Lebel B, Bousquet J. Experimental models in rhinitis. Clin Exp Allergy. 1999;29(Suppl 3):72–6.
35. Likert R. A technique for the measurement of attitudes. Arch Psychol. 1932;22(140):55.
36. Bousquet PJ, Combescure C, Neukirch F, Klossek JM, Mechin H, Daures JP, et al. Visual analog scales can assess the severity of rhinitis graded according to ARIA guidelines. Allergy. 2007;62(4):367–72.

37. Demoly P, Bousquet PJ, Mesbah K, Bousquet J, Devillier P. Visual analogue scale in patients treated for allergic rhinitis: an observational prospective study in primary care: asthma and rhinitis. Clin Exp Allergy. 2013;43(8):881–8.
38. Lebel B, Bousquet J, Morel A, Chanal I, Godard P, Michel FB. Correlation between symptoms and the threshold for release of mediators in nasal secretions during nasal challenge with grass-pollen grains. J Allergy Clin Immunol. 1988;82(5 Pt 1):869–77.
39. Linder A. Symptom scores as measures of the severity of rhinitis. Clin Allergy. 1988;18(1):29–37.
40. Hoffmann HJ, Santos AF, Mayorga C, Nopp A, Eberlein B, Ferrer M, et al. The clinical utility of basophil activation testing in diagnosis and monitoring of allergic disease. Allergy. 2015;70(11):1393–405.
41. MacGlashan DW Jr. Basophil activation testing. J Allergy Clin Immunol. 2013;132(4):777–87.
42. Osguthorpe JD. In vitro allergy testing. Int Forum Allergy Rhinol. 2014;4(Suppl 2):S46–50.
43. Wide L, Bennich H, Johansson SG. Diagnosis of allergy by an in-vitro test for allergen antibodies. Lancet. 1967;2(7526):1105–7.
44. Bousquet J, Lebel B, Dhivert H, Bataille Y, Martinot B, Michel FB. Nasal challenge with pollen grains, skin-prick tests and specific IgE in patients with grass pollen allergy. Clin Allergy. 1987;17(6):529–36.
45. Bryant DH, Burns MW, Lazarus L. The correlation between skin tests, bronchial provocation tests and the serum level of IgE specific for common allergens in patients with asthma. Clin Allergy. 1975;5(2):145–57.
46. Niederberger V, Stübner P, Spitzauer S, Kraft D, Valenta R, Ehrenberger K, et al. Skin test results but not serology reflect immediate type respiratory sensitivity: a study performed with recombinant allergen molecules. J Invest Dermatol. 2001;117(4):848–51.
47. Norman PS, Lichtenstein LM, Ishizaka K. Diagnostic tests in ragweed hay fever. A comparison of direct skin tests, IgE antibody measurements, and basophil histamine release. J Allergy Clin Immunol. 1973;52(4):210–24.
48. Pauli G, Bessot JC, Thierry R, Lamensans A. Correlation between skin tests, inhalation tests and specific IgE in a study of 120 subjects allergic to house dust and Dermatophagoïdes pteronyssinus. Clin Allergy. 1977;7(4):337–45.
49. Perera MG, Bernstein IL, Michael JG, Johansson SG. Predictability of the radioallergosorbent test (RAST) in ragweed pollenosis. Am Rev Respir Dis. 1975;111(5):605–10.
50. Petersson G, Dreborg S, Ingestad R. Clinical history, skin prick test and RAST in the diagnosis of birch and timothy pollinosis. Allergy. 1986;41(6):398–407.
51. Purohit A, Laffer S, Metz-Favre C, Verot A, Kricek F, Valenta R, et al. Poor association between allergen-specific serum immunoglobulin E levels, skin sensitivity and basophil degranulation: a study with recombinant birch pollen allergen bet v 1 and an immunoglobulin E detection system measuring immunoglobulin E capable of binding to Fc epsilon RI. Clin Exp Allergy. 2005;35(2):186–92.
52. Stenius B, Wide L, Seymour WM, Holford-Strevens V, Pepys J. Clinical significance of specific IgE to common allergens. I. Relationship of specific IgE against Dermatophagoides spp. and grass pollen to skin and nasal tests and history. Clin Allergy. 1971;1(1):37–55.
53. Witteman AM, Stapel SO, Perdokc GJ, Sjamsoedin DHS, Jansen HM, Aalberse RC, et al. The relationship between RAST and skin test results in patients with asthma or rhinitis: a quantitative study with purified major allergens. J Allergy Clin Immunol. 1996;97(1):16–25.
54. Alcocer M, Yman L. Chapter 9.14: Allergy. In: Wild D, editor. The immunoassay handbook. 4th ed. Oxford: Elsevier; 2013. p. 857–67.
55. Johansson SG, Yman L. In vitro assays for immunoglobulin E. Methodology, indications, and interpretation. Clin Rev Allergy. 1988;6(2):93–139.
56. Zetterström O, Johansson SG. IgE concentrations measured by PRIST in serum of healthy adults and in patients with respiratory allergy. A diagnostic approach. Allergy. 1981;36(8):537–47.
57. Lloyd M. Interpretation of IgE-mediated allergy tests (RAST). Curr Allergy Clin Immunol. 2015;28:90–4.

11 Allergen Extract Production and Standardization

Edward G. Brooks

Introduction

Allergen extracts contain the allergenic proteins necessary for allergen testing and immunotherapy. Much work has been done to characterize those major allergenic proteins that drive allergenic sensitization and subsequently desensitization. Levels of allergenic proteins deemed most important may vary from lot to lot and between different species. Standardization is the process by which the potency, purity, and consistency of allergenic extracts are evaluated and regulated. Allergen extracts derived from diverse natural sources and diverse manufacturers are inherently variable in their qualitative and quantitative composition. It is a challenge to balance the variability and ensure batch-to-batch and between-manufacturer consistency. Standardization at every level of production has been an ongoing process for many years and as a result the quality of allergen extracts available in the United States is continually improving.

E. G. Brooks (✉)
Department of Pediatrics, Division of Immunology and Infectious Disease, The University of Texas Health Science Center at San Antonio, San Antonio, TX, USA
e-mail: brookse@uthscsa.edu

Regulatory Framework in the United States

Regulation of manufactured allergen extracts originally began with the Hygienic Laboratory of the Public Health and Marine Hospital Service, which in 1930 became the National Institutes of Health (NIH) and biologics were regulated in the Division of Biologics Standards [1]. In 1972, biologics regulation moved to the US Food and Drug Administration (FDA), and are regulated by the FDA Title 21 of the Code of Federal Regulations (21 CFR) under the Public Health Service Act (PHS Act), as drug products under the Federal Food, Drug and Cosmetics Act (FD&C Act) and good manufacturing process (cGMP) (21 CFR part 680). Additional regulations under General Biological Products Standards (21 CFR Part 610) also apply to allergenic extracts.

The Center for Biologics Evaluation and Research (CBER) is the center within the FDA that regulates biological products for human use (https://www.fda.gov/about-fda/fda-organization/center-biologics-evaluation-and-research-cber). Within CBER, recommendations regarding allergen products are conducted at the Office of Vaccines Research and Review, Division of Bacterial, Parasitic & Allergenic Products (Director, Jay E. Slater, MD). CBER convenes the Allergenic Products Advisory Committee (APAC) composed of outside experts and stake-

C. Damask et al. (eds.), *Allergy in Otolaryngology Practice*,
https://doi.org/10.1007/978-3-031-93455-1_11

holders and provides advice to the Commissioner of Food and Drugs (https://www.fda.gov/advisory-committees/allergenic-products-advisory-committee/roster-allergenic-products-advisory-committee).

Regulations

Regulations include (1) considerations for source materials, manufacturing, and process controls, (2) limits on extraneous allergenic substances during the manufacturing process and in culture media used in production. Specific testing requirements include (1) requirements for lot release, (2) sterility, (3) identity and constituent materials (ingredients and preservative content), (4) stability, and (5) potency.

Requirements for pollen include specific identification of source materials and a 1.0% limit on detectable foreign materials (21 CFR 680.1). In practice, identification is accomplished through macroscopic examination of the pollinating plants and microscopic identification of collected pollen grains. Foreign materials are detected by light microscopy. The manufacturing and propagation records of each lot of source material must be maintained (21 CFR 680.2). Records for pollen source materials include the name of the collector and the date, time, and geographic location of collection. Records also include documentation of collection, cleaning, delipidation steps, and identity and potency testing.

Extracts, in which a potency standard and test(s) have been established, are identified as "standardized" (Table 11.1). To ensure standard-

Table 11.1 Standardized extracts in the United States

	Labeling	Potency testing	Identity testing	Additional testing
Short ragweed	Amb a 1 units	Amb a 1 RID (ELISA[a])		
Cat hair	BAU/ml	Fel d 1 RID (ELISA)	IEF	Protein
Cat pelt	10–19.9 Fel d U/mL = 10,000 BAU/mL		Fel d 2 IEF	
Dermatophagoides pteronysinus	AU/ml	cELISA[b]		Protein
Dermatophagoides farinae				
Timothy grass	BAU/ml	cELISA	IEF	Protein
Perennial rye				
Bermuda grass				
Redtop grass				
June				
Orchard				
Meadow fescue				
Sweet vernal				
Wasp	mcg protein	Hyaluronidase and phospholipase activity		Ves v 5 (electrophoresis)
Honey bee (Apis)				
Wasp (Polistes)				
White faced hornet (Vespa)				
Yellow hornet (Vespa)				
Yellow jacket (Vespula)				
Mixed vespid (Vespa + Vespula)				

[a]Sandwich ELISA in development will become the new standard potency measure for Amb a 1 and Fel d 1
[b]cELISA-competition ELISA, BAU-bioequivalent allergy units, AU-allergy units, PEG

ized reagents, CBER maintains a program to provide reference standards and serum pools to manufacturers for potency testing. The vast majority of extracts are classified as "nonstandardized" and have no potency requirements. Nonstandardized extracts are measured in units of weight/volume (w/v) of protein (Lowry method) or protein nitrogen units (PNUs) (Kjeldahl method) and are also exempt from stability (21 CFR 211.166) and identity testing (21 CFR 680.3). w/v units = amount of allergenic source material added to the extracting fluid. For example, a 1:20 w/v extract indicates that the solution contains the extractable material from 1 g of raw material added to each 20 ml of extracting fluid. PNU represent the quantification of the amount of protein in 20 ml extract, as measured by a protein nitrogen assay.

Nonstandardized extracts in 50% glycerin are assigned an expiration date of 6 years from the time of extraction and is divided into a maximum of 3 years for manufacturer storage and 3 years for final vial dating (21 CFR, Section 610.53). Non-glycerinated products expire in 3 years, divided into 18 months for manufacturer storage and 18 months for vial dating. Guidelines for compounded sterile preparations (CSP) that include allergen treatment vials prepared in physician offices have been put forth by USP (USP 797) and adopted by FDA (https://go.usp.org/Proposed_2021_Revisions_795_797). The new rules delineate specific sterile procedures encompassing the facility or area of compounding as well as procedures and personal protective equipment (PPE). The expiration date or by-use date (BUD) under USP 797 for compounded allergen preparations is set at 1 year from date of preparation or the earliest expiration date of allergen extracts used in preparation of treatment vials. Expiration dates for diagnostic tests (such as for skin prick and intradermal testing) and dilutions of immunotherapy treatment vials have not been studied extensively and thus there are no specific guidelines other than the expiration dates of the individual extracts, except where indicated by specific manufacturers (such as dilutions of venom extracts). Loss of potency and reduced stability of lower extract concentrations (> 1:1000 v/v) may result from adsorption of proteins to glass vials. The addition of human serum albumin to the vials may reduce this effect [2].

Allergen Extract Production

Standardization of allergen extracts derived from natural sources is challenging due to the high complexity in the collection and/or growth of source materials and variability in the extraction and purification process and variability of measures of potency, identity, and protein content. Overall composition includes allergenic and nonallergenic proteins, components of the collection, growth and extraction process, and other production contaminants.

Pollen extracts are produced from numerous anemophilous (wind-pollinated) species and some Entomophilous (insect-pollinated) species. Pollens are collected using several methods: vacuuming, cutting and drying, and water-setting [1]. Pollens may be vacuumed directly from cultivated plants (such as weeds and grasses). Pollens may be collected by cutting the branches, catkins, or flowers and drying on paper. Sometimes the pollen must be separated from the flowers or catkins by grinding. Water setting is performed by placing freshly cut flowers into containers of water, the pollen is collected on paper as the flowers pollinate. After collection, pollens are cleaned by successive sieves to remove particulates, washed with organic solvents to remove contaminants and to dissolve the lipid cuticle surrounding most pollens (delipidation) and then dried.

Several source materials from mammals contain different levels of allergenic proteins [3]. Urine and saliva contain more than hair, dander, and pelt, but extracts are currently produced from hair or pelt. Hair is collected from live animals, defatted with acetone, and then separated by sieving, filtering, and drying. The proteins are then extracted from phosphate-buffered saline (1:40 wt/vol), dialyzed, sterile filtered, frozen, and freeze-dried. Many known animal allergens contain lipocalins, and small amounts of the α-1,3-galactose (alpha-gal) allergens may be present in cat and dog dander extracts. Avian feather extracts contain allergens originating from urine, stool, and dander, as well as resident mite allergens that may cross-react with house dust mite [4, 5]. Specific requirements for mammalian and avian source materials include (1) animal care, (2) overall health and immunization status, and (3) freedom from specific diseases (21 CFR 680.1). For example, cattle must originate from sources documented to be free of bovine spongiform encephalopathies.

The major dust mite species (*Dermatophagoides farinae* and *Dermatophagoides pteronyssinus*) represent a major allergen around the world. Their diet consists of exfoliated human skin and other organic debris, and thus are found in high concentrations in beds, carpeting, furniture, and clothing [6]. *Blomia tropicalis* may be found in tropical homes at densities equal to *Dermatophagoides*. Storage mites are found in stored grain, barn dust, and hay. The major allergens of dust mite can be found in the bodies and feces [7]. Extracts are derived from mite bodies grown in the laboratory but can also contain fecal pellets, mite bodies, mite parts, egg cases, and skin casts. Different mite allergens vary in origin. Many are digestive enzymes present in salivary glands and gut cells and concentrate in fecal pellets. Mites bodies are collected, washed, defatted, and extracted in aqueous buffer. After extraction, residual proteins derived from the culture medium should be below defined limits. Allergen extracts in sublingual tablets contain defined fractions of whole bodies and fecal material.

Venom extracts from hornets, paper wasps, and yellow jackets are extracted from the dissected venom sacs. Venom from honeybees is produced by electrical stimulation, which produces purer venom and is more efficient than collecting the venom sac [8]. The amounts of major allergens, hyaluronidase and phospholipase, are quantified by their enzyme activities and vespid antigen 5 (Ves v 5) by immunoassay. Fire ant venom proteins are purified from whole-body extracts but contain significant concentrations of nonallergenic proteins.

Respirable particles from caddis fly, midge, and cockroach species contain potent allergens. For insects that cause inhalant allergy, extracts are produced from the whole body. Caddis fly (Trichoptera) allergen is a hemocyanin-like protein that cross-reacts with other invertebrate allergens found in arthropods and mollusks [9]. The allergenic activity of midges, or lake flies, resides in the hemoglobin (erythrocruorin) molecules [10]. Cockroach allergens from *Blattella germanica* (German cockroach) and *Periplaneta americana* (American cockroach) are found in whole bodies, cast skins, and fecal pellets [11–13]; some allergenic proteins are produced in the gut [14]. Cockroach allergen extracts are prepared from whole bodies and undergo delipidation, crushing, sieving, and aqueous extraction.

Common allergenic fungi include *Alternaria, Cladosporium, Aspergillus, Fusarium, Epicoccum, Penicillium, Candida,* and *Trichophyton* genera as well as multiple genera from *Basidiomycetes* and *Ascomycetes*. Fungal extracts are produced from laboratory cultures using well-defined seed cultures derived from established culture collections such as the American Type Culture Collection (ATCC). However, genetic variability among fungal strains is high and the ideal culture conditions are unknown and thus not standardized across different manufacturers [15]. As such, the allergen composition and IgE binding capacity of fungal extracts vary widely [16]. 21 CFR 680.1 specifies quality control requirements for mold source materials. These regulations address specific requirements during each step of the mold production process from seed cultures through harvesting. Mold manufacturers are required to maintain written Standard Operating Procedures that will ensure the (1) identity, maintenance, and storage of cultures, (2) processing, and (3) limits on contaminates (21 CFR 610.18).

Extractions are performed in aqueous solutions [1]. Slightly alkaline buffers such as bicarbonate buffer (pH 8) are usually preferred. Conditions for extraction have been optimized to account for allergenic protein variables such as heat-lability or protease-sensitivity and may be performed either at lower temperatures or in the presence of glycerin. To prevent microbial contamination, phenol may be present. Processing times are controlled as they may affect total protein recovery and denaturation. Dialysis or ultrafiltration may be used to remove low-molecular-weight substances. Quality control testing including potency testing for standardized extracts is performed on bulk extracts to ensure quality, safety, and sterility.

Sterilization is accomplished by filtration through a 0.2 μm filter (21 CFR 610.12) and tested using validated methods outlined by the United States Pharmacopeia (USP). Allergen extracts in multiple-dose vials must contain a preservative unless the extract contains 50% or more v/v glycerin (21 CFR 610.15). Most manufacturers use phenol (0.2–0.5%) as a preservative with or without glycerin. Allergen extracts for sublingual tablets are not required to be sterile but are required to meet limits for microorganism contamination (USP 61 and 62). Sterile-filtered extracts are stored at 2–8 °C or freeze-dried.

Allergen Extract Potency

Potency standards vary among allergens. Some are based on the content of one or two major allergenic proteins. Standardization for ragweed is based on Amb a 1 content measured by radial immunodiffusion assay (RID) but will be changed to enzyme-linked immunosorbent assay (ELISA) [17]. Cat hair extracts are/will be standardized to Fel d 1 content by RID or ELISA. Since 20% of individuals allergic to cats were found to be sensitized to non-Fel d 1 proteins such as albumin (Fel d 2) measured by isoelectric focusing (IEF). IEF was added as a requirement for cat pelt extracts, since they contain larger amounts of albumin [18]. Venom potency is based on levels of enzymatic activity of hyaluronidase and phospholipase A2.

When data do not sufficiently support assigning potency to a few dominant allergens, as is the case for mite and grass pollen extracts, CBER uses a measure of "overall allergenicity." To assign units of overall potency or allergenicity, a method was developed called the "**I**ntra**D**ermal dilution for **50** mm sum of **E**rythema determines bioequivalent **AL**lergy units" (BAU) (ID50EAL) [19, 20]. It entails intradermal testing with dilutions of a reference extract and calculating the sum of the longest and the midpoint orthogonal diameters of erythema (ΣE) at each dilution. The mean dose producing a 50 mm ΣE (D_{50}) from at least 15 highly allergic individuals is calculated [21]. Extracts with a mean D_{50} = 14 were arbitrarily assigned the value of 100,000 BAU/mL. Subsequent comparisons of similar extracts are made by a variant analysis of $ID_{50}EAL$ testing called the "parallel-line bioassay" and may require 100 subjects [20, 22, 23].

Since skin testing is not feasible for routine lot evaluation, surrogate in vitro potency assays that correlate with the $ID_{50}EAL$ have been developed [19]. For dust mite and grass pollens, the surrogate test is a competition ELISA (cELISA) that measures inhibition by the newly manufactured test extract to binding of IgE from reference allergic sera to a reference extract for grass pollen and mites [24]. The cELISA can be engineered to detect the loss of specific allergens as well as overall potency [25]. Acceptable lots of grass and mite extract must fall within the 98% confidence limits of the reference standard in cELISA testing and thus can range from 65% to 150% of relative potency compared to the standard [26].

Grass pollen extracts are measured in BAU; For mites, "allergy unit" (AU), which is equivalent to BAU, was originally assigned and has been retained. Potency units for short ragweed pollen extracts were originally assigned based on their Amb a 1 content as units of Amb a 1, with 1 unit of Amb a 1 equivalent to 1 mg of Amb a 1. While $ID_{50}EAL$ testing showed that 350 Amb a 1 units/mL is equivalent to 100,000 BAU/mL, the original Amb a 1 units labeling has been retained. Cat extracts were originally standardized based on their Fel d 1 content as AU/mL. $ID_{50}EAL$ testing resulted in the assignment of 10,000 BAU/mL to cat extracts containing 10–19.9 Fel d 1 U/mL [27]. While Venom extract potency is based on enzymatic activity, the extracts are labeled according to their total protein content.

In addition to determining the potency of these allergen extracts, manufacturers are expected to confirm the "identity" of some standardized extracts. This is achieved by isoelectric focusing (IEF), which separates proteins based on their isoelectric points [28]. The IEF patterns identify known allergens and contaminants and is important for safety and lot-to-lot variation for grass pollen and cat hair and pelt extracts.

Potency of lots of extract are allowed to vary between 50% and 150%, except mites and grass extracts, where a range of 50–200% is allowed [29]. Extracts must maintain this potency range for the duration of their shelf life [30]. This range is required given the variability between batches of starting material and variability in potency assays. Similar to the determination of total allergenic activity, the determination of the total protein content (w/v or PNU) in a range of 50%–150% is allowed. Therefore, substantial variation regarding the potency of an allergen product is possible where a new lot is being given to a patient.

Conclusion

Allergen extracts are subjected to numerous rigorous regulatory standards at every level of their production. The inherent nature of the natural source materials and processes results in a range of efficacy based on the presence of the major and minor allergenic proteins and glycoproteins as well as extraneous and irrelevant constituents. As the science proceeds, the FDA has a continuous and rigorous review process allowing for continued guidelines, recommendations, and regulations to improve the quality and efficacy of allergen extracts [31].

References

1. Bridgewater JL, Slater JE, Rabin RL. Preparation and standardization of allergen extracts. In: Middleton's allergy: principles and practice. 9th ed. Elsevier Press; 2020. p. 467–78.
2. Nelson HS, Ikle D, Buchmeier A. Studies of allergen extract stability: the effects of dilution and mixing. J Allergy Clin Immunol. 1996;98:382–8.
3. Fernandez-Caldas E, Cases B, El-Qutob D, et al. Mammalian raw materials used to produce allergen extracts. Ann Allergy Asthma Immunol. 2017;119:1–8.
4. Colloff MJ, Merrett TG, Merret J, et al. Feather mites are potentially an important source of allergens for pigeon and budgerigar keepers. Clin Exp Allergy. 1997;27:60–7.
5. Kilpio K, Makinen-Kiljunen S, Haahtela T, et al. Allergy to feathers. Allergy. 1998;53:159–64.
6. Carnés J, Iraola V, Cho SH, Esch RE. Mite allergen extracts and clinical practice. Ann Allergy Asthma Immunol. 2017;118(3):249–56.
7. Erban T, Harant K, Hubert J. Detailed two-dimensional gel proteomic mapping of the feces of the house dust mite Dermatophagoides pteronyssinus and comparison with D. Farinae: reduced trypsin protease content in D. Pteronyssinus and different isoforms. J Proteome. 2017;162:11–9.
8. Plunkett G, Jacobson RS, Golden DBK. Hymenoptera venoms used to produce allergen extracts. Ann Allergy Asthma Immunol. 2017;118:649–54.
9. Kagen RM. Insect allergens: characterizations and partial sequencing of a caddis fly hemoglobin aeroallergen. J Allergy Clin Immunol. 1990;85:152.
10. Baur H, et al. Structure, antigenic determinants of some clinically important insect allergens: chironomid hemoglobins. Science. 1986;233:351–4.
11. Menon P, Menon V, Hilman B, et al. Skin test reactivity to whole body and fecal extracts of American (Periplaneta americana) and German (Blattella germanica) cockroaches in atopic asthmatics. Ann Allergy. 1991;67:573–7.
12. Richman PG, Khan HA, Turkeltaub PC, Malveaux FJ, Baer H. The important sources of German cockroach allergens as determined by RAST analyses. J Allergy Clin Immunol. 1984;73(5 Pt 1):590–5.
13. Yun YY, et al. Comparison of allergenic components between German cockroach whole body and fecal extracts. Ann Allergy Asthma Immunol. 2001;86(5):551–6.
14. Arruda LK, Vailes LD, Mann BJ, Shannon J, Fox JW, Vedvick TS, Hayden ML, Chapman MD. Molecular cloning of a major cockroach (Blattella germanica) allergen, Bla g 2. Sequence homology to the aspartic proteases. J Biol Chem. 1995;270(33):19563.
15. Esch RE. Manufacturing and standardizing fungal allergen products. J Allergy Clin Immunol. 2004;113:210–5.

16. Wurth MAA, Hadadianpour DJ, Horvath J, Daniel O, Bogdan K, Goleniewska A, Pomés RG, Hamilton RS, et al. Human IgE mAbs define variability in commercial aspergillus extract allergen composition. JCI Insight. 2018;3(20)
17. Rabin RL. Proposed Change of Potency Assay to be used by CBER for Standardized Short Ragweed Pollen and Cat Allergen Extracts. Presented at; Allergenic Products Advisory Committee, 18 March 2009.; Available from https://wayback.archive-it.org/7993/20170111224206/http://www.fda.gov/AdvisoryCommittees/CommitteesMeetingMaterials/BloodVaccinesandOtherBiologics/AllergenicProductsAdvisoryCommittee/ucm129361.htm
18. Turkeltaub PC, Matthews J. Determination of compositional differences (CD) among standardized cat extracts by in vivo methods. J Allergy Clin Immunol. 1992;89:292. https://doi.org/10.1016/0091-6749(92)90393-G.
19. Turkeltaub PC. Biological standardization of allergenic extracts. Allergol Immunopathol (Madr). 1989;17:53–65.
20. Turkeltaub PC. Biological standardization. Arb Paul Ehrlich Inst Bundesamt Sera Impfstoffe Frankf A M. 1997;91:145–56.
21. Slater JE, James R, Pongracic JA, Liu AH, Sarpong S, Sampson HA, Satinover SM, Woodfolk JA, Mitchell HE, Gergen PJ, Eggleston PA. Biological potency of German cockroach allergen extracts determined in an inner city population. Clin Exp Allergy. 2007;37(7):1033–9.
22. Turkeltaub PC. In vivo methods of standardization. Clin Rev Allergy. 1987;4:371–87.
23. Turkeltaub PC, Anderson MC, Baer H. Relative potency (RP), compositional differences (CD), and assignment of allergy units (AU) to mite vaccines (Dp and Df) assayed by parallel line skin test (PLST). J Allergy Clin Immunol. 1987;79:235.
24. Slater JE, Gam AA, Solanki MD, Burk SH, May FM, Pastor RW. Statistical considerations in the establishment of release criteria for allergen vaccines in the USA. Arb Paul Ehrlich Inst Bundesamt Sera Impfstoffe Frankf A M. 1999;93:47–55.
25. Dobrovolskaia E, Gam A, Slater JE. Competition ELISA can be a sensitive method for the specific detection of small quantities of allergen in a complex mixture. Clin Exp Allergy. 2006;36:525–30.
26. Lin Y, Miller CA. Standardization of allergenic extracts: an update on CBER's standardization program. Arb Paul Ehrlich Inst Bundesamt Sera Impfstoffe Frankf A M. 1997;91:127–30.
27. Matthews J, Turkeltaub PC. The assignment of biological allergy units (AU) to standardized cat extracts. J Allergy Clin Immunol. 1992;89(292)
28. Yunginger JW. Allergenic extracts: characterization, standardization and prospects for the future. Pediatr Clin N Am. 1983;30:795–805.
29. U.S. Food and Drug Administration. Guidance for reviewers: potency limits for standardized dust mite and grass allergen vaccines – a revised protocol. 2000. https://www.fda.gov/downloads/BiologicsBloodVaccines/GuidanceComplianceRegulatoryInformation/Guidances/Allergenics/UCM078624.pdf
30. Slater JE, Pastor RW. The determination of equivalent doses of standardized allergen vaccines. J Allergy Clin Immunol. 2000;105:468–74.
31. Goodman RE, Chapman MD, Slater JE. The allergen: sources, extracts, and molecules for diagnosis of allergic disease. J Allergy Clin Immunol Pract. 2020;8:2506–14.

12 Inhalant Allergy Panels: What Allergens Should Be Tested?

David Danis and Michael Platt

Clinical History

Allergy evaluation begins with a comprehensive history which will help determine the appropriate allergy testing panel. A detailed inquiry into a patient's environmental exposures and timing of symptoms is essential to determining the testing panel and clinical context for interpretation of results. Exposures at home and in the workplace, including animals, molds, dust, and geographical regions of living and travel can help identify causative allergens. Patients may also describe specific exposures which trigger symptoms, although these exposures may not be the cause of their symptoms. For example, patients may misinterpret pollen on pines trees as an allergy to pines rather than oak pollen which may disperse to pine trees [1]. Patients who report an allergy to cut grass may be allergic to a mold in the cut grass or other pollens which are aerosolized by a lawn mower rather than the grass pollen. The presence of pets, pests, or visible mold in their environment should warrant careful consideration with testing.

Information about seasonal variations in symptoms may be helpful in determining causative allergens based on the geographic allergome of a region. Pollen is the reproductive germinal cells produced by various plants, including grass, trees, and weeds, and are often the causative allergen for seasonal rhinoconjunctivitis symptoms. [1] The seasonal variations in symptoms may be helpful in narrowing down potential allergens. Trees generally pollinate in the spring. Angiosperms, which are deciduous flowering trees, produce more potent allergenic pollen than gymnosperms, or coniferous trees, with the Cypress family being one exception within the gymnosperms.

Highest concentrations of grass pollen will usually occur in the summer months. The most important allergen-producing grasses in North America are within the Pooideae, Cloridoideae, Panicoideae, Arundinoideae, and Bambusoideae subfamilies, with geographic variations in grass species. Finally, most weed pollen will rise in concentration in the fall months, with Asteraceae, Amaranthaceae, and Chenopodaceae families being the most important in North America.

A history consistent with year-round symptoms points to other allergens including dust

D. Danis
Department of Otolaryngology - Head and Neck Surgery, Boston University School of Medicine, Boston, MA, USA
e-mail: ddanis@tuftsmedicalcenter.org

M. Platt (✉)
Department of Otolaryngology- Head and Neck Surgery, Boston University School of Medicine, Boston, MA, USA

Boston Medical Center, Boston, MA, USA
e-mail: miplatt@bu.edu

C. Damask et al. (eds.), *Allergy in Otolaryngology Practice*,
https://doi.org/10.1007/978-3-031-93455-1_12

mites, animal epidermals, and insects, such as cockroaches. Molds are also present year-round in the environment, however, there may be times of increased aerosolized mold spores if the temperature and humidity promote mold growth and dispersion.

A social history including workplace exposures, family and friend contacts, and travel are important considerations. Some allergen exposures can occur from inadvertent contact with a co-worker or family member who happens to carry dander on clothing. The symptomatology when traveling to alternate regions can also clue clinicians to a possible allergen.

Locale Factors

Geography

To distinguish distributions of allergenic plants throughout the United States, the country has been divided into 11 distinct pollen regions: Northern Forest, Eastern Agricultural, Southeast Coast, Subtropical Florida/Caribbean, Central Plains, Rocky Mountains, Great Basin, Arid Southwest, Northwest Coast, California Coast, and Tropical Hawaii [1]. Understanding these geographic distributions of allergens can allow physicians to provide accurate and helpful testing in their region of practice.

In the Northeastern United States, trees can pollenate into the summer. This extended allergenic season can have implications for allergenic species in the area. For example, although the Pinaceae (pine) family typically produces poorly allergenic pollen, the pitch pine (*Pinus rigida*) may produce allergenic pollen in the Northeastern coastal United States. The pitch pine pollenates at the end of the tree pollen season, after the pollination of other members of the Pinaceae family. The continued exposure to pine pollen throughout the spring may cause eventual sensitization and allergy symptoms to pitch pine pollen, as it peaks at the end of the tree pollen season. The Aceraceae family of trees, which includes maples, are prevalent in the Northeast and coastal United States and produce allergenic pollen. Finally, the genera *Baccharis*, which consists of large, woody shrubs with thistle-like flowers and antigenic pollen, are prevalent in coastal regions, especially in Cape Cod, Massachusetts, and near the Columbia River in the Northwestern United States. Prevalent allergenic pollens in the Eastern United States include the white oak (*Quercus alba*) and northern red oak (*Quercus rubra*), as well as the mulberry tree (Moraceae family).

The Southeastern United States possesses many unique potent pollens, including pecan trees (Juglandaceae family) and jasmine trees (Oleaceae family). Within Florida, *eucalyptus* genus, ornamental Australian pines (*casuarina*), commercial date palm (*Phoenix dactylifera*), and wall pellitory (*Parietaria*) may produce allergenic pollen. Also, in Florida, grasses can pollenate perennially, which may produce an atypical presentation of pollen allergy.

In the Southern and Southwestern United States, some trees can pollenate in the fall and winter rather than the spring. For example, members of the Ulmaceae family, which includes elms and hackberries (*Celtis*), pollenate and can produce allergy symptoms in the fall rather than in the spring. Also, the mountain cedar (*Juniper ashei*) produces highly allergenic pollen in Texas and the Southwestern United States. Walnuts (Juglandaceae family) produce allergenic pollen in the Southern and Western United States. Other allergenic species in the Southwestern United States include the olive tree (Oleaceae family) in urban areas, the mulberry (Moraceae family), and Acacia genus, which produces pollen perennially. Finally, the genera *Baccharis* produces allergenic pollen in Colorado and Nebraska.

California is another region of the United States where certain species of plants may need to be included in screens due to their high prevalence of allergenicity. For example, ornamental Australian pines (*casuarina*), commercial date palms (*Phoenix dactylifera*), jasmine trees, elms, and hackberries may be considered in screening. In Southern California, there are higher prevalences of *eucalyptus*, and grass pollen can be produced perennially.

Climate and Humidity

Climate and humidity can be significant contributors to allergen content in a particular area and must be considered when determining testing panels. In general, climate conditions can have profound impacts on pollen concentrations, as colder climates may lead to shorter growing seasons [2]. Dust mites, which are microscopic arthropods that live in mattresses, rugs, and fabric furniture and feed on human and animal dander, can produce strong allergic responses. These creatures require humidity greater than 50% (75% humidity promoting optimal growth) and temperatures of 25–30 °C, and cannot survive in arid or high-altitude conditions [3]. The two main species of dust mites are *Dermatophagoides farina* and *Dermatophagoides pternoyssinus*, with the latter being more dependent on high humidity to survive. Understanding humidity requirements for dust mites can have clinical implications, as dehumidifying homes may provide some symptomatic relief in dust mite allergy [4].

Molds are a class of fungi which are also more prevalent in humid environments, as mold species need adequate moisture to grow. The most common allergenic molds include *Alternaria, Aspergillus, Cladosporium, Epicoccum, Fusarium, Helminthosporium, Mucor, Penicillium, Phoma,* and *Rhizopus*. Ziska et al. found an increase in the ragweed pollen season at latitudes where there was lengthening of the frost-free period due to global warming [5]. A nationwide allergy study conducted by Quest Diagnostics found that ragweed sensitization rates have increased by 15% and mold sensitization rates have increased by 14% from 2007 to 2011 [6]. One possible explanation for these increases in ragweed and mold sensitization rates is that global warming has led to a more humid and temperate climate throughout the United States, leading to increased ragweed and mold growth and subsequent increased sensitization to these species [6]. Global warming will likely cause a northern migration of tree species in the United States, [7] so distributions of tropical and subtropical tree species may increase in the United States, increasing the importance of their pollens as potential allergens.

Animal Exposures

One cause of inhalant allergy is exposure to animal dander, which includes proteins from an animal's hair, skin, feathers, or saliva [1]. Common animal exposures that may cause allergic responses include domestic animals (cats, dogs, birds, rodents), farm and occupational animals (horses, cattle, sheep, birds), and laboratory animals (rodents) [8]. For example, cats produce highly allergenic proteins, and 28% of homes in the United States have domestic cats [9]. The major antigenic protein produced by cats is Fel d 1, a small, buoyant protein produced by sebaceous gland secretions. While less allergenic than cats, [10] dog dander can also produce allergic responses. The antigens in dog dander are more varied than in cats, and certain breeds of dogs can be more or less antigenic [1]. Obtaining a thorough occupational history may reveal frequent contact with livestock on a farm, work with birds, or laboratory work with rodents, all of which can produce antigenic dander. For example, rodent dander can produce a strong allergic response, and it is also very chemically stable, resulting in the potential for significant buildup of the allergen. Contact with friends and family members who own a pet can result in an unknowing exposure and trigger of pet dander.

Practical Considerations

Allergy Panel Size

The use of allergen panel screens has been reported but is not commonplace today. Screens would have a representation of allergens in each class: pollens of 1–2 trees, 1–2 grasses, and 1–2 weeds, as well as at least 2 families of molds, dust mites, and cat epidermals. In North America, panels which cover the majority of clinically relevant allergens range in size from 24 to 40 antigens. In the Pan-European GA2LEN skin test study III, 8 allergens were needed to detect sensitization in more than 95% of patients, but all 18 allergens tested were needed to detect sensitization in 100% of patients [11]. While increasing panel size may seem to offer more clinical benefits, false-positive results and clinically insignificant findings including a positive test without clinical exposure can confound the interpretation of the results. The usefulness of inhalant allergy testing includes confirmation of diagnosis, institution of avoidance measures, and consideration of immunotherapy. These treatment options are only relevant for those allergens to which a patient is exposed. While there is some variability in testing panel size in different regions of the United States, overly extensive panel sizes become less cost-effective and confuse results with false-positive tests.

Cross-reactivities

Distantly related or unrelated species may have conserved antigens, resulting in cross-reactivity of one antibody toward these antigens from different species. One benefit of understanding cross-reactivities among allergenic species is predicting if other allergens will produce a response given a positive allergen test. This can be helpful when counseling a patient on specific allergens to avoid. One example of clinically significant cross-reactivities is oral allergy syndrome, where inhalant allergens cross-react with food proteins from different species. A common cross-reactivity is among the inhalant birch pollen and fruits and nuts, such as hazelnuts, potatoes, apples, carrots, or celery [12].

Another benefit of cross-reactivity is the capability of reducing the size of an allergen testing panel. If two similar species or antigens have significant cross-reactivity, just one of the antigens can be included in the test. Testing for cross-reactive species can result in less cost-effective panels and higher dose exposure to an antigen which could trigger an adverse reaction. Testing and treatment panels can be limited to minimize cross-reactive species. Generally, one representative from each highly cross-reactive family is needed.

Trees and weeds have less cross-reactivity among families, subfamilies, and genera; however, there can be significant cross-reactivity within a genus of trees. For example, trees of the Aceraceae family, which include maples, show significant cross-reactivity, so the box elder (*Acer negundo*) is usually selected as the representative maple in testing, as this species is the most allergenic and widespread in the United States [1]. Similarly, the Salicaceae family (cottonwoods, poplars, aspens, willows) has good cross-reactivity, so clinicians will use the poplar as a representative species, as the highest percentage of individuals are sensitized to this species [1].

Grass pollen tends to be the most cross-reactive of plants, and just one species is usually needed to determine sensitivity to pollen from a subspecies. The three most important grass subfamilies in inhalant allergy are the Pooideae subfamily, the Panicoideae subfamily, and the Chloridoideae subfamily. The most common allergens in the Pooideae subfamily are rye, blue, brome, fescue, June, orchard, saltgrass, and timothy grasses, and timothy grass is often the representative species. Since members of the Pooideae subfamily are such potent allergens, it is important to only test one representative species to prevent antigen overload. Allergenic species in the Panicoideae subfamily include bahia, barnyard, crabgrass, gamma, Johnson, and St. Augustine grasses. Bahia grass is generally selected as the representative species, as it includes unique antigens, but Johnson grass may need to be tested separately, as it has incomplete cross-reactivity. Finally, the representative species of the Chloridoideae subfamily is generally Bermuda grass.

Weed pollen tends to have variable cross-reactivity within their three important families: Asteraceae, Amaranthaceae, and Chenopodaceae. The Asteraceae family contains ragweed (*Ambrosia*), the most common allergen in many parts of the United States. All 17 species of ragweed have complete cross-reactivity, as well as cross-reactivity with the allergenic *Iva* (marsh elders) and *Xanthium* (cocklebur) genera [1]. Short ragweed is generally the representative species in testing. However, other species within the Asteraceae family may need to be tested individually. There is strong cross-reactivity within the Amaranthaceae family, which includes waterhemps, pigweeds, careless weed, amaranths, *Tidestromia*, and cultivated flowering cockscomb (*Celiosa*). Finally, the Chenopodaceae family includes 22 genera which show little cross-reactivity, except for the *Atriplex* genus, which includes saltbush, shadscale, spearscale, and wingscale.

Other inhalant allergens, including mold, animal dander, dust mites, and cockroaches, tend to have less cross-reactivity among species. For example, the most common cockroaches in the United States, American cockroaches (*Periplaneta americana*) and German cockroaches (*Blattella germanica*), have some cross-reactivity, but American cockroaches produce enough unique antigens to require their own testing. The two main species of dust mites, *Dermatophagoides farina* and *Dermatophagoides pternoyssinus,* have distinct antigens in their fecal particles and decomposing mite bodies that they are usually tested separately [9]. Molds are generally not cross-reactive and need to be tested individually to determine sensitization.

Financial Considerations

When developing an allergen panel, it is important to consider the cost of testing. The American Academy of Allergy Asthma & Immunology reports that the cost to a patient for in vivo testing, such as skin prick testing, generally ranges from $60 to $300, and that IgE in vitro allergy testing can cost from $200 to $1000. Insurances will generally cover in vivo testing if there is a medical indication, but patients may still be subject to deductible charges. In addition to the patient's allergy testing costs, clinicians must consider their own costs of allergy testing. One study evaluating the cost-effectiveness of inhalant allergies found that an intradermal testing screen of 14 allergens with 6 serial dilutions and 2 controls cost a total of $159.02, with an estimated fixed cost of $6.00 [13]. Clinicians will need to purchase and store allergen extracts, testing controls, and items used for testing from antigen suppliers. Allergen extracts should be refrigerated at 2–8 °C, as changes in temperature can be detrimental to their potency in testing. One study evaluating allergen extract stability found that elevated temperatures to 40 °C for 3–6 days caused a loss of allergen content in aqueous extracts but not glycerinated extracts, and that freezing aqueous extracts can decrease potency significantly [14]. Improper storage or infrequent usage of allergen extracts can result in increased waste and decreased cost-effectiveness of allergy testing. Cost-effective care would include limiting testing panels to clinically relevant antigens and avoiding testing redundant cross-reactive species.

Where to Find Allergy Panel Information

When determining specific allergens to include in a panel, clinicians may look for resources on local prevalence of common allergens. Catalogs from antigen suppliers can provide a list of standardized extracts that can be used for testing, as well as common screening panels that are used in clinical practice in a particular region. Flora maps and pollen surveys from agricultural services and Universities may also provide information on prevalence and concentrations of allergenic pollens. For example, the American Academy of Allergy Asthma and Immunology publishes pollen and mold levels, entitled National Allergy Bureau™, on its website (https://www.aaaai.org/global/nab-pollen-counts?ipb=1). However, there are limitations to these data, as there can be significant local variations in pollen concentrations, even within a city. For example, in the city and county of Zagreb, Croatia, the northern and western regions had high sensitizations to birch pollen, while southern and eastern regions showed high sensitizations to ambrosia [15]. Publications, such as journal articles and textbooks, may provide additional information on regional variations in inhalant allergens. In 1983, Lewis et al. published a comprehensive textbook on distributions of allergenic pollen titled *Airborne and Allergenic Pollen of North America* [16]. Finally, clinicians can use pollen counters to determine current pollen concentrations and pollen trends at the locations of their practices. Some of these pollen counters can be used by patients, providing individualized exposures to potential allergens based on their daily activities.

Conclusion

Inhalant allergy testing can provide useful information to help patients avoid triggers and provide clinicians with desensitization treatment plans. The selection of allergens for testing should include a detailed history of exposures and symptoms in conjunction with relevant geographic and environmental factors which determine possible causative triggers for allergic disease. A cost-effective panel selection should involve consideration of the appropriate allergens which are representative of the environment and clinically plausible while reducing cross-reactive species.

References

1. Krouse JH, editor. Allergy and immunology: an otolaryngic approach. Lippincott Williams & Wilkins; 2002.
2. Wise SK, et al. International consensus statement on allergy and rhinology: allergic rhinitis. Int Forum Allergy Rhinol. 2018;8(2):85.
3. Miller JD. The role of dust mites in allergy. Clin Rev Allergy Immunol. 2019;57(3):312–29.
4. Arlian LG, et al. Reducing relative humidity is a practical way to control dust mites and their allergens in homes in temperate climates. J Allergy Clin Immunol. 2001;107(1):99–104.
5. Ziska L, et al. Recent warming by latitude associated with increased length of ragweed pollen season in Central North America. Proc Natl Acad Sci. 2011;108(10):4248–51.
6. Kaufman HW, Odeh MA, Bost WH, Ragothaman P. Allergies across America. Health Trends Allergy Report 2011, p 1–40.
7. Lafleur B, et al. Response of northeastern north American forests to climate change: will soil conditions constrain tree species migration? Environ Rev. 2010;18:279–89.
8. Wallace DV, et al. The diagnosis and management of rhinitis: an updated practice parameter. J Allergy Clin Immunol. 2008;122(2):S1–S84.
9. Thien FCK, et al. Indoor allergens and IgE-mediated respiratory illness. Immunol Allergy Clin N Am. 1994;14(3):567–90.
10. Knysak D. Animal aeroallergens. Immunol Allergy Clin N Am. 1989;9(2):357–64.
11. Bousquet P-J, et al. GA2LEN skin test study III: minimum battery of test inhalent allergens needed in epidemiological studies in patients. Allergy. 2009;64(11):1656–62.
12. Dreborg S, Foucard T. Allergy to apple, carrot and potato in children with birch pollen allergy. Allergy. 1983;38(3):167–72.
13. Lewis AF, Franzese C, Stringer SP. Diagnostic evaluation of inhalant allergies: a cost-effectiveness analysis. Am J Rhinol. 2008;22(3):246–52.
14. Plunkett GA, Schell M. Allergen extract stability following short term temperature variations. J Allergy Clin Immunol. 2010;125(2):AB37.
15. Toth I, et al. Micro-regional hypersensitivity variations to inhalant allergens in the city of Zagreb and Zagreb County. Coll Antropol. 2011;35(2):31–7.
16. Lewis WH, Vinay P, Zenger VE. Airborne and allergenic pollen of North America. Johns Hopkins University Press; 1983.

Allergy Skin Testing 13

Andrew Vaughn

Background

Allergy skin testing aims to elicit specific IgE-mediated responses to different allergens through an immediate wheal and flare reaction. This wheal and flare response is mediated by mast cell degranulation that occurs due to exposure to the allergen. Initial erythema occurs due to increases in vascular permeability with the progression of the erythema via a neural-related axonal response. Whealing subsequently develops due to the aggregation of transudative fluid. It is this whealing response that is measured during allergy skin testing. Within 5 min following allergen injection histamine and tryptase are released with peak responses seen at 30 min.

Aeroallergen testing can be performed via in vivo or in vitro testing (to be discussed separately). In vivo, or skin testing, can be performed with a variety of techniques including skin prick testing, intradermal dilutional testing, or a combination of the two techniques. Historically in vivo techniques have included scratch testing, but this is nearly historical as it lacks sensitivity, specificity, and is less comfortable for patient [1]. Skin testing relies on the histamine-mediated wheal and flare response. A histamine control is placed which allows for clinician determination of normal response to histamine followed by application of different antigen (via skin prick or intradermal dilutional testing) with measurement of wheal. The concentration of histamine injected does not necessarily correlate with the wheal response. With all allergic testing it should be noted that a positive response denotes allergy sensitization but does not confirm allergic disease (which should be correlated with clinical symptoms).

Skin prick testing (SPT) has a sensitivity of 85–87% and specificity of 79–86% for allergic rhinitis. In regard to allergic asthma the sensitivity of skin prick testing is possibly as high as 98% [2, 3]. SPT is usually performed either on the volar forearm or back. The forearm is more convenient for testing but less accurate than the upper back or lower back [4]. SPT is advantageous in some circumstances due to the rapidity of results, relative safety profile, and specificity of the results in showing a sensitization. Conversely, SPT is limited by its negative predictive value and starting point conversion for subcutaneous immunotherapy. In general, intradermal dilutional testing is used when clinical suspicion requires a higher degree of sensitivity than that which is seen from skin prick testing.

A. Vaughn (✉)
Lake Cumberland Medical Associates ENT, Medical Clinic in Somerset, Somerset, KY, USA

C. Damask et al. (eds.), *Allergy in Otolaryngology Practice*,
https://doi.org/10.1007/978-3-031-93455-1_13

Indications

Allergy skin testing should be considered when guided by patient history and physical examination with a reasonable suspicion of atopic disease with specific triggers. The aim of allergy testing should be to correlate sensitization to particular aeroallergens and these patient symptoms. This can aid in the diagnosis of specific allergies and for initiation of immunotherapy.

Preparation

There are several classes of medications that will affect the normal wheal and flare response required for accurate allergy skin testing. A thorough medication reconciliation should occur prior to allergy skin testing and counseling should occur before planned skin testing (Table 13.1).

Antihistamines

The most commonly used medications in the atopic patients are antihistamines. Additionally, certain antihistamines may be used for non-allergic issues including as sleep aids (Diphenhydramine, commonly) and anxiolysis (Hydroxyzine) Antihistamines are also responsible for the most inaccurate results of skin testing. Antihistamines act to stabilize H1 receptors (termed inverse agonism) of mast cells preventing histamine release and normal wheal and flare response [5]. This inverse agonism generally fades by 72 h of last administration and conventional recommendation is to hold these medications for at least this long prior to skin testing. A more conservative approach would be to discontinue 1 week prior to testing (particularly with Loratadine). A blunted response from antihistamines should be suspected by a lack of skin reactivity to a histamine control. A lack of reactivity to this control should warrant further inquiry into recent medication use, additional counseling, and delay of skin testing. Antihistamines may also be applied topically, either via spray to the nasal mucosa (Azelastine, Olopatadine) or as an ophthalmic preparation (Levocabastine Ophthalmic, Olopatadine ophthalmic). Intranasal antihistamines are felt to have a similar effect as oral antihistamines and should be discontinued 72 h prior to skin testing, although this is debated [4, 6]. Ophthalmic preparations are felt to have little effect on wheal and flare response and do not require discontinuation [6].

Table 13.1 When to stop selected medication classes prior to allergy skin testing

Medication	When to discontinue
First-generation antihistamine (H1)	3 days
Second-generation antihistamine (H1)	3–7 days
H2 blockers	2 days
Intranasal antihistamines	3 days
Ophthalmic antihistamines	Discontinuation unnecessary
Tricyclic antidepressants	7 days
Leukotriene antagonists	Discontinuation unnecessary
Beta-blockers	5 days
Omalizumab (anti-IgE)	4–6 months
Oral and intranasal corticosteroids	Discontinuation unnecessary
Benzodiazapines	7 days
SSRIs/SNRIs	Discontinuation unnecessary

Beta2-Receptor Antagonists

Beta-blockers (Propranolol, Metoprolol, Atenolol, among others) may enhance whealing response by decreasing intracellular cyclic AMP (cAMP) which lowers the threshold for mast cell and basophil degranulation [7, 8]. This effect is often minimal but more importantly, beta-blockers lead to increased difficulty in the treatment of anaphylaxis and systemic reactions to testing. Epinephrine is first-line therapy for anaphylactic reactions and has a mechanism of action by acting on smooth muscle beta receptors, both in bronchioles and arterioles leading to vasoconstriction and bronchodilation to increase mean arterial pressure and improve respiration. Should a practitioner find themselves in an unfortunate circumstance of severe systemic reaction in a patient taking a beta antagonist, Glucagon has been shown effective in these circumstances in raising mean arterial blood pressures through strong inotropism [9]. Concurrent beta-blocker use is a relative contraindication for skin testing and should be stopped 5 days prior to testing. If the patient is unable to discontinue for testing and should warrant strong consideration for in vivo testing [10]. H2 antihistamines (Cimetidine, Famotidine, Ranitidine) have been shown to have a more modest suppression of skin reactivity. These are recommended be stopped 2 days prior to testing [11–13]. Proton pump inhibitors (PPIs) do not require cessation prior to skin testing [14].

Antidepressants/Anti-psychotics/Benzodiazepines

Tricyclic antidepressants (Amitriptyline, Nortriptyline, Doxepin) are a class of medications used to treat depression, migraines, and less commonly, urticaria. These medications have known antihistamine and anti-muscarinic properties and were originally developed for this use. Studies have shown blunting of wheal and flare response for several days, to both SPT and IDT, after the last administration of TCAs and the current recommendation is avoidance for 7 days prior to skin testing [15]. This same recommendation applies to Tetracyclic antidepressants (Mirtazapine), which have effect on whealing response. Quetiapine is an atypical antipsychotic that is also commonly used as a sleep aid. This medication has significant antihistamine properties and has been shown to suppress histamine controls in a majority of patients. This effect tends to disappear after about 5 days [14]. Benzodiapines (Clonazepam, Diazampam, Alaprazolam) may affect skin testing and should be discontinued 1 week prior to testing [14].

Corticosteroids. Oral corticosteroids have been shown to have no effect on skin testing [16, 17]. Intranasal corticosteroids have very low levels of systemic absorption and can also be assumed to not effect wheal and flare response during allergy skin testing [18]. However, prolonged topical steroids do reduce skin test responses in the affected area [19]. Therefore, patients should be counseled to avoid the use of topical corticosteroids in the desired skin prick testing area.

Biologics. Omalizumab is humanized monoclonal anti-IgE antibody. It currently holds FDA approval for the treatment of allergic asthma, poorly controlled despite inhaled corticosteroids. Administration of Omalizumab results in a rapid decrease in serum-free IgE levels that blunts allergic response. Allergen-specific IgE remains intact, leaving in vitro testing options as a viable option. Multiple studies have shown Omalizumab blunts the response to skin prick testing for up to 1 year, but testing may be performed 6 weeks following last administration [20, 21].

Leukotriene receptor antagonists [22, 23] (Montelukast), mast cell stabilizers [24] (Cromolyn sodium), inhaled beta 2 agonists [25], selective serotonin reuptake inhibitors (SSRIs), and selective norepinephrine reuptake inhibitors (SNRIs) [14] are safe to continue through skin testing and also present no challenges to the normal wheal and flare response.

Special consideration should be paid to food and inhalant allergy cross reactivity as this can enhance the whealing response. This is based on the observation that certain food and inhalant allergens share similar epitopes [26] (Table 13.2). It has also been noted that skin reactivity displays seasonality. A "priming" of circulating IgE is thought to occur when aeroallergens are "in season" that can result in exaggerated responses dur-

Table 13.2 Common cross-reacting food and aeroallergens

Inhalant allergen	Food allergen
Birch (Bet v1)	Apple, cherry, apricot, pear, peach, plum, almond, hazelnut, mango, kiwi, strawberry
Birch (Bet v2)	Cherry, pear
Mugwort	Mango
Latex	Avocado, Banana, kiwi, chestnut
Dust mite	Crustaceans
Cat	Pork meat
Grass	Melon, watermelon, kiwi, orange
Ragweed	Melon, watermelon, cantaloupe, banana

ing testing [27]. The age of the patient should also be considered when interpreting whealing responses. Pediatric (particularly <2 years of age) patients tend to be less reactive to skin challenges. This is thought to be related to lower concentrations of cutaneous mast cells and lower cumulative exposure to allergens [28]. Elderly patients may also be less reactive and have less suitable skin surface available for testing related to degenerative and actinic changes.

Contraindications

Dermatographism

In some patients the physical action of intradermal needle placement or skin prick can produce a wheal and flare response. This condition is referred to as dermatographism meaning literally "to write on skin." It is the most common physical urticarial that effects approximately 5% of the atopic population and has a prevalence of 1.5% of the total population. Incidence tends to peak in the second and third decades of life. Presence of dermatographism precludes allergy skin testing as a whealing response is expected from the act of touching the skin with a needle [29].

Uncontrolled Asthma

Asthma is a nearly ubiquitous finding in patients who have suffered fatal reactions to both allergy skin testing and immunotherapy administration. A majority of these patients were poorly controlled with FEV1 less than 70% of its predicted value [4]. Poor asthma control should warrant consideration of in vitro testing.

Atopic Dermatitis

Atopic dermatitis, or eczema, is a chronic cutaneous manifestation of atopy, characterized by pruritic, erythematous, raised lesions that tend to occur on the face, neck, arms, and legs. Active atopic dermatitis limits area where skin tests may be applied, and in vitro testing should be considered if adequate area is not available.

Office Setup

Allergy testing and immunotherapy administration requires a fair amount of space and equipment. Treatment areas should have adequate area for counterspace, refrigeration, a sink, and a table or chair for patient testing. This is possible in most existing Otolaryngology exam rooms, provided they are equipped with a sink. Most practices have a separate mixing area for treatment vials as there are very specific requirements, which are outlined in USP 797, regarding compounding of allergy concentrate in office.

Equipment

Stock solutions of allergy extract (1:20 weight to volume) should be obtained specific to your region. These should include a seasonal profile of allergens that cover the major allergens the patient would be exposed to. Perennial allergen concentrates should also be part of the testing armamentarium. Concentrates should be refrigerated (2–8 degrees Celsius) to maintain potency with daily checks to ensure this process.

Several different types of syringes are needed for injection and mixing. These are commercially available with needle pre-attached to syringe to minimize dead space and subsequent wasting of costly concentrate solution. Mixing syringes are typically larger bore than the other types used (23 gauge with 1/2″ needle). Intradermal testing needles are generally 27 gauge with a short 3/8″ needle and a short bevel. The needles used for administration of immunotherapy are typically 26 gauge with 1/2″ needle with a long bevel. Sterile vials for mixing patient treatment vials are necessary to hold concentrate for testing. These are available both as an empty vial or prefilled with a diluent (either glycerin or phenolated normal saline). Diluents available include normal

Table 13.3 Suggested anaphylaxis supplies

Sphymomanometer
Oxygen
Bag-valve mask
Laryngoscope, endotracheal tubes
IV fluids, tubing
ACLS medications
Epinephrine (ampule or auto-injectable)
Automatic electronic defibrillator (AED)
Antihistamines
Corticosteroids
Inhalers/nebulizers

saline, serum albumin, phenolated normal saline (most common), or glycerin. Normal saline is rarely used due to lack of preservative properties limiting shelf life. For skin testing, the concentrates are usually organized on a treatment board to facilitate testing in a methodical fashion. These treatment boards are usually acrylic or plastic and arranged with wells (6 × 10) to hold vials for a five-fold dilution.

Peak flow testing may be useful in monitoring a patient's respiratory status before skin testing and immunotherapy administration.

Severe systemic response supplies. Basic medical supplies should be available in office for dealing with anaphylactic emergencies that may arise during skin testing (see Table 13.3). This may be organized into a crash cart. Commercial options with supplies are available with premade anaphylaxis kits and subscription services for expiring medications.

Personnel

It is important to understand that regulations vary from state to state regarding who may perform skin prick testing. Overall however, the Physician provides direct supervision of the testing and should remain in the office while testing is being performed in order to manage emergencies. Adequate training should be provided to staff on safe administration and management of emergencies. Training courses exist for office staff on the administration of skin testing and administration of immunotherapy.

References

1. Seidman MD, Gurgel RK, Lin SY, Schwartz SR, Baroody FM, et al. Clinical practice guideline: allergic rhinitis. Otolaryngol Head Neck Surg. 2014;151
2. Gungor A, Houser SM, Aquino BF, Akbar I, Moinuddin R, Mamikoglu B, et al. A comparison of skin endpoint titration and skin-prick testing in the diagnosis of allergic rhinitis. Ear Nose Throat J. 2004;83(1):54–60.
3. Krouse JH, Sadrazodi K, Kerswill K. Sensitivity and specificity of prick and intradermal testing in predicting response to nasal provocation with timothy grass antigen. Otolaryngol Head Neck Surg. 2004;131(3):215–9.
4. Bernstein DI, Wanner M, Borish L, Liss GM. Twelve-year survey of fatal reactions to allergen injections and skin testing: 1990-2001. J Allergy Clin Immunol. 2004;113(6):1129–36.
5. Leurs R, Church MK, Taglialatela M. H1-antihistamines: inverse agonism, anti-inflammatory actions and cardiac effects. Clin Exp Allergy. 2002 Apr;32(4):489–98.
6. Agarwal MK, Vijayan VK, Vermani M. Effect of azelastine nasal spray on histamine- and allergen-induced skin wheal response in patients with allergic rhinitis. J Asthma. 2008;45(7):548–51.
7. Mark Duffy S, Cruse G, Lawley WJ, Bradding P. B 2 -Adrenoceptor regulation of the K + channel iK Ca 1 in human mast cells. FASEB J. 2005;19(8):1006–8.
8. Coop CA, Schapira RS, Freeman TM. Are ACE inhibitors and Beta-blockers dangerous in patients at risk for anaphylaxis? J Allergy Clin Immunol Pract. 2017;5(5):1207–11. https://doi.org/10.1016/j.jaip.2017.04.033.
9. Zaloga G, Delacey W, Holmboe E, Chernow B. Glucagon and anaphylaxis. Ann Intern Med. 1986;105(1):65–6.
10. Lieberman P, Nicklas RA, Randolph C, Oppenheimer J, Bernstein D, Bernstein J, et al. Anaphylaxis – a practice parameter update 2015. Ann Allergy Asthma Immunol. 2015;115(5):341–84. https://doi.org/10.1016/j.anai.2015.07.019.
11. Cohen SH, Kagen SL. Cimetidine and allergy skin testing. Ann Intern Med. 1982;96(6):787.
12. Miller J, Nelson HS. Suppression of immediate skin tests by ranitidine. J Allergy Clin Immunol. 1989;84(6 PART 1):895–9.
13. Kupczyk M, Kupryś I, Bocheńska-Marciniak M, Górski P, Kuna P. Ranitidine (150 mg daily) inhibits wheal, flare, and itching reactions in skin-prick tests. Allergy Asthma Proc. 2007;28(6):711–5.
14. Shah KM, Rank MA, Davé SA, Oslie CL, Butterfield JH. Predicting which medication classes interfere with allergy skin testing. Allergy Asthma Proc. 2010;31(6):477–82.
15. Karnineni Rao MD, Prem Menon MD, Bettina Hilman MD, et al. Duration of the suppressive effect of tricyclic antidepressants on histamine-induced

wheal-and-flare reactions in human skin. J Allergy Clin Immunol. 1988;82(5):752–7.
16. Lopez-Campos C, Rincon-Castaneda CB, Cano-Rios P, Martinez-Ordaz VA, Velasco-Rodriguez VM. Is the histamine skin test inhibited by prednisone? Arch Med Res. 1998;29(1):63–5.
17. Slott RI, Zweiman B. A controlled study of the effect of corticosteroids on immediate skin test reactivity. J Allergy Clin Immunol. 1973;54:4.
18. Demoly P. Safety of intranasal corticosteroids in acute rhinosinusitis. Am J Otolaryngol Head Neck Med Surg. 2008;29(6):403–13.
19. Andersson M, Pipkorn U. Inhibition of the dermal immediate allergic reaction through prolonged treatment with topical glucocorticosteroids. J Allergy Clin Immunol. 1987;79(2):345–9.
20. Ong YE, Menzies-Gow A, Barkans J, Benyahia F, Ou TT, Ying S, et al. Anti-IgE (omalizumab) inhibits late-phase reactions and inflammatory cells after repeat skin allergen challenge. J Allergy Clin Immunol. 2005;116(3):558–64.
21. Corren J, Shapiro G, Reimann J, Deniz Y, Wong D, Adelman D, et al. Allergen skin tests and free IgE levels during reduction and cessation of omalizumab therapy. J Allergy Clin Immunol. 2008;121(2):506–11.
22. Hill SL, Krouse JH. The effects of montelukast on intradermal wheal and flare. Otolaryngol Head Neck Surg. 2003;129(3):199–203.
23. Simons FER, Johnston L, Gu X, Simons KJ. Suppression of the early and late cutaneous allergic responses using fexofenadine and montelukast. Ann Allergy Asthma Immunol. 2001;86(1):44–50. https://doi.org/10.1016/S1081-1206(10)62354-X.
24. Ting S, Zweiman B, Lavker RM. Cromolyn does not modulate human allergic skin reactions in vivo. J Allergy Clin Immunol. 1983;71(1 PART):12–7.
25. Spector SL. Effect of a selective beta2 adrenergic agonist and theophylline on skin test reactivity and cardiovascular parameters. J Allergy Clin Immunol. 1979;64(1):23–8.
26. Faber MA, van Gasse AL, Decuyper II, Sabato V, Hagendorens MM, Mertens C, et al. Cross-reactive aeroallergens: which need to cross our mind in food allergy diagnosis? J Allergy Clin Immunol Pract. 2018;6(6):1813–23. https://doi.org/10.1016/j.jaip.2018.08.010.
27. Choi IS, Lee SS, Myeong E, Lee JW, Kim WJ, Jin J. Seasonal variation in skin sensitivity to aeroallergens. Allergy Asthma Immunol Res. 2013;5(5):301–8.
28. Bock S. Diagnostic Evaluation. Pediatrics. 2003;111(6):1638–44.
29. Bhute D, Doshi B, Pande S, Mahajan S, Kharkar V. Dermatographism. Indian J Dermatol Venereol Leprol. 2008;74:177.

Skin Prick, Intradermal, and Blended Techniques

14

Duncan C. Watley and Farrah N. Siddiqui

History of Skin Testing

Introducing allergens into the skin has been utilized for the past 150 years to identify the source of environmental allergy. Blackley first performed skin scratch testing in 1872, in which he abraded his own arm with a needle, applied grass pollen to the area, and covered the wound with a bandage. This resulted in intense local inflammation and is thought to represent the first scientifically based allergy test [1]. In 1908 Koch and von Pirquet introduced the tuberculin skin test which paved the way for Cooke to develop the first intradermal allergen skin testing in 1915 [2, 3]. In this seminal work published in the early "Laryngoscope", Dr. Cooke identified the wheal and flare reactions caused by intradermally injecting prepared pollen extracts. He also correctly identified polysensitization in patient's suffering from Hay Fever. Work on skin testing continued throughout the early 1900s, including recognition of the wheal and flare reaction with skin prick by Sir Thomas Lewis in 1926 [4]. Dr. Jack Pepys popularized skin prick testing for the diagnosis of allergen sensitization in the 1970s [5].

D. C. Watley (✉) · F. N. Siddiqui
Department of Otolaryngology, The University of Texas Medical Branch, Galveston, TX, USA
e-mail: fnsiddiq@utmb.edu

Pathophysiology of Inhalant Allergy and Mechanics of Skin Testing

The Th2 adaptive immune system, through the production of IgE, forms the basis of atopy. Dendritic cells in the nasal epithelium capture allergens, leading to differentiation of Th2 cells [2, 6]. These Th2 cells secrete IL-4, IL-5, and IL-13, thus encouraging B cells to produce IgE [6–9]. IgE interacts with mast cells and basophils in the nasal epithelium, leading to degranulation and release of histamine, resulting in rhinorrhea, congestion, and itching [9]. This IgE-mediated response translates as a visible reaction on the skin, thus forming the basis behind skin testing [9]. Antigen presenting Langerhans cells process aeroallergens, resulting in production of specific IgE, followed by degranulation of mast cells and basophils. The release of histamine leads to a wheal and flare which can then be measured during skin prick (SPT), intradermal testing, and modified quantitative testing (MQT).

Skin Prick Testing (SPT)

Skin prick testing has been the primary means for diagnosing aeroallergen sensitization for the past 100 years [10]. The procedure involves applying a small amount of antigen solution to either the

C. Damask et al. (eds.), *Allergy in Otolaryngology Practice*,
https://doi.org/10.1007/978-3-031-93455-1_14

skin or the end of a sharp applicating device and puncturing the epidermis. After 20 minutes, the test is interpreted based on the classic wheal and flare of local histamine release in the skin. SPT is performed either using a single antigen applying device or multiple-prick device. Single-prick devices can be used in two ways. In the first method, antigen solution is first applied to the skin with a dropper or syringe and then the prick device, often a Burrow's needle, is then utilized to superficially puncture the epidermis through the solution. Alternatively, the device can be dipped into the allergen extract first, then used to prick the skin. Examples of single-prick devices include: Burrow's needle, Greer® Pick® (Stallergenes-Greer), Duotip-Test® II (Lincoln Diagnostics, Inc.) (Fig. 14.1). Multi-prick devices allow the application of up to 10 different antigens at once, spaced far enough from one another to allow for easy interpretation of results. Examples of multi-prick devices include: Skintestor OMNI™ (Stallergenes-Greer), Multi-Test® II (Lincoln Diagnostics, Inc.), ComforTen® (Hollister-Stier Laboratories), and Quintest® (Hollister-Stier Laboratories) (Fig. 14.2). Both single-prick and multi-prick testing devices are available in generic versions. Single-prick devices can be utilized to confirm controls prior to starting testing or to confirm a few allergen sensitivities. Larger testing panels are more efficiently done and technically more reproducible through multi-prick testing.

Skin Prick Testing Controls

Prior to initiation of skin testing, positive and negative controls are applied to the skin to ensure the results of testing will be representative of true responses. The positive control used is full-strength histamine dihydrochloride (6 mg/mL) or histamine phosphate (1 mg/ml), which is applied using either a single or multi-prick device [10]. A normal positive control test results in the classic wheal and flare response. Individual patient's skin can be variably responsive to testing and some patients may display false positive results to testing. The classic example of this is the dermatographic patient in which even minor trauma to the skin will result in large wheal and flare reactions (Fig. 14.3). To differentiate false positive from true positive results, a negative control is also placed with each allergy test. 50% glycerin in normal saline is utilized for the negative control. A normal negative control result will not cause a large wheal and flare response. A smaller

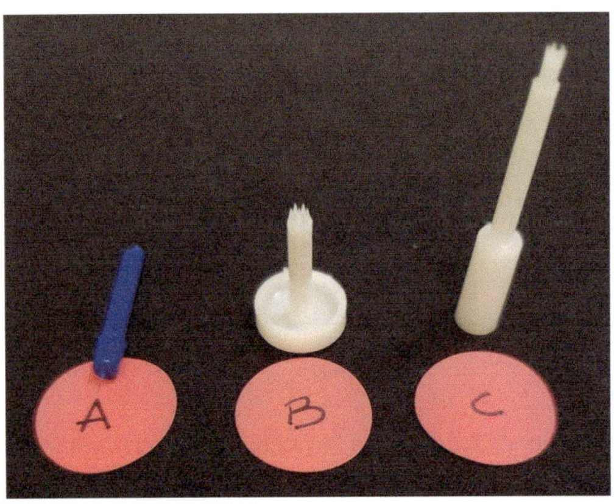

Fig. 14.1 Single-prick applicators from 3 different manufacturers

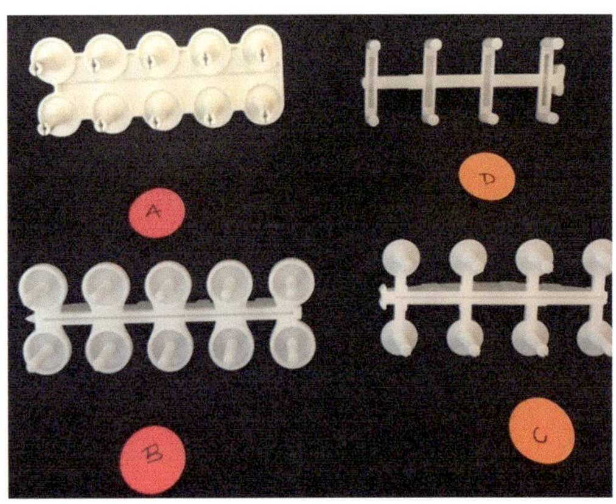

Fig. 14.2 Multi-prick applicators from 4 different manufacturers

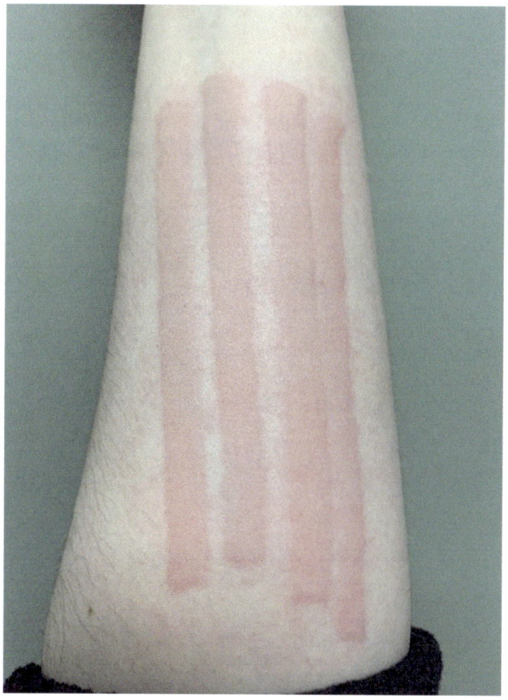

Fig. 14.3 Classic dermatographic response to mechanical trauma

wheal may form due to local skin trauma, but this negative control wheal should be at least 3 mm smaller than the histamine wheal for the test to be validated.

Body Surface Selection

Skin testing can be performed on various surfaces of the body including the volar surface of the forearm, anterior thigh, and the upper back. Testing on the forearm for children is technically more challenging due to decreased surface area, and thus the upper back or anterior thigh is usually selected. Some evidence exists for decreased skin sensitivity in the pediatric and geriatric populations [11, 12]. This is thought to be due to proportional reduction in capillary and mast cell density with skin thickness decline [13, 14]. Testing on these populations is theoretically more accurate on areas of the body with thicker skin such as the upper back or thigh. The overall sensitivity and specificity of skin prick testing positivity with clinical symptoms of allergy is approximately 80% [2, 15, 16].

Patient Instructions Prior to Testing

Many medications and medical conditions can alter the efficacy or safety of allergy skin testing. A thorough discussion on this topic can be found in. Specifically, allergy skin testing is contraindicated in pregnant women, patients taking a beta-blocker, severe cardiopulmonary disease, active urticaria at test sites, and in poorly controlled asthmatics [17]. We advise patients to continue their asthma inhalers surrounding testing, and to avoid testing in an active asthma flare. Additionally, many medications need to be stopped prior to testing (Table 14.1). If appropriate, patients can be provided with instructions on how to apply topical anesthetic cream to the skin along with a prescription for the medication.

Multi-Prick SPT Technique

1. Gather equipment/supplies including the following:
   (a) Stock allergens (concentrate in 50% glycerin).
   (b) Controls (histamine & glycerin).
   (c) Applicator device (8 vs. 10 test devices).

Table 14.1 Common medications that may affect skin testing

Medication	Timeline of discontinuation prior to skin testing
Oral H1 blockers	7–10 days
Tricyclic antidepressants	14 days
Intranasal H1 blockers	2–3 days
Ocular antihistamines	1–2 days
Topical steroids/topical tacrolimus (on skin testing site)	3–4 weeks
Omalizumab	6 months
Benzodiazepines **controversial**	7 days
Oral H2 blockers **controversial**	3 days

   (d) Skin wheal measuring device, skin marker.
   (e) Forms to record results, timer.
   (f) Alcohol pads.
   (g) Personal protective equipment including gloves, gown, mask, goggles.
   (h) Anaphylaxis/emergency kit.
2. Optional: 1 h prior to patient coming to clinic for testing have them apply local anesthetic (EMLA or similar) cream to the volar surface of the forearms as well as the upper arms.
3. Clean the area with alcohol and allow to dry.
4. Mark the skin with washable pen: Identify each 8 or 10 test battery with A, B, C, D, etc. Make sure to space these apart by 2 cm. Within each battery, number the tests appropriately to indicate the location of each puncture. Utilize a standardized approach to marking sites such as: the #1 test is in the 1 o'clock position with the following numbers recorded in a clockwise fashion.
5. Take the multi-prick device from the antigen well and firmly apply to skin with corresponding numbered boxes. The test should be firm enough to cause mild discomfort but should not pierce the skin to cause bleeding. If done properly, the impression of the tip of the skin prick device will be visible on the skin. A small amount of residual antigen will likely remain following removal of the multi-test. Do not wash this away, and do not allow the patient to move the arm to avoid cross-contamination.
6. Evaluate the wheal and flare response to each test after 20 min (Fig. 14.4). The most accurate way to measure each individual test is to use an objective measuring aid and record the diameter of each wheal in mm. The wheal is specifically the raised portion of the skin response which should be differentiated from the flare, which is the erythematous discoloration of surrounding skin. Palpating the wheal helps in the evaluation along with the actual visual inspection. Occasionally, small areas of raised skin will radiate from the main wheal, called pseudopods. Their dimension should be included in the measurement of the wheal. Mark your results clearly in a table, either directly in the electronic medical record or in written form, including control and test results of wheals measured in mm.

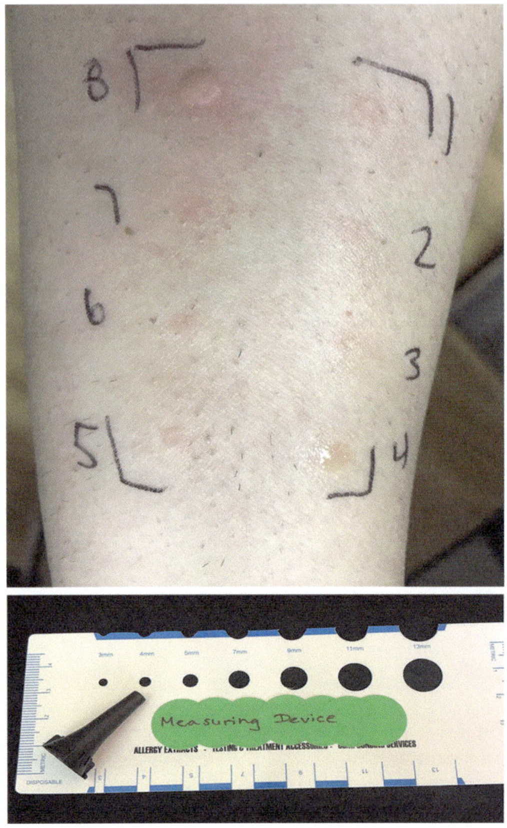

Fig. 14.4 Top: Multi-prick testing numbered in clockwise fashion with #8 showing positive result with wheal size of 7 mm, while the rest are all negative. Bottom: Wheal measuring device alongside 4 mm otoscope speculum

Intradermal Skin Testing

Direct injection of antigen into the dermis of the skin can be used by the otolaryngologic allergist to not only diagnose allergic sensitization to a wide variety of antigens, but can also be injected in a series of dilutions to approximate a starting concentration for immunotherapy. The technique involves utilizing a short beveled needle to inject both positive and negative control solution, as well as antigen into the dermis creating a mechanical wheal. Approximately 0.01 to .05 mL of solution is injected creating a 4 mm wheal. This wheal is reexamined and measured following a 10-min waiting period. This waiting period is critical to ensure that an IgE-mediated wheal and flare reaction has enough time to occur, thus decreasing risk of false negative results. The skin surface selected is generally the volar forearm, with option for the upper arm and back.

A negative testing result is indicated if the wheal fails to grow larger than 5 mm. The initial 4 mm wheal grows slightly during the 10-min waiting period through diffusion of solution through surrounding dermis to a size of 5 mm. A positive testing result is indicated if the wheal grows to a size larger than which would be typically expected from simple diffusion of the solution. A 2 mm growth, or a wheal size of 7 mm represents a positive testing result.

Intradermal Testing Controls

Controls are used to ensure testing results represent true sensitization. Histamine base 0.1 mg/mL is used as the positive control [18]. The normal skin response to a positive control is a growth of the wheal by 2 mm, so it should grow from 5 mm to at least 7 mm.

Two negative controls are used to reduce the risk of false positive results. Phenolated normal saline (PNS) is used as the test antigens are preserved in this. A second glycerin (#2 dilution from 50% glycerin stock) control is also utilized since this is the preservative used in the concentrate extracts as well as in the subcutaneous immunotherapy treatment vials. The normal skin response to a negative control is no growth of the 5 mm wheal. Patients may have sensitivity to glycerin which can be suspected after repeated positive wheals to the glycerin control. Patients with whealing responses to negative controls are poor candidates for skin testing and should undergo in vitro testing.

Single Intradermal Testing

A single intradermal test can be utilized to confirm sensitivity to an allergen after skin prick testing and is useful in medication and venom allergy practice. It can also be used as part of a blended technique, known as modified quantitative testing (MQT).

Single Intradermal Testing Technique

1. Clean the skin surface either on the volar forearm, upper arm, or upper back with an alcohol swab.
2. Use a washable marker to mark controls and allergens to be tested and space these at least 2 cm apart.
3. Draw up 0.01–05 mL of the prepared solution into an allergy testing syringe. Tense the skin with the non-dominant hand and while keeping the syringe and needle mostly parallel to the skin. Shallowly inject the solution into the dermis creating a 4 mm wheal. It is helpful to have the bevel pointed downward to fully insert the bevel into the skin using the shortest distance but many will perform this in the bevel up position as well. Additionally, the bevel down technique provides the operator increased levels of occupational safety and will not lead to inadvertent spraying of solution into the eyes [18]. If injected solution spills from the injection site while pressing the syringe plunger the needle bevel was likely not completely within the skin. This is not harmful, continue advancing the needle until it is completely covered and continue plunging the syringe to create a 4 mm wheal. Measure the wheal to ensure it is the correct size with the pre-made wheal sizing tool. Creating an exact 4 mm wheal is challenging

and often takes practice to perfect. When first learning to perform this skill, it is helpful to use a 4 mm ear speculum to indent the skin where you will place the injection to give yourself a guide (section "Intradermal skin testing"). If the wheal disappears during the 10-min waiting period, the injection was likely into the subcutaneous layers of the skin instead of the dermis.

4. Wait 10 min then measure and record the wheal size using a measuring device. Mark your results clearly in a table either in directly in the electronic medical record or in written form, included control and test results in mm.

Intradermal Dilutional Testing (IDT)

This skin testing method utilizes a series of intradermal tests at increasing five-fold dilutions to identify a whealing endpoint for a given antigen which can then be used as a safe starting dose for subcutaneous immunotherapy [19, 20]. This process uses a 1:5 dilutional series, injecting from weakest (dilution #6) to strongest (generally stops at dilution #2). The endpoint is the first positive (7 mm or greater) wheal that is followed by a confirmatory wheal of the next stronger dilution that grows at least 2 mm larger (Fig. 14.7). In the occasion that the next stronger dilution produces the same size of wheal or a wheal <2 mm larger testing continues until a higher concentration results in a wheal 2 mm larger. It is common for the confirmatory wheal to grow by 3–4 mm. A complete normal series could include wheals of 5 mm, 8 mm, 10 mm, in which the 8 mm wheal represents the endpoint.

Otolaryngologic allergists first create a testing board made up of five-fold dilutions, with #1 being a five-fold dilution of the concentrate and #6 being the weakest dilution. These dilutions are created in phenolated saline thus are not as well-preserved as glycerin-containing extracts. This testing board needs to be replenished every 6 weeks to maintain antigen integrity.

IDT Testing Board Technique: Five-Fold Dilution

1. Clean the top of all vials with alcohol swabs and let dry prior to creating dilutions.
2. For the 1:5 dilution method, prefill the vials accordingly with 4 mL of PNS.
3. Draw up 1 mL of concentrated antigen, which is designated 1:20 weight per volume (w/v) using the 1 mL syringe and inject into the 5 mL prefilled vial, creating a 1:5 dilution. Gently pull up and plunge the mixture multiple times in the syringe and push it back into the vial to make sure it is well mixed. Label this vial for that antigen with the designator dilution #1.
4. Repeat step 3 for the next dilution using 1 ml of the #1 dilution and place it into the next prefilled vial, again mixing it well. This vial will be labeled dilution #2.
5. Continue this process by placing 1 ml of the newly created dilution into the prefilled 4 ml of PNS, so that dilutions #3, #4, #5 and #6 are incrementally created (Fig. 14.5).
6. Place the testing board in the refrigerator set at 2–8 degrees Celsius for optimal storage and to preserve antigens. Unlike skin prick testing allergens which are preserved in 50% glycerin, the IDT testing board needs to be replenished every 6–8 weeks.

IDT Technique

1. Equipment/supplies:
   (a) A series of syringe and needle combination with intradermal style needle bevel.
   (b) Gloves, washable skin marker, paper recording sheet or EMR recording sheet, alcohol swabs.
   (c) Positive control: histamine base.
   (d) Phenolated saline negative control.
   (e) Glycerin negative control.
   (f) Testing board (see section "IDT testing board technique: Five-fold dilution").

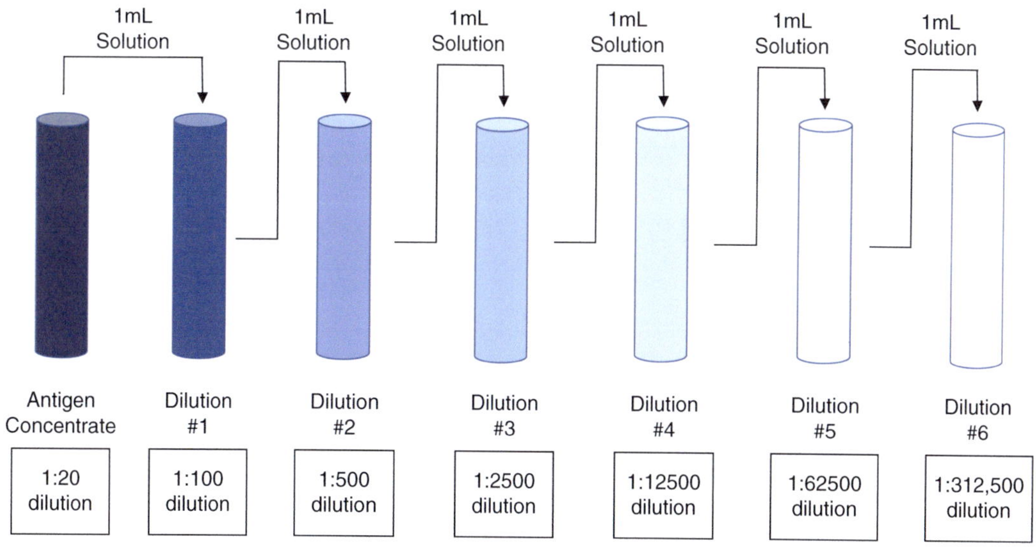

Fig. 14.5 Dilution series

(g) Wheal measuring device.
(h) Anaphylaxis emergency supplies described in another chapter.

2. This technique is best done on the upper arm for ease of injection, patient comfort, and also space to inject many dilutions. Clean the skin surface of the upper arm with an alcohol swab.
3. Use a washable marker to clearly mark controls, then in a grid fashion, mark all test allergens in the y axis and the dilutions starting from #6 decreasing to #2 in the horizontal x axis with each test spaced 2 cm apart (see Fig. 14.6).
4. Perform series of intradermal tests for the three controls (as described in section "Intradermal testing controls") and then each allergen (as described in section "Intradermal dilutional testing (IDT)"). The allergens are tested beginning from the weakest dilution (#6) and after measuring these results in 10 minutes, then the next stronger dilution (#5) is applied.
5. Continue applying the dilutional series in this fashion until you have seen a positive wheal followed by a confirmatory wheal. A positive wheal grows by 2 mm and the confirmatory wheal then grows by another 2 mm at the next stronger dilution (see Fig. 14.7 for special considerations).
6. To improve patient comfort and test efficiency, clinical practice varies with this technique in the hands of an experienced operator. In non-brittle patients, some physicians may choose to start with a stronger concentration (starting with #5 or #4), some may inject multiple concentrations at once (placing #6 and

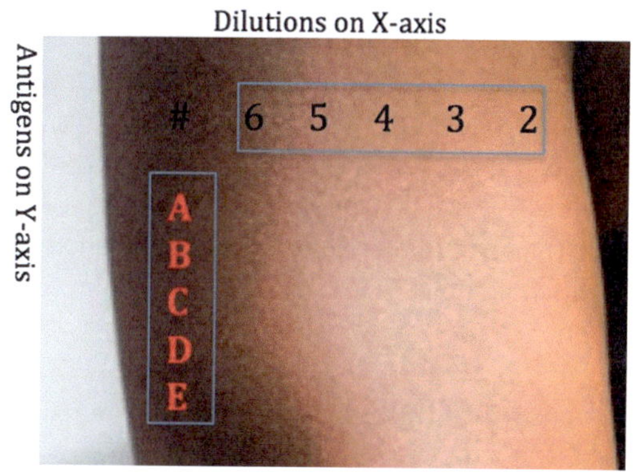

Fig. 14.6 IDT grid. X axis: indicates decreasing dilution number (weakest dilution to most concentrated solution). Y axis: different antigens labeled A through E

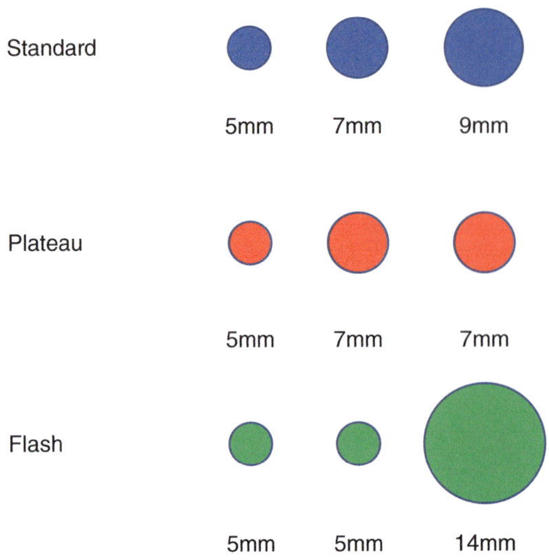

Fig. 14.7 Abnormal wheel responses

#5), while others may inject every other concentration (placing #6, #4, #2) then extrapolating results.

7. Mark your results clearly in a table either directly in the electronic medical record or in written form, including both control and test results in mm.

Abnormal Whealing Phenomena in IDT

A "plateau phenomenon" infrequently occurs where there is a positive wheal at low concentration but all stronger concentrations applied to produce a confirmatory wheal result in the same size. The endpoint in this situation is the first positive wheal (Fig. 14.7).

A "flash phenomenon" is an abnormal result in which the wheal of the next larger concentration grows much larger than expected (Fig. 14.7). If this occurs, no endpoint can be calculated for this particular antigen and testing will need to be repeated during a second session 4–7 days later. Testing for other antigens, however, can continue [18].

Modified Quantitative Technique (MQT)

MQT blends intradermal and skin prick allergy testing to efficiently determine an endpoint for specific antigens. This process marries the time efficiency of skin prick testing with the sensitivity of intradermal testing to establish a safe starting concentration of antigen for subcutaneous immunotherapy [21]. SPT is first performed, and wheal responses are evaluated at 20 minutes. SPT wheals of 9 mm or larger are automatically assigned endpoint #6 while wheals that are 2 mm or smaller are evaluated by #2 single intradermal test. SPT wheals of 3–8 mm are followed by #5 single intradermal test to establish the final endpoint (Fig. 14.8). The skin testing controls are the same as previously described in the skin prick and intradermal skin testing sections of this chapter.

1. Repeat steps 1–4 in the SPT Instruction section of this chapter for the various antigens you plan to test.
2. Wait 20 min for the wheals to form and record their diameter.
3. Place intradermal dilutions of the antigens being tested as follows:
   (a) SPT wheal <3 mm place a #2 intradermal dilution.
   (b) SPT wheal 3-8 mm place a #5 intradermal dilution.
   (c) SPT wheal ≥9 mm the automatic endpoint is a #6 dilution which represents the starting concentration for immunotherapy, alternatively a #6 dilution could be placed to confirm the endpoint.
4. If a #2 IDT dilution was placed continue as follows:
   (a) If the wheal is ≥7 mm then an endpoint of #3 is assigned.
   (b) If the wheal is ≤6 mm it is a negative test.
5. If a #5 IDT dilution was placed continue as follows:
   (a) If the wheal ≤6 mm the endpoint is #4.

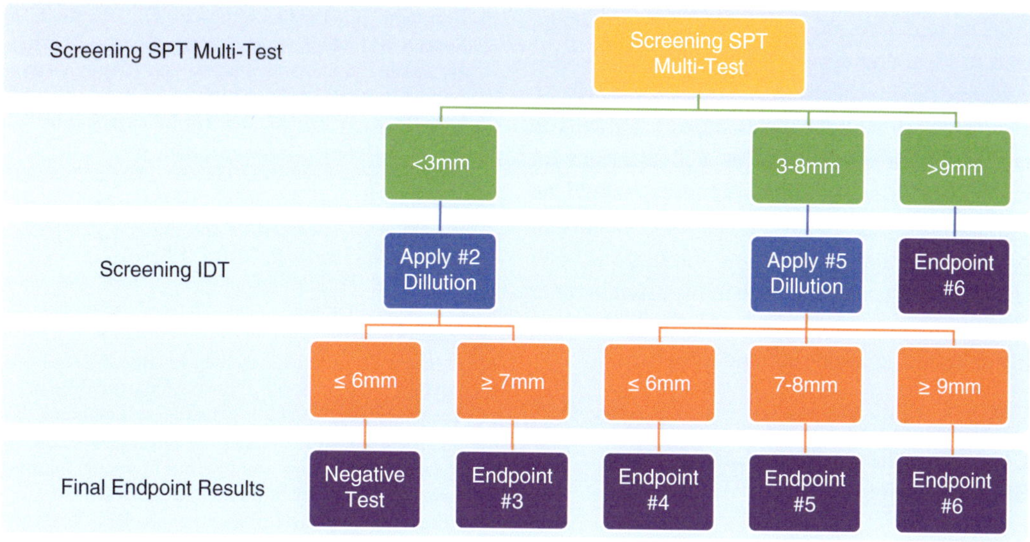

Fig. 14.8 Modified quantitative testing (MQT) algorithm

  (b) If the wheal is 7–8 mm the endpoint is #5.
  (c) If the wheal is ≥9 mm the endpoint is #6.
6. Mark your results clearly in a table either directly in the electronic medical record or in written form, including both control and test results in mm.

Technical Considerations in Skin Testing

It is imperative that all controls and antigen extracts are stored properly and checked often for expiration dates. This is especially true with aqueous extracts preserved in phenolated saline without glycerin, which is the case for the testing board utilized in intradermal testing. These should be refrigerated at 2–8 degrees Celsius and replenished at least every 6–8 weeks. Skin prick testing extracts are preserved in 50% glycerin and have a longer expiration (2–3 years) but should still be refrigerated in the same fashion. In multi-prick testing, it is important to make sure that the wells are filled enough so the device is sufficiently submerged such that the right quantity of test antigen is applied with each epicutaneous application. When applying skin prick tests, it is important to not cause any bleeding as this may lead to traumatic whealing and confound the test. When applying intradermal tests, it is imperative to practice making 4 mm intradermal wheals which are not too superficial. Technical errors during skin testing can make the test invalid. Finally, if a patient has already decided to pursue sublingual immunotherapy then a quantitative endpoint is not as helpful and completion of skin prick testing alone is appropriate.

Safety Considerations in Skin Testing

Both the patient and physician testing are potentially at risk during the skin testing process. It is imperative to wash the patient's skin adequately with soap and water and alcohol prior to testing to reduce the risk of skin infection. Additionally, the physician must wear adequate personal protective equipment including gloves and eye protection. Allergy testing during the sars-cov2 pandemic has intensified the need for personal protection for clinic employees to include masks, gowns, and advanced eye protection. Testing during the pandemic is more easily done on the patient's forearm, upper arm, and upper thigh instead of the back, as it is easier for patients to wear their masks properly.

Although rare, all forms of skin testing can lead to local and systemic reactions; hence, epinephrine and other safety measures must be available (see Anaphylaxis Chapter). Patients at higher risk for anaphylaxis, as well as those with inadequate skin whealing responses, should be evaluated through specific IgE testing. Details on patient selection, medication interactions, and allergy emergencies are further discussed in other chapters and need to be understood prior to starting skin testing in one's clinical practice.

Considerations After Completing Skin Testing

It is important to evaluate the skin test results in the context of the patient's presentation. A positive test result signifies sensitivity, but not necessarily atopy if the patient does not have relevant history or symptoms. Similarly, a negative result needs to be interpreted with caution if the patient has consistent symptoms around that allergen. Skin testing provides the otolaryngic allergist with a wealth of opportunity to tailor treatment of the atopic patient including pharmacotherapy, immunotherapy, and environmental modification.

References

1. Blackley C. Experimental researches on the cause and nature of catarrhus aestivus (hay-fever or hay-asthma). London: Balliere, Tindall and Cox; 1873. p. 34–8.
2. Shulman ST. Clemens von Pirquet: a remarkable life and career. J Pediatr Infect Dis Soc. 2017;6:376–9.
3. Cooke RA. The treatment of hay fever by active immunization. Laryngoscope. 1915;25:108–12.
4. Lewis T, Zotterman Y. Vascular reactions of the skin to injury. J Physiol. 1927;62:280–8.
5. Pepys J. Skin testing. Br J Hosp Med. 1975:412–20.
6. Bernstein IL, Li JT, Bernstein DI, Hamilton R, Spector SL, Tan R, et al. Allergy diagnostic testing: an updated practice parameter. Ann Allergy Asthma Immunol. 2008;100:S1–S148.
7. Kleinjan A, Willart M, van Rijt LS, Braunstahl G-J, Leman K, Jung S, et al. An essential role for dendritic cells in human and experimental allergic rhinitis. J Allergy Clin Immunol. 2006;118:1117–25.
8. Chaplin DD. Overview of the immune response. J Allergy Clin Immunol. 2010;125:S345.
9. Abbas AK. Basic immunology: functions and disorders of the immune system. 6th ed. Philadelphia, PA: Elsevier; 2020.
10. Franzese C. Skin prick testing. In: Handbook of otolaryngic allergy. 1st ed. Thieme Medical Publishers.
11. Yuenyongviwat A, Koonrangsesomboon D, Sangsupawanich P. Comparison of skin test reactivity to histamine on back and forearm in young children. Asian Pac J Allergy Immunol. 2012;30:301–5.
12. Bordignon V, Burastero SE. Age, gender and reactivity to allergens independently influence skin reactivity to histamine. J Investig Allergol Clin Immunol. 2006;16:129–35.
13. Nelson HS, Knoetzer J, Bucher B. Effect of distance between sites and region of the body on results of skin prick tests. J Allergy Clin Immunol. 1996;97:596–601.
14. Alexander HL, McConnell FS. The variability of skin reactions in allergy. J Allergy. 1930;2:23–33.
15. Peltier J, Ryan MW. Comparison of intradermal dilutional testing, skin prick testing, and modified quantitative testing for common allergens. Otolaryngol Head Neck Surg. 2007;137:246–9.
16. Fornadley JA. Skin testing for inhalant allergy. Int Forum Allergy Rhinol. 2014;4:S41–5.
17. Wise SK, Lin SY, Toskala E, Orlandi RR, Akdis CA, Alt JA, et al. International consensus statement on allergy and rhinology: allergic rhinitis. Int Forum Allergy Rhinol. 2018;8:108–352.
18. Franzese C. Intradermal skin testing. In: , Handbook of otolaryngic allergy. 1st ed. Thieme Medical Publishers.
19. Cox L, Nelson H, Lockey R, Calabria C, Chacko T, Finegold I, et al. Allergen immunotherapy: a practice parameter third update. J Allergy Clin Immunol. 2011;127:S1–S55.
20. Watley DC, Haroun KB, Siddiqui FN. Controversies in skin testing for allergic rhinitis. Curr Otorhinolaryngol Rep. 2020;8:175–84.
21. Krouse JH, Mabry RL. Skin testing for inhalant allergy 2003: current strategies. Otolaryngol Head Neck Surg. 2003;129:S33–49.

In Vitro Specific IgE Testing

15

Jennifer N. Shehan and Christopher D. Brook

Introduction

Currently, immunoglobulin E (IgE) is the most commonly accepted biomarker to evaluate for a variety of allergic conditions. The rise of IgE for a specific antigen demonstrates a sensitization to the antigen, and so clinical suspicion of an allergic sensitization may be confirmed by identifying the allergen-specific IgE antibodies in vivo or in vitro. Aforementioned tests used in allergy diagnostics are in vivo methods and include the skin prick test (SPT), intradermal test, and patch test. In vitro tests utilize molecular-based assays to identify a circulating IgE.

In vitro allergen assays include the following:

1. Total IgE assay.
2. Serum IgE assays against specific allergen antibodies including radioallergosorbent testing (RAST) and enzyme-linked immunosorbent assays (ELISA).
3. Basophil Activation Test (BAT).

J. N. Shehan
Department of Otolaryngology, Boston Medical Centre, Boston, MA, USA
e-mail: Jennifer.shehan@bmc.org

C. D. Brook (✉)
Division of Otolaryngology, Head & Neck Surgery, Beth Israel Deaconess Medical Centre, Harvard Medical School, Boston, MA, USA

This chapter describes the relevance, indications, interpretation, and characteristics of in vitro testing for environmental allergens affecting otolaryngologic patients.

Relevance of in vitro Testing

Identification and confirmation of a causative allergen sensitization is essential in managing allergic symptoms and conditions. Typically, a group of potential allergens may be distilled based on history and physical exam alone [1]. Any identified temporal association between symptoms and a specific allergen can lead to testing. Molecular-based allergy diagnosis is helpful in the selection of immunotherapy, evaluation of cross-reactivity, and assessment of reaction to various allergens [2]. While in vivo testing evaluates for a limited number of specific allergens with standardized extracts, in vitro testing can identify sensitization to a larger number of allergens with a one-time sample. Additionally, in vitro testing can be helpful in identifying a patient's sensitization to subset or family of molecules. This allows for broader, more comprehensive testing. Not only is this helpful in understanding a patient's allergy prognosis, but it is also useful in identifying prevention strategies. Testing results are helpful for management of symptoms through avoidance and pharmacologic

C. Damask et al. (eds.), *Allergy in Otolaryngology Practice*,
https://doi.org/10.1007/978-3-031-93455-1_15

treatment methods. In vitro testing is useful when immunotherapy is prescribed to patients, especially those with respiratory allergies or comorbidities [3]. Specific antigen sensitivity allows for tailoring the immunotherapy to the specific antigen even within a family of allergens.

When in vitro IgE tests were first introduced in 1967, there was initial concern for the validity of the tests [4]. Since that time, laboratory methods and systems have improved with increased diagnostic accuracy and reduced labor and costs [5]. Currently, in vitro and in vivo methods have been shown to have comparable results [6]. In vivo testing, specifically SPT, remains the most commonly used diagnostic method for allergen sensitization.

Indications Versus Skin Testing

Skin tests are the most reliable and cost-effective allergen sensitization identification methods, but there are still clear indications for serologic-based testing [4].

Indications [3]

- *Equivocal* in vivo *or skin testing:* When skin testing does not yield clear results, serum testing can lead to clear, identifiable test results.
- *Anaphylaxis during the* in vivo *testing process:* Although it is rare, skin testing is aborted in patients with any signs of a type 1 hypersensitivity reaction. In this event, in vitro testing can be used to test for sensitivities without risk of a systemic reaction.
- *Severe asthma:* Skin testing has the risk of inducing an asthma exacerbation, thus, in vitro testing can be used without this risk.
- *Eczema, psoriasis, or other existing skin condition:* Skin testing has the risk of temporarily worsening underlying skin conditions.
- *Dermatographia:* Patients with dermatographia yield false positive and inaccurate skin testing, as they respond to non-allergen-specific tactile trauma when tested.
- *Infants or young children*: In vitro tests require only one needle prick, which is more tolerable than skin testing. This allows for earlier testing in children, which can lead to earlier prevention of allergen exposure and earlier treatment.
- *Pre-existing medication requirements*: Patients who are not able to discontinue medications which are contraindicated in skin testing may be considered for in vitro evaluation.

In Vitro Methods

Total IgE Assays

The total IgE test is a comprehensive quantitative measurement of IgE in an individual's blood. Initially, the amount of total IgE in the blood was thought to be a reliable measure of allergy status. However, any number of factors can affect the total value. IgE levels are variable based on age and sex, and children generally have lower IgE levels, as their immunoglobulins increase with age and exposures up to 15 years. Individuals with atopic disorders such as asthma typically have higher baseline IgE levels. Additionally, IgE levels increase with parasitic infections, multiple myeloma, primary immunodeficiencies, and aspergillosis, to name a few [4].

Total serum IgE is particularly useful in patients with atopic diagnoses such as asthma or allergic bronchopulmonary aspergillosis. A baseline level allows for monitoring when these patients are treated with monoclonal anti-IgE antibody therapy with omalizumab [7]. For environmental allergies, this method has been found to be less useful than other molecular-based testing.

Serum-Specific IgE Assays

In vitro testing identifies IgE specific to allergens through individual reagents (singleplex) or with a pre-identified panel, which are tested simultaneously (multiplex). There are currently more than 130 allergenic molecules available for in vitro testing [2]. With the purification of allergens, singleplex assays have increased in sensitivity, specificity, and diagnostic accuracy, and both qualitative and quantitative assays are available. A qualitative assay measures negative versus positive results. Quantitative assays reveal the amount of allergen-specific IgE antibody concentration within the sample, which can be helpful given the variable amount of total IgE.

Of note, panels between adults and children, environmental and food, and among geographic locations have proven to be different. It is recommended that individual allergists establish their own panels based on their patient population [4].

One of the most common methods for identifying serum-specific IgE sensitization is radioallergosorbent test (RAST). The antigen is bound to a solid carrier and then introduced to human serum. If the serum has IgE to the antigen, they will bind to the antigen-carrier compound. Next, a radiolabeled anti-human IgE is then added as a marker to detect the specific antigen. As a result, the quantity of bound radiolabeled anti-human IgE is measured, and the radioactivity is seen as proportional to the serum IgE for the specific allergen [7]. RAST was initially a brand name, but is now used to describe the method for testing.

A more widely used method today is enzyme-linked immunosorbent assays (ELISA). The antigen of interest is coated on the assay, and the patient's serum containing IgE is introduced to the antigen. Next, an enzyme-linked antibody for the specific IgE is introduced. Finally, a substrate is added to the sample to produce an enzymatic reaction with color formation proportional to the amount of specific antibody in the sample [8]. ELISA has been shown to have same diagnostic abilities as RAST and offers advantages including higher specificity, good accuracy and precision, high reproducibility, decreased costs, and ease of performance. It is now used widely as an alternative to RAST [9].

Despite advancements, the role of specific IgE testing remains limited, and it serves as a tool to confirm a clinical diagnosis in conjunction with a patient's history and physical exam.

Basophil Activation Test (BAT)

Basophils are effector cells within the allergen sensitization and reaction system. They have a similar reaction to antigen exposure as mast cells; the cells have a high affinity for IgE receptors, and thus carry IgE on their surfaces. The BAT uses flow cytometry to evaluate specific receptors on the surfaces of basophils that increase in a hypersensitivity reaction [10]. The patient's sample is combined with a specific allergen, and the BAT is used to measure an in vitro response to that allergen. In IgE-mediated allergies, the BAT can reproduce the immediate-type allergic reactions in the test tube. This is useful clinically to diagnose specific IgE-mediated allergic conditions and monitor patients' response to immunotherapy. Overall BAT has a higher specificity and lower sensitivity than allergen-specific IgE testing and SPT.

With BAT, both drug and environmental allergens can easily be tested, and they can be used to monitor response to standard allergy treatment and immunotherapy. BAT cannot be used in patients who are considered non-responders. There are 5–20% of patients who have no basophilic response measured by the IgE receptor despite various stimulants used. Additionally, BAT requires fresh blood, is not readily available among laboratories, requires complex testing setup, and is not standardized [11].

Clinical Significance of Specific IgE Results

Positive Test

A positive specific IgE test denotes the patient has been exposed to the allergen and must be interpreted as a quantitative not qualitative measurement. Specific cut-off points are used to determine the probability of allergen sensitization and reaction at any given quantity. The higher the concentration of the specific IgE, the higher probability an individual is allergic or will have a clinical reaction to the specific allergen [12]. Standardized cut-off points have been established by the various assay suppliers. It is important to note that cut-off points are distinct for various allergens and among populations. Ultimately, the results should be correlated with a patient's history.

Negative Test

Conversely, a low specific IgE level denotes there is a low probability a patient will have a clinical reaction to that allergen. These patients should consider causes other than IgE-mediated allergy to understand their symptoms.

Advantages [2]

- One-time serum or plasma sample required.
- Many allergens can be tested for at once.
- Can monitor sensitization, which may be useful in a patient undergoing immunotherapy.
- High sensitivity, which decreases when testing is performed as a multiplex assay.
- Results are not affected by medications or skin reactivity.

Disadvantages [12]

- More variability in inter-assay results.
- Cross-reactivity between different allergen sources can yield false or clinically irrelevant positives.
- Potential interference between IgE and other types of immunoglobulins, giving faulty results.
- Results are delayed compared to SPT.
- Cost prohibits ability to test unlimited number of allergens.
- Does not predict the severity of a clinical reaction to an antigen.

How Can It Be Used to Select a Safe Starting Dose for Immunotherapy

Both in vivo and in vitro testing can be used to effectively initiate avoidance therapy and immunotherapy. In vitro testing allows for quantitative information of an individual's pre-existing sensitization to an allergen, while skin testing allows for a patient's exposure reaction to a particular antigen. In vitro testing is seen as an equivalent method to skin testing for establishing a baseline for immunotherapy initiation [13, 14]. Immunotherapy may be initiated based on in vitro testing with the understanding that a patient is more sensitive to certain antigens than others, and thus should receive a lower starting dose than recommended if necessary [8]. Immunotherapy may be initiated in accordance with the American Academy of Otolaryngic Allergy (AAOA) guidelines using the class minus 1 convention, which is based on in vitro testing [13]. This will be discussed in later sections.

Practicalities

To carry out specific IgE testing, a practitioner's laboratory needs the ability to run RAST or ELISA assays. This typically requires purchasing specific, predetermined commercial assays. The test is a two-step assay, which can be completed in less than 4 h. Standard laboratories which have the ability to run ELISA also are also able to perform this technique. This is typically achievable with standard laboratories as institutions with inpatient components or diagnostic laboratories. Practitioners who are solely in an outpatient setting may need to send patients to a similar facility for testing. Each laboratory needs certification from the Clinical Laboratory Improvement Amendments (CLIA), which monitors quality standards for laboratory testing performed on human specimens for the purpose of diagnosis, prevention, or treatment of a specific disease.

Conclusion

In vitro assays should only be used for diagnosis in environmental allergic disease for patients who have a high clinical suspicion or who have clear indications in favor of in vivo testing. When used, clinical history is the most important guiding factor.

References

1. Pawankar R, Canonica GW, Holgate S, Lockey R, Blaiss M. World allergy organization white book on allergy: update 2013 executive summary. Milwaukee: World Allergy Organization; 2013. p. 20.
2. Canonica GW, Ansotegui IJ, Pawankar R, Schmid-Grendelmeier P, van Hage M, Baena-Cagnani CE, et al. A WAO – ARIA – GA^{2}LEN consensus document on molecular-based allergy diagnostics. World Allergy Organ J. 2013;6:17.
3. Melioli G, Savi E, Crivellaro MA, Passalacqua G. Potential of molecular based diagnostics and its impact on allergen immunotherapy. Asthma Res Pract. 2016;2(1):9.
4. Ansotegui IJ, Melioli G, Canonica GW, Caraballo L, Villa E, Ebisawa M, et al. IgE allergy diagnostics and other relevant tests in allergy, a world allergy organization position paper. World Allergy Organ J. 2020;13(2):100080.
5. Cox L, Williams B, Sicherer S, Oppenheimer J, Sher L, Hamilton R, et al. Pearls and pitfalls of allergy diagnostic testing: report from the American College of Allergy, asthma and immunology/American Academy of allergy, asthma and immunology specific IgE test task force. Ann Allergy Asthma Immunol. 2008;101(6):580–92.
6. Hamilton RG, Matsson PN, Hovanec-Burns DL, Van Cleve M, Chan S, Kober A, et al. Analytical performance characteristics, quality assurance and clinical utility of immunological assays for human IgE antibodies of defined allergen specificities. (CLSI-ILA20-A3). J Allergy Clin Immunol. 2015;135(2):AB8.
7. Makhija M, O'Gorman M. Chapter 31: common in vitro tests for allergy and immunology. Allergy Asthma Proced. 2012;1:108–11.
8. Platt MP, Wulu JA. Rational approach to allergy testing. Otolaryngol Clin N Am. 2017;50(6):1103–10.
9. Negrini AC, Troise C, Voltolini S. ELISA in diagnosis of respiratory allergy.: a comparison with RAST and skin tests. Allergy. 1985;40(4):238–41.
10. Hemmings O, Kwok M, McKendry R, Santos AF. Basophil activation test: old and new applications in allergy. Curr Allergy Asthma Rep. 2018;18(12):77.
11. Hoffmann HJ, Knol EF, Ferrer M, Mayorga L, Sabato V, Santos AF, et al. Pros and cons of clinical basophil testing (BAT). Curr Allergy Asthma Rep. 2016;16(8):56.
12. Lloyd M. Interpretation of IgE mediated allergy tests (RAST). Clin Immunol. 2015;28(2):5.
13. Kaffenberger TM, Dedhia RC, Schwarzbach HL, Mady LJ, Lee SE. Comparative effectiveness of allergy testing method in driving immunotherapy outcomes: allergy testing method and immunotherapy outcomes. Int Forum Allergy Rhinol. 2018;8(5):563–70.
14. Emanuel IA. In vitro testing for allergy diagnosis. Otolaryngol Clin N Am. 2003;36(5):879–93.

16 Molecular Allergology and Component Resolved Diagnosis

Michael S. Benninger and Gary A. Falcetano

Introduction

Allergic disease is a highly prevalent disease with a number of clinical manifestations that can include allergic rhinitis and sinusitis, allergic dermatologic disorders, allergic conjunctivitis, allergic laryngitis, chronic cough, asthma, and food-related symptoms. It is difficult to identify true prevalence rates in that diagnosis may not be confirmed, studies may be looking at only one of the allergic diseases and many studies rely on survey responses. When looking at allergic rhinitis, for example, reported prevalence ranges from 10% to 30% in adults and up to 40% in children [1]. There is also evidence that allergies may be increasing particularly in Western countries with the global prevalence of asthma has been reported from 10% to 18% [2]. Conservative estimates from the CDC suggest In the United States, this prevalence has been estimated to be approximately 8.4%, with 7.7% in adults and 9.5% in children [3] In the United States alone, the economic burden of asthma-related medical expenses, lost work and school time, and deaths was estimated to be $80 billion yearly [4].

The diagnosis of allergic disease relies on a classical history based on the patient's perception of specific exposures resulting in symptoms with confirmation by allergy testing or response to treatment. Allergy testing can be performed either through skin tests or in-vitro (blood) testing for specific IgE directed against potential allergens [3]. Clinical guidelines for allergic rhinitis developed by the American Academy of Otolaryngology-Head and Neck Surgery recommend that clinicians should perform and interpret, or refer to a clinician who can perform and interpret, specific IgE (skin or blood) allergy testing for patients with a clinical diagnosis of AR who do not respond to empiric treatment, or when the diagnosis is uncertain, or when knowledge of the specific causative allergen is needed to target therapy [5].

Allergy testing, whether skin or blood, can be expensive and is associated with some minor morbidity. Test positivity rates may vary based on the level of suspicion of the ordering provider, the prevalence of specific allergen disease, and the type of clinical practice. Individual allergens can be pursued based on specific symptoms or panels of allergens can be ordered to assess sensitization to a wider range of suspected allergens,

M. S. Benninger (✉)
Department of Otolaryngology-Head and Neck Surgery, Cleveland Clinic Lerner College of Medicine, Head and Neck Institute, The Cleveland Clinic, Cleveland, OH, USA
e-mail: Benninm@ccf.org

G. A. Falcetano
ImmunoDiagnostics Division, U.S. Clinical Affairs Manager – Allergy, Portage, MI, USA
e-mail: Gary.falcetano@thermofisher.com

C. Damask et al. (eds.), *Allergy in Otolaryngology Practice*,
https://doi.org/10.1007/978-3-031-93455-1_16

these may be additionally grouped by geography. There is also some subjectivity in interpretation of skin test response and the relationship between symptoms and the level of response in both skin and IgE bleed testing may be unpredictable.

In an effort to try to refine a cost-effective allergy test panel, Bousquet and colleagues looked at large numbers of skin allergy tests in an effort to identify which tests were highly positive and what size panel might be able to identify the majority of positive allergens. They tested 3034 patients of which 1996 (68.2%) were sensitized to at least one allergen, and identified eight allergens (grass pollen, Dermatophagoides pteronyssinus, birch pollen, cat dander, Artemisia, olive pollen, Blatella, and Alternaria) that allowed them to detect more than 95% of sensitized subjects. These studies did overlap a number of European countries which suggested that there were some differences observed between countries, but despite this only 13 allergens were needed to identify all sensitized subjects [6]. Although there have been studies evaluating the prevalence of food allergies [7], there have not been many that have looked at positivity rates of allergy testing for foods.

Benninger et al. evaluated large numbers of specific IgE tests finding that evaluated of the 125,190-potential inhalant/respiratory allergens, the most common positive antigens were dog (24%), cat (23%), dust mites (23% for both D pteronyssinus and D farina), and June grass (21%). Of the 23,438 potential individual food responses, the most common positive allergen tests were milk (18%), peanut (17%), wheat (16%), and egg whites (15%). Most of the results were in Classes 1–3, although there were still notable very high Class 5 and 6 Class responses. It was found that there was wide variability of positive in-vitro allergy tests, and the likelihood of a positive in allergen panels can be estimated. Evaluating such rates will help to further identify the most and least common allergens and will help to cost-effectively refine allergy assessment panels [8].

There has been ongoing debate as to whether skin testing or in-vitro specific IgE testing are better for patient care, but it is becoming clearer that they are equivalent in relationship to sensitivity and specificity. ICAR: Allergic Rhinitis 2018 confirmed this equivalence, noting that sIgE shows excellent correlations with both nasal provocation testing (NPT) and skin prick testing (SPT) in the diagnosis of AR. ICAR: Allergic Rhinitis 2018 noted that there is good evidence to show that sIgE is, in many ways, equivalent to SPT [9].

ICAR: Allergic Rhinitis 2018 also helped to clarify the potential role of specific IgE testing in the management of allergic patients, noting that serum IgE testing offers several benefits. The safety profile of serum IgE testing is the best of all available allergy tests as the risk of anaphylaxis is nonexistent. Furthermore, the use of skin testing is limited in the presence of certain medical conditions. In patients where skin testing is contraindicated or potentially impacted by medications, sIgE testing offers a safe and effective option for determining the presence of sensitization as a biomarker of IgE-mediated hypersensitivity and confirming specific allergen triggers [9].

One of the major issues with skin or specific IgE testing is that the test positivity may recognize immune reaction to a specific protein, but that protein may be present in more than one allergen and the testing may be identifying a cross-reactivity rather than the original sensitization. Therefore, the treatment strategies avoidance, pharmacotherapy, or immunotherapy may not necessarily be designed to truly select for the preferred targeted allergen. Recent developments and refinements of blood testing allow for a more specific approach to identifying specific allergens by evaluating the specific allergen components, mostly proteins, unique to each specific allergen. This evaluation is referred to as component resolved diagnostics (CRD) or component testing. This chapter will discuss the use of CRD in the evaluation and treatment of allergic disease.

The Basics of Component Resolved Diagnostics

An allergen contains thousands of molecules but only a few of these molecules are allergenic to humans. Each allergen has a number of components which are generally proteins and each of these allergens has different characteristics which may impact the effects of sensitization. Species-specific components are in general unique to the allergen and can be evaluated to determine if the sensitization is specific and unique to that allergen. Since many of these proteins can be found in multiple allergens it is the specificity of the unique component(s) that helps to determine if a person is truly sensitized to that allergen. Furthermore, each of these components has specific characteristics which impact the effects of sensitization. Sensitization to cross-reactive components may suggest that the sensitivity noted in traditional whole extract-based allergy testing may be from one of these cross-reacting components and not to the specific proteins of those allergens. The ability to identify components that are unique to an allergen or that may be cross-reactive to other allergens helps to identify the true sources of sensitization.

In 1991 it was first shown that recombinant allergens could be used for the in-vitro diagnosis of allergy [10]. The first studies used immunoblot to make this assessment. The mRNA is isolated from a particular allergen source. This is then cloned, and a specific DNA sequence is produced. The sequence is then identified for its specific allergen structure and utilized in the diagnosis of the specific allergen that causes sensitization [11]. Each of the allergen components can be evaluated to determine if the patient is sensitized to the allergen-specific protein or one of the cross-reacting components.

The ability of component analysis allows for the determination of the allergen-specific component or cross-reacting component and thereby allows for the assessment of the true sensitization. Since skin testing and specific IgE testing may be positive due to the cross-reacting proteins, a positive test may not determine true symptomatic sensitization. In addition, specific components may induce different clinical responses, depending on the specific characteristics which can affect the consequences of sensitization. Although this chapter could identify hundreds of ways that specific component assessment can be used for the refinement of allergy diagnosis, we will highlight only three: food allergy (particularly peanut and tree nut), pet allergy, and an example of the use of component analysis to identify symptomatic sensitivity in cross-reacting allergens from different unique pollen sources.

Food Allergy: Component Resolved Diagnostics

Food allergy tends to be very common, even more so in the pediatric population. The most common food allergies are milk, peanut, tree nut, wheat, egg white, soybean, fish, shellfish, and sesame [8, 16]. Since certain components such as profilins and cross-reactive carbohydrate determinants (CCDs) are ubiquitous in nature, it is often difficult with standard testing to be sure that the clinical symptoms correlate with the skin or sIgE test results. Component testing can be useful in such circumstances to identify the true sensitization.

Probably the most dramatic of the specific component characteristics is with foods where stability or lability of foods once they are processed in the gut impacts the clinical symptoms. Stability of allergens depends on several factors, including the molecular weight of the proteins, hydrophilicity, and the contact surface. Allergens that enter through the respiratory tract can be low molecular weight and can have low stability. Allergens have more difficulty crossing the skin barrier. Those that enter via the digestive tract are exposed to proteases and food processing, therefore they need to have high stability to not be broken down [12]. Disulfide bonds contribute to protein stability; these disulfide bonds help to create a three-dimensional structure where IgE binding is preserved, resulting in resistance to proteolytic enzyme degradation [12]. Egg is particularly sensitive to degradation not only in the GI tract but also with cooking; many egg-allergic patients do not have a clinical reaction to extensively heated/cooked eggs. Assessing for the presence of allergen component proteins that are resistant to heat degradation such as ovomucoid in the egg and casein in milk can aid in the diagnosis of those patients who will not tolerate egg and milk in any form including extensively heated foods like muffins and cakes.

Peanut and Tree Nuts

The diagnosis of peanut and tree nut allergy can range from straightforward to complex. As with any allergy diagnosis, the history, physical examination, and prevalence in the specific population must guide the selection and interpretation of diagnostic testing.

Whole extract testing for peanut and tree nut-specific IgE by either SPT or in vitro serological assay is routinely employed as the primary method of assessing relevant IgE antibody response. Correlated with a clear history of a systemic reaction, this may be all that is necessary to confirm a clinical allergy to peanut or tree nuts [11].

Often however, the history is unclear, and additional diagnostics may be helpful in reaching an ultimate diagnosis. The availability of single molecular peanut and tree nut allergen components has added additional diagnostic specificity and often provides a basis to predict, on a more individual level, a patient's potential clinical response to ingestion to the suspected food [11, 12]. Understanding the properties of these individual components can inform clinical management and further diagnostic procedures such as whether an oral food challenge (OFC) should be performed [11]. When used appropriately, component resolved peanut diagnostics can help clinicians to evaluate the risks involved, potentially increasing the number of low-risk OFCs, eventually leading to "de-labeling" of an allergy diagnosis. Alternatively, the components can also indicate when a high-risk situation exists, potentially reducing the number of positive OFCs performed [11]. For clinicians that do not perform OFCs themselves, this information can inform appropriate referrals to those specialists that do.

As detailed in Fig. 16.1, peanut and tree nut allergen component families can be considered on a stratified "risk ramp" with heat and digestion stable proteins being associated with the greatest risk of systemic reactions [11].

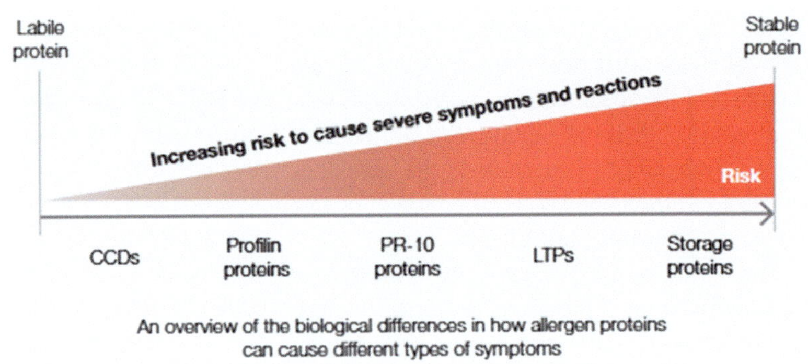

Fig. 16.1 Reproduced with permission from Thermo Fisher Scientific

Seed Storage Proteins

Allergen components demonstrating the highest risk of clinical reactions are the seed storage proteins [12]. Tree nuts and legumes, such as peanuts, contain storage proteins such as 2S albumins and 7S and 11S globulins, these are predominantly "species-specific" and demonstrate the least cross-reactivity with proteins found in other plant foods and pollens. Storage proteins are highly abundant in plant foods and are resistant to denaturing by both heat and digestive enzymes [11]. Examples of storage proteins associated with the highest risk of clinical reactions are the members of the 2S albumin family; Ara h 2, Ara h 6 in the peanut, Ana o 3 in cashew, Cor a 14 in hazelnut, Ber e 1 in brazil nut, and Jug r 1 in walnut. These 2S albumins have all been identified as significantly predictive of clinical reactions to their related foods [12].

Non-specific Lipid Transfer Proteins (nsLTPs/LTPs)

Non-specific lipid transfer proteins also known as LTPs present some unique challenges from a clinical standpoint when attempting to evaluate their ability to cause systemic symptoms in sensitized patients. They are typically considered to be of variable risk. Patients sensitized to LTPs, such as Ara h 9 in peanut and Cor a 8 in hazelnut, may exhibit symptoms ranging from pollen-food (oral allergy) syndrome to anaphylaxis. Like storage proteins they are highly abundant in plant foods and are resistant to denaturing by both heat and digestive enzymes [11]. Unlike storage proteins however, their location is not restricted to seed tissues, but ubiquitously expressed throughout the plant [11].

LTPs mostly exhibit a high degree of cross-reactivity with homologous LTPs in other plant foods and pollens. This cross-reactivity with pollens is thought to promote the sensitization and subsequent development of associated plant food allergy [11].

Geographic location appears to play a unique role in allergic responses for patients sensitized to LTPs. Populations in Mediterranean countries seem to represent the highest prevalence of LTP-related clinical food allergy [11].

PR-10 Proteins

The remaining allergen components have decreasing levels of clinical significance, from Ara h 8 in the peanut and Cora a 1 in hazelnuts, which are pathogenesis-related (PR-10) proteins that are homologous to Fagales family of pollens (e.g., Birch.) Ara h 8 and Cor a 1 are labile and can be denatured by digestive enzymes making systemic symptoms from sensitization to them unlikely. Those individuals that do exhibit symptoms related to PR-10 proteins have symptoms that are typically confined to the oropharynx and this is commonly referred to as "food-pollen syndrome" or "oral allergy syndrome." The PR-10 family of proteins is very cross-reactive, and this cross-reactivity often accounts for clinically insignificant whole allergen extract positive assays of PR-10 containing plant foods such as peanuts and tree nuts in patients that are sensitized to pollen proteins such as Birch Bet v 1 a homologous protein to Ara h 8 and Cor a 1 in peanuts and hazelnuts respectively [13].

Cross-Reactive Carbohydrate Determinates and Profilins

Other peanut and tree nut allergen components that are highly cross-reactive with pollens and typically are not associated with symptoms of clinical allergy, include profilins and cross-reactive carbohydrate determinants (CCDs.) Profilins and CCDs are ubiquitous in nature and are present in all plants and pollens. Both CCDs

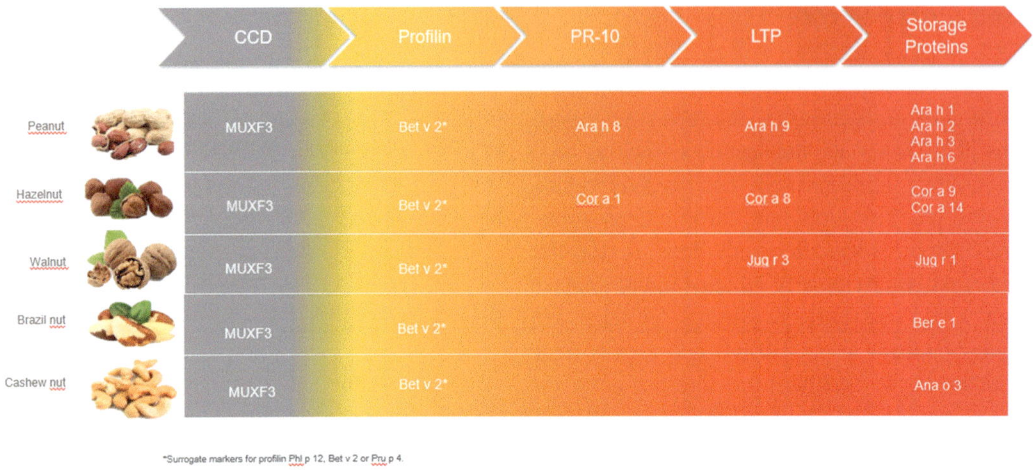

Fig. 16.2 Reproduced with permission from Thermo Fisher Scientific

and profilins are labile molecules that are denatured by digestive enzymes [11, 13].

The structures of profilins are highly conserved within different species. This allows the assessment of sensitizations to be accomplished by assaying a single representative allergen such as Bet v 2 in birch pollen or Phl p 12 in Timothy grass pollen as surrogates for the entire profilin family. Similarly assessing for a single cross-reactive carbohydrate marker such as MUXF3 allows for a thorough assessment of CCD sensitizations from pollens and plant food sources [11].

Figure 16.2 displays the most commonly utilized and commercially available peanut and tree nut allergen components in the risk ramp format discussed previously.

Furry Animals

Pet allergies, particularly dogs and cats, are among the most common allergies. Many patients who test positive for dog also test positive for cat and they can also test positive for horse. Although patients may be truly sensitized to all three of these, at times it is the cross-sensitization of nonspecific components that do not cause symptoms that result in the positive testing. The primary allergenic lipocalins for dog is Can f 1 and Can f 2, Fel d 1 and Fel d 4 for cat and Equ c 1 for horse as shown in Fig. 16.3. The use of specific component testing can be used to define the true sensitization.

In the case of a patient where the symptomatic true animal sensitivity is not clear and where there is a positive skin or in vitro sIgE test, component analysis can be used to clarify which animals the patient is truly allergic to. The example in Fig. 16.4 shows a suspected allergy to dog with positive testing also to horse and cat. By identifying the animal-specific components and going through an elimination process, the true sensitizing allergy can be identified.

One of the interesting phenomena in pet dog dander allergy is that up to 40% of dog allergic patients are monosensitized to the prostate protein Can f 5, and if this is identified as the only protein, the patient could tolerate a female dog or a dog that was neutered before maturation. A clinical benefit of assessing pet allergen components is the ability to better predict both the development of future disease and the severity of disease as well. In a population-based longitudinal study from Sweden, Asarnoj and colleagues demonstrated that the more individual cat or dog allergen components a child was sensitized to at age 4 years, the greater the likelihood of develop-

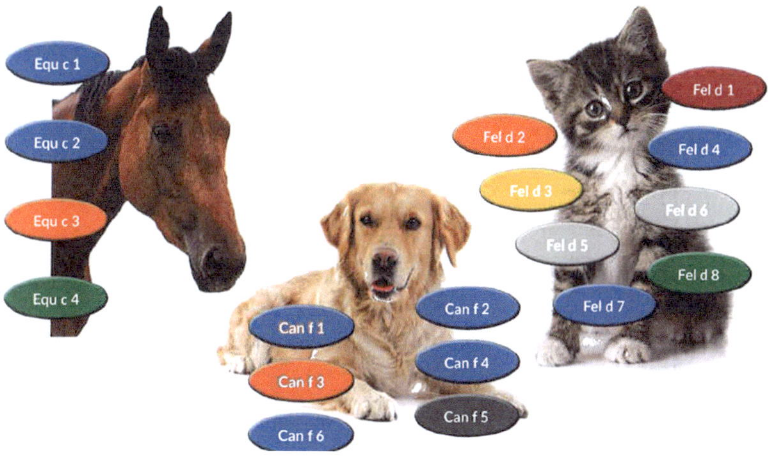

Fig. 16.3 Known components for horse, dog, and cat [11]

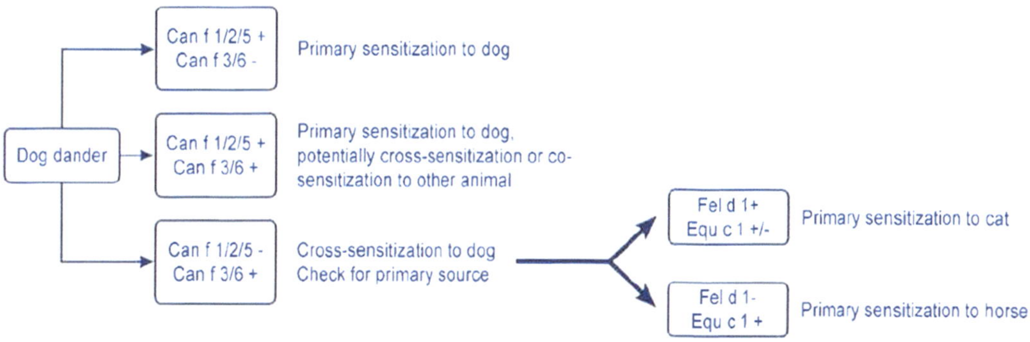

Fig. 16.4 The value of the use of specific component analysis in a patient with a positive IgE test for dog dander [11]

ing clinical disease by age 16 years [17]. Additional researchers, such as Patelis and Konradsen and colleagues, have demonstrated a similar relationship with an increasing number of furry animal component allergen sensitizations being correlated with increasing severity of disease [18, 19]. This additional information allows clinicians to base their management recommendations on the risks involved in continued animal exposure and may determine how proscriptive advice such as pet avoidance or immunotherapy should be.

With sophisticated analysis, the true sensitizations related to furry animals can be assessed. Such an algorithm can also be set up for any allergen grouping, such as trees, grasses, or weeds.

Using Component Analysis to Identify Allergy in Cross-Reactivity Among Types of Allergens

One of the problems in identifying the true sensitization in individuals who are polysensitized is that many components within an allergen are common among many allergens. This is particularly true for the profilin, polcalcin, and cross-reactive carbohydrate determinants. A very good example is mugwort, birch, and Timothy grass. The allergens come from three different allergen groups: weeds, tree, and grass. A positive skin or invitro sIgE test may be positive to all of them due to the shared profilin and polcalcin found in all of them. Specific components for Timothy

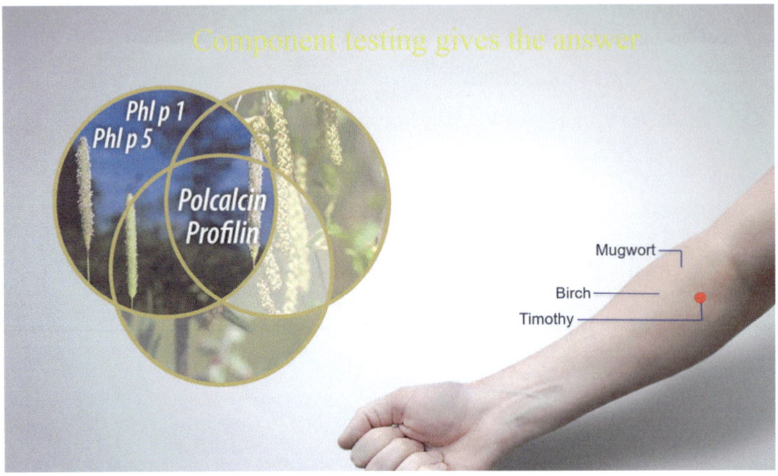

Fig. 16.5 Positive test to Phl p 1 and Phl p 5 identify the sensitizing allergen as Timothy [11]

include Phl p 1 and Phl p 5. If these are positive, but species-specific components to mugwort and birch are not identified, then the true sensitivity is to Timothy grass as demonstrated in Fig. 16.5.

Using Component Testing to Refine Allergy Assessment

Component testing can be valuable in determining the true sensitizing allergen, refining specific treatment, and determining the best antigens for immunotherapy. The use of component testing is probably less valuable in monosensitized patients, but can be invaluable in polysensitized individuals. The more positive tests that there are by skin or sIgE testing, the more likely that some of these may be due to cross-sensitization. Therefore, the utility of molecular component testing becomes more valuable in the management of their allergic disease. It is also more valuable where the risks of exposure on clinical symptoms is high such as in peanut allergy, where the risk of anaphylaxis can be assessed as shown in Fig. 16.6 [13].

This approach to testing can also be used where the abundance of molecules in whole extract is low or when the stability of a single allergen is low. In such cases molecular assessment can be especially useful. Molecular testing can also be adopted to transform an allergy practice. If an individual has symptomatic allergic disease, skin tests or in vitro sIgE testing can be obtained. If they are monosensitized or there are few positive tests, and the individual is symptomatic to these allergens, then avoidance, pharmacotherapy or immunotherapy can be initiated. If, however, the individual is polysensitized or sensitized to allergens that impart a high clinical risk, then molecular component testing can be performed to identify the true allergens and initiate treatment accordingly.

As component testing becomes easier to perform, utilizing large numbers of components and becomes less expensive, then it is foreseeable that component testing at the outset and then working backward to whether or not the patient is symptomatic to the identified allergens, could be the best approach. In some cases, it can even be used to identify at risk patients prior to significant symptomatology. An example of this is that children who test positive to Bet v 1 (birch) at an early age are more likely to have more significant respiratory symptoms by age 16 years [14]. With the development of micro-array chips where multiple components can be assessed with only a few drops of blood, the ability to identify allergic disease simply and efficiently has become a reality [15].

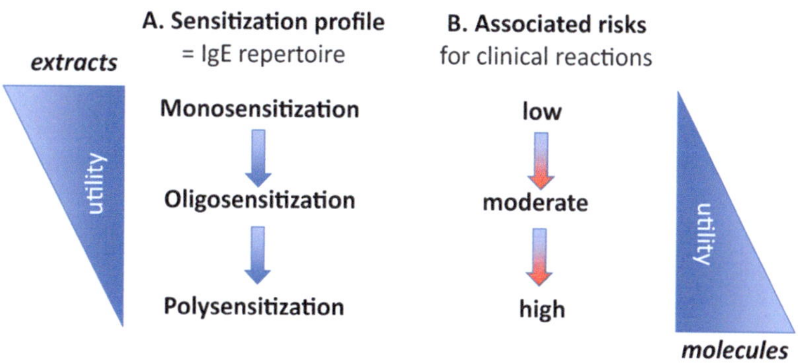

Fig. 16.6 Utility of molecular testing in patients who are polysensitized or those with risk for high clinical reactions [11]

References

1. McCrory DC, Williams JW, Dolor RJ, et al. Management of allergic rhinitis in the working-age population. Evid Rep Technol Assess (Summ). 2003;67:1–4.
2. Andersson M. Emerging treatments for allergic rhinitis. Expert Opin Emerg Drugs. 2003;8:63–9.
3. Centers for Disease Control and Prevention. Asthma facts – CDC'S National Asthma Control Program Grantees. Atlanta: U.S. Department of Health and Human Services, Centers for Disease Control and Prevention; 2013.
4. Nurmagambetov T, Kuwahara R, Garbe P. The economic burden of asthma in the United States, 2008-2013. Ann Am Thorac Soc. 2018;15(3):348–56. https://doi.org/10.1513/AnnalsATS.201703-259OC.
5. Seidman MD, Gurgel RK, Lin SY, Schwartz SR, Baroody FM, et al. Clinical practice guideline: allergic rhinitis. Otolaryngol Head Neck Surg. 2015;152(1S):S1–4.
6. Bousquet PJ, Burbach G, Heinzerling LM, EdenharterG BC. GA2LEN skin test study III: minimum battery of test inhalent allergens needed in epidemiological studies in patients. Allergy. 2009;64:1656–62.
7. Sampson HA. Update on food allergy. J Allergy Clin Immunol. 2004;113:805–8019.
8. Benninger MS, Grafmiller K, Yong V, Daly T. Relationship between specific atopic diseases and in-vitro allergic sensitivities. ENT J. 2018;97:296–322.
9. Wise SK, Lin SY, Toskala E, et al. International consensus statement on allergy and rhinology: allergic rhinitis. Int Forum Allergy Rhinol. 2018;8:108–352.
10. Valenta R, Duchene M, Vrtala S, et al. Receombinant allergens for immunoblot diagnosis of tree-pollen allergy. J Allergy Clin Immunol. 1991;88:889–94.
11. Matricardi PM, Klein-Tebbe J, Hoffman HJ, Valenta R, Ollert M. EAACI molecular allergology: user's guide. Pediatr Allergy Immunol. 2016;27(Suppl 23):1–250.
12. Pekar J, Ret D, Untersmayr E. Stability of allergens. Mol Immunol. 2018;100:14–20.
13. Steering Committee Authors; Review Panel Members. A WAO – ARIA – GA^{2}LEN consensus document on molecular-based allergy diagnosis (PAMD@): update 2020. World Allergy Organ J. 2020;13(2):100091. https://doi.org/10.1016/j.waojou.2019.100091.
14. Westman M, Lupinek C, et al. Early childhood IgE reactivity to pathogenesis-related class 10 proteins predicts allergic rhinitis in adolescence. J Allergy Clin Immunol. 2014;135:1199–206.
15. Lupinek C, Wollman F, Baar A. Advances in allergen-microarray technology for diagnosis and monitoring of allergy: the MeDALL allergen chip. Methods. 2014;106:106–19.
16. FDA (n.d.). https://www.fda.gov/food/food-labeling-nutrition/food-allergies
17. Asarnoj A, Hamsten C, Wadén K, Lupinek C, Andersson N, Kull I, Curin M, Anto J, Bousquet J, Valenta R, Wickman M, van Hage M. Sensitization to cat and dog allergen molecules in childhood and prediction of symptoms of cat and dog allergy in adolescence: a BAMSE/MeDALL study. J Allergy Clin Immunol. 2016;137(3):813–21.e7. https://doi.org/10.1016/j.jaci.2015.09.052.
18. Patelis A, Gunnbjornsdottir M, Alving K, Borres MP, Högman M, Janson C, Malinovschi A. Allergen extract vs. component sensitization and airway inflammation, responsiveness and new-onset respiratory disease. Clin Exp Allergy. 2016;46(5):730–40. https://doi.org/10.1111/cea.12607.
19. Konradsen JR, Nordlund B, Onell A, Borres MP, Grönlund H, Hedlin G. Severe childhood asthma and allergy to furry animals: refined assessment using molecular-based allergy diagnostics. Pediatr Allergy Immunol. 2014;25(2):187–92. https://doi.org/10.1111/pai.12198.

Part IV

Immunotherapy

Edited by Christine Franzese

Immunologic Changes and Efficacy of Immunotherapy

17

Alissa Kanaan and Mary Catherine Brown

Introduction

Treatment of allergic rhinitis/conjunctivitis and allergic asthma is aimed to alleviate symptoms such as itchy, sneezy, runny, and blocked up nose, as well as to improve control of asthma. Allergen avoidance is always recommended as an initial form of treatment when a sole triggering antigen can be identified and avoided appropriately. This can be achieved with the use of dust mite covers, HEPA filters, or pet removal for indoor allergens. Pharmacotherapy is a next step in the treatment paradigm and consists of the use of oral or intranasal medication such as antihistamines, decongestants, or steroids. When both of these measures fail at offering symptom control, immunotherapy—administered subcutaneously or sublingually—offers the only chance for a "cure" by modifying the immunologic response of the patient.

A. Kanaan (✉) · M. C. Brown
South Florida ENT Associates, Miami Lakes, FL, USA
e-mail: akanaan@uams.edu; Mcbrown4@uams.edu

Aim of Immunotherapy

Allergen immunotherapy, for the treatment of allergic rhinitis, was introduced in the early 1900s by Noon [1]. It consists of exposing the allergic patient to gradually increasing doses of an offending allergen. This subsequently alleviates the symptoms that occur from exposure to that specific allergen by mechanisms such as the production of specific antibodies, the alteration of the T-cell response [2], and other mechanisms that will be further discussed in this chapter.

Indications for the treatment of allergic rhinitis and asthma with immunotherapy include failure of pharmacotherapy such as antihistamines or topical therapy to control symptoms, patients who do not wish to take long-term medication for symptom control, undesirable side effects of these medications, and year-round exposure to allergens requiring continuous treatment [3–5]. Benefits versus risks should be evaluated in every case and a specialist assessment is required prior to the initiation of immunotherapy [2]. Since the treatment consists of regular dosing and frequent escalation, patient compliance and commitment to the treatment is necessary to achieve successful results.

Relative and absolute contraindications to SCIT include patients on beta-blockers, those with uncontrolled or severe asthma, or those with a history of anaphylaxis with immunotherapy.

C. Damask et al. (eds.), *Allergy in Otolaryngology Practice*,
https://doi.org/10.1007/978-3-031-93455-1_17

Mechanisms of Action of Immunotherapy

The immune response is mostly regulated by cytokines that stimulate or inhibit effector T cells [6–9]. In a brief summary, Th1 cells are responsible for cell-mediated immunity, including cytotoxicity, inflammation, and delayed-type hypersensitivity by secreting IL-2, TNF-β, and IFN-γ. Th2 cells, on the other hand, regulate eosinophilia and antibody responses by secreting IL-4, IL-5, and IL-13 [10]. Allergy involves the activation of the Th2 pathway in predisposed individuals, and is associated with elevation of serum levels of allergen-specific IgE, eosinophilia, and mast cell activation. While IL-4 and IL-13 are responsible for IgE production, IL-5 increases eosinophil survival [11, 12].

The immune response works by the activation of the serum antibody response and the T lymphocyte responses peripherally and in the tissues [13].

Serum antibody response consists of an increase in the formation of IgG1, IgG4, and IgA levels [14]. Specific IgG4 was found to be detectable in the serum 60 days after initiation of treatment in specific venom and dust mite studies [15, 16].

These IgG antibodies compete with IgE receptors on mast cells, basophils, and other IgE receptor presenting cells, thus blocking the effect of IgE, such as the release of histamine by basophils and suppressing allergen-specific T cell responses [17]. Allergen-specific IgG4 elevation has been shown to be temporally related to symptom improvement, gradually falling after discontinuation of immunotherapy.

Early studies about the T lymphocyte response demonstrated a shift away from a Th2 response to a Th1 response causing a reduction in the proliferative response to the allergen in patients treated by inhalant and venom immunotherapy [15, 18] (Fig. 17.1). A more highly consistent finding is

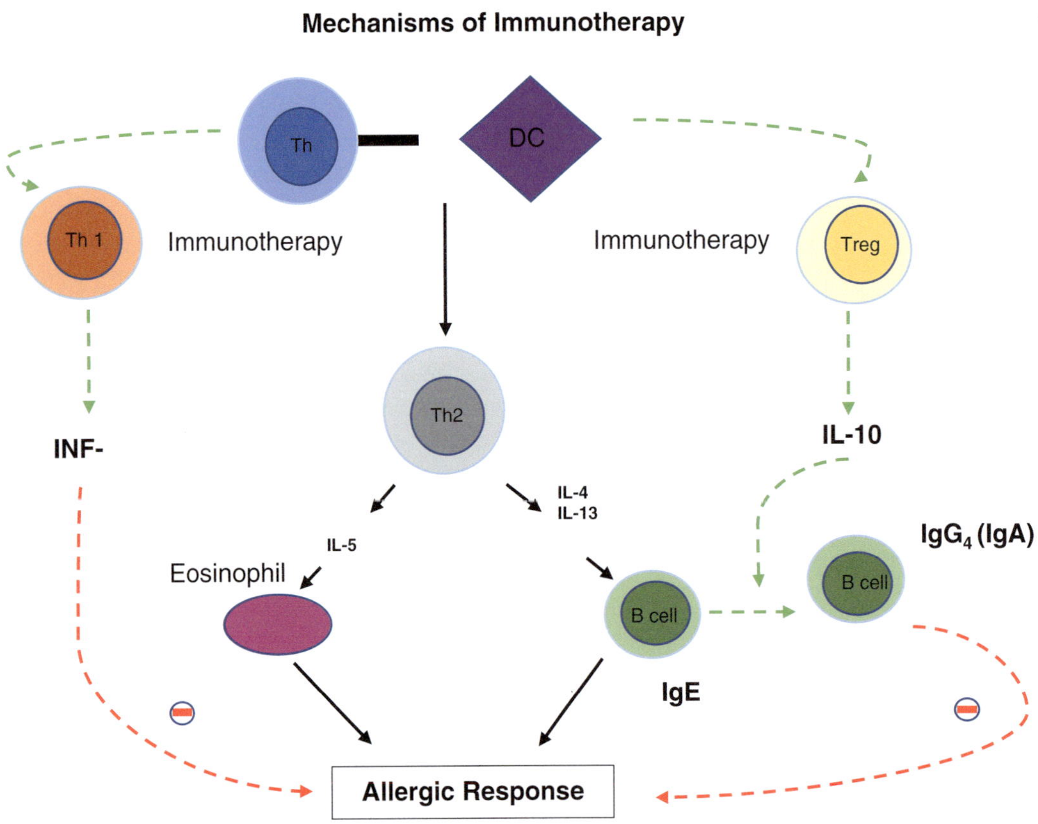

Fig. 17.1 Proposed mechanisms of immunotherapy in which there is a shift from Th2 to Th1 response. This modulation results in increased production of IL-10 and INF-γ which ultimately dampens the allergic response. *DC* dendritic cell

the presence of peripheral blood T cells that produce IL-10. IL-10-secreting T cells are prevalent in a healthy immune response [19]. The Treg cells control the allergen-specific immune response on several levels whether directly or indirectly by suppressing mast cells, basophils, and eosinophils, thus increasing the production of IL-10 and TGF-β. IL-10, in turn, inhibits IgE and enhances the production of IgG4, whereas TGF-β increases IgA production.

Several studies have shown the importance of IL-10 in immunotherapy response regardless of the immunotherapy method utilized. Whether administered orally, such as in peanut allergy [20], subcutaneously [21] or sublingually, immunotherapy was shown to increase IL-10 and decrease allergy symptoms during exposure to the offending allergen, eventually leading to tissue remodeling in the inflamed skin, nose, and lungs. The end result of immunotherapy was the restoration of a tolerant T-cell response similar to that seen in healthy individuals.

Mechanisms of Immunotherapy

Efficacy of Immunotherapy

How Do We Measure the Efficacy of Immunotherapy?

When determining the efficacy of immunotherapy, it is important to consider both subjective and objective criteria. From the patient's perspective, quality of life is arguably the most important indicator of the success or failure of a particular intervention. This can be evaluated by assessing changes in symptomatology and/or the need for allergy medication after treatment [22, 23]. As providers, we also have to consider at what point these patient-derived measures translate to clinically significant changes. Conversely, we can also quantify the success of immunotherapy by monitoring changes in various parameters such as immunologic changes, provocation tests, skin reactivity, and lung function during and after treatment [23]. However, it is also critical to determine if improvements in these objective measures translate to clinical improvement for patients.

Given that there is substantial variability in how we quantify and assess the efficacy of immunotherapy, there has been a push to standardize outcome measures and use validated tools so that accurate comparisons can be made across studies. Furthermore, research has been directed at determining at what point therapeutic benefit translates to clinical significance [24, 25]. In 2012, the World Allergy Organization developed a total combined score (TCS), reflecting medication use and symptoms, to assess clinical benefit. A 20% mean reduction in score was proposed as a clinically significant benefit [26].

The US Food and Drug Administration (FDA) has stipulated that two criteria must be met before allergy immunotherapy can be approved. The first criterion states that the TCS must demonstrate an average relative difference of 15% compared with placebo. The second states that the upper limit of the 95% confidence interval around the point estimate (i.e., the smallest estimated treatment effect) must be at least 10% different from the placebo group, to demonstrate a clear separation between active treatment and placebo.

Appropriate Indications

When contemplating immunotherapy as a potential treatment option, it is important to address several questions. First, does my patient have a condition that will benefit from immunotherapy? Second, is the allergen clinically significant? Third, have other measures been maximized? Finally, is current management suboptimal? [27].

We know that patients with seasonal or perennial allergic rhinitis with or without conjunctivitis and seasonal or perennial allergic asthma can possibly benefit from immunotherapy [28]. Allergies related to multiple antigens including grass, tree birch, weed pollen, animal dander, cockroach, dust mites, and mold have successfully been treated with subcutaneous immunotherapy (SCIT) [27]. However, we must ensure that the patient has symptoms when they are exposed to the specific allergen and that there are high levels of specific IgE confirmed through serum or skin testing. Once the aforementioned conditions are met, patients must complete adequate trials of environmental and pharmacologic treatments for symptom management. If patients still have suboptimal control of symptoms after an appropriate observation period and other etiologies such gastroesophageal reflux disease and chronic rhinosinusitis have been ruled out, immunotherapy should be considered [27, 29].

Efficacy of Subcutaneous Immunotherapy

Subcutaneous immunotherapy is a well-established form of immunotherapy for the management of allergic disease. It involves the injection of carefully titrated doses of allergen at scheduled intervals. When addressing the efficacy of SCIT, it is important to understand that significant practice variability exists across the globe. In addition to practice and treatment variability related to dosing, duration, and schedule, studies vary widely in defining outcome measures of efficacy such as symptoms, medication use, or 20% reduction in TCS. Therefore, it has been challenging to make direct comparisons across studies regarding the efficacy of immunotherapy.

For instance, in the United States, allergists often administer mixtures of allergens to which a patient is sensitive. Conversely, patients in Europe typically only receive injections with the one or two allergens that cause the most symptoms. The majority of research has focused on the efficacy of single antigen therapy. Therefore, it is difficult to say whether treatment with more than 2 allergens is beneficial [30] or possibly detrimental [31–33], due to a dilutional effect. Additional confounding factors include the composition of allergen extracts, dosing, and preparation of extracts. These topics will be discussed in greater detail in subsequent chapters.

There are a number of randomized controlled trials that demonstrate the efficacy of SCIT in the management of allergic rhinitis. In 2007, a meta-analysis by Calderon et al. looked at 51 double-blind, placebo-controlled randomized trials that included both adults and children who were treated for seasonal pollen allergies. Patients received treatment anywhere from 3 days to 3 years and had an average of 18 injections. This analysis found that patients experienced a significant reduction in both symptoms and medication usage [34].

A study comparing SCIT to glucocorticoid therapy in patients with allergic rhinoconjunctivitis found that SCIT was roughly equivalent to a nasal steroid spray in reducing the need for rescue medications [35]. It is thought that the combination of these two therapies may have an additive effect and represent the best treatment for allergic rhinitis.

Abramson et al. conducted a Cochrane Review that analyzed 88 randomized controlled trials investigating the effect of SCIT on allergic asthma. The various trials included house dust mite, pollen, animal dander, Cladosporium mold, and multiple other allergens. This review found that there was an overall reduction in symptoms, medication use, and bronchial hyperactivity [36] The National Institute of Health conducted a study that examined the safety and efficacy of immunotherapy on allergic asthma related to ragweed allergy. Interestingly, this study looked at both subjective and objective criteria and found that symptoms, peak expiratory flow rates, and skin provocation sensitivity were all improved when compared to placebo after immunotherapy [37]. Given the growing body of evidence supporting SCIT for the treatment of asthma, the National Asthma Education and Prevention Program (NAEPP) recommends that immunotherapy be used in addition to standard medical therapy for allergic asthma [38].

Unfortunately, we are unable to predict the long-term efficacy of immunotherapy after

SCIT is discontinued. Typically, patients are counseled that they may continue to see benefit for several years after treatment. In the event that a patient's symptoms relapse, it is possible to initiate treatment again, however, we have yet to identify a biomarker that reliably predicts how a patient will respond after treatment is discontinued [39]. The limited studies that have been conducted thus far indicate that long-term outcomes are multifactorial and related to patient age and the extent and type of allergic disease [40–42].

Efficacy of Sublingual Immunotherapy

Sublingual immunotherapy (SLIT) can be offered in a dissolvable tablet or in an aqueous/liquid form. In the United States, the tablets are the only form of sublingual allergen immunotherapy that is approved by the FDA. These tablets can be self-administered at home, once daily, and come in a standard dose based on prior optimal dosing studies. In practice, however, it is advisable to have the patient trial the first dose under medical supervision and be monitored in clinic for 30 minutes after administration.

Sublingual Drops

The sublingual aqueous form can also be self-administered in the form of drops placed under the tongue and held there for a few minutes and then swallowed. They are not FDA approved and thus incur an out-of-pocket expense due to lack of cost coverage by insurance companies. Lin et al. reviewed 63 randomized controlled trials and concluded that there is "moderate grade level evidence" to support effectiveness [43]. The authors did, however, find an improvement in symptoms score, need for medication, and quality of life. They also did not find any reports of severe adverse events or anaphylactic reactions. A similar review was conducted in children, the evidence was again moderate for allergic rhinitis and conjunctivitis but of high quality for asthma scores [44]. These reviews are limited given the lack of standardization, ability to accurately comment on clinical meaningful improvement, and appropriate dosing. Further studies are needed to elucidate these details.

Sublingual drops contain the same allergen extracts as those used in SCIT. Patient compliance is necessary as dosing is on a daily basis as opposed to weekly injections with SCIT.

Absolute and relative contraindications for SLIT include severe, uncontrolled asthma, acute asthma exacerbation, eosinophilic esophagitis, a history of anaphylaxis or hypersensitivity to any ingredients. It is recommended to temporarily hold therapy if the patient develops oral inflammation such as thrush, ulcers, or wounds.

Sublingual Tablets

There are 4 sublingual immunotherapy tablets available on the market in the United States: Odactra, Oralair, Grastek, and Ragwitek [45–47].

Oralair contains Timothy, Orchard, Perennial Rye, Kentucky Blue, and Sweet Vernal grasses. The patient should have positive allergy test to any of the 5 grasses to receive this treatment. Grastek is a Timothy grass sublingual tablet. Patients can be treated with Grastek if they test positive for Timothy or to a cross-reactive grass species such as Orchard, Sweet Vernal, Meadow Fescue, Perennial Rye, Kentucky Blue/June, or Redtop. Ragwitek is a short ragweed pollen tablet for patients who test positive to ragweed.

Typically, tablets are held under the tongue until they completely dissolve and patients are instructed not to swallow for at least 1 min afterwards. Common side effects include oral itching, ear itching, throat irritation, and mouth edema. Oralair, Grastek, and Ragwitek can be started in patients aged 5–65 years of age.

Odactra is available for house dust mite treatment. It contains 12 standardized-quality house dust mite (SQ-HDM) units of HDM allergen and is indicated in patients 18–65 years of age, who tested positive for *Dermatophagoides farinae* or *D. pteronyssinus*. Similar administration techniques and contraindications apply to the use of Odactra as the pollen tablets [48].

A systematic review by Radulovic et al. reviewed 60 randomized trials comparing sublingual immunotherapy (drops and tablets) to placebo for allergic rhinitis. Fifteen of these trials included children. Their results showed symptom control and less medication required compared to placebo. No cases of anaphylaxis or patients requiring epinephrine were reported [49]. A meta-analysis conducted in 2014 by Devillier et al. made indirect comparisons between SLIT tablets and standard pharmacotherapy. They concluded that grass pollen SLIT tablets had a greater clinical impact than second-generation antihistamines and montelukast. However, when compared to corticosteroids, the clinical impact was similar. Interestingly, the same study found that SLIT tablets were superior to pharmacotherapy for management of perennial allergic rhinitis related to house dust mites [50].

In 2015, a systematic review was conducted that included all randomized trials through 2014 that compared grass pollen SLIT tablets to placebo. They found modest, yet significant, improvement in both symptom and medication scores related to allergic rhinoconjunctivitis [51]. A large multinational randomized double-blind trial found that 12 unit SLIT ragweed tablets resulted in a statistically significant reduction (24%) in TCS. This number is clinically meaningful based on the World Health Organization cutoff of 20% for TCS [52]. A large randomized trial of over 1400 patients age 12 and older investigated house dust mite allergic rhinitis, with or without either conjunctivitis and/or asthma, after 1 year of treatment with daily SLIT. The primary endpoint of TCS and medication rhinitis score was reduced by 17% [53].

SLIT has been shown to be safe for patients with allergic rhinitis, with or without conjunctivitis, and concomitant mild-moderate asthma. However, there is not sufficient evidence that shows SLIT is an effective treatment for persistent, poorly controlled allergic asthma [54].

Preventative Treatment

A meta-analysis was conducted in 2017 examining the preventative effects of immunotherapy including both subcutaneous and sublingual routes. This analysis looked at a total of 32 studies and concluded there was a decreased risk of patients with allergic rhinitis developing asthma in the short term (less than 2 years). This study also investigated the long-term risk of developing asthma, preventing the first allergic disease in sensitized but asymptomatic individuals, and preventing sensitization to new allergens. Although the general trend indicated there may be some benefit the results were not statistically significant [55].

SLIT Versuus SCIT

There are many considerations when deciding which immunotherapy to initiate for patients. One group conducted an indirect meta-analysis that compared the efficacy of SCIT versus SLIT in treating seasonal allergic rhinitis from grass pollen and found that SCIT is more effective in controlling symptoms and reducing medication use [56]. However, both modalities have demonstrated efficacy in treating allergic disease, and the final decision may come down to patient preference and practical considerations (Table 17.1).

Table 17.1 Comparison of SCIT vs SLIT

SCIT	SLIT
Pros FDA approved for wider variety of injections Covered by insurance Once weekly dosing	Pros Fewer side effects No injections Can be administered at home
Cons Injections Must be administered by health care provider Increased risk of adverse reactions	Cons Patient is held accountable for all dosing Requires daily dose Out-of-pocket expense

Summary

The precise mechanism by which immunotherapy works within the human body is controversial. Research has shown there appears to be a shift from a Th2 to Th1 response, increased production of IL-10, and increased Treg activity.

In appropriately selected patients, both SCIT and SLIT represent effective treatments for reducing both symptoms and medication usage in patients with allergic rhinitis with or without conjunctivitis. Additionally, SCIT has been shown to be an effective treatment for allergic asthma, and the NAEPP recommends this treatment in addition to standard medical therapies.

Although SCIT has been shown to be slightly more effective, some practical considerations and side effect profiles may make SLIT a preferable choice for certain patients. Either treatment option requires a significant time commitment to therapy for optimal results. Finally, further research is needed to investigate the efficacy of the aqueous form of SLIT in the United States.

References

1. Noon L. Prophylactic inoculation against hay fever. Lancet. 1911;1:1572–3.
2. Bousquet J, Lockey R, Malling HJ. Allergen immunotherapy: therapeutic vaccines for allergic diseases a WHO position paper. J Allergy Clin Immunol. 1998;102(4):558–62.
3. Report of a WHO/IUIS Working Group. The current status of allergen immunotherapy (hyposensitisation). Allergy. 1989;44:369–79.
4. Current Status of Allergen Immunotherapy. Shortened version of a World Health Organisation/International Union of Immunological Societies Working Group Report. Lancet. 1989;1:259–61.
5. Malling H, Weeke B. Position paper of the European academy of allergy and clinical immunology. Allergy. 1993;48(suppl 14):9–35.
6. Mosmann TR, Sad S. The expanding universe of T-cell subsets: Th1, Th2 and more. Immunol Today. 1996;17:138–46.
7. Romagnani S. Lymphokine production by human T cells in dis-ease states. Annu Rev Imunol. 1994;12:227–57.
8. Abbas AK, Murphy KM, Sher A. Functional diversity of helper T lymphocytes. Nature. 1996;383:787–93.
9. Paul WE, Seder RA. Lymphocyte responses and cytokines. Cell. 1994;76:241–51.
10. Kapsenberg ML, Jansen HM, Bos JD, Wierenga EA. Role of type 1 and type 2 T helper cells in allergic diseases. Curr Opin Immunol. 1992;4:788–94.
11. Spiegelberg HL, Beck L, Kocher HP, Fanslow WC, Lucas AH. Role of interleukin-4 in human immunoglobulin E formation in hu-PBL-SCID mice. J Clin Invest. 1994;93:711–7.
12. Hamelmann E, Gelfand EW. IL-5-induced airway eosinophilia – the key to asthma? Immunol Rev. 2001;179:182–91.
13. Till SJ, Francis JN, Nouri-Aria K, Durham SR. Mechanisms of immunotherapy. J Allergy Clin Immunol. 2004;113(6):1025–34.
14. Gehlhar K, Schlaak M, Becker W, Bufe A. Monitoring allergen immunotherapy of pollen-allergic patients: the ratio of allergen-specific IgG4 to IgG1 correlates with clinical outcome. Clin Exp Allergy. 1999;29:497–506.
15. Jutel M, Akdis M, Budak F, Aebischer-Casaulta C, Wrzyszcz M, Blaser K, et al. IL-10 and TGF-beta cooperate in the regulatory T cell response to mucosal allergens in normal immunity and specific immunotherapy. Eur J Immunol. 2003;33:1205–14.
16. Muller U, Akdis CA, Fricker M, Akdis M, Blesken T, Bettens F, et al. Successful immunotherapy with T-cell epitope peptides of bee venom phospholipase A2 induces specific T-cell anergy in patients allergic to bee venom. J Allergy Clin Immunol. 1998;101:747–54.
17. Garcia BE, Sanz ML, Gato JJ, Fernandez J, Oehling A. IgG4 blocking effect on the release of antigen-specific histamine. J Investig Allergol Clin Immunol. 1993;3:26–33.
18. Jutel M, Pichler WJ, Skrbic D, Urwyler A, Dahinden C, Muller UR. Bee venom immunotherapy results in decrease of IL-4 and IL-5 and increase of IFN-gamma secretion in specific allergen-stimulated T cell cultures. J Immunol. 1995;154:4187–94.
19. Akdis M, Verhagen J, Taylor A, et al. Immune responses in healthy and allergic individuals are characterized by a fine balance between allergen-specific T regulatory 1 and T helper 2 cells. J Exp Med. 2004;199:1567–75.
20. Jones SM, Pons L, Roberts JL, Scurlock AM, Perry TT, Kulis M, Shreffler WG, Steele P, Henry KA, Adair M, et al. Clinical efficacy and immune regulation with peanut oral immunotherapy. J Allergy Clin Immunol. 2009;124:292–300.
21. Mobs C, Slotosch H, Loffler T, Jakob M, Hertl W. Pfutzner birch pollen immunotherapy leads to differential induction of regulatory T cells and delayed helper T cell immune deviation. J Immunol. 2010;184:2194–203.
22. Cox LS, Larenas Linnemann D, Nolte H, Weldon D, Finegold I, Nelson HS. Sublingual immunotherapy: a comprehensive review. J Allergy Clin Immunol. 2006;117(5):1021–35. https://doi.org/10.1016/j.jaci.2006.02.040.
23. Leatherman BD, Owen S, Parker M, Chadwick S, Fornadley JA, Colson D, Fass P. Sublingual immu-

notherapy: past, present, paradigm for the future? A review of the literature. Otolaryngol Head Neck Surg. 2007;136(3 Suppl):S1–20. https://doi.org/10.1016/j.otohns.2006.11.057.
24. Casale TB, Canonica GW, Bousquet J, Cox L, Lockey R, Nelson HS, Passalacqua G. Recommendations for appropriate sublingual immunotherapy clinical trials. J Allergy Clin Immunol. 2009;124(4):665–70. https://doi.org/10.1016/j.jaci.2009.07.054.
25. Canonica GW, Bousquet J, Casale T, Lockey RF, et al. Sublingual immunotherapy: world allergy organization position paper 2009. Allergy. 2009;64(Suppl 91):1–59. https://doi.org/10.1111/j.1398-9995.2009.02309.x.
26. Canonica GW, Baena-Cagnani CE, Bousquet J, Bousquet PJ, Lockey RF, Malling HJ, Passalacqua G, Potter P, Valovirta E. Recommendations for standardization of clinical trials with allergen specific immunotherapy for respiratory allergy. A statement of a world allergy organization (WAO) taskforce. Allergy. 2007;62(3):317–24. https://doi.org/10.1111/j.1398-9995.2006.01312.x.
27. Cox L, Nelson H, Lockey R, Calabria C, Chacko T, Finegold I, Nelson M, Weber R, Bernstein DI, Blessing-Moore J, Khan DA, Lang DM, Nicklas RA, Oppenheimer J, Portnoy JM, Randolph C, Schuller DE, Spector SL, Tilles S, Wallace D. Allergen immunotherapy: a practice parameter third update. J Allergy Clin Immunol. 2011;127(1 Suppl):S1–55. https://doi.org/10.1016/j.jaci.2010.09.034.
28. Omnes LF, Bousquet J, Scheinmann P, Neukirch F, Jasso-Mosqueda G, Chicoye A, Champion L, Fadel R. Pharmacoeconomic assessment of specific immunotherapy versus current symptomatic treatment for allergic rhinitis and asthma in France. Eur Ann Allergy Clin Immunol. 2007;39(5):148–56.
29. Nelson HS. Multiallergen immunotherapy for allergic rhinitis and asthma. J Allergy Clin Immunol. 2009;123(4):763–9. https://doi.org/10.1016/j.jaci.2008.12.013.
30. Calderón MA, Cox L, Casale TB, Moingeon P, Demoly P. Multiple-allergen and single-allergen immunotherapy strategies in polysensitized patients: looking at the published evidence. J Allergy Clin Immunol. 2012;129(4):929–34. https://doi.org/10.1016/j.jaci.2011.11.019.
31. Johnstone DE. Study of the role of antigen dosage in the treatment of pollenosis and pollen asthma. AMA J Dis Child. 1957;94(1):1–5. https://doi.org/10.1001/archpedi.1957.04030020003001.
32. Johnstone DE, Crump L. Value of hyposensitization therapy for perennial bronchial asthma in children. Pediatrics. 1961;27:39–44.
33. Johnstone DE, Dutton A. The value of hyposensitization therapy for bronchial asthma in children – a 14-year study. Pediatrics. 1968;42(5):793–802.
34. Calderon MA, Alves B, Jacobson M, Hurwitz B, Sheikh A, Durham S. Allergen injection immunotherapy for seasonal allergic rhinitis. Cochrane Database Syst Rev. 2007;24(1):CD001936. https://doi.org/10.1002/14651858.CD001936.
35. Rak S, Heinrich C, Jacobsen L, Scheynius A, Venge P. A double-blinded, comparative study of the effects of short preseason specific immunotherapy and topical steroids in patients with allergic rhinoconjunctivitis and asthma. J Allergy Clin Immunol. 2001;108(6):921–8. https://doi.org/10.1067/mai.2001.119743.
36. Abramson MJ, Puy RM, Weiner JM. Injection allergen immunotherapy for asthma. Cochrane Database Syst Rev. 2010;8:CD001186. https://doi.org/10.1002/14651858.CD001186.
37. Creticos PS, Reed CE, Norman PS, Khoury J, Adkinson NF Jr, Buncher CR, Busse WW, Bush RK, Gadde J, Li JT. Ragweed immunotherapy in adult asthma. N Engl J Med. 1996;334(8):501–6. https://doi.org/10.1056/NEJM199602223340804.
38. NIH. National Asthma Education and Prevention Program: Expert Panel Report III: Guidelines for the diagnosis and management of asthma. Bethesda, MD. National Heart, Lung, and Blood Institute, 2007. (NIH publication no. 08–4051). www.nhlbi.nih.gov/guidelines/asthma/asthgdln.htm. Accessed Apr 23 2009.
39. Jacobsen L, Nüchel Petersen B, Wihl JA, Løwenstein H, Ipsen H. Immunotherapy with partially purified and standardized tree pollen extracts. IV. Results from long-term (6-year) follow-up. Allergy. 1997;52(9):914–20. https://doi.org/10.1111/j.1398-9995.1997.tb01251.x.
40. Naclerio RM, Proud D, Moylan B, Balcer S, Freidhoff L, Kagey-Sobotka A, Lichtenstein LM, Creticos PS, Hamilton RG, Norman PS. A double-blind study of the discontinuation of ragweed immunotherapy. J Allergy Clin Immunol. 1997;100(3):293–300. https://doi.org/10.1016/s0091-6749(97)70240-9.
41. Durham SR, Walker SM, Varga EM, Jacobson MR, O'Brien F, Noble W, Till SJ, Hamid QA, Nouri-Aria KT. Long-term clinical efficacy of grass-pollen immunotherapy. N Engl J Med. 1999;341(7):468–75. https://doi.org/10.1056/NEJM199908123410702.
42. Des Roches A, Paradis L, Knani J, Hejjaoui A, Dhivert H, Chanez P, Bousquet J. Immunotherapy with a standardized Dermatophagoides pteronyssinus extract. V. Duration of the efficacy of immunotherapy after its cessation. Allergy. 1996;51(6):430–3. https://doi.org/10.1111/j.1398-9995.1996.tb04643.x.
43. Lin SY, Erekosima N, Kim JM, Ramanathan M, Suarez-Cuervo C, Chelladurai Y, Ward D, Segal JB. Sublingual immunotherapy for the treatment of allergic rhinoconjunctivitis and asthma: a systematic review. JAMA. 2013;309(12):1278–88. https://doi.org/10.1001/jama.2013.2049.
44. Kim JM, Lin SY, Suarez-Cuervo C, Chelladurai Y, Ramanathan M, Segal JB, Erekosima N. Allergen-specific immunotherapy for pediatric asthma and rhinoconjunctivitis: a systematic review. Pediatrics. 2013;131(6):1155–67. https://doi.org/10.1542/peds.2013-0343.

45. FDA. Prescribing information for Oralair is available at http://www.fda.gov/downloads/BiologicsBloodVaccines/Allergenics/UCM391580.pdf
46. MERCK. Prescribing information for Grastek http://www.merck.com/product/usa/pi_circulars/g/grastek/grastek_pi.pdf
47. MERCK. Prescribing information for Ragwitek is available at http://www.merck.com/product/usa/pi_circulars/r/ragwitek/ragwitek_pi.pdf
48. FDA. https://www.fda.gov/downloads/BiologicsBloodVaccines/Allergenics/UCM544382.pdf
49. Radulovic S, Wilson D, Calderon M, Durham S. Systematic reviews of sublingual immunotherapy (SLIT). Allergy. 2011;66(6):740–52. https://doi.org/10.1111/j.1398-9995.2011.02583.x.
50. Devillier P, Dreyfus JF, Demoly P, Calderón MA. A meta-analysis of sublingual allergen immunotherapy and pharmacotherapy in pollen-induced seasonal allergic rhinoconjunctivitis. BMC Med. 2014;12:71. https://doi.org/10.1186/1741-7015-12-71.
51. Di Bona D, Plaia A, Leto-Barone MS, La Piana S, Di Lorenzo G. Efficacy of grass pollen allergen sublingual immunotherapy tablets for seasonal allergic Rhinoconjunctivitis: a systematic review and meta-analysis. JAMA Intern Med. 2015;175(8):1301–9. https://doi.org/10.1001/jamainternmed.2015.2840.
52. Creticos PS, Maloney J, Bernstein DI, Casale T, Kaur A, Fisher R, Liu N, Murphy K, Nékám K, Nolte H. Randomized controlled trial of a ragweed allergy immunotherapy tablet in north American and European adults. J Allergy Clin Immunol. 2013;131(5):1342–9. https://doi.org/10.1016/j.jaci.2013.03.019.
53. Nolte H, Bernstein DI, Nelson HS, Kleine-Tebbe J, Sussman GL, Seitzberg D, Rehm D, Kaur A, Li Z, Lu S. Efficacy of house dust mite sublingual immunotherapy tablet in North American adolescents and adults in a randomized, placebo-controlled trial. J Allergy Clin Immunol. 2016;138(6):1631–8. https://doi.org/10.1016/j.jaci.2016.06.044.
54. Normansell R, Kew KM, Bridgman AL. Sublingual immunotherapy for asthma. Cochrane Database Syst Rev. 2015;8:CD011293. https://doi.org/10.1002/14651858.CD011293.
55. Kristiansen M, Dhami S, Netuveli G, Halken S, Muraro A, Roberts G, Larenas-Linnemann D, Calderón MA, Penagos M, Du Toit G, Ansotegui IJ, Kleine-Tebbe J, Lau S, Matricardi PM, Pajno G, Papadopoulos NG, Pfaar O, Ryan D, Santos AF, Timmermanns F, Wahn U, Sheikh A. Allergen immunotherapy for the prevention of allergy: a systematic review and meta-analysis. Pediatr Allergy Immunol. 2017;28(1):18–29. https://doi.org/10.1111/pai.12661.
56. Di Bona D, Plaia A, Leto-Barone MS, La Piana S, Di Lorenzo G. Efficacy of subcutaneous and sublingual immunotherapy with grass allergens for seasonal allergic rhinitis: a meta-analysis-based comparison. J Allergy Clin Immunol. 2012;130(5):1097–107. https://doi.org/10.1016/j.jaci.2012.08.012.

SCIT Vial Preparation and Dosing

18

Jennifer A. Villwock and Matthew Ryan

Key Points

- Subcutaneous immunotherapy is a potentially disease-modifying therapy that is effective for the treatment of allergic rhinitis, allergic conjunctivitis, and allergic asthma.
- The decision to proceed with allergen immunotherapy should be a shared decision, taking into account individual patient factors such as disease severity, efficacy of avoidance measures and pharmacological therapy, and patient preferences.
- Injections should be given under medical supervision in settings that are equipped to manage life-threatening anaphylaxis.

Introduction

It has been over a century since immunotherapy was first used at St Mary's Hospital in London and yet many of the basic principles described by Noon and Freeman still remain valid today [1]. In 1911, subcutaneous immunotherapy (SCIT) with Timothy pollen extract was demonstrated to be effective in reducing hay fever symptoms. The use of SCIT gradually increased, remaining the only mode of administration for more than 70 years, and its use was progressively extended to include other allergens. Frankland and Johnstone established in the 1950s and 1960s that SCIT is an effective form of treatment [2, 3].

Among the various therapeutic options for allergic disorders, allergen-specific immunotherapy (AIT) has the unique potential to induce desensitization and long-lasting tolerance. Over the past century, SCIT has been practiced by the same method employed by Noon, injections at weekly intervals of progressively greater concentrations of extract followed by a period of maintenance injections for years. However, SCIT over the years has evolved in different ways in individual practices across the world, leading to distinct philosophic approaches to treatment.

In more recent years, well-controlled clinical trials have confirmed the effectiveness of SCIT in both seasonal and perennial allergic rhinitis [4]. There is however a wide range of clinical practice and a variety of strongly held opinions about the best way to perform SCIT. For example, American allergists tend to treat for all sensitivities identified as clinically relevant on skin testing, whereas in Europe, patients are normally

J. A. Villwock (✉)
Department of Otolaryngology – Head and Neck Surgery, University of Kansas Medical Center, Kansas City, KS, USA
e-mail: jvillwock@kumc.edu

M. Ryan
Department of Otolaryngology-Head and Neck Surgery, University of Texas Southwestern Medical Center, Dallas, TX, USA
e-mail: matthew.ryan@utsouthwestern.edu

C. Damask et al. (eds.), *Allergy in Otolaryngology Practice*,
https://doi.org/10.1007/978-3-031-93455-1_18

only treated with a single allergen. Furthermore, American allergists use mixtures of extracts which are prepared from bulk vials, whereas in Europe, their allergen is supplied directly from the manufacturer. The basic goals and principles of SCIT are similar worldwide, but the differences are in the details [5].

Clinical Efficacy and Evidence of Disease Modification

The clinical efficacy of immunotherapy has been expanded upon in great detail in Chap. 18, *Immunologic Changes and Efficacy of Immunotherapy*, in this book. The clinical efficacy of SCIT has been supported by numerous clinical trials and meta-analyses [6]. The majority of the double-blind placebo-controlled studies that have demonstrated the efficacy of SCIT in allergic rhinitis and asthma have been conducted with single allergen extracts.

In monosensitized patients, SCIT has been shown to decrease the rate of development of new sensitizations [7]. A large, retrospective cohort study by Schmitt et al. demonstrated that AIT prevented the onset of asthma in patients with AR in a real-world setting [8]. Persistence of clinical improvement after discontinuation of SCIT has also been demonstrated. In a clinical trial, Durham et al. demonstrated that SCIT for grass-pollen allergy for 3–4 years induced prolonged clinical remission accompanied by a persistent alteration in immunologic reactivity [9]. SCIT is typically administered for 3–5 years and produces continuing relief of symptoms for years after discontinuation.

Multi Versus PAUCI

Polysensitization, which is sensitization to more than one allergen, is a common feature in patients with allergic rhinitis (AR) [10]. Polysensitization is an immunologic phenomenon that is epidemiologically as well as clinically relevant [11]. Polysensitization is generally more prevalent than monosensitization with 12.8–25.3% of the participants in the first European Community Respiratory Health Survey being polysensitized [12]. The National Health and Nutrition Examination Surveys reported that 38.8% of US participants were polysensitized [13]. The majority of patients consulting otolaryngologists in the United States are polysensitized.

Polysensitization has been proposed to be a risk factor for subsequent development of allergic diseases, especially allergic asthma. This has been demonstrated in several longitudinal birth cohort studies including the Multicenter Allergy Study in Germany, the Manchester Asthma and Allergy Study in the UK, and the Barn Allergy Milieu Stockholm Epidemiology study in Sweden [14–17]. There is also suggestion that polysensitization may influence the clinical expression of disease with more severe allergic expression in patients with greater number of sensitizations [18]. Asthma is more likely to be associated with AR in polysensitized patients than in monosensitized patients [16].

A polysensitized patient however does not necessarily have polyallergy. Polyallergy is a documented, causal relationship between exposure to two or more specific, sensitizing allergens and the subsequent occurrence of relevant clinical symptoms of allergy [16]. Approximately 50–80% of patients seeking treatment for respiratory allergies are polysensitized, demonstrating response to 2 or more allergens on skin prick testing or in vitro specific-IgE testing [19, 20]. Otolaryngologists must use this information along with a patient's clinical history to determine whether a patient is truly polyallergic or symptomatic due to 2 or more clinically relevant allergens. Allergen immunotherapy treatment strategies for the polysensitized patient vary between the United States and Europe. The European approach involves treating the single or the 2 most clinically relevant allergen(s), whereas patients in the US are usually treated for all potential clinically relevant allergens [21–23].

Polysensitization

In the United States, prevalence of allergic sensitization in the general population has been estimated in three National Health and Nutrition Examination Surveys (NHANES) [19, 24–26]. In NHANES II (1976–1980) and III (1988–1994) allergy testing was conducted by skin prick tests, whereas NHANES 2005–2006 measured sIgE levels in serum. The NHANES 2005–2006 provides the largest and most recent nationally representative data on IgE-mediated sensitization in the US population [27]. Participants aged 6 years and older were tested for 19 sIgE antibodies and those aged 1–5 years were tested for 9 sIgE antibodies. The NHANES 2005–2006 not only tested a greater number of allergens across a wider age range than the prior studies, but also provided quantitative information on the extent of allergic sensitization [27]. The threshold for a positive test, which was considered indicative of sensitization, was specific IgE value ≥0.35 kUA/L. In the children aged 6 years and older, 44.6% tested positive to at least one of the 19 allergens and 36.2% of children aged 1–5 years old were sensitized to at least one of the 9 allergens tested [27]. The overall prevalence of sensitization did not differ significantly by census region, but there were regional differences for individual allergens and allergen types noted [27].

In NHANES III, 10,863 individuals between the ages of 6 and 59 years old underwent skin prick testing (SPT) with one or more positive SPTs present in 54.3% of those tested individuals. Forty percent of those tested were sensitized to at least one outdoor allergen. Of those having a positive skin prick test result, 71.3% were sensitive to more than one allergen with the median number of positive responses being three [19]. In another study assessing data obtained from the Asthma Clinical Research Network trials, 1338 US subjects with mild to moderate asthma underwent skin prick testing with 12 allergens or allergen mixes. Ninety-five percent of the subjects demonstrated at least 1 positive skin test response. Of these, 14% had positive reactions to 1 or 2 allergens and 81% had positive reactions to 3 or more allergens [28]. Skin prick testing was conducted in 11,355 individuals for nine aeroallergens in the first European Community Respiratory Health Survey with over 40% of that population demonstrating a positive skin prick test result with 53% being polysensitized [20].

There is an evolution of allergy at the clinical level from birth into adulthood, which has also been demonstrated at the level of sensitization. In a cross-sectional, observational study by Melioli et al., the evolution of the IgE repertoire was analyzed. This study documented that atopic infants are often initially monosensitized, sensitization to only one class of allergens, but soon tend to become sensitized to other allergens over time [29]. This increasing number of sensitizations seems to characterize the natural history of the allergic patient and may represent a typical evolution of allergy [30]. Thus suggesting that polysensitization increases with age. In the French ODISSEE study, the prevalence of polysensitization increased with age; 54% of children under 11 years were polysensitized, 61.7% of adolescents, and 64.8% of adults [31]. In a retrospective study conducted by Purello-D'Ambrosio et al. assessing the prevention of new sensitizations in monosensitized subjects treated with specific immunotherapy, after 4 years, 68% of those previously monosensitized had become polysensitized and after 7 years, the prevalence of polysensitization had increased to 77% [32].

Immunotherapy in Polysensitized Patients

Some studies have suggested that there may be a difference between mono- and polysensitized patients in their clinical and immunologic responses to allergens. A study of 130 Korean children by Kim et al. examined the differences between monosensitized and polysensitized individuals noting that symptom scores and total IgE levels were significantly higher in the polysensitized group than those in the monosensitized group [27].

Allergen-specific immunotherapy is the only allergen-driven therapy for AR and asthma because of its ability to diminish allergic symptoms and reduce the use of medications by inducing clinical and immunologic tolerance to the causal allergen. However, polysensitization may represent a crucial obstacle surrounding the choice of the allergen extract to be used for immunotherapy [17]. A series of real-life, multicenter, observational studies, termed POLISMAIL (Polysensitization Impact on Immunotherapy), was conducted to elucidate the clinical relevance of polysensitization [33]. These studies also aimed to evaluate not only characteristics of polysensitized AR patients, but also the behavior of the allergists treating them. A single allergen extract was used in two-thirds of patients, whereas a mix of two allergens was chosen in the remaining one-third. Both groups demonstrated improvement in the severity grade of AR and QoL, thus demonstrating that immunotherapy with one or two allergen extracts can achieve significant improvement in polysensitized patients.

The efficacy of grass SLIT tablets in monosensitized and polysensitized patients has been examined. There was no difference in efficacy between those sensitive only to grass and those polysensitized when both were treated with a 5-grass SLIT tablet [34, 35] or a Timothy-SLIT tablet [30].

Polysensitization Versus Polyallergy

It is common practice in the United States to treat polysensitized patients by combining multiple extracts to treat all sensitizations. An analysis of prescriptions for SCIT written by US allergists and submitted to an extract laboratory (Greer Laboratories, Lenoir, NC, USA) was performed and determined that the average SCIT preparation contains a mean of eight unrelated allergen extracts per prescription [36]. The prevailing approach in Europe is to treat the most clinically significant allergen(s) by using extracts that contain 1, or at most 2, allergens. The Allergen Immunotherapy: A Practice Parameter Third Update emphasizes that allergen immunotherapy preparations should contain only clinically relevant allergens in line with the European philosophy [37]. Summary Statement 73 from the Allergen Immunotherapy Practice Parameter specifically states that the selection of the components of an allergen immunotherapy extract should be based on a careful history in correlation with positive allergy skin test results or serum specific IgE antibodies (Cox2011).

The difference in treatment approaches between the United States and Europe pivots on the debate of whether a polysensitized patient is actually polyallergic. Symptom intensity and duration, unavoidable allergen exposure, and impact on quality of life all play a role when determining which allergen(s) to treat. In some patients with multiple allergen sensitizations, even a detailed history may not completely elucidate which allergens are clinically significant. Another often cited reason for treatment with multiple allergens in the United States is the significant investment of time required for SCIT, due to in-office administration and monitoring after each injection. This fact often makes it difficult for US physicians to justify treating only one allergen if there is a possibility that the patient may still remain symptomatic from another allergen after completing immunotherapy for just a single allergen.

Clinical Indications

Allergen-specific immunotherapy is indicated in patients with allergic rhinitis, allergic conjunctivitis, and/or allergic asthma who also have evidence of specific IgE antibodies to clinically relevant allergens and exhibit symptoms upon exposure to those relevant allergens. Individuals with allergic rhinitis, allergic conjunctivitis, or allergic asthma who may be potential candidates for immunotherapy include those who: have symptoms that are not well controlled by pharmacological therapy or avoidance measures; require high doses of medication, multiple medications, or both to maintain control of their disease; experience adverse effects of medications; are unable to avoid triggering allergens; or wish to avoid the long-term use of pharmacological therapy. Cox Jaci 2011 parameters Other potential candidates include those with coexisting

Table 18.1 Subcutaneous Immunotherapy: indications, contraindications, and special considerations

Indications	Patients with allergic rhinitis, allergic conjunctivitis, and/or allergic asthma who also have evidence of specific IgE antibodies to clinically relevant allergens and exhibit symptoms upon exposure to those relevant allergens
	Patients who are unable to avoid triggering allergens
	Patients who do not achieve symptom control with pharmacotherapy and environmental controls/avoidance measures
	Patients who are unable to tolerate pharmacotherapy/have undesirable side effects with pharmacotherapy
	Patients who require high doses of medication, multiple medications, or both to maintain control of their disease
	Patients who do not want to be long-term/ongoing pharmacotherapy
Relative and absolute contraindications	
	Patients with uncontrolled asthma
	Patients with significant cardiovascular disease
	Patients on beta-blockers
	Patients with a history of noncompliance or who are mentally or physically unable to communicate clearly may be poor candidates for immunotherapy as this would make it difficult for the patient to report signs and symptoms suggestive of anaphylaxis
Special considerations	
	Children <6 years of age
	Pregnancy
	Elderly patients
	Patients with immunodeficiencies, malignancy, and autoimmune diseases

allergic rhinitis and asthma as well as possible prevention of asthma in patients with allergic rhinitis. These individuals also need to understand the risks and limitations of treatment along with the commitment required to be compliant with the course of treatment (Table 18.1).

Practical Considerations

Patient Selection

The decision to proceed with allergen-specific immunotherapy should be a shared decision agreed upon by the otolaryngologist and the patient, taking into account individual patient factors such as the degree to which symptoms can be reduced by avoidance measures and pharmacological therapy, the amount and type of medication required to control symptoms, and the adverse effects of pharmacological treatment as well as risks associated with SCIT. Before initiating immunotherapy, patients should understand its benefits, risks, and costs. Counseling should also include the expected onset of efficacy and duration of treatment, as well as the risk of anaphylaxis and importance of adhering to the immunotherapy schedule.

Furthermore, patients who opt for SCIT should be cooperative and compliant. Patients with a history of noncompliance or who are mentally or physically unable to communicate clearly may be poor candidates for immunotherapy as this would make it difficult for the patient to report signs and symptoms suggestive of anaphylaxis. There is no specific upper or lower age limit for initiating allergen immunotherapy. The risk/benefit assessment must be evaluated in every situation, although comorbid medical conditions that could increase immunotherapy risk are often present in the elderly, there is no absolute upper age limit for initiation of immunotherapy.

Allergen immunotherapy in asthmatic patients should not be initiated unless the patient's asthma is stable with pharmacotherapy as patients with severe or uncontrolled asthma are at increased risk for systemic reactions with immunotherapy injections.

Special Considerations

Pregnancy

As always, the otolaryngologist must be aware of the benefits versus potential risks of immunotherapy, but this is especially true in pregnant patients. Allergen immunotherapy is typically not initiated during pregnancy because of concerns about the potential adverse effects of systemic reactions and their resultant treatment on the fetus, mother, or both. However, it can be safely continued in women who have been on treatment prior to becoming pregnant. Discontinuation of immunotherapy should be considered if the pregnancy occurs during the build-up phase and the patient is receiving a dose unlikely to be therapeutic.

Beta-Blockers

There are 3 potential components of risk that can be influenced by beta-blockers during allergen immunotherapy administration. Reactions might be [1] more frequent, [2] more severe, and [3] refractory to treatment. Concomitant use of beta-blockers and allergen immunotherapy should be carefully considered from an individualized risk-benefit standpoint. Beta-blockers can enhance mediator release and thus potentially intensify pulmonary, cardiovascular, and cutaneous end-organ effects of these mediators. Furthermore, epinephrine might be less efficacious or epinephrine might also paradoxically worsen anaphylaxis by facilitating unopposed a-adrenergic and vagotonic effects. A cautious attitude should be adopted by the otolaryngologist regarding the concomitant use of beta-blockers and SCIT. In patients taking beta-blockers for whom an acceptable medication alternative is not available, withholding immunotherapy may be the most prudent management option.

Immunodeficiency and Autoimmune Disorders

Concern about the safety of allergen immunotherapy in patients with autoimmune disorders has been raised in the past, however there is no substantive evidence that such treatment is harmful in these patients. As with all patients, the benefits and risks of allergen immunotherapy must be assessed on an individual basis including patients with HIV infection, other immunodeficiencies, or autoimmune disorders. Immunotherapy can be considered in patients with immunodeficiency and autoimmune disorders.

Contraindications

Allergen-specific immunotherapy is contraindicated in patients with medical conditions that increase the patient's risk of dying from treatment-related systemic reactions, such as those with severe or poorly controlled asthma or significant cardiovascular diseases (e.g., unstable angina, recent myocardial infarction, significant arrhythmia, and uncontrolled hypertension). Beta-blocker use is a relative contraindication since these agents can amplify the severity of the reaction and make the treatment of systemic reactions more difficult.

Mixing SCIT

Once it has been determined that the patient is suitable for immunotherapy, the otolaryngologist will use extracts of clinically relevant allergens for immunotherapy treatment vials. Allergen extracts are commercially available for most of the commonly recognized allergens. When possible, standardized extracts should be utilized to prepare treatment vials since the efficacy and safety of immunotherapy are dependent on the quality of the allergen extracts used. In choosing the components for a clinically relevant allergen immunotherapy extract, the otolaryngologist must also be familiar with local and regional aerobiology and indoor and outdoor allergens, paying special attention to potential allergens in the patient's own environment.

Subcutaneous immunotherapy should be administered by trained staff in a facility with an appropriate observation area, facilities for vial storage at 2–8 °C, and ability for resuscitation measures. Injections should only be administered when a provider, who is trained in the management of anaphylaxis, is present. Furthermore, in-office compounding of individual treatment sets for allergen immunotherapy should follow the standards developed by USP for preparing compounded sterile medications [38].

At each immunotherapy injection, a record should be made of the date, dose, and volume administered. Any immediate (0–30 min) local or systemic reactions recorded. Also, any delayed local or systemic reactions following the previous injection should be recorded at the subsequent visit. At every visit, epinephrine should be immediately available. The patient should be monitored for at least 30 min following injections. The patient should be well, without significant concomitant allergen exposure and their asthma should be under good control. The time interval since the last immunotherapy injection and any reaction to previous injections should be verified. The dose of immunotherapy selected should double checked. In general, injections are given in the upper outer surface of the arm by subcutaneous route.

Injections should be postponed in the presence of respiratory infection, intercurrent illness, active asthma, or symptoms due to significant concomitant allergen exposure. Dosage reduction according to standard guidelines should be performed in relation to previous systemic or large local reactions, during increased allergen exposure and if there is an extended time interval since the previous administration.

Management of Adverse Events

In general, some local swelling following injections is to be expected. No treatment is required other than reassurance, although occasionally the use of an antihistamine may be indicated. Systemic reactions should be promptly recognized and treated. Epinephrine administered intramuscularly (in a dose of 0.01 mg/kg of a 1:1000 [1 mg/mL] solution to a maximum of 0.5 mg in adults and 0.3 mg in children) into the anterolateral thigh is the first-line treatment for anaphylaxis [39]. In general, if in doubt, give epinephrine, which is more effective when administered early during a systemic reaction. Greater detail on the management of adverse reactions can be found in Chap. 22, *Adverse Reactions in Immunotherapy*, in this book.

All practices offering immunotherapy should have detailed standard operating procedures and regular review of practice and staff training in immunotherapy procedures and the early recognition and treatment of adverse events. Patients should be supplied with information sheets which detail the benefits and risks of immunotherapy and detailed information on practical aspects of immunotherapy.

Injection Schedules

Typically, patients receive a course of injections, starting with a very low dose of allergen and building up gradually until a plateau or maintenance dose is achieved. Maintenance injections are then given at 4- to 6-week intervals for 3–5 years. The updosing phase is generally given as a series of weekly injections, but several alternative induction regimens have been tried, some giving several doses on each day and then waiting a week before giving a further series of injections (cluster protocol), whereas others give the whole series of incremental injections in a single day (rush protocol).

Rush

Several variations have been suggested, including "rush" and "semirush" protocols, in which the incremental phase of the regime is compressed by giving several injections on the same day with 30–60 min intervals. Rush protocols typically reduce the number of injections to eight over a period of 1–3 days [40, 41]. The chief drawback to these protocols is the increased likelihood of side effects, but this must be weighed against the ability to achieve protection within a few days or weeks, which may be particularly useful in patients with Hymenoptera allergy.

Cluster

With cluster immunotherapy, two or three injections (at increasing doses) are given sequentially in a single day of treatment on non-consecutive days. Cluster protocols achieve maintenance doses in 3–6 weeks [42].

Combination with Biologics

Anti-Immunoglobulin E (Anti-IgE)

The potential for anaphylactic reactions with SCIT has been a safety concern. There has been a suggestion for the role of omalizumab in patients with a high risk of systemic reactions to SCIT, such as in children with severe allergic asthma. In a study by Lambert et al., omalizumab pretreatment and subcutaneous AIT led to good safety and tolerability [43]. In another study by Casale et al., a fivefold decrease in anaphylaxis risk was observed in subjects who received pre-treatment with omalizumab with a rush schedule of subcutaneous AIT in 159 patients with allergic rhinitis caused by ragweed pollen [44].

Future Strategies

Concerns about systemic reactions with SCIT have led to investigations into methods to reduce the allergenicity of extracts and also investigation into ways to slow the absorption of extracts after injection.

In the past, the development of more effective, safe, and easy-to-manufacture vaccines for SCIT had been limited by the poor quality of natural allergen extracts. Progress made in the field of molecular allergen characterization has allowed for better standardization of allergen extracts and has afforded the opportunity for individualized treatment which can be tailor-made according to individual sensitivities [45]. There have been published trials of recombinant allergens for immunotherapy. In a randomized controlled trial by Pauli et al., a recombinant Bet v 1 product was shown to be efficacious with numerically similar results compared to a purified Bet v 1 extract and the standardized crude Birch extract in tree pollen allergy [46].

Novel adjuvants to delay absorption or modify T lymphocyte responses are being investigated. One of the first methods used to delay absorption was precipitation with alum; a commercially available aluminum-precipitated ragweed extract is an example that is widely used in Europe [47]. In a clinical trial by Nelson et al., therapy with aluminum-precipitated extract resulted in far fewer local and systemic reactions, and higher mean extract doses were obtained using this preparation [48].

Summary

Subcutaneous allergen immunotherapy is highly effective, particularly in patients with seasonal allergic rhinitis. Suppression of late-phase responses and long-term disease remission are seen in conjunction with clinical efficacy. Studies have demonstrated lasting benefit after an adequate course of SCIT. SCIT has been used for over a century and will continue to be the gold standard against which other novel approaches will be compared in the future.

References

1. Freeman J. Vaccination against hay fever: report of results during the first three years. Lancet. 1914;1:1178–80.
2. Frankland AW, Augustin R. Prophylaxis of summer hay fever and asthma: controlled trial comparing crude grass pollen extracts with isolated main protein component. Lancet. 1954;1:1055–7.
3. Johnstone DE, Dutton A. The value of hyposensitization therapy for bronchial asthma in children: a 14-year study. Pediatrics. 1968;42:793–802.
4. Dhami S, Nurmatov U, Arasi S, et al. Allergen immunotherapy for allergic rhinoconjunctivitis: a systematic review and meta-analysis. Allergy. 2017;72(11):1597–631.
5. Frew AJ. Allergen immunotherapy. J Allergy Clin Immunol. 2010;125(2 Suppl 2):S306–13.
6. Compalati E, Penagos M, Tarantini D, et al. Specific immunotherapy for respiratory allergy: state of the art according to current meta-analyses. Ann Allergy Asthma Immunol. 2009;102:22e28.

7. Purello-D'Ambrosio F, Gangemi S, Meredino RA, et al. Prevention of new sensitizations in monosensitized subjects submitted to specific immunotherapy or not. A retrospective study. Clin Exp Allergy. 2001;31:1295–302.
8. Schmitt J, Schwarz K, Stadler E, Wüstenberg EG. Allergy immunotherapy for allergic rhinitis effectively prevents asthma: results from a large retrospective cohort study. J Allergy Clin Immunol. 2015;136(6):1511–6.
9. Durham SR, Walker SM, Varga EM, Jacobson MR, O'Brien F, Noble W, Till SJ, Hamid QA, Nouri-Aria KT. Long-term clinical efficacy of grass-pollen immunotherapy. N Engl J Med. 1999;341(7):468–75.
10. Ciprandi G, Incorvaia C, Puccinelli P, Soffia S, et al. Polysensitization as a challenge for the allergist: the suggestions provided by the Polysensitization impact on allergen immunotherapy studies. Expert Opin Biol Ther. 2011;11(6):715–22.
11. Ciprandi G, Melioli G, Passalacqua G, Canonica GW. Immunotherapy in polysensitized patients: new chances for the allergists? Ann Allergy Asthma Immunol. 2012;109(6):392–4.
12. Bousquet PJ, Castelli C, Daures JP, Heinrich J, Hooper R, Sunyer J, et al. Assessment of allergen sensitization in a general population-based survey (European Community respiratory health survey I). Ann Epidemiol. 2010;20:797–803.
13. Arbes SJ Jr, Gergen PJ, Elliott L, Zeldin DC. Prevalences of positive skin test responses to 10 common allergens in the US population: results from the third National Health and nutrition examination survey. J Allergy Clin Immunol. 2005;116:377–83.
14. Illi S, et al. Perennial allergen sensitisation early in life and chronic asthma in children: a birth cohort study. Lancet. 2006;368(9537):763–70.
15. Custovic A, Sonntag HJ, Buchan IE, Belgrave D, Simpson A, Prosperi MC. Evolution pathways of IgE responses to grass and mite allergens throughout childhood. J Allergy Clin Immunol. 2015;136(6):1645–52.e8.
16. Simpson A, Lazic N, Belgrave DC, Johnson P, Bishop C, et al. Patterns of IgE responses to multiple allergen components and clinical symptoms at age 11 years. J Allergy Clin Immunol. 2015;136(5):1224–31.
17. Westman M, Lupinek C, Bousquet J, Andersson N, Pahr S, Baar A, et al. Mechanisms for the development of allergies consortium. Early childhood IgE reactivity to pathogenesis-related class 10 proteins predicts allergic rhinitis in adolescence. J Allergy Clin Immunol. 2015;135:1199–206.
18. Ciprandi G, Alesina R, Ariano R, Aurnia P, Borrelli P, Cadario G, et al. Characteristics of patients with allergic polysensitization: the POLISMAIL study. Eur Ann Allergy Clin Immunol. 2008;40(3):77–83.
19. Nelson HS, Makatsori M, Calderon MA. Subcutaneous immunotherapy and sublingual immunotherapy: comparative efficacy, current and potential indications, and warnings – United States versus Europe. Immunol Allergy Clin N Am. 2016;36:13–24.
20. Pepper AN, Calderón MA, Casale TB. Sublingual immunotherapy for the polyallergic patient. J Allergy Clin Immunol Pract. 2017;5(1):41–5.
21. Calderón MA, Cox L, Casale TB, Moingeon P, Demoly P. Multiple-allergen and single-allergen immunotherapy strategies in polysensitized patients: looking at the published evidence. J Allergy Clin Immunol. 2012;129:929–34.
22. Tabatabaian F, Casale TB. Selection of patients for sublingual immunotherapy (SLIT) versus subcutaneous immunotherapy (SCIT). Allergy Asthma Proc. 2015;36:100–4.
23. Cox L, Jacobsen L. Comparison of allergen immunotherapy practice patterns in the United States and Europe. Ann Allergy Asthma Immunol. 2009;103:451–9.
24. Salo PM, Calatroni A, Gergen PJ, Hoppin JA, et al. Allergy-related outcomes in relation to serum IgE: results from the National Health and nutrition examination survey 2005–2006. J Allergy Clin Immunol. 2011;127:1226–35.
25. Gergen PJ, Turkeltaub PC. The association of individual allergen reactivity with respiratory disease in a national sample: data from the second National Health and nutrition examination survey, 1976–80 (NHANES II). J Allergy Clin Immunol. 1992;90:579–88.
26. Gergen PJ, Turkeltaub PC, Kovar MG. The prevalence of allergic skin test reactivity to eight common aeroallergens in the U.S. population: results from the second National Health and nutrition examination survey. J Allergy Clin Immunol. 1987;80:669–79.
27. Kim KW, Kim EA, Kwon BC, Kim ES, et al. Comparison of allergic indices in monosensitized and polysensitized patients with childhood asthma. J Korean Med Sci. 2006;21:1012–6.
28. Craig TJ, King TS, Lemanske RF Jr, Wechsler ME, et al. Aeroallergen sensitization correlates with PC(20) and exhaled nitric oxide in subjects with mild-to-moderate asthma. J Allergy Clin Immunol. 2008;121(3):671–7.
29. Melioli G, Marcomini L, Agazzi A, Bazurro G, et al. The IgE repertoire in children and adolescents resolved at component level: a cross-sectional study. Pediatr Allergy Immunol. 2012;23(5):433–40.
30. Nelson H, Blaiss M, Nolte H, et al. Efficacy and safety of the SQ- standardized grass allergy immunotherapy tablet in mono- and polysensitized subjects. Allergy. 2013;68:252–5.
31. Didier A, Chartier A, Démonet G. Specific sublingual immunotherapy: for which profiles of patients in practice? Midterm analysis of ODISSEE (observatory of the indication and management of respiratory allergies [rhinitis and/or conjunctivitis and/or allergic asthma] by specific sublingual immunotherapy). Rev Fr Allergol. 2010;50:426–33.
32. Purello-D'Ambrosio F, Gangemi S, Merendino RA, et al. Prevention of new sensitizations in monosensitized subjects submitted to specific immunotherapy or not. A retrospective study. Clin Exp Allergy. 2001;31:1295–302.

33. Ciprandi G, Incorvaia C, Puccinelli P, et al. The POLISMAIL lesson: sublingual immunotherapy may be prescribed also in polysensititized patients. Int J Immunopathol Pharmacol. 2010;23:637e640.
34. Malling H-J, Montagut AM, Patriarca G, et al. Efficacy and safety of 5-grass pollen sublingual immunotherapy tablets in patients with different clinical profiles of allergic rhinoconjunctivitis. Clin Exp Allergy. 2009;39:387–93.
35. Cox LS, Casale TB, Nayak AS, et al. Clinical efficacy of 300IR 5-gass pollen sublingual tablet in a US study: the importance of allergen-specific serum IgE. J Allergy Clin Immunol. 2012;130:1327–34.
36. Esch RE. Specific immunotherapy in the U.S.A.: general concept and recent initiatives. Arb Paul Ehrlich Inst Bundesamt Sera Impfstoffe Frankf AM. 2003;94:17–22.
37. Cox L, Nelson H, Lockey R, Calabria C, Chacko T, Finegold I, et al. Allergen immunotherapy: a practice parameter third update. J Allergy Clin Immunol. 2011;127:S1–55.
38. USP. https://www.usp.org/compounding/general-chapter-797. Accessed 4 Feb 2021.
39. Shaker MS, Wallace DV, Golden DBK, Oppenheimer J, et al. Anaphylaxis-a 2020 practice parameter update, systematic review, and grading of recommendations, assessment, development and evaluation (GRADE) analysis. J Allergy Clin Immunol. 2020;145(4):1082–123.
40. Bousquet J, Hejjaoui A, Dhivert H, Clauzel AM, Michel FB. Immunotherapy with a standardized Dermatophagoides pteronyssinus extract. Systemic reactions during the rush protocol in patients suffering from asthma. J Allergy Clin Immunol. 1989;83(4):797–802.
41. Sharkey P, Portnoy J. Rush immunotherapy: experience with a one-day schedule. Ann Allergy Asthma Immunol. 1996;76(2):175–80.
42. Tabar AI, Echechipía S, García BE, Olaguibel JM, et al. Double-blind comparative study of cluster and conventional immunotherapy schedules with Dermatophagoides pteronyssinus. J Allergy Clin Immunol. 2005;116(1):109–18.
43. Lambert N, Guiddir T, Amat F, Just J. Pre-treatment by omalizumab allows allergen immunotherapy in children and young adults with severe allergic asthma. Pediatr Allergy Immunol. 2014;25(8):829–32.
44. Casale TB, Busse WW, Kline JN, Ballas ZK, et al. Omalizumab pretreatment decreases acute reactions after rush immunotherapy for ragweed-induced seasonal allergic rhinitis. J Allergy Clin Immunol. 2006;117(1):134–40.
45. Valenta R, Campana R, Focke-Tejkl M, Niederberger V. Vaccine development for allergen-specific immunotherapy based on recombinant allergens and synthetic allergen peptides: lessons from the past and novel mechanisms of action for the future. J Allergy Clin Immunol. 2016;137(2):351–7.
46. Pauli G, Larsen TH, Rak S, Horak F, et al. Efficacy of recombinant birch pollen vaccine for the treatment of birch-allergic rhinoconjunctivitis. J Allergy Clin Immunol. 2008;122(5):951–60.
47. Frew AJ, et al. Efficacy and safety of specific immunotherapy with SQ allergen extract in treatment-resistant seasonal allergic rhinoconjunctivitis. J Allergy Clin Immunol. 2006;117:319–25.
48. Nelson HS. Long-term immunotherapy with aqueous and aluminum-precipitated grass extracts. Ann Allergy. 1980;45(6):333–7.

19 SLIT: Aqueous Preparation and Dosing

Katie M. Phillips

Sublingual Immunotherapy

There are two types of sublingual immunotherapy (SLIT) currently available in clinical practice which include sublingual self-dissolving allergen tablets and sublingual allergen extract liquid drops. While oral immunotherapy was first proposed in the early 1900s, it was not until the 1980s that the first SLIT clinical trials using specific allergens were undertaken. It then took three more decades for the World Allergy Organization to propose SLIT as a feasible alternative to subcutaneous immunotherapy (SCIT), which was the standard of care in regard to immunotherapy at the time. This late adoption of SLIT is likely secondary to the heterogeneity of study design and dosing regimens in the early SLIT clinical trials. These early trials were for the most part completed in Europe and used the same glycerinated-saline allergen extracts prescribed for SCIT and therefore sublingual allergen extract liquid drops were the first type of SLIT popularized, mainly in Europe. With more rigorous study design and landmark double-blind placebo-controlled clinical trials, SLIT gained more popularity in both Europe and the United States (US). Subsequently, the dissolving sublingual tablet was designed for specific allergens and has also increased in acceptance with recent Federal Drug Administration (FDA) approval in the US in 2014. See Table 19.1 for a list of SLIT products with evidence-based regimens.

SLIT works by decreasing allergen sensitivity via promoting immune tolerance and decreasing the inflammatory reaction to the specific allergen via multiple mechanisms with the goal of reducing allergy symptoms during SLIT and after therapy is completed. The following paragraph briefly describes the overall mechanism of action of SLIT, however many details are yet to be elucidated. When SLIT is placed sublingually, the allergen is taken up by the dendritic cells within the oral mucosa, cleaved into smaller peptides and then presented to T cells which produces a systemic immune response with both an early and later response. The early response includes a decrease in mast cells and basophil degranulation. A later adaptive response via both the humoral and cellular immune system includes an increase in allergen-specific IgG4 and concomitant decrease in allergen-specific IgE as well as an overall decrease in T helper type 2-dependent inflammation and suppression of B cell isotype switching to IgE [1].

To use SLIT, patients are instructed to hold either the tablet under their tongue until the tablet dissolves or hold the solution under their tongue for a specified time period and then swallow the

K. M. Phillips (✉)
Otolaryngology – Head & Neck Surgery, University of Cincinnati, Cincinnati, OH, USA

C. Damask et al. (eds.), *Allergy in Otolaryngology Practice*,
https://doi.org/10.1007/978-3-031-93455-1_19

Table 19.1 Sublingual immunotherapy products with evidence-based regimens

Allergen extract	Manufacturer	Buildup period	Maintenance dose	Dosing regimen
5-grass [7, 8]	ALK-Abello	No	5 drops of 25 BU/ml, 5x/week	Coseasonal
Ragweed [9, 10]	Greer laboratories, Inc.	Yes (rapid)	2 options: 50 Amb a 1-U daily OR 48 Amb a 1-U, daily	Pre and Coseasonal
House dust mite [11, 12]	ALK-Abello	Yes	1.12 ug of group 1 HDM allergen, 0.56 ug of group 2 HDM allergen, BID	Year round
House dust mite [11, 12]	Anallergo	Yes	5 drops 10,000 RAST/mL 3x/week	Year round
Birch tree [13, 14]	Stallergenes S. A.	Yes	300 IR daily	Pre and Coseasonal
Birch tree [13, 14]	HAL allergy B.V.	Yes	5 drops of 40,000 AUN/mL daily	Pre and Coseasonal
Japanese Cedar Pollen [15]	Torii Pharmaceutical Co, Ltd.	Yes	2000 JAU daily	Pre and Coseasonal
Cat Dander [16]	Laboratorios LETI, S.L.	Yes	0.51 ug/ml fed d1 daily	Year round
Mold (Alternaria) [17, 18]	Anallergo	Yes	5 drops 10,000 RAST units QOD	Pre and Coseasonal
Mold (Alternaria) [17, 18]	ALK-Abello	No	1 vial daily (cumulative monthly dose 3.6 ug/month)	Year round

remaining substance. The advantages to SLIT over SCIT include the ability to self-administer at home after the first dose, no need for injections, and the relatively lower risk of anaphylaxis. Listed disadvantages include higher cost as more allergen is often used in product formation, difficulty with daily compliance, decreased ability to treat the polysensitized patient, and perceived decreased efficacy relative to SCIT although there are few head-to-head trials with inconclusive results at this time.

The indications for SLIT vary by country. In the US, SLIT is approved for seasonal allergic rhinitis or allergic rhinoconjunctivitis for patients monosensitized to grasses or ragweed or in perennial allergic rhinitis or rhinoconjunctivitis for patients monosensitized to house dust mite products. In contrast, US practitioners often use SCIT in patients who have clinical sensitivity to multiple aeroallergens. In Europe, in addition to allergic rhinitis or rhinoconjunctivitis (seasonal or perennial), house dust mite-associated allergic asthma also serves as an indication for SLIT [2]. Contraindications to SLIT include severe or uncontrolled asthma, eosinophilic esophagitis, hypersensitivity to an ingredient with the formulation or previous severe local reaction to SLIT. Patients are also recommended to temporarily stop SLIT in the setting of an asthma exacerbation or oral mucosal injury such as thrush, lichen planus, or mucosal laceration.

One unique aspect of the liquid formulation of SLIT includes the ability to combine multiple different allergens to treat the multi-sensitized or pauci-sensitized allergic patient. While not FDA-approved or verified with large clinical trials for this use, some practitioners will combine multiple liquid SCIT extracts in one vial to treat a patient's corresponding allergen sensitivities. The dosing regimen, amount of each allergen to include, safety, and efficacy has not been well elucidated for this method. In contrast, SLIT tablets contain only one allergen and therefore are used for the mono-sensitized allergic patient. Interestingly, there is increasing evidence that the decrease in allergic immune response to one particular allergen may have cross-reactivity with other allergens in the multi-sensitized patient and therefore immunotherapy to one particular allergen may still be of use to the multi-sensitized patient.

SLIT: Liquid Preparation

This section will focus on the allergen extract liquid drops and the following section will address sublingual allergen tablets.

While liquid regimens and preparations have been proposed, there are currently no US FDA-approved liquid formulations. Yet, the "off-label" use of sublingual liquid drops is practiced in the US, with a recent survey of US allergists reporting that 23.4% use both FDA-approved SLIT tablets and SLIT drops (using extract that is FDA approved for SCIT) and 8% of surveyed US allergists reporting use of only SLIT drops [3]. Although the SCIT drops are FDA approved for SCIT, the safety and effective dose for SLIT of each product has not been rigorously studied and therefore not recommended by the FDA or the American Academy of Allergy, Asthma & Immunology/American College of Allergy, Asthma & Immunology Joint Task Force [4]. In contrast in Europe, SLIT in both tablet and liquid form has been used over the last three to four decades. Yet despite this long-term use in Europe, there is variability within methods of administration, types of products used, the specific dosing recommended, and indications for use. Specific guidelines have been made in an attempt to address this heterogeneity [5]. In regard to other areas of the world, the World Allergy Organization put out a position paper with an update in 2013, which describes the global status of SLIT and includes several clinical guidelines from various countries around the world [6].

To speak further to heterogeneity among various SLIT liquid products, it is important to note manufacturers often use in-house assays which are not standardized across the industry and thus report dosing in different units often unique to the manufacturer. Additionally, each allergen extract may have different inherent properties which impact development of the product and stability in liquid form thus introducing more variability among extracts. Finally, most dosing is based on the randomized clinical trial which showed safety and efficacy and therefore is also not standardized across different extracts. With this in mind, the following sectioning outlining different products will have different units of measures and dosing protocols based on the clinical trials which showed efficacy and safety for each product.

Specific Products

Please refer to Table 19.1 which outlines the products listed below.

Grass Extract

This is a liquid formation made by ALK-Abello (Horsham, Denmark) which contains five grass allergens including orchard (Dactylis glomerata), perennial rye (Lolium perenne), meadow fescue (Fetuca pratensis), timothy (Phleum pretense), and Kentucky blue grass (Poa pratensis) in an aqueous solution. The recommended dosing is a single maintenance dose of 5 drops of 25 Biologic unit (BU)/mL (0.5 ug/mL) five times per week during pollen season for 3 years [7]. This recommendation is based on a randomized control trial published in 2004 which randomized 113 children (ages 5–14) with allergic rhinoconjunctivitis with sensitivity limited to grass pollen to once daily grass liquid extract drops via SLIT during pollen season for 3 years versus standard symptomatic medical therapy. The authors found the control group had a higher risk (relative risk (RR) 3.8, 95% confidence interval, 1.5–10.0) of developing asthma relative to the SLIT group after 3 years of coseasonal SLIT therapy [8].

Ragweed Pollen

A glycerinated liquid formulation of ragweed extract made by Greer Laboratories, Inc. (Lenoir, NC, USA) has been included in two large studies with slightly different dosing. The first study was a phase III randomized, placebo-controlled trial of adult patients with allergic rhinoconjunctivitis sensitized to ragweed who were randomized to using 50 Ambrosia artemisiifolia 1-unit (Amb a 1-U) starting approximately 8–16 weeks prior to ragweed season and continuing through ragweed season versus placebo. The group using the ragweed extract SLIT had improved symptom and medication scores at the end of the season relative to the placebo group. The occurrence of adverse events was similar between the two groups with all local site reactions being transient and self-limited and no anaphylaxis occurring in either group [9]. In a second study, adult patients with ragweed-induced allergic rhinoconjunctivitis were randomized to a placebo group, a medium-dose extract group (4.8 Amb a 1-U) or a high-dose extract group (48 Amb a 1-U) administered 8–10 weeks prior to ragweed season. Both treatment groups had a 15% reduction in symptom scores compared to placebo during the ragweed season, but the difference was not statistically significant. In subsequent analysis of covariance, where preseasonal symptoms were corrected for, the authors found the mean daily symptom scores and medication scores were significantly reduced in the high-dose treatment group relative to the placebo group. Adverse events were similarly reported among the three groups but oral-mucosal adverse events occurred more commonly in the treatment groups [10].

House Dust Mite

Long-term efficacy of liquid house dust mite allergen SLIT has been shown in 2 prospective trials following children and adults for 10 and 15 years respectively, although the product and dosing was different between the two trials [11, 12]. The first trial followed children with allergic rhinitis sensitive to house dust mites and compared a group who underwent SLIT for 5 years versus a group controlled with medical therapy during the same time frame. The SLIT regimen was an extract of Dermatophagoides pteronyssinus and Dermatophagoides farina in equal proportion (Alk-Abello, Horsham, Denmark) which included a 30-day induction phase with gradual increase in the dose until reaching a maintenance dose. The maintenance dose was 1.12 ug of group 1 mite allergen and 0.56 ug of group 2 allergen to be taken twice weekly. At the end of 5 years, those in the SLIT group had improvement in asthma severity and decreased use of asthma medication relative to their baseline and upon 5 more years of follow-up without SLIT these findings remained consistent. In contrast, the medical therapy group did not see a change in baseline from the beginning of the study in regard to asthma severity and use of asthma medication [11]. The other long-term prospective trial evaluated adults with allergic rhinitis and bronchial hyperreactivity with or without over asthma monosensitized to dust mites and divided the participants into four groups including those undergoing medical management only and those undergoing either 3, 4 or 5 years of SLIT therapy. These participants were then followed for 15 years. The SLIT formulation was a glycerinated solution (Anallergo, Florence, Italy) with a 50-day build-up phase, followed by a maintenance regimen of 5 drops from a vial containing 10,000 radioallergosorbent test (RAST) units/mL 3 times per week for a mean cumulative dose per year of 390 ug of Der p1/Der p 2 (about 10 times greater than the corresponding SCIT course). The authors found no relevant change in the control group. In the 3-year SLIT group, clinical benefit was noted up to 7 years while in the 4 and 5-year SLIT group, clinic benefit persisted up to 8 years. A second course of SLIT was given after decrease in clinical benefit and return of clinical benefit was noted more rapidly relative to the first course of SLIT. Objective clinical measures paralleled clinical benefit scores [12].

Birch Tree Pollen

There have been two large double-blind, placebo-controlled, multi-institutional studies evaluating liquid birch pollen extract SLIT with two different formulations. The first study randomized adults with allergic rhinoconjunctivitis monosensitized to birch pollen to receive 300 Index of reactivity (IR) birch pollen sublingual solution daily versus placebo starting 4 months prior to pollen season and to continue through pollen season for two consecutive pollen seasons in a pre- and co-seasonal manner. The liquid extract was provided by Stallergenes S.A. (Antony, France). Of note, there was a 12-day build-up period of daily dose escalation with the following regimen: 1, 2, 4, 6, 8, 10, 30, 60, 120, 180, 240, and 300 IR/day. After the second pollen season, the symptom scores were significantly lower in the treatment group (30.6% reduction) relative to the placebo group. The local side effects were well tolerated in the treatment group without report of anaphylaxis [13]. The second study mentioned is a phase III trial which investigated the safety and efficacy of sublingual liquid birch pollen extract (40,000 allergy units native (AUN)/mL made by HAL Allergy B.V., Leiden, Netherlands) in adults with allergic rhinoconjunctivitis with or without asthma monosensitized to birch pollen. The birch pollen (Betula verrucosa [Bet v 1]) content of the product was 0.4 mg/mL as measured by the EDQM-Bet v 1 reference preparation. Participants were randomized to SLIT versus placebo and received treatment 3–6 months prior to pollen season and continued during the season. There was a brief build-up period where patients started with 1 drop of the solution and increased by 1 drop daily until reaching the maintenance dose of 5 drops daily. In the treatment group, there was a significant and clinically relevant (32%) reduction in total symptom and medication score relative to placebo. The birch pollen extract SLIT was also noted to be well tolerated with a good safety profile in the treatment group [14].

Japanese Cedar Pollen

The most common cause of allergic rhinoconjunctivitis in Japan is attributed to Japanese cedar pollen. A phase III randomized, double-blind, placebo-controlled multi-institutional study was performed to evaluate the efficacy and safety of an oral solution of Japanese cedar pollen made by Cedartolen, Torii Pharmaceutical Co, Ltd. (Tokyo, Japan). Adult participants with allergic rhinoconjunctivitis monosensitized to Japanese cedar pollen were randomized to receive either daily SLIT with a maintenance dose of 2000 Japanese allergy units (JAU)/day or placebo starting 4 months prior to the predicted allergy season and continued until the end of the second allergy season. There was an initial build-up period of 2 weeks where the dose was escalated from 40 JAU/day to 2000 JAU/day. The total nasal symptom and medication score was significantly lower ($p < 0.0001$) in the SLIT group relative to placebo by 18% and 30% reduction in the first and second season respectively. The SLIT was noted to be well tolerated without recorded anaphylaxis [15].

Cat Dander

Group 1 major cat allergen (Fel d 1) is the major cat allergen, and of those with cat allergy, approximately 80% are sensitized to Fel d1. A relatively small ($n = 50$) randomized, double-blind, placebo-controlled trial was performed to evaluate cat dander extract (Laboratorios LETI, S.L., Barcelona, Spain). Cat allergic participants with allergic rhinoconjunctivitis with or without asthma were randomized to cat extract SLIT (0.51 ug/mL Fed d1) for 1 year versus placebo. There was a build-up phase with an accumulated dose of 1.7 ug of Fel d 1 over a several-week period until the maintenance dose was reached (0.51 ug/mL/day). The active treatment group showed marked reduction (62%) in symptoms based on a natural exposure challenge test, a reduced peak expiratory flow response to cat exposure, and an improvement in skin test reactivity to standardized cat extract. No significant changes in these primary outcomes were observed in the placebo group. Of note, only 66% of participants ($n = 33$) were able to complete the study. No local or systemic reactions were reported and none of the 17 withdrawals were triggered by an adverse reaction [16].

Mold (Alternaria Extract)

Two relatively small trials have been conducted evaluating SLIT for Alternaria sensitivity using two different products. The first trial is a randomized double-blind, placebo-controlled trial of adolescents and adults ($n = 27$) with allergic rhinitis with or without intermittent asthma monosensitized to Alternaria randomized to SLIT versus placebo for 10 months. Those in the SLIT group were started on a buildup phase of 15 days starting with 1 drop from the 100 RAST units vial of Alternaria major allergen (Alt a 1) made by Anallergo (Firenze, Italy) and up-titrated until the maintenance dose (5 drops of 10,000 RAST units) was taken on alternate days for 10 months. The content of Alt a 1 was 1.5 ug/mL in the 10,000 RAST unit vial. Those in the treatment group had a significant improvement in symptoms, reduction in medication, decrease in skin prick reactivity, and specific Alt a 1 IgE level increase. These changes were not observed in the placebo group. Minimal adverse reactions were reported with no report of anaphylaxis [17]. The other trial used SLITOne Alternaria alternata made by ALK-Abello (Horsham, Denmark). This study was a randomized, parallel group study ($n = 52$) of adults with allergic rhinitis with or without mild to moderate asthma monosensitized to Alternaria who were divided 2:1 into a treatment group who received SLIT (1 vial per day without a buildup period for 3 years) and a control group who were treated with standard of care. The SLIT product contained Alt a 1 as the major allergen. The cumulative monthly dose was 3.6 ug/month. After 3 years, the treatment group had significant improvement in patient-reported visual analog scale of symptoms and rescue medication use relative to the control group. Mild and transient adverse treatment effects were reported in the treatment group without reported anaphylaxis [18].

References

1. Sahin E, Bafaqeeh SA, Gulseven S, et al. Mechanism of action of allergen immunotherapy. Am J Rhinol Allergy. 2016;30(5):1–3.
2. Virchow JC, Backer V, Kuna P, et al. Efficacy of a house dust mite sublingual allergen immunotherapy tablet in adults with allergic asthma: a randomized clinical trial. JAMA. 2016;315:1715–25.
3. Sivam A, Tankersley M. American College of Allergy, asthma, and immunology immunotherapy and diagnostics committee. Perception and practice of sublingual immunotherapy among practicing allergists in the United States: a follow-up survey. Ann Allergy Asthma Immunol. 2019;122(6):623–9.
4. Greenhawt M, Oppenheimer J, Nelson M, et al. Sublingual immunotherapy: a focused allergen immunotherapy practice parameter. Ann Allergy Asthma Immunol. 2017;118(3):276–82.
5. Muraro A, Roberts G, Halken S, et al. EAACI guidelines on allergen immunotherapy: executive statement. Allergy. 2018;73(4):739–43.
6. Canonica GW, Cox L, Pawankar R, et al. Sublingual immunotherapy: world allergy organization position paper 2013 update. World Allergy Organ J. 2014;7(1):6.
7. Jin JJ, Li JT, Klimek L, Pfaar O. Sublingual immunotherapy dosing regimens: what is ideal? J Allergy Clin Immunol Pract. 2017;5(1):1–10.
8. Novembre E, Galli E, Landi F, et al. Coseasonal sublingual immunotherapy reduces the development of asthma in children with allergic rhinoconjunctivitis. J Allergy Clin Immunol. 2004;114:851–7.
9. Creticos PS, Esch RE, Couroux P, et al. Randomized, double-blind, placebo-controlled trial of standardized ragweed sublingual-liquid immunotherapy for allergic rhinoconjunctivitis. J Allergy Clin Immunol. 2014;133:751–8.
10. Skoner D, Gentile D, Bush R, Fasano MB, McLaughlin A, Esch RE. Sublingual immunotherapy in patients with allergic rhinoconjunctivitis caused by ragweed pollen. J Allergy Clin Immunol. 2010;125(660–6):666.e1–4.
11. Di Rienzo V, Marcucci F, Puccinelli P, et al. Long lasting effect of sublingual immunotherapy in children with asthma due to house dust mite: a 10-year prospective study. Clin Exp Allergy. 2003;33:206–10.
12. Marogna M, Spadolini I, Massolo A, Canonica GW, Passalacqua G. Long lasting effects of sublingual immunotherapy according to its duration: a 15-year prospective study. J Allergy Clin Immunol. 2010;126:969–75.

13. Worm M, Rak S, de Blay F, et al. Sustained efficacy and safety of a 300IR daily dose of a sublingual solution of birch pollen allergen extract in adults with allergic rhinoconjunctivitis: results of a double blind, placebo-controlled study. Clin Transl Allergy. 2014;4:7.
14. Pfaar O, Bachert C, Kuna P, et al. Sublingual allergen immunotherapy with a liquid birch pollen product in patients with seasonal allergic rhinoconjunctivitis with or without asthma. J allergy Clin Immunool. 2019;142(3):970–7.
15. Okamoto Y, Okubo K, Yonekura S, et al. Efficacy and safety of sublingual immunotherapy for two seasons in patients with Japanese cedar pollinosis. Int Arch Allergy Immunol. 2015;166:177–88.
16. Álvarez-Cuesta E, Berges-Gimeno P, Mancebo EG, Fernández-Caldas E, Cuesta-Herranz J, Casanovas M. Sublingual immunotherapy with a standardized cat dander extract: evaluation of efficacy in a double blind placebo controlled study. Allergy. 2007;62:810–7.
17. Cortellini G, Spadolini I, Patella V, et al. Sublingual immunotherapy for Alternaria-induced allergic rhinitis: a randomized placebo-controlled trial. Ann Allergy Asthma Immunol. 2010;105:382–6.
18. Pozzan M, Milani M. Efficacy of sublingual specific immunotherapy in patients with respiratory allergy to Alternaria alternata: a randomised, assessor-blinded, patient-reported outcome, controlled 3-year trial. Curr Med Res Opin. 2010;26:2801–6.

Sublingual Immunotherapy: Tablets

20

Katie M. Phillips

Sublingual Immunotherapy Tablets

While the concept of allergic immunotherapy has been around for about a century, the first clinical trials of specific allergens using sublingual immunotherapy (SLIT) did not come about until the 1980s. Currently, in the United States (US), four sublingual immunotherapy (SLIT) tablets have FDA approval for treating seasonal allergic rhinitis, in those sensitized to ragweed and grasses, and in perennial allergic rhinitis in those sensitized to house dust mites. SLIT tablets are often used for patients monosensitized to one of the above-mentioned allergens, whereas subcutaneous immunotherapy (SCIT) is often for the polysensitized allergic patients. The first dose, and subsequent 30 min after taking the first dose, is observed in the office setting and then patients are able to do the remainder of their doses at home. Patients are instructed to place the tablet under the tongue and let it completely dissolve, with specific instructions to not swallow for 1 min. In the case of oral inflammation or mucosal defects, patients are instructed to stop their SLIT until oral mucosa is healed. Contraindications for SLIT tablets in the US include severe or uncontrolled asthma, eosinophilic esophagitis or history of severe systemic allergic reactions. Additionally, when prescribing SLIT tablets in the US, practitioners must also prescribe an epinephrine autoinjector with the tablets for the rare case of anaphylaxis [1].

Prescribing practices and patterns are similar in Europe with some exceptions. House dust mite SLIT tablets are used in allergic asthma in Europe. Additionally, throughout Europe there are different national preferences for products and therapeutic options including SLIT and SCIT based on region as well as different payer authorizations based on country [1]. The World Allergy Organization put out a position paper with an update in 2013, which describes the global status of SLIT and includes several clinical guidelines from various countries around the world [2]. Table 20.1 lists the commercially available sublingual tablets as of 2020.

Single-Grass Pollen Tablet

This product is named GRASTEK and is made by ALK-Abello (Horsham, Denmark) and is indicated in people ages 5–65 for patients with allergic rhinitis or allergic rhinoconjunctivitis sensitized to Timothy grass or cross-reactive grass pollens. The tablet contains 2800 Bioequivalent Allergy units (BAUs) and is dosed once daily with the intention to start at least

K. M. Phillips (✉)
Otolaryngology – Head & Neck Surgery, University of Cincinnati, Cincinnati, OH, USA

C. Damask et al. (eds.), *Allergy in Otolaryngology Practice*,
https://doi.org/10.1007/978-3-031-93455-1_20

Table 20.1 Commercially available sublingual tablets

Allergen extract	Manufacturer	Buildup period	Maintenance dose	Dosing regimen
Single grass (GRASTEK)	ALK-Abello	No	2800 BAU daily (15 mcg of Phl P 5) [3]	Pre and Coseasonal
5-grass (ORALAIR)	Stallergenes S.A.	Yes (only in children 5–17)	300 IR daily [7] (20–25 mcg of group 5 allergen)	Pre and Coseasonal
Ragweed (RAGWITEK)	ALK-Abello	No	12 Amb a 1-U daily (12 mcg) [12]	Pre and Coseasonal
House dust mite (ODACTRA, ACARIZAX, MITICURE)	ALK-Abello	No	12 SQ (15 mcg of Der 1 and 15 mcg of Der 2) [15]	Year round
House dust mite (ACTAIR)	Stallergenes S.A.	Yes	300 IR daily (16mcg of Der P1 68 mcg of Der F1) [18]	Year round
Japanese cedar pollen (CEDARCURE)	Torii Pharmaceutical Co, Ltd.	Yes	5000 JAU daily [21]	Pre and Coseasonal

12 weeks prior to the expected onset of grass pollen season with continuation throughout the season. The tablet can be used for three consecutive pollen seasons. Adverse reactions have been reported in ≤5% of patients and include ear pruritus, oral pruritus, tongue pruritus, mouth edema and throat irritation [3]. This information was based on several clinical trials, three of which focused on efficacy and safety of the 2800 BAU dose, and will be highlighted here.

The first study discussed is a phase III randomized, double-blind, placebo-controlled trial which included adults with allergic rhinoconjunctivitis with or without asthma polysensitized to grass and compared those in the active treatment group who underwent single-grass pollen SLIT tablet for 3 years to placebo with follow up for 2 years after completion of SLIT and found a reduced total symptom and medication score and long-lasting significant effect on allergen-specific antibody response in the treatment group relative to the placebo group. Participants started the sublingual tablets 4–8 months prior to the grass pollen season and continued for 3 subsequent years until the end of the third grass pollen season [4]. Next, a study of children (ages 5–16) with rhinoconjunctivitis with or without asthma were enrolled in a randomized, double-blind, placebo-controlled trial where participants were given either a placebo tablet or single grass pollen SLIT tablets. Tablets were started 8–23 weeks prior to grass pollen season and continued throughout the season. Total symptom and medication scores were reduced in the treatment group relative to placebo without serious adverse events related to treatment reported [5]. The last study highlighted was a large (n = 1501) randomized, double-blind, placebo-controlled trial which included children and adults from North America and again confirmed the results of the prior two studies discussed [6].

5-Grass Tablet

This product is named ORALAIR and is made by Stallergenes S.A. (Antony, France) and is indicated in 5–65-year-old people with the diagnosis of allergic rhinitis with or without conjunctivitis sensitized to grass pollen. The tablet contains mixed grass pollen allergen extract including Sweet Vernal, Orchard, Perennial Rye, Timothy, and Kentucky Blue Grass. In children aged 5–17, the dosing includes a buildup phase with 100 index of reactivity (IR) on day 1, two tablets of 100 IR on day 2 and then on day 3 patients achieve maintenance daily dosing of 300 IR. In adults (age 18–65), patients are immediately started on the maintenance daily dosing of 300 IR without a buildup period. The manufacturer reports the 300 IR tablet contains approximately 25 ug of the major group 5 allergens. It is recommended to start the tablet 4 months before the expected onset of each grass pollen season and continuing the tablet through the pollen season. Adverse reactions are reported in ≤5% and include oral pruritus, throat irritation, ear pruritus, mouth edema, tongue pruritus, cough, asthma, oropharyngeal pain, tonsillitis, and oral paresthesia [7]. This information was based on data from several clinical trials, some of which are highlighted below.

A randomized, double-blind, placebo-controlled study of 278 children (age 5–17) with allergic rhinoconjunctivitis sensitized to grass were randomized to SLIT versus placebo which was initiated 4 months prior to grass pollen season and continued throughout the season. The buildup period was 3 days, starting at 100 IR and building to 300 IR at day 3. At the end of season, those in the treatment group had significant improvement in total symptom and medication score relative to the placebo group with generally mild to moderate adverse events reported [8]. Next a group looked at safety and efficacy of this tablet in adults in the 2 years following 3 years of SLIT therapy. A randomized, double-blind, placebo-controlled, parallel group study ($n = 633$) evaluated adults with allergic rhinoconjunctivitis sensitized to grass and divided participants into a group using 300 IR 5-grass tablet SLIT initiated 4 months prior to grass pollen season, initiated 2 months prior to grass pollen season and placebo for 3 years in a discontinuous pre- and co-seasonal protocol. Participants were then followed for two more years after discontinuation of treatment. No build-up phase when initiating SLIT was used. During the first post-treatment year, both treatment groups showed efficacy with significant difference versus placebo in the total symptom and rescue medication score. However, in the second year post-treatment, only the group who started SLIT 4 months prior to pollen season showed significant differences in symptom and rescue medication use scores relative to placebo [9]. Other studies showed similar efficacy and safety with level I evidence of the 5-Grass tablet SLIT [10, 11].

Ragweed Pollen Tablet

This product is named RAGWITEK and made by ALK-Abello (Horsham, Denmark). RAGWITEK is indicated in adults ages 18 to 65 with allergic rhinitis with or without conjunctivitis with confirmed hypersensitivity to ragweed pollen allergen. The recommended dose is 1 tablet daily which contains 12 Ambrosia artemisiifolia 1-unit (Amb a 1-U) to start 12 weeks before ragweed pollen season and continue through the season. Adverse events are reported ≤5% and include throat irritation, oral pruritus, ear pruritus, oral paresthesia, mouth edema, and tongue pruritus [12]. FDA product approval was based on several clinical trials with two of the pertinent trials which focus on safety and efficacy summarized here.

The first is a large ($n = 784$) randomized, double-blind, placebo-controlled trial of adults with allergic rhinoconjunctivitis induced by ragweed pollen which randomly assigned adults to 4 groups including, placebo, 1.5, 6, or 12 Amb a 1-U SLIT tablets. No build-up phase was given and participants started therapy approximately 16 weeks prior to ragweed pollen season and continued for 52 weeks. During ragweed season, participants in the 6 and 12 Amb a 1-U groups saw significant reduction in total symptom and medication scores relative to placebo, with greater reduction in the 12 Amb a 1-U group. Treatment was well tolerated in all groups without systemic adverse events reported and therefore authors concluded the 12 Amb a 1-U dose was effective and well tolerated [13]. A subsequent study pooled data from four randomized, double-blind, placebo-controlled trials investigating the ragweed pollen sublingual tablet to better understand safety and tolerability of the various doses studied. Across all 4 trials (n = 757, 198, 454, 1058), adult participants with allergic rhinoconjunctivitis induced by ragweed pollen allergen were randomized to placebo or 1.5, 6, or 12 Amb a 1-U SLIT tablets. Treatment-related adverse events were more common in the 6 and 12 Amb a 1-U groups and were primarily limited to local site reactions in the first days of treatment. One systemic anaphylactic reaction did occur leading to a published rate of anaphylaxis of 0.06% [14].

House Dust Mite Tablet

There are currently two house dust mite allergen extract SLIT tablets on the market globally, however only ODACTRA has US FDA approval.

ODACTRA is a product made by ALK-Abello (Horsham, Denmark) and contains house dust mite allergen extract including both dermatophagoides farina and dermatophagoides pteronyssinus. Of note, this product is marketed under the name ACARIZAX in Europe and Australia and MITICURE in Japan. In the US, this tablet is approved for adults (18–65) with allergic rhinitis with or without conjunctivitis provoked by house dust mites. In Europe and Australia, this product also has an indication to treat allergic asthma induced by house dust mites in addition to allergic rhinoconjunctivitis. The recommended dosing is 1 tablet daily without a buildup period. Each tablet contains 12 standardized quality (SQ) house dust mite allergen extract. Adverse reactions are reported in ≤10% of subjects and include throat irritation, itching in the mouth, itching in the ear, swelling of uvula, swelling of the lips, swelling of the tongue, nausea, tongue pain, throat swelling, tongue ulceration, stomach pain, mouth ulcer, and taste alteration [15]. Several clinical trials led to development and approval of this tablet and this section will highlight two of these pertinent studies.

The first study is a large (n = 992) randomized, double-blind, placebo-controlled phase III trial which evaluated adults with house dust mite-induced allergic rhinitis and divided participants into 1 year of treatment with placebo, 6 SQ house dust mite allergen extract SLIT or 12 SQ house dust mite allergen extract SLIT. Both the 6SQ SLIT and 12SQ SLIT group saw significant improvement in the absolute reduction in combined rhinitis score compared to placebo. The 12SQ SLIT group also had significant reductions in all secondary endpoints of the study including reduction in combined rhinitis and medication score, improved quality of life and reduced rhinoconjunctivitis score. Both treatment groups reported good tolerance of the SLIT therapy [16]. The following study highlights the efficacy of house dust mite SLIT in allergic asthma. Virchow et al. conducted a large (n = 834) randomized, double-blind, placebo-controlled study of adults with house dust mite-induced allergic asthma and allergic rhinitis. Patients were randomized to treatment with placebo versus house dust mite allergen SLIT (either 6SQ or 12SQ) in addition to an inhaled corticosteroid and short-acting beta2 agonist. In both SLIT treatment groups, there was a significant reduction in risk of moderate or severe asthma exacerbation compared to placebo, but no significant change in asthma quality of life or asthma control questionnaires relative to placebo. There were no reported severe systemic allergic reactions reported [17]. This study, along with other clinical trials, led to the adoption of house dust mite allergen SLIT for allergic asthma in Europe but not in the US.

The other house dust mite allergen extract sublingual tablet is named ACTAIR and is made by Stallergenes S.A (Antony, France). The tablet is indicated for ages 12 to 65 in the setting of allergic rhinoconjunctivitis induced by house dust mites. The product contains a mixture of dermatophagoides farina and dermatophagoides pteronyssinus. There is a recommended build-up period of 3 days. The initial dose is 100 IR which is uptitrated to 200 IR on the second day and then 300 IR on the third day. The maintenance dose is then 300 IR to be taken daily for 1 year. This product is currently approved in Japan, Australia, South Korea, and New Zealand [18]. One of the initial trials of safety and efficacy for this sublingual tablet is a large (n = 509) randomized, double-blind, placebo-controlled trial of adults with house dust mite associated allergic rhinitis. Participants were divided into 1 year of treatment with either placebo or house dust mite allergen SLIT with either the 300 IR or 500 IR dose. Follow-up continued for 1 year after cessation of immunotherapy. Both SLIT treatment groups had significant reduction in symptom scores relative to placebo both at the cessation of immunotherapy and at the subsequent year follow-up compared to placebo. Adverse events were similar for both treatment groups and limited to local site reactions [19]. A subsequent randomized, double-blind, placebo-controlled trial in Japan was extended to adolescents (ages 12–18) in addition to adults (ages 18–65) with similar results of safety and efficacy of both the 300IR and 500 IR house dust mite extract sublingual tablets [20].

Japanese Cedar Pollen Tablet

The most common cause of allergic rhinoconjunctivitis in Japan is attributed to Japanese cedar pollen. CEDARCURE is a new sublingual tablet made by Torii Pharmaceutical Co, Ltd. (Tokyo, Japan). This tablet is approved in Japan for allergic rhinoconjunctivitis induced by Japanese Cedar pollen. There is a build-up phase of 1 week where patients take a dose of 2000 Japanese allergy units (JAU)/day and then transition to the maintenance dose of 5000 JAU/day [21].

Several clinical trials led to the recommended dosing and approval for this medication including the study highlighted here. This was a large (n = 1042) randomized, double-blind, placebo-controlled study of patients (aged 5–64) with allergic rhinitis induced by Japanese Cedar pollen. Participants were divided into four groups including placebo as well as 3 groups undergoing SLIT at different doses (2000, 5000, and 10,000 JAU/day) with a brief build-up period. Therapy was started 6 months before the Japanese Cedar pollen allergy season. All three treatment groups saw significant reduction in total symptom and medication scores during peak symptom season in the first season. After this first season, 5000 JAU/day was determined to be the optimal dose when balanced between efficacy and tolerated adverse events. Participants in the placebo and 5000 JAU/day groups continued the study and were subdivided into four groups (placebo to stay in placebo, placebo to go active therapy, active therapy to placebo, and active therapy to active therapy) for therapy to continue 2 more years and then observed for 2 years after cessation of SLIT. Those in the treatment group continued to show significant reduction in total symptom and medication scores relative to placebo during the follow-up period. The study confirmed the 5000 JAU/day tablet has good efficacy and safety over a 3-year treatment period [22].

Areas of Future Study

The field of SLIT has changed dramatically over the last decade with 4 sublingual tablets now FDA approved in the US, yet there is much more on the horizon with many areas of active study. With many US practitioners already using liquid allergen extracts for SLIT and approval in Europe, further study of liquid products in the US is ongoing. Additionally, work is being done to understand how food allergies, which are quite prevalent in the US, can be treated with SLIT [23]. Another area of active study involves patients with polyallergy. It has been reported that in patients with allergies, nearly 80% have multiple allergen sensitivities and therefore would benefit from desensitization to more than one allergen. Investigative studies as well as small studies of safety are being done to understand if patients can tolerate simultaneous treatment with two SLIT tablets or multiple allergens in liquid forms of SLIT [24, 25]. Finally, understanding how SLIT and SCIT compare in efficacy, safety, and appropriate patient selection can lead to better personalized care for patients and continues to be an active area of study.

References

1. Mahler V, Esch RE, Kleine-Tebbe J, et al. Understanding differences in allergen immunotherapy products and practices in North America and Europe. J Allergy Clin Immunol. 2019;143(3):813–28.
2. Canonica GW, Cox L, Pawankar R, et al. Sublingual immunotherapy: world allergy organization position paper 2013 update. World Allergy Organ J. 2014;7(1):6.
3. FDA. GRASTEK (R) (Timothy Grass Pollen Allergen Extract) tablet for sublingual use prescribing information. Available from: http://www.fda.gov/downloads/BiologicsBloodVaccines/Allergenics/UCM393184.pdf. Accessed 27 Mar 2020.
4. Durham SR, Emminger W, Kapp A, et al. SQ-standardized sublingual grass immunotherapy:

confirmation of disease modification 2 years after 3 years of treatment in a randomized trial. J Allergy Clin Immunol. 2012;129:717–725.e5.
5. Bufe A, Eberle P, Franke-Beckmann E, Funck J, Kimmig M, Klimek L, et al. Safety and efficacy in children of an SQ-standardized grass allergen tablet for sublingual immunotherapy. J Allergy Clin Immunol. 2009;123:167–73.
6. Maloney J, Bernstein DI, Nelson H, Creticos P, Hebert J, Noonan M, et al. Efficacy and safety of grass sublingual immunotherapy tablet, MK-7243: a large randomized controlled trial. Ann Allergy Asthma Immunol. 2014;112:146–53.
7. FDA. ORALAIR(R) (Sweet Vernal, Orchard, Perennial Rye, Timothy, and Kentucky Blue Grass Mixed Pollens Allergen Extract) tablet for sublingual use prescribing information. Available from: https://www.fda.gov/media/87935/download. Accessed 27 Mar 2020.
8. Wahn U, Tabar A, Kuna P, et al. Efficacy and safety of 5-grass-pollen sublingual immunotherapy tablets in pediatric allergic rhinoconjunctivitis. J Allergy Clin Immunol. 2009;123:160–166.e3.
9. Didier A, Malling HJ, Worm M, Horak F, Sussman GL. Prolonged efficacy of the 300IR 5-grass pollen tablet up to 2 years after treatment cessation, as measured by a recommended daily combined score. Clin Transl Allergy. 2015;5:12.
10. Cox LS, Casale TB, Nayak AS, et al. Clinical efficacy of 300IR 5-grass pollen sublingual tablet in a US study: the importance of allergen-specific serum IgE. J Allergy Clin Immunol. 2012;130:1327–34.
11. Didier A, Worm M, Horak F, et al. Sustained 3-year efficacy of pre- and coseasonal 5-grass-pollen sublingual immunotherapy tablets in patients with grass pollen-induced rhinoconjunctivitis. J Allergy Clin Immunol. 2011;128:559–66.
12. FDA. RAGWITEK(R) (Short Ragweed Pollen Allergen Extract) tablet for sublingual use prescribing information. Available from https://www.fda.gov/media/88712/download. Accessed 27 Mar 2020.
13. Creticos PS, Maloney J, Bernstein DI, et al. Randomized controlled trial of a ragweed allergy immunotherapy tablet in North American and European adults. J Allergy Clin Immunol. 2013;131:1342–9.
14. Nolte H, Amar N, Bernstein DI, et al. Safety and tolerability of a short ragweed sublingual immunotherapy tablet. Ann Allergy Asthma Immunol. 2014;113:93–100.e3.
15. FDA. ODACTRA(R) (House Dust Mite allergen extract) tablet for sublingual use prescribing information. Available from https://www.fda.gov/media/103380/download. Accessed on 27 Mar 2020.
16. Demoly P, Emminger W, Rehm D, Backer V, Tommerup L, Kleine-Tebbe J. Effective treatment of house dust mite-induced allergic rhinitis with 2 doses of the SQ HDM SLIT-tablet: results from a randomized, double-blind, placebo controlled phase III trial. J Allergy Clin Immunol. 2016;137:444–451.e8.
17. Virchow J, Backer V, Kuna P, Prieto L, Nolte H, Vilessen HH, et al. Efficacy of a house dust mite sublingual allergen immunotherapy tablet in adults with allergic asthma: a andomized clinical trial. JAMA. 2016;315:1715–25.
18. MEDSAFE. Product information: ACTAIR 100 IR and 300 IR sublingual tablets. Available from https://www.medsafe.govt.nz/Profs/Datasheet/a/Actairtab.pdf. Accessed on 27 Mar 2020.
19. Bergmann KC, Demoly P, Worm M, et al. Efficacy and safety of sublingual tablets of house dust mite allergen extracts in adults with allergic rhinitis. J Allergy Clin Immunol. 2014;133:1608–14.
20. Okamoto Y, Fujieda S, Okano M, Yoshida Y, Kakuda S, Masuyama K. House dust mite sublingual tablet is effective and safe in patients with allergic rhinitis. Allergy. 2017;72(3):435–43.
21. TORII. Product information: CEDARCURE(R) Japanese Cedar Pollen Sublingual tablet. Available from: https://www.torii.co.jp/en/release/2018/20180524_E.pdf. Accessed on 27 Mar 2020.
22. Gotoh M, Yonekura S, Imai T, et al. Long-term efficacy and dose-finding trial of Japanese cedar pollen sublingual immunotherapy tablet. J Allergy Clin Immunol Pract. 2019;7(4):1287–97.
23. Scurlock AM. Oral and sublingual immunotherapy for treatment of IgE-mediated food allergy. Clin Rev Allergy Immunol. 2018;55(2):139–52.
24. Maloney J, Berman G, Gagnon R, et al. Sequential treatment initiation with Timothy grass and ragweed sublingual immunotherapy tablets followed by simultaneous treatment is well tolerated. J Allergy Clin Immunol Pract. 2016;4(2):301–309.e2.
25. Ortiz AS, McMains KC, Laury AM. Single vs multi-allergen sublingual immunotherapy in the polysensitized patient: a pilot study. Int Forum Allergy Rhinol. 2018;8(4):490–4.

Adverse Reactions in Immunotherapy

21

Haidy Marzouk, Rohan Patel, and Amanda Gemmiti

Introduction

Advances over time with regard to allergy immunotherapy have been impressive and have created dramatic improvements in patients' allergy symptoms and quality of life. It is the only disease-modifying intervention and as such has gained much interest and support [2]. However, as with any form of medical intervention, there are risks associated with such intervention. Efficacy of allergy immunotherapy has been strongly validated in the literature with reduction in allergic symptoms and rescue medication of 30–40% during treatment and 20–30% two years following treatment, with a reported overall adverse event rate of ranging from 20–80% for local reactions and < 1% for systemic reactions [3–5]. Having an in-depth understanding of the different adverse reactions and risks associated with allergy immunotherapy is crucial not only to their diagnosis and management, but also to their prevention. Moreover, discussion of the types of adverse events and their likelihood is important when setting up an allergy practice, patient selection, and the discussion to obtain informed consent.

Education regarding allergy adverse reactions is not only limited to the medical provider, but should also include office staff and the patient. Preparing the office with the appropriate medical equipment, educating staff members on an office protocol to handle an allergy emergency, and counseling patients on signs and symptoms of immunotherapy adverse events along with auto-injectable epinephrine training can mean the difference between life and death in a case of anaphylaxis. Immunotherapy is a treatment for a non-fatal disease process that can have the rare but real possibility of a fatal adverse event. To date, there have been no fatalities with sublingual immunotherapy. However, anaphylaxis with subcutaneous immunotherapy is still a very real concern despite its decline from earlier decades. Data from 2008–2013 showed an overall 1.9% incidence of systemic reaction, 0.2% being considered anaphylactic in nature with 4 patient mortalities identified from SCIT during this time frame [6].

Overall, adverse reactions due to allergy immunotherapy can be separated into two broad categories: non-IgE-mediated and IgE-mediated adverse reactions (Fig. 21.1). The most common non-IgE-mediated adverse reaction is a vasova-

H. Marzouk (✉)
Otolaryngology-Head and Neck Surgery, SUNY Upstate Medical Center and Saint Joseph's Health, Syracuse, NY, USA
e-mail: MARZOUKH@upstate.edu

R. Patel · A. Gemmiti
Otolaryngology-Head and Neck Surgery, SUNY Upstate Medical Center, Syracuse, NY, USA

C. Damask et al. (eds.), *Allergy in Otolaryngology Practice*,
https://doi.org/10.1007/978-3-031-93455-1_21

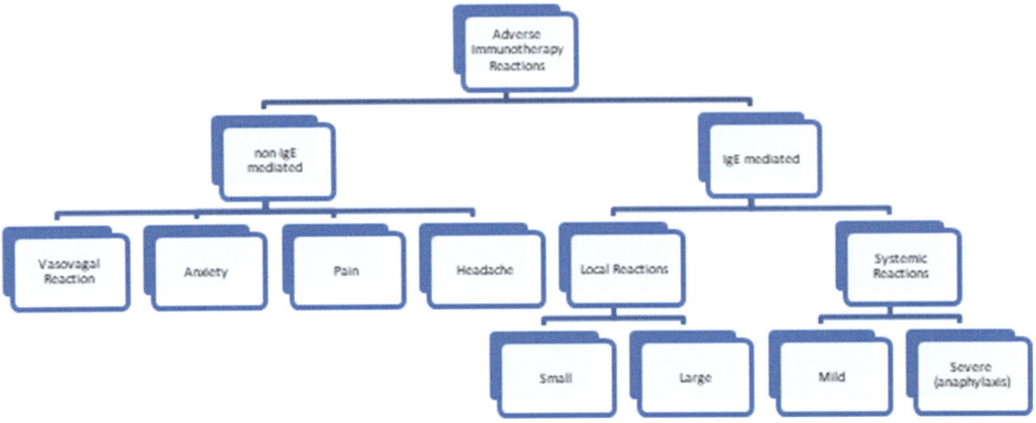

Fig. 21.1 Types of adverse reactions with allergy immunotherapy

gal event. Differentiating a vasovagal event from anaphylaxis is critical and time-sensitive with regard to prognosis and outcome. However, at times distinguishing the two can be challenging. Below we will provide key features of both, their differentiating features, and their various management strategies. Other non-IgE-mediated reactions include headache, anxiety, pain at the injection site, infections, and will be discussed briefly. IgE-mediated adverse reactions to immunotherapy can be further categorized between local reactions, mild systemic reactions, and anaphylaxis. Each of these has similar pathophysiology, but differ in manifestations, severity, and management. Some of these manifestations are immediate and some are delayed. Moreover, there are risk factors associated with increased incidence of IgE-mediated adverse events as well as factors that make these events more refractory to treatment.

Sublingual immunotherapy also carries with it a risk of adverse events that are unique from subcutaneous immunotherapy, although the overall safety profile of sublingual immunotherapy has been shown to be more favorable [3]. Literature regarding the efficacy of sublingual immunotherapy has been validated, although the evidence regarding its efficacy compared to subcutaneous immunotherapy is more heterogeneous [3]. Sublingual immunotherapy adverse reactions also carry with them a unique set of considerations given that the vast majority of treatment occurs outside of the office setting. Patient education and counseling under these circumstances is even more critical, and management strategies and prevention literature is more sparse. As the FDA continues to approve increasing forms of immunotherapy, including the recent approval of oral immunotherapy for peanut allergy, understanding the prevention, diagnosis, and management of adverse reactions with sublingual immunotherapy will play an increasing role in practice [7].

Below we will begin to explore the various adverse reactions of allergy immunotherapy in greater detail.

Non-IgE-Mediated Adverse Reactions

Vasovagal Events

Patients may experience non-allergic reactions following immunotherapy that can resemble anaphylaxis. Vasovagal episodes are syncopal or near-syncopal events caused by dysregulation of blood pressure leading to decreased cerebral perfusion that may result in a transient loss of consciousness [8]. Symptoms include hypotension with bradycardia and prodromic lightheadedness, sweating, dyspnea, abdominal discomfort, vision changes, and pallor. Similarly, patients experiencing anaphylactic shock may also demonstrate

	Vasovagal	Anaphylaxis
Heart Rate	Bradycardia	Tachycardia
Blood Pressure	Normal or low	Hypotension
Skin Color	Pallor	Flushed
Itching	No Urticaria	Urticaria
Pulmonary	No Wheezing	Wheezing

Fig. 21.2 Vasovagal episode versus anaphylaxis

hypotension, lightheadedness, dyspnea, and syncope; among other similar symptoms as found in vasovagal episodes. Vasovagal syncope is often triggered by painful stimuli, emotional stress, and fear of bodily injury, all of which may be involved in the administration of SCIT.

At a time when a patient is feeling ill after the administration of immunotherapy, it is critical to be able to quickly differentiate between a vasovagal episode and anaphylaxis. Quickly differentiating the two and managing them appropriately makes a large difference in outcome for the patient. Anaphylaxis is a serious condition that necessitates acute intervention, and vasovagal episodes are often self-resolving. Systemic allergic reactions often are associated with pruritis, hives, wheezing, skin flushing, and oropharyngeal edema; these symptoms would not be expected during a vasovagal episode. Vasovagal episodes commonly present with bradycardia and pallor whereas tachycardia and flushing are seen in anaphylaxis. Figure 21.2 provides a chart helping to differentiate anaphylaxis from vasovagal episodes.

Once the diagnosis of a vasovagal episode is confirmed, treatment should initially involve placing the patient in the supine position, head down, placing an ice pack on the forehead or back of the neck, smelling salts if necessary, isotonic fluids, and crossing the lower extremities. Many patients need reassurance during this time as the episodes usually self-resolve [9].

Other Non-IgE-Mediated Adverse Events

Other non-IgE-mediated adverse events that can occur during immunotherapy include headache, anxiety, and pain at the injection site. One could consider infection as a possible adverse reaction to subcutaneous immunotherapy as well as the possibility of vial contamination. However, studies have found this risk to be minimal to nonexistent [10]. Epstein et al. reported that no infections occurred in 17.3 million injection visits for SCIT between 2014 and 2016. The milder adverse events mentioned above can be treated symptomatically. However, if these events recur frequently, consideration may be given to ceasing immunotherapy.

IgE-Mediated Adverse Reactions

Pathophysiology

With the goal of tolerance, increasing concentrations of allergens are presented to an atopic patient in hopes of instigating an immunologic change to reduce allergic symptomatology. This conversion requires an upregulation of Th1, Treg, and IgG-mediated response over the predominant Th2 and IgE response among many other immunologic changes [11]. By providing slowly increasing concentrations of allergens over an extended period of time, every patient undergoing immunotherapy is at risk for having an adverse reaction.

Atopic patients undergoing immunotherapy already have an immune system that is predisposed to hypersensitivity. This includes populations of allergen-specific IgE attached to mast cells and basophils and a population of Th2 cells. Upon presentation with an antigen, the antigen is taken up by antigen-presenting cells such as macrophages, dendritic cells, or Langerhans cells. These cells process the antigen and present them to T helper cells. In an atopic individual with a predominant Th2 cell response, IL-4, IL-5, and IL-13 are released when the CD4+ cell is activated. These cytokines have a vast diversity of activity. Of importance to the allergic response, they promote further Th2 growth and differentiation, B-cell growth, promotion of IgE isotype class switching, activation and recruitment of mast cells and eosinophils, among other signals. This activation not only promotes downstream signaling which results in allergic symptomatology but also promotes continued Th2 and IgE responses with later activation.

IgE is unique from other immunoglobulin classes in that it requires crosslinking upon antigen presentation to initiate its signaling cascade. Once activated, mast cells and basophils release the contents of their secretory granules which contain preformed immunomodulators and cytokines. Histamine, serotonin, and cytokines such as IL-4 and TNF-a are some of the chemicals immediately released from these cells. Mast cells and basophils also form and release lipid mediators upon activation such as thromboxanes, prostaglandins, and leukotrienes which are involved in a more delayed response.

The severity of response is dependent on the local or systemic activation of the immune response and can be seen as an early (minutes) or late response (6–48 h) [12]. Symptoms of tingling, pruritus, erythema, warmth, rhinorrhea, nasal congestion, hives, acute asthma attacks, abdominal pain, nausea, vomiting, and anaphylaxis can be seen as a response to these immunomodulators. These substances act on a variety of broadly dispersed receptors. They act on smooth muscle cells (bronchoconstriction), vasculature (increased permeability, vasodilation, edema, hypotension), nasal mucosa (rhinorrhea, sneezing), and serve as receptors for pruritus and visceral hypernociception.

A basic understanding of the allergic response is important for clinicians administering immunotherapy as to promptly recognize and treat possible adverse reactions during a patient's treatment course.

Risk Factors for Adverse Events

As clinicians providing immunotherapy, it is useful to be able to stratify patients at increased risk of adverse effects or reduced effectiveness of immunotherapy. Much of our knowledge base regarding risk of adverse reaction with immunotherapy comes from post-event data. Multiple agencies and task forces have compiled guidelines regarding relative and absolute contraindications to immunotherapy due to high risk of severe adverse reactions. Across multiple guidelines, various diseases or characteristics are considered risk factors for patients planning on initiating immunotherapy [13]. Furthermore, there are differences in what are considered relative and absolute risks. This delineation is made with the intention of stratifying patients into groups where risks outweigh benefits and one in which further disease control or caution should be taken prior to therapy initiation. The variability and overall lack of high-quality research to evaluate these questions leaves the clinician responsible to properly evaluate a patient's candidacy for treatment.

Relative contraindications for aeroallergen treatment with immunotherapy included partially controlled asthma, autoimmune disorders in remission, B-blockers, cardiovascular disease, patient age between 2–5 years, HIV with CD4+ >250, psychiatric/mental health disorders, chronic infections, immunodeficiencies, and use of immunosuppressive drugs [14]. Absolute contraindications for immunotherapy included uncontrolled asthma, active/nonresponding autoimmune disorders, malignancies, initiation during pregnancy, patient age less than 2 years, and AIDS [14]. The recommendations for VIT (venom immunotherapy) differed from aeroallergen immunotherapy slightly in that malignancies and ACE inhibitors were felt to be relative contraindications and B-blocker and cardiovascular disease were felt to not be significant risk factors [14]. Figure 21.3 summarizes the risk factors and contraindications for immunotherapy.

Immunotherapy for treatment of asthma has been well studied with evidence of improvements in symptoms, lung function, bronchial reactivity, and reduction in medication requirements [15]. However, the level of control is an important factor in assessing the safety profile of immunotherapy in this population of patients. Bousquet et al. found that during prospective trial assessing maintenance SCIT on asthmatics, 73.3% of patients with an FEV1 < 80% had severe systemic reactions compared to 12.6% of patients with an FEV1 > 80% [16]. Consequently, it was recommended that peak flow testing prior to each

Fig. 21.3 Risk factors for adverse reactions during immunotherapy. *A* absolute contraindication, *R* relative contraindication, *No* no contraindication

Risk Factor	Immunotherapy Aeroallergen	Immunotherapy Venom
Asthma (uncontrolled)	A	A
Asthma (controlled)	R	R
Autoimmune disorder (remission)	R	R
Autoimmune disorder (active/nonresponsive to treatment)	A	A
Malignancies	A	R
Pregnancy (initiation)	A	A
B Blockers	R	No
ACE inhibitors	No	R
Cardiovascular disease	R	No
Age 2-5 yrs	R	R
Age <2 yrs	A	A
HIV	R	R
AIDS	A	A
Psychiatric/mental health disorders	R	R
Immunodeficiencies	R	R
Immunosuppressants	R	R
Chronic infection	R	R

therapy be done to evaluate a patient's current level of control. Therapy should be held for patients with a reduction of 20% from their personal best peak flow value [17]. SLIT therapy was found to have an improved safety profile for asthmatics making it a possible safer alternative to treatment in this subgroup of patients [18].

Immunotherapy in patients with autoimmune diseases is one of the more poorly understood interactions with the majority of concerns presented as case reports or case series. There are no controlled studies to guide our level of concern or decisions on therapy usage and progression. There are various reports raising concerns regarding the development of autoimmune disease with the initiation of immunotherapy. Reported diseases included Sjogren's disease, vasculitis, pericarditis, multiple sclerosis, rheumatoid arthritis, and scleroderma [19–24]. The autoimmune/inflammatory syndrome induced by adjuvants is a theory that attempts to explain these possible reactions but is as of yet unproven [25]. The theory describes the interaction between various adjuvants, such as silicone, tetramethylpentadecane, pristane, and aluminum, among others, and their interaction with the immune system to create the broad and vague symptoms seen in the syndrome. Aluminum, as was mentioned, is one such additive described which correlates this theory to aluminum-based immunotherapy. Though some of these adjuvants have been shown to produce autoimmunity in animal or human models, there have been equivalent conflicting data with no definitive proof to the validity of this theory.

There is similarly weak evidence evaluating the effects of immunotherapy in patients with malignancy. The basis of contraindication of allergen immunotherapy in patients with malignancy stems from a safety and ethical basis. There have been no reported data on the interaction of allergen immunotherapy in patients with malignancies or the effectiveness of rescue medication in this population either. A study evaluating VIT in patients with malignancy found no difference in rates of effectiveness, adverse effects, and general long-term symptom control against reported rates in patients without malignancies [26]. Given these findings, malignancies are only a relative contraindication for patients who may benefit life-saving VIT.

B-blockers and ACE inhibitors are widely used medications for a variety of common diseases. The concern regarding these medications stems from their physiologic changes to an individual's ability to adequately compensate to an anaphylactic reaction or respond to emergency treatment. Studies have found that a concentration of 80x the standard dose of epinephrine would be needed to overcome the actions of β receptor blockade [27]. Furthermore, under a system with beta-adrenergic receptor blockage, epinephrine would activate unopposed alpha-adrenergic receptors resulting in hypertension, reflex bradycardia, and bronchoconstriction. Despite these concerns, it was found that patients taking b-blockers were not at an increased risk of severity or number of adverse reactions during venom subcutaneous immunotherapy [28, 29]. Similarly, there is a concern that patients on ACE inhibitors will have a depressed response to severe hypotension from anaphylaxis, citing its inhibition of the renin-angiotensin system (RAS) [30]. Though some studies do not show ACE inhibitors to be a risk factor for severe systemic reactions, one study identified patients on ACE inhibitors to be at an increased risk of anaphylaxis (odds ratio 2.26) when undergoing venom immunotherapy [31].

Certain patient demographics, such as young age and pregnancy, have also been considered risk factors for adverse events. This is largely due to lack of good quality data, though also due to difficulty in the ability to assess affects or concerning symptoms in these at-risk populations. Children pose a host of difficulties, partially from a standpoint of cooperation, but also limitations in the ability to describe and communicate potential symptomatic reactions that may or may not require treatment. Despite this, studies have shown no difference between local reaction occurrences in children 2–5 years of age compared to their older counterparts [32]. Several studies have reported low incidence, < 0.1/1000, of adverse reactions in children undergoing SLIT [33, 34]. In pregnancy, the risk stems from the unknown effects of immunotherapy or potential emergency treatment on the fetus. Systemic stimulation from epinephrine administration would result in placental vasoconstriction, uterine contractions leading to maternal and fetal hypoxemia which increases the risk of premature labor, miscarriage, morbidity, and mortality [35]. Despite this risk, multiple studies have found immunotherapy initiated or continued during pregnancy had no increase in risk to the fetus as compared to the general population [36]. In fact, atopic women who did not undergo immunotherapy seemed to have increased incidence of miscarriage, toxemia, or prematurity [37, 38].

Local Reactions

Despite being careful and selective with regard to patient characteristics, history, and compliance, adverse reactions to immunotherapy are a very real possibility. As a patient progresses through their journey of immunotherapy, they are regularly being exposed to allergens either during escalation therapy or maintenance. Adverse reactions can occur with any one of these exposures and recognition and treatment of these reactions must be taken seriously. Although anaphylaxis, the most severe reaction that can occur, is very rare, local reactions are more common and are very likely to happen during a patient's course through desensitization.

The symptomatology of a local reaction may differ depending on the modality of immunotherapy, such as oral, subcutaneous, or sublingual. Generally, local reactions may take the form of oropharyngeal pruritus, perioral rash, localized edema, or injection site erythema/pruritus. Oral immunotherapy is one such method known to be associated with a large number of local reactions; Pajno et al. found an increased relative risk of 2.14 in patients treated with oral immunotherapy [39]. SCIT in comparison, has reported local reactions in 26–86% of patients occurring in 0.7–4% of injections [4]. A single-center experience over 10 years found slightly reduced values with 11.9% of patients having had local reactions, occurring in approximately 0.38% of injections most frequently during escalation therapy [40]. SCIT therapy has also been reported to result in more severe reactions, though uncommon. SLIT, alternatively, has been cited to be a relatively safer method of immunotherapy in that it elicits less frequent or severe systemic reactions though the frequency of local reactions varies. Studies have reported local reactions during SLIT to be between 71%–84% [41, 42]. In another report, it was estimated that SLIT therapy results in 2.7 reactions in 1000 administrations with 0.056% of these reactions being considered severe [43]. In another trial of 1500 patients treated with SLIT, it was reported that 79% of patients had local reactions, 6% of whom discontinued treatment due to the severity of the local reaction [44]. Meta-analysis by Calderon et al. subdivided patients with local reactions requiring treatment. They found that of 907 patients, 92% did not require treatment while 10% of 208 patients did require treatment for local reactions. In a smaller study of 72 patients comparing SLIT versus SCIT, local adverse reactions were only seen in the SCIT population with equal treatment efficacy [45]. Despite the higher frequency of local reaction rates, there has not been any evidence to indicate that local reactions predict systemic reactions or that dose alterations alter the risk of systemic reactions [46–48].

Treatment of local reactions can vary depending on the severity of the reaction. Small local reactions (< 2.5 cm) can be observed or treated symptomatically with topical or oral antihistamines or topical steroids for the comfort of the patient. In addition, an icepack on the area can be helpful in relieving discomfort. Large local reactions may require similar measures as smaller reactions in addition to the option of adjusting the immunotherapy dose at the next visit and consideration of premedication in certain situations. Studies have found premedicating patients to prevent local reactions may be effective in accelerated immunotherapy schedules. For instance, several studies have demonstrated H1 blockers given 15–120 min prior to each injection during rush and cluster protocols decrease the rate of local reactions [49, 50]. Premedicating with the leukotriene antagonist montelukast was found to delay onset and decrease the size of local reactions during rush venom immunotherapy in a 2007 study [51]. However, premedicating has not been found to be an effective intervention to prevent local reactions in patients undergoing conventional immunotherapy schedules [47, 52].

Several studies have shown that dose adjustments following local reactions do not change the rate of future local or systemic reactions [25, 46, 52]. However, a 2007 study that surveyed over 750 allergists found that most, 91.9%, do make dose adjustments following local reactions. The most common rationales clinicians shared regarding dose adjustments were the ideas that local reactions were directly related to noncompliance and risk of both future local and systemic reactions [53].

Studies have not demonstrated that individual local reactions increase the risk of systemic reactions to immunotherapy [46, 48]. However, there does appear to be a positive correlation between frequent, large local reactions and the incidence of systemic reactions over the course of therapy [54]. A 2007 retrospective study found that patients with a history of a systemic reaction from immunotherapy had a 4 times greater incidence of large local reactions than patients who had never experienced a systemic reaction [55]. Although it has not been shown that dose reductions prevent future local or systemic reactions, for patients with multiple large local reactions (>2.5 cm) or a local reaction that is larger than the patient's palm, clinicians may consider altering the therapy schedule to be a more gradual increase.

Systemic Reactions

Mild Systemic Reactions

Systemic reactions are rare following immunotherapy but are potentially very dangerous. Systemic allergic reactions to immunotherapy can range from mild, such as generalized urticaria, to severe, including anaphylaxis. Based on several high-powered studies, there is relative agreement that the overall incidence of systemic reactions is about 0.2%, or 2 in 1000 patients with severe and anaphylactic reactions being even more rare [56]. Clinical manifestations include generalized urticaria, oropharyngeal swelling, wheezing, abdominal pain, nausea, and vomiting.

Following administration of SCIT, most severe hypersensitivity reactions occur within 30 minutes. It is therefore recommended that clinicians require patients to remain in a medical setting for a minimum of 30 min after injection [52]. About 30–50% of less severe systemic reactions, such as urticaria, wheezing, and stridor, are delayed, or occur greater than 30 minutes following injection [57]. However, since serious reactions occur within 30 minutes, it is not indicated to monitor the patient in the clinic or office for greater than 30 minutes [58].

Anaphylaxis

Anaphylaxis is a serious, generalized hypersensitivity reaction that is life-threatening and occurs suddenly after exposure to a provoking allergen [59]. In 2006, the WAO established criteria for diagnosing an anaphylactic reaction in the clinical setting [60]. Figure 21.4 outlines the criteria which aimed to simply and quickly allow for accurate diagnosis. Anaphylaxis presents acutely with skin and/or mucosal involvement including hives, oral edema, or pruritis. Decreased blood pressure and/or respiratory compromise including wheezing, dyspnea, or hypoxemia can be seen. Symptoms of gastrointestinal distress such as diarrhea, vomiting, or abdominal pain are also frequently associated with anaphylaxis. Eighty percent of patients with systemic adverse reactions present with cutaneous findings and it was therefore estimated that 80% of cases can be diagnosed from criteria 1 [60]. Categories 2 and 3 are based on increasingly vague symptoms or lack of cutaneous findings though with increased suspicion due to suspected allergen exposure.

In 2010, a universal grading system for immunotherapy systemic reactions was established by an international Joint Task Force organized by the World Allergy Organization. The purpose of this 5-grade grading system was designed to be used by clinicians and researchers practicing SCIT to better classify systemic reactions and study the effects of different immunotherapy formulations and administration methods. Figure 21.5 further elaborates the classification system [56]. Higher grading indicates more severe symptoms. These increase from symptomatology affecting a single organ to multiorgan effects with increasing effect on lower and upper respiratory systems.

Anaphylaxis is highly likely when any one of the following 3 criteria are fulfilled:

1. Acute onset of an illness (minutes to several hours) with involvement of the skin, mucosal tissue, or both (eg, generalized hives, pruritus or flushing, swollen lips-tongue-uvula)
   AND AT LEAST ONE OF THE FOLLOWING
   a. Respiratory compromise (eg, dyspnea, wheeze-bronchospasm, stridor, reduced PEF, hypoxemia)
   b. Reduced BP or associated symptoms of end-organ dysfunction (eg, hypotonia [collapse], syncope, incontinence)
2. Two or more of the following that occur rapidly after exposure *to a likely allergen for that patient* (minutes to several hours):
   a. Involvement of the skin-mucosal tissue (eg, generalized hives, itch-flush, swollen lips-tongue-uvula)
   b. Respiratory compromise (eg, dyspnea, wheeze-bronchospasm, stridor, reduced PEF, hypoxemia)
   c. Reduced BP or associated symptoms (eg, hypotonia [collapse], syncope, incontinence)
   d. Persistent gastrointestinal symptoms (eg, crampy abdominal pain, vomiting)
3. Reduced BP after exposure to *known allergen for that patient* (minutes to several hours):
   a. Infants and children: low systolic BP (age specific) or greater than 30% decrease in systolic BP*
   b. Adults: systolic BP of less than 90 mm Hg or greater than 30% decrease from that person's baseline

Fig. 21.4 Clinical criteria for diagnosis anaphylaxis—reproduced with permission [60]

Grade 1	Grade 2	Grade 3	Grade 4	Grade 5
*Symptom(s)/sign(s) of 1 organ system present** **Cutaneous** Generalized pruritus, urticaria, flushing, or sensation of heat or warmth† **or** Angioedema (not laryngeal, tongue or uvular) **or** **Upper respiratory** Rhinitis - (eg, sneezing, rhinorrhea, nasal pruritus and/or nasal congestion) **or** Throat-clearing (itchy throat) **or** Cough perceived to originate in the upper airway, not the lung, larynx, or trachea **or** **Conjunctival** Erythema, pruritus or tearing **Other** Nausea, metallic taste, or headache	*Symptom(s)/sign(s) of more than 1 organ system present* **or** **Lower respiratory** Asthma: cough, wheezing, shortness of breath (eg, less than 40% PEF or FEV_1 drop, responding to an inhaled bronchodilator) **or** **Gastrointestinal** Abdominal cramps, vomiting, or diarrhea **or** **Other** Uterine cramps	**Lower respiratory** Asthma (eg, 40% PEF or FEV_1 drop NOT responding to an inhaled bronchodilator) **or** **Upper respiratory** Laryngeal, uvula, or tongue edema with or without stridor	**Lower or upper respiratory** Respiratory failure with or without loss of consciousness **or** **Cardiovascular** Hypotension with or without loss of consciousness	Death

Fig. 21.5 World Allergy Organization SCIT systemic reaction grading system. Reproduced with permission [56]

Another temporal pattern of immunotherapy reactions are biphasic anaphylactic reactions. These reactions are defined as onset of symptoms after symptomatic resolution of the initial reaction. Recurrence of symptoms is usually within 24 hours and is less severe than the initial reaction. There is not a known association between symptoms associated with the initial reaction and likelihood of developing a biphasic response. A 2009 prospective study demonstrated that biphasic reactions occur in 23% of patients who suffered a systemic reaction after immunotherapy injections and occurred more frequently in women as well as in patients who required greater than one dose of epinephrine to resolve the initial reaction [61]. These findings support patient counseling regarding biphasic reactions however, prescribing epinephrine following a systemic reaction is not necessarily indicated given the low severity of the biphasic reaction, and the decision is at the discretion of the provider [52].

Treatment of Systemic Reactions

Although extremely rare, anaphylaxis is a potentially deadly adverse event that can occur following the administration of allergy immunotherapy. Several practices have been found to reduce the risk of anaphylaxis as well as manage it appropriately. Preventative measures include optimizing asthma control, and avoiding dosing errors. Early initiation and escalation of treatment for systemic reaction is critical to outcome. Office preparedness with regard to equipment and staffing can be lifesaving for a patient having a severe systemic reaction.

Asthma is a significant risk factor for adverse events to immunotherapy. It is therefore recommended that asthma be well controlled prior to initiation of immunotherapy and asthmatics be evaluated for recent exacerbations of symptoms prior to administration of immunotherapy [52]. Studies suggest that premedicating with H1 antihistamines may reduce the risk of systemic reactions in not only rush and cluster, but also conventional immunotherapy schedules [62]. A concern regarding the use of antihistamines prior to immunotherapy is that the initial symptoms of a severe systemic reaction may be masked. As evidence supporting this concern is lacking, current guidelines encourage the use of H1 antihistamines during conventional immunotherapy [52]. Several studies have demonstrated a decreased rate of both systemic and local reactions with combination therapy involving premedication with H1 and H2 antihistamines as well as glucocorticoids during accelerated cluster build-up protocols [63, 64]. Notably, allergists typically only administer these premedication combinations during accelerated immunotherapy schedules. Omalizumab may also be considered as a premedication prior to cluster or rush immunotherapy. This IgE monoclonal antibody decreased the risk of anaphylaxis during rush immunotherapy by five-fold in a 2006 controlled trial [65]. Additionally, a prospective trial involving 250 patients found that premedication with omalizumab decreased the rate of systemic reactions during cluster immunotherapy by half [66]. Hurst et al. reported that the most common risk factors for anaphylaxis during immunotherapy were escalation of immunotherapy, presence of active asthma, and the first dose of a new vial [67]. Based on the results of a 2006 survey, dosing errors and providing immunotherapy during peak pollen season were the most commonly stated associations to adverse reactions [68]. Dosing errors are best avoided with providing education to all staff involved in administering immunotherapy, developing and maintaining a uniform labeling system for dilutions, and confirming patient identity [52]. Conflicting data exists regarding whether systemic reactions occur more frequently during pollen seasons. However, dose adjustments during pollen season are not generally required as several high-powered, prospective studies did not demonstrate an association [69, 70]. However, it remains common for allergists to choose to decrease maintenance doses during peak pollen season.

Early recognition and prompt initiation of treatment is imperative for successful management of anaphylaxis. Clinical staff should be educated on how to identify patients experiencing anaphylaxis and a plan for management should be implemented. The 2015 practice parameter update for managing anaphylaxis in the office setting provides suggested equipment for an "anaphylaxis emergency cart" to be stationed in the clinic [71] (Fig. 21.6).

Prompt administration of epinephrine is the most important intervention in the management of severe systemic allergic reactions. Epinephrine

Anaphylaxis emergency cart

Basic supplies	Airway & intravenous fluid support equipment	Medications
First line: required supplies and priority medications		
Written emergency protocol	Bag-valve-mask, self-inflating with reservoir (eg, Ambu bag) for adult and child*	Epinephrine 1:1,000 3 ampules or 1 multidose vial
Flow chart for recording times and events	Disposable face masks (infant, toddler, child, adult)	O_2 E-cylinder 2 and wrench; >1,100 psi
Stethoscope	Oropharyngeal airways: 6, 7, 8, 9, 10 cm	0.9% normal saline (2 1-L bags)
Sphygmomanometer, blood pressure cuffs (infant, child, adult, obese adult)	Nasal pharyngeal airway: 6,7,8, 9 mm	Albuterol inhalational solution 0.5%
Watch or clock	O_2 extension tubing	Glucagon 1 mg/mL (2 vials)
Gloves, preferably without latex*	O_2 nasal cannula	
Synthetic tape	Macro-drip administration set (10–15 drops/mL) and connection tubing	
Alcohol swabs	Intravenous pole or suitable substitute	
Tourniquets	Pulse oximeter	
Indwelling intravenous catheters (gauge 14, 16, 18, 20, 22)	Twin-jet nebulizer, face mask, tubing	
Intravenous butterfly needles (gauge 19, 21, 23)		
Syringes (1, 10, 20 mL)		
Needles 1–2 inches, 18, 21, 23 gauge		
Macro-drip administration sets		
Extension tubing		
T-connectors		
3-way stopcocks		
Arm boards (2–4 sizes)		
Second line: supplies and medications		
Automated external defibrillator	Laryngeal mask airways (sizes 2, 3, 4, 5)	Diphenhydramine 50 mg/mL intravenously
	suction machine and tubing	Cetirizine 10-mg tablets, 5 mg/tsp liquid
	cardiac arrest backboard	Ranitidine 25 mg/mL intravenously
		Methylprednisolone 125-mg vial
		Prednisone 5- or 10-mg tablets, prednisolone syrup 15 mg/tsp
Third line: supplies and medications		
Electrocardiograph and supplies	Equipement for intubation (for remote areas only)	Dopamine 200 mg/5 mL intravenously (1 ampule)
	5% dextrose in water 500 mL (for dopamine infusion)	Atropine 0.5 mg/mL intravenously

Fig. 21.6 Adverse reaction office toolkit—permission obtained [71]

is to be administered intramuscularly in the outer thigh at the first signs of anaphylaxis. A quantity of 0.2–0.5 mL (or 0.01 mg/kg for children, maximum 0.3 mg per dose) of 1:1000 dilution of aqueous epinephrine should be given every 5 min as symptoms persist [52]. Patients who do not demonstrate a full response to epinephrine therapy or those with severe systemic symptoms should be immediately transferred to an emergency department [71].

Ongoing assessments of the patient's airway, breathing, circulation, and mental status are to be conducted. To promote systemic circulation, the patient should be placed in the supine position and cardiopulmonary resuscitation, supplemental oxygen, nebulized beta-2 agonists, and intravenous fluids are to be started if deemed necessary. Antihistamines (both H1 and H2 blockers) and corticosteroids may be considered as adjunctive interventions in the setting of anaphylaxis. Dopamine administration can be considered for refractory cases. Patients on beta blockers with resistant systemic reactions may also be assisted with the administration of glucagon [71]. It is left to the practitioner's judgment to determine the duration and level of observation for which the patient needs to be directly monitored following an episode of anaphylaxis. However, a period of observation in a monitored setting is recommended [71].

Adverse Events Related to Sublingual Immunotherapy (SLIT)

In addition to the advantages of self-administration outside of the office setting and lack of an injection, sublingual immunotherapy has a better safety profile than subcutaneous immunotherapy as systemic reactions are very rare and, to date, there are no reported fatalities secondary to SLIT [72].

Adverse events related to SLIT primarily involve local reactions, which are relatively common and are graded based on severity using a 3-grade scale [72] shown in Fig. 21.7. Improvement in symptoms is frequently noted with continued therapy. Incidence of local reactions does not appear to be related to the presence of build-up dosing [52]. The most common local reaction is oral pruritus. Oral pruritus typically occurs with the first dose of SLIT in about 40% of patients [73]. The pruritic symptoms tend to self-resolve within an hour. Oral edema is another common side effect that about one in ten patients experience within a week of the first dose of SLIT [74]. If significant swelling is present, epinephrine should be considered. There is also a possible association between SLIT and eosinophilic esophagitis. A 2014 meta-analysis found 2.7% of patients undergoing SLIT developed

World Allergy Organization Grading System for SLIT Local Reactions[a]

Symptom/sign	Grade 1: mild	Grade 2: moderate	Grade 3: severe	Unknown severity
Pruritus/swelling of mouth, tongue, or lip; throat irritation, nausea, abdominal pain, vomiting, diarrhea, heartburn, or uvular edema	• Not troublesome AND • No symptomatic treatment required AND • No discontinuation of SLIT because of local side effects	• Troublesome OR • Requires symptomatic treatment AND • No discontinuation of SLIT because of local side effects	• Grade 2 AND • SLIT discontinued because of local side effects	Treatment is discontinued, but there is no subjective, objective, or both description of severity from the patient/physician.

Each local AE can be early (<30 minutes) or delayed.

Fig. 21.7 Local reaction grading system—permission obtained [72]

eosinophilic esophagitis, with resolution of the condition upon discontinuation of SLIT in most cases [75]. Although local hypersensitivity reactions to SLIT are not usually severe, the high incidence of these reactions validates the need for patient counseling.

What's Next…

Since gaining FDA approval in 2014, SLIT therapy has been increasingly popular in the United States secondary to its convenience, safety profile, and efficacy [76]. Although there have only been very rare reports of SLIT-associated anaphylaxis, its administration outside of the medical setting has led to discussion whether an epinephrine auto-injector (EAI) should be concurrently prescribed. Portnoy and Cox address this debate in a 2017 article [77]. The authors note that 14% of SCIT systemic reactions occur after the 30-minute window following injections when patients have left the office, but EAI is not often prescribed for patients receiving SCIT [78]. The article also suggests taking into account the high cost associated with prescribing autoinjectors to each patient undergoing SLIT. While considering the extremely low risk of anaphylaxis secondary to SLIT, the authors suggest prescribing EAI is left to the clinician's judgment [77]. The package insert for SLIT-Tablets in the US does specify that clinicians prescribe auto-injectable epinephrine, instruct, and train patients on its appropriate use, and instruct patients to seek immediate medical care upon its use [82].

Another topic on the horizon of immunotherapy is the treatment of food allergies with oral immunotherapy (OIT). As was mentioned previously, the FDA recently approved Palforzia ™ as oral immunotherapy for children with severe peanut allergies. Phase 3 clinical trial by the PALISADE group demonstrated that 67.2% of children (ages 4 to 17) in the active treatment group were able to ingest 600 mg of peanut protein at exit interview without dose-limiting symptoms [79]. This is compared to 4% in the placebo treatment group. Despite its success and approval to diminish life-threatening allergic reactions, 98.7% of patients had adverse reactions during the intervention period. Patients in the active group had higher incidence of adverse effects compared to placebo with reported severity as 34.7% for mild, 59.7% for moderate, and 4.3% for severe [79]. A meta-analysis of oral immunotherapy for peanut allergies similarly showed an increased risk of anaphylactic and non-anaphylactic adverse effects in patients undergoing escalation or maintenance therapy. They reported an increased risk of anaphylaxis with a risk ratio of 3.12, increased frequency of anaphylaxis with risk ratio of 2.72, and increased epinephrine use with a risk ratio of 2.21 [80]. Despite its benefit for desensitization to reduce lethal reactions, the high risk of adverse reactions during oral immunotherapy is the reason for clinicians to be vigilant and attentive when treating pediatric patients for peanut allergies. The protocol for managing such adverse reactions will likely be a subject of discussion in the future.

Lastly, biologics have become increasingly popular in the armamentarium of treatment options for T2-mediated diseases like asthma, but also chronic rhinosinusitis and are predicted to be increasingly given by otolaryngologists as adjuvant treatment options for patients. However, like other immune modifying agents, they carry their own safety profiles and reported adverse reactions that include, but are not limited to anaphylaxis, injection site reactions, conjunctivitis, arthralgia, and others [81–83]. Diagnosis and management of adverse reactions with biologics are topics for future research and discussion.

Summary

Immunotherapy stands to significantly benefit patients with severe allergies. With its disease-modifying effects and ability to reduce the need for rescue medication, immunotherapy is a mainstay in the standard of care for allergies failing environmental controls and medical therapy. Despite its benefits, risks of adverse effects during therapy initiation, escalation, or maintenance carry significant concerns to both providers and patients. Of most particular significance is the clinician's and office staff's ability to quickly recognize adverse reactions and to administer appropriate treatment. Office preparation is also paramount. Responsiveness and preparedness are vital. Fortunately, severe systemic reactions are far less common, however, delayed recognition or treatment can be lethal and therefore requires vigilance on the part of staff and clinicians as well. A clinician may want to stratify patients that are high risk of having an adverse effect. Unfortunately, there is a lack of high-quality evidence in many of these areas of interest and therefore is largely dependent on a clinician's judgment to determine the risks and benefits of immunotherapy for each individual patient. Adequate preparedness and clinician judgment will be essential as more high-quality data regarding the rates and severity of adverse reactions to immunotherapy become available.

References

1. Oktemer T, et al. Clinical efficacy of immunotherapy in allergic rhinitis. American J Rhinol Allergy. 2016;30(5):4–7.
2. Frew AJ. Allergen immunotherapy. J Allergy Clin Immunol. 2010;125:306–13.
3. Durham S, Penagos M. Sublingual or subcutaneous immunotherapy for allergic rhinitis? J Allergy Clin Immunol. 2016;137:339–49.
4. Nelson B, Dupont L, Reid M. Prospective survey of local and systemic reactions to immunotherapy with pollen extracts. Ann Allergy. 1986;45:331–4.
5. Epstein T, Liss G, Murphy-Berendts K, et al. AAAI and ACAAI surveillance study of subcutaneous immunotherapy, year 3: what practices modify the risk of systemic reactions? Ann Allergy Asthma Immunol. 2013;110:274–8.
6. Epstein T, Liss G, Murphy-Berendts K, et al. Risk factors for fatal and nonfatal reactions to subcutaneous immunotherapy. Ann Allergy Asthma Immunol. 2016;116:354–9.
7. FDA Approves First Drug for Treatment of Peanut Allergy for Children. Food and Drug Administration. 2020. https://www.fda.gov/news-events/press-announcements/fda-approves-first-drug-treatment-peanut-allergy-children. Access 16 March 2020.
8. Jeanmonod R, Silberman M. Vasovagal Episode. StatPearls Publishing; 2019.
9. Aydin M, Salukhe T, Wilke I, et al. Management and therapy of vasovagal syncope: a review. World J Cardiol. 2010;2:308–15.
10. Epstein T, Liss G, Murphy-Berendts K, et al. AAAA/ACAAI subcutaneous immunotherapy surveillance study (2013-2017): fatalities, infections, delayed reactions, and use of epinephrine autoinjectors. J Allergy Clin Immunol Pract. 2019;7:1996–2003.
11. Matsuoka T, Shamji MH, Durham SR. Allergen immunotherapy and tolerance. Allergol Int. 2013;62:403–13.
12. Galli S, Tsai M, Piliponsky A. The development of allergic inflammation. Nature. 2008;454:445–54.
13. Pitsios C, Tsoumani M, et al. Contraindications to immunotherapy: a global approach. Clin Transl Allergy. 2019;9:9.
14. Pitsios C, Demoly P, Bilo M, et al. Clinical contraindications to allergen immunotherapy: an EAACI position paper. European J Allergy Clin Immunol. 2015;70:897–909.
15. Abramson MJ, Puy RM, Weiner JM. Injection allergen immunotherapy for asthma. Cochrane Database Syst Rev 2010;8.
16. Bousquet J, Hejjaoui A, et al. Immunotherapy with a standardized Dermatophagoides Pteronyssinus extract: systemic reaction during the rush protocol in patients suffering from asthma. J Allergy Clin Immunol. 1989;83:797–802.
17. Alvarez-Cuesta E, Bousquet J, et al. Standards for practical allergen-specific immunotherapy. Allergy. 2006;82:1–20.
18. Garcia-Robaina J, Inmaculada S, et al. Successful Management of Mite- Allergic Asthma with modified extracts of Dermatophagoides Pteronyssinus and Dermatophagiodes Farinae in a double-blind, placebo-controlled study. J Allergy Clin Immunol. 2006;118:1026–32.
19. Turkcapar N, Kinikli G, et al. Specific immunotherapy-induced Sjogren's syndrome. Rheumatol Int. 2005;26:182–4.
20. Taylor R. Hypersensitivity Vasculitis occurring in a patient receiving immunotherapy. J Allergy Clin Immunol. 1991;87:889–90.
21. Quirce S, Fernandez M, Losada E, et al. Recurrent pericarditis: a rare complication of allergen immunotherapy. Allergy. 1992;47:343–5.
22. Nakajima H, Ohtsuka S, Nishina T, et al. Multiple sclerosis after allergen-specific immunotherapy and influenza vaccination. Eur Neurol. 2003;50:248–9.
23. Ghoreschi K, Fischer J, Biedermann T. Manifestation of rheumatoid arthritis during subcutaneous allergen-specific immunotherapy with bee venom. J Allergy Clin Immunol. 2012;130:1438–9.
24. Maciel M, Morfin C. Scleroderma related to specific immunotherapy. A report of a case. Rev Alerg Mex. 2009;56:136–45.
25. Perricone C, Colafrancesco S, Mazor RD, et al. Autoimmune/inflammatory syndrome induced by adjuvants (ASIA) 2013: unveiling the pathogenic, Clinical and Diagnostic Aspects. J Autoimmun. 2013;47:1–16.
26. Aeberhard J, Haeberli G, Muller U, et al. Specific immunotherapy in hymenoptera venom allergy and

concomitant malignancy: a retrospective follow-up focusing on effectiveness and safety. J Investig Allergol Clin Immunol. 2017;27:370–7.
27. Hiatt W, Wolfel E, Stoll S, et al. Beta-2 adrenergic blockade evaluated with epinephrine after placebo, atenolol, and Nadolol. Clin Pharmacol Ther. 1985;37:2–6.
28. Muller U, Haeberli G. Use of Beta-blockers during immunotherapy for hymenoptera venom allergy. J Allergy Clin Immunol. 2005;115:606–10.
29. Hepner M, Ownby D, Anderson J, et al. Risk of systemic reactions in patients taking Beta-blocker drugs receiving allergen immunotherapy injections. J Allergy Clin Immunol. 1990;86:407–11.
30. Hermann K, Ring J. The renin-angiotensin system in patients with repeated anaphylactic reactions during hymenoptera venom Hyposensitization and sting challenge. Int Arch Allergy Immunol. 1997;112:251–6.
31. Rueff F, Przybilla B, Muller U, et al. Predictors of severe systemic anaphylactic reactions in patients with hymenoptera venom allergy: importance of baseline serum Tryptase-a study of the European academy of Allergology and clinical immunology interest group on insect venom hypersensitivity. J Allergy Clin Immunol. 2009;12:1047–54.
32. Rodriguez SO. Sublingual immunotherapy in allergic rhinitis and asthma in 2–5-year-old children sensitized to mites. Rev Alerg Mex. 2008;55:71–5.
33. Rienzo V, Minelli M, Musarra A, et al. Post-marketing survey on the safety of sublingual immunotherapy in children below the age of 5 years. Clin Exp Allergy. 2005;35:560–4.
34. Agostinis F, Tellarini L, Canonica G, et al. Safety of sublingual immunotherapy with a monomeric Allergoid in very young children. Allergy. 2005;60:133.
35. Simons F, Schatz M. Anaphylaxis during pregnancy. J Allergy Clin Immunol. 2012;130:597–606.
36. Okyham P, Kim H, Ellis A. Allergen immunotherapy in pregnancy. Allergy Asthma Clin Immunol. 2015;11:11.
37. Metzger W, Turner E, Patterson R. The safety of immunotherapy during pregnancy. J Allergy Clin Immunol. 1978;61:268–72.
38. Shaikh W. A retrospective study on the safety of immunotherapy in pregnancy. Clin Exp Allergy. 1993;23:857–60.
39. Pajno G, Fernandez-Rivas M, Arasi S, et al. EAACI guidelines on allergen immunotherapy: IgE- mediated food allergy. Allergy. 2018;73:799–815.
40. Nacaroglu H, Erdem S, Sumer O, et al. Local and systemic reactions to subcutaneous allergen immunotherapy: ten years' experience in a pediatric clinic. Ann Allergy Asthma Immunol. 2016;116:349–53.
41. Maloney J, Berman G, Gagnon R, et al. Sequential treatment initiation with Timothy grass and ragweed sublingual immunotherapy tablets followed by simultaneous treatment is well tolerated. J Allergy Clin Immunol Pract. 2016;4:301–9.
42. Nolte H, Bernstein D, Helson H, et al. Efficacy of house dust mite sublingual immunotherapy tablet in north American adolescents and adults in a randomized, placebo-controlled trial. J Allergy Clin Immunol. 2016;138:1631–8.
43. Cox L, Larenas D, Nolte H, et al. Sublingual immunotherapy: a comprehensive review. J Allergy Clin Immunol. 2006;117:1021–35.
44. Maloney J, Bernstein D, Nelson H, et al. Efficacy and safety of grass sublingual immunotherapy tablet, MK-7243: a large randomized controlled trial. Ann Allergy Asthma Immunol. 2014;112:146–53.
45. Atta A, Amer R, Mesbah A, et al. Sublingual versus subcutaneous immunotherapy as regards efficacy and safety in respiratory allergic patients. Egypt J Immunol. 2019;26:65–75.
46. Tankersley M, Butler K, Butler W, et al. Local reactions during allergen immunotherapy do not require dose adjustment. J Allergy Clin Immunol. 2000;106:840–3.
47. Calabria C, Coop C, Tankersley M. The LOCAL study: local reactions do not predict local reactions in allergen immunotherapy. J Allergy Clin Immunol. 2009;124:739–44.
48. Kelso J. The rate of systemic reactions to immunotherapy injections is the same whether or not the dose is reduced after a local reaction. Ann Allergy Asthma Immunol. 2004;92:225–7.
49. Reimers A, Hari Y, Müller U. Reduction of side-effects from Ultrarush immunotherapy with honeybee venom by pretreatment with fexofenadine: a double-blind, placebo-controlled rrial. Allergy. 2000;55:483–7.
50. Nielsen L, Johnsen C, Mosbech H, et al. Antihistamine premedication in specific cluster immunotherapy: a double-blind, placebo-controlled study. J Allergy Clin Immunol. 1996;97:1207–13.
51. Wöhrl S, Gamper S, Hemmer W, et al. Premedication with Montelukast reduces local reactions of allergen immunotherapy. Int Arch Allergy Immunol. 2007;144:137–42.
52. Cox L, Nelson H, Lockey R, et al. Allergen immunotherapy: a practice parameter third update. J Allergy Clin Immunol. 2011;127:S1–S55.
53. Coop C, Tankersley M. Dose adjustment practices among allergists for local reactions to immunotherapy. Ann Allergy Asthma Immunol. 2007;99:77–81.
54. Calabria C, Stolfi A, Tankersley M. The REPEAT study: recognizing and evaluating periodic local reactions in allergen immunotherapy and associated systemic reactions. Ann Allergy Asthma Immunol. 2011;106(1):49–53.
55. Roy S, Sigmon J, Olivier J, et al. Increased frequency of large local reactions among systemic reactors during subcutaneous allergen immunotherapy. Ann Allergy Asthma Immunol. 2007;99(1):82–6.
56. Cox L, Larenas-Linnemann D, Lockey R, et al. Speaking the same language: the world allergy organization subcutaneous immunotherapy systemic reaction grading system. J Allergy Clin Immunol. 2010;125:569–74.

57. Greenberg M, Kaufman C, Gonzalez G, et al. Late systemic-allergic reactions to inhalant allergen immunotherapy. J Allergy Clin Immunol. 1988;82:287–90.
58. DaVeiga S, Liu X, Caruso K, et al. Systemic reactions associated with subcutaneous allergen immunotherapy: timing and risk assessment. Ann Allergy Asthma Immunol. 2011;106(6):533–7.
59. Simons F, Ardusso L, Bilo M, et al. World allergy organization guidelines for the assessment and Management of Anaphylaxis. World Allergy Organ J. 2011;4:13–37.
60. Sampson H, Munoz-Furlong A, Campbell, et al. Second symposium on the definition and Management of Anaphylaxis: summary report—second National Institute of allergy and infectious disease/Food Allergy and Anaphylaxis Network symposium. J Allergy Clin Immunol. 2006;117:391–7.
61. Scranton S, Gonzalez E, Waibel K. Incidence and characteristics of biphasic reactions after allergen immunotherapy. J Allergy Clin Immunol. 2009;123:493–8.
62. Ohashi Y, Nakai Y, Murata K. Effect of pretreatment with fexofenadine on the safety of immunotherapy in patients with allergic rhinitis. Ann Allergy Asthma Immunol. 2006;96:600–5.
63. Portnoy J, Bagstad K, Kanarek H, et al. Premedication reduces the incidence of systemic reactions during inhalant rush immunotherapy with mixtures of allergenic extracts. Ann Allergy. 1994;73:409–18.
64. Dietrich J, Moore L, Nguyen, et al. Imported fire ant hypersensitivity: a 1-day rush immunotherapy schedule without premedication. Ann Allergy Asthma Immunol. 2009;103:535–6.
65. Casale T, Busse W, Kline J, et al. Omalizumab pretreatment decreases acute reactions after rush immunotherapy for ragweed-induced seasonal allergic rhinitis. J Allergy Clin Immunol. 2006;117:134–40.
66. Massanari M, Nelson H, Casale T, et al. Effect of pretreatment with Omalizumab on the tolerability of specific immunotherapy in allergic asthma. J Allergy Clin Immunol. 2010;125:383–9.
67. Hurst D, Gordon B, Fornadley J, et al. Safety of home-based and office allergy immunotherapy: a multicenter prospective study. Otolaryngol Head Neck Surg. 1999;121:553–61.
68. Amin H, Liss G, Bernstein D. Evaluation of near-fatal reactions to allergen immunotherapy injections. J Allergy Clin Immunol. 2006;117:169–75.
69. Tinkelman D, Cole W, Tunno J. Immunotherapy: a one-year prospective study to evaluate risk factors of systemic reactions. J Allergy Clin Immunol. 1995;95:8–14.
70. Lin M, Tanner E, Lynn J, et al. Nonfatal systemic allergic reactions induced by skin testing and immunotherapy. Ann Allergy. 1993;71:557–62.
71. Lieberman P, Nicklas RA, Randolph C, et al. Anaphylaxis—a practice parameter update 2015. Ann Allergy Asthma Immunol. 2015;115:341–84.
72. Passalacqua G, Baena-Cagnani C, Bousquet J, et al. Grading local side effects of sublingual immunotherapy for respiratory allergy: speaking the same language. J Allergy Clin Immunol. 2013;132:93–8.
73. Bernstein D, Kleine-Tebbe J, Nelson H, et al. SQ house dust mite sublingual immunotherapy tablet subgroup efficacy and local application site reaction duration. Ann Allergy Asthma Immunol. 2018;121:105–10.
74. Nelson H, Nolte H, Creticos P, et al. Efficacy and safety of Timothy grass allergy immunotherapy tablet treatment in north American adults. J Allergy Clin Immunol. 2011;127:72–80.
75. Lucendo A, Arias A, Tenias J. Relation between eosinophilic esophagitis and Oral immunotherapy for food allergy: a systematic review with meta-analysis. Ann Allergy Asthma Immunol. 2014;113:624–9.
76. Linkov G, Toskala E. Sublingual immunotherapy: what we can learn from the European experience. Curr Opin Otolaryngol Head Neck Surg. 2014;22:208–10.
77. Portnoy J, Cox L. Is the benefit from prescribing epinephrine autoinjectors for sublingual immunotherapy worth the cost? Lessons learned from clinical trials. J Allergy Clin Immunol Pract. 2017;5:90–1.
78. Fitzhugh D, Bernstein D. Should epinephrine autoinjectors be prescribed to all patients on subcutaneous immunotherapy? J Allergy Clinical Immunol Pract. 2016;4(5):862–7.
79. Vickery B, Vereda A, Casale T, et al. AR101 Oral immunotherapy for Peanut allergy. N Engl J Med. 2018;379:1991–2001.
80. Chu K, Wood R, French S, et al. Oral immunotherapy for Peanut allergy (PACE): a systematic review and meta-analysis of efficacy and safety. Lancet. 2019;393:2222–32.
81. Rathinam K, Abraham J, Vijayakumar T. An evidence based review of Dupilumab in the treatment of moderate to severe asthma. Curr Ther Res. 2019;91:91.
82. ALK-Abelló Inc. (2017). ODACTRA™ house dust mite (Dermatophagoides farinae and Dermatophagoides pteronyssinus) allergen extract tablet for sublingual use: highlights of prescribing information. Hørsholm, Denmark.Gevaert P, Saenz R, Corren J, Han JK, Mullol J, Lee SE, ow RA, Zhao R, Howard M, Wong K, Islam L, Ligueros-Saylan M, Omachi TA, Bachert C. Long-term efficacy and safety of omalizumab for nasal polyposis in an open-label extension study. J Allergy Clin Immunol. 2022;149(3):957–65.
83. Han JK, Bachert C, Fokkens W, Desrosiers M, Wagenmann M, Lee SE, Smith SG, Martin N, Mayer B, Yancey SW, Sousa AR, Chan R, Hopkins C, SYNAPSE study investigators. Mepolizumab for chronic rhinosinusitis with nasal polyps (SYNAPSE): a randomised, double-blind, placebo-controlled, phase 3 trial. Lancet. Respir Med. 2021;9(10):1141–53.

Part V

Asthma

Edited by Cecelia Damask

Basics and Epidemiology of Asthma

22

Michael Parker

Introduction

Asthma is a chronic inflammatory condition that affects the airway and lungs of more than 25 million Americans [1], and approximately 235 million individuals globally [2]. The inflammation of asthma can be quite variable with regard to the presentation of the disease, the triggers provoking the inflammatory process and in the response of the lungs and lower airway to that provocation. Inflammation of the airway is frequently not site-specific and patients seeking medical attention in the Otolaryngologist's office with complaints and symptoms related to inflammation of the upper aerodigestive tract frequently have symptoms and findings of lower airway inflammation as well. This observation of the potential for disseminated airway inflammation contributes to the need for Otolaryngologists to have an awareness and understanding of asthma, its clinical presentation and management. Warning signs of asthma can vary from mild to minimal symptoms of wheezing and cough with minimal patient awareness of airway inflammation to severe and persistent symptoms of airway inflammation, which in some cases can result in life-threatening airway compromise. Asthma is most frequently classified based on a combination of symptom frequency and severity, with frequency ranging from intermittent to persistent episodes and symptom severity varying from mild to severe. Asthma can also be classified based on the variables leading to the provocation of airway inflammation. Allergic asthma, seasonal asthma, nocturnal asthma, exercise-induced asthma, and viral/URI-induced asthma have all been well described as types of asthma classified by inciting events. Treatment of asthma begins with identifying and minimizing provoking events, acutely reversing the airway compromise, and lessening the inflammatory changes that occur.

Pathophysiology and Definition of Asthma

Asthma is a heterogeneous, noncommunicable inflammatory condition of the airway below the level of the larynx, marked by episodes of airway hyperresponsiveness and inflammation resulting in narrowing of the airway [3]. These episodes of airway inflammation are associated with recurrent symptoms of wheezing, coughing, chest tightness, and shortness of breath, although the symptoms can vary significantly based on the patient's age and comorbidities. During an asthmatic event, the patient's airway becomes

M. Parker (✉)
Department of Otolaryngology and Communication Sciences, State University of New York Upstate Medical University, Syracuse, NY, USA

C. Damask et al. (eds.), *Allergy in Otolaryngology Practice*,
https://doi.org/10.1007/978-3-031-93455-1_22

inflamed, narrowed, and swollen, and can be associated with excess mucus production, all making it more difficult to breath. Several variables have been linked to the etiology of airway stimulation and irritation with the most frequent variables increasing the risk of asthma including the patient's age, the presence of allergies, and associated viral upper respiratory tract infections.

This airway hyperresponsiveness results in an exaggerated bronchoconstrictor response. Over time, repetitive events of airway inflammation and hyperresponsiveness can result in airway remodeling. This airway remodeling can include structural changes to both the large and small airways. These changes include subepithelial fibrosis, increased smooth muscle activity, and hypertrophy of mucosal glandular activity with increased secretions. This epithelial remodeling has been demonstrated in all degrees of asthma severity [4].

Burden of Disease

Asthma affects 1 in 13 people in the United States based on Centers for Disease Control and Prevention (CDC) data, with 8.4 percent of children and 7.7 percent of adults carrying the diagnosis [1]. The distribution of asthma across the United States population varies, with asthma being more common in children than in adults, and among children, boys are more commonly affected than girls [1]. In adults however, women are more commonly diagnosed than men [1]. There is also evidence of ethnic/racial variability with asthma. With asthma deaths in the United States three times more likely in African Americans [2], while the prevalence of the disease in the United States is highest among Puerto Ricans compared to all other ethnic groups [2]. These differences in racial and ethnic subpopulations are highly connected with poverty, urban air quality, poor patient education, and diminished health care opportunity [3].

Asthma places a significant burden on the health care system in the United States, with 9.8 million doctor's office visits, 1.8 million emergency department visits, and 188,968 discharges from hospital inpatient care annually in the United States [1]. Mortality associated with asthma is also significant, with approximately 10 Americans dying every day from the disease (3564 deaths from asthma in 2017) [2]. Asthma also creates a significant economic burden, with the economic cost of asthma care in the United States costing more than $81.9 billion annually including medical costs and lost work and school days [5].

The heterogenicity of asthma makes it difficult to use population-based studies to define the true incidence of the disease so an epidemiologic definition of asthma has also been developed to define clinically important asthma [6]. In the epidemiologic definition of asthma, "current asthma" is defined as bronchial hyperresponsiveness in the presence of wheezing within the past twelve months. If bronchial hyperresponsiveness testing is not available, the patient's or parent's reports of a physician's diagnosis of airway hyperresponsiveness remain the standard [7].

Questionnaires have also been used to assess asthma prevalence in varied populations, but these questionnaires are often burdened with intrinsic problems and biases. Two examples of clinical asthma questionnaires include the Tasmanian Asthma Survey and the International Study of Asthma and Allergies in Children. When questionnaires are used in combination with bronchial hyperresponsiveness, the specificity of the data collection is high but the sensitivity of the data remains low resulting in difficulties with accurate reporting of asthma in a specific population [8].

Global variation of asthma has also been observed, with some of this variability possibly being attributed to the use of different definitions of the disease and different tools to measure the disease [9], with environmental exposures and genetic predisposition also playing some role [10].

Patient Symptoms and Classification of Disease Severity

Symptoms of asthma can vary widely among patients, from mild and intermittent symptoms causing minimal patient awareness to severe incapacitating and persistent inflammation causing significant airway compromise. The most common symptoms associated with asthma include wheezing, cough, chest tightness, and shortness of breath. The patient's age can also be a variable with regard to presenting symptoms of asthma with young children occasionally being diagnosed only after repeated hospitalizations for bronchitis and pneumonia [11], while adults often modify their behavior to avoid or minimize activity which might provoke an asthmatic attack [12].

The National Asthma Education and Prevention Program (NAEPP) has used the patient's frequency and severity of symptoms to classify a patient's asthma to be either intermittent, mild persistent, moderate persistent, or severe ersistent [13]. This classification system is based on symptoms before treatment, and a patient's classification can change over time. It is also possible for a person with any category of asthma to have a severe asthmatic attack.

The diagnosis of intermittent asthma is used when the symptoms of asthma occur fewer than 2 days a week and do not interfere with normal activities of the patient and nighttime symptom frequency is fewer than two days a month. Lung function is normal between events and tests of airway function, discussed in another chapter, are typically normal when the patient is not having an attack.

The diagnosis of persistent asthma can be divided into three categories, mild persistent, moderate persistent, and severe persistent disease, with disease severity, and frequency of symptoms increasing from mild to severe classification. Mild persistent asthma is characterized by symptoms occurring on more than two days in a week but not daily. Attacks interfere with normal daily activities and nighttime symptoms occur three to four times a month. Lung function tests are also normal for mild persistent asthma when the person is not having an attack. The diagnosis of moderate persistent asthma is made when symptoms occur daily and inhaled short-acting rescue medications are used every day. Moderate persistent asthmatics have nighttime symptoms that occur at least one time per week, but do not occur nightly. Lung function tests are abnormal (60% -80% of expected value). Severe persistent asthma occurs when symptoms occur throughout each day and severely limit daily physical activities. Nighttime symptoms occur frequently in severe asthma, often occurring every night, with lung function tests often 60% or less than expected [3].

Classification of disease severity in asthma is fundamental to proper disease management, with greater pharmacotherapeutic intervention recommended as disease severity increases.

Types of Asthma and Asthma Triggers

Besides classifying disease based on severity and frequency, asthma can also be classified by the type of inciting event that provokes airway inflammation and hyperresponsiveness. These inciting events or asthma triggers are not necessarily related to severity of disease or frequency of attacks. Allergic asthma, respiratory tract infection-induced asthma, exercise-induced asthma, non-allergic or irritant-induced asthma also known as occupational asthma, and gastroesophageal reflux-provoked asthma have all been well described [3, 13].

Allergic asthma is triggered by inhaling allergens such as airborne pollens, dust mites, mold spores, or animal dander. The reaction that occurs is similar to the allergic events that occur in the nose and upper respiratory tract in allergic rhinitis. Allergens bind to antigen-specific IgE on sensitized mast cells in the airway mucosa, triggering mast cell degranulation and release of mediators which provoke inflammatory changes and airway constriction. Allergic asthma is the most common form of asthma [15].

Asthma triggered by respiratory infections compose a frequent etiology for an asthmatic exacerbation in susceptible individuals. A variety of infectious agents have been implicated as triggers of asthmatic events including rhinovirus associated with the common cold, influenza, sinus infections, and pneumonia [14]. Rhinitis and sinusitis (rhinosinusitis) are also commonly associated with asthma exacerbations and patients with rhinosinusitis are more likely to develop asthma than those without the disease [15].

Non-allergic asthma is used to describe asthma which is triggered by some form of airway irritation in susceptible individuals. The specific airway trigger and mechanism of inflammation is non-allergic and not infectious but has the potential to result in comparable degrees of airway compromise, hyperresponsiveness, and inflammation.

Exercise induced asthma, also known as exercise induced bronchospasm, can occur in allergic asthmatics as an additional trigger or it can occur in isolation, occurring more commonly in high-level athletes. Signs and symptoms of exercise-induced bronchoconstriction usually begin during or soon after beginning exercise [17]. Symptoms include coughing, wheezing, shortness of breath, chest tightness, fatigue during exercise, and poorer-than-expected athletic performance. Factors contributing to an increased probability of triggering exercise-induced bronchospasm include cold air, dry air, failure to warm-up, chemical exposures, such as chlorine in swimming pools, and air pollution [14].

Occupational asthma is defined as airway inflammation which occurs in the work environment with exposures to an allergic or non-allergic stimulant that triggers airway hyperreactivity. Occupational asthma should be considered in an adult with new-onset asthma, and is typically caused by inhaling fumes, gases, particulates, or other potentially harmful substances related to workplace exposures [16]. Occupational asthma is typically divided into high-molecular-weight stimulants and low-molecular-weight stimulants. The high-molecular-weight compounds include animal, insect, fish and shellfish, flours and cereals, enzymes, and natural rubber latex, while the low-molecular-weight compounds include chemicals (e.g., formaldehyde, diisocyanates, and incomplete antigens or haptens) [14, 18].

Gastroesophageal reflux disease (GERD) has been identified as a potential trigger for asthma and is a common comorbidity associated with severe and difficult to treat asthma [19]. Several proposed mechanisms for asthma activation have been suggested in patients with GERD and they include an increase in vagal tone related to exposure of the esophagus to acid [20], heightened bronchial reactivity [21], and microaspirations [22]. For asthmatic patients who experience worsening asthma symptoms associated with an episode of gastroesophageal reflux, such as an asthma exacerbation associated with eating a high-fat meal or an increased use of a rescue inhaler associated with heartburn symptoms, concomitant treatment of the suspected GERD is indicated to help control the airway inflammation [22].

Extremes of temperature and humidity have been shown to trigger an asthmatic response and have been shown to worsen the severity of exercise-induced asthma [23]. Inhalation of dry, cold air can trigger bronchoconstriction in predisposed individuals during exercise. While the exact mechanism is unclear, it may be related to the airway's attempt to condition the cold dry air by adding increased blood flow to the airway to help in heating and humidifying the inspired air. It is postulated that this increased blood flow results in airway narrowing and the production of increased airway turbulence, increasing airway inflammation [24].

Obstructive sleep apnea (OSA) is common chronic condition and can occur in combination with asthma or produce symptoms that mimic nocturnal asthma [25]. Nocturnal awakenings often associated with a perception of shortness of breath are common place in OSA patients. Appropriate diagnostic testing for sleep apnea is warranted for patients with nocturnal symptoms of asthma who have nocturnal exacerbations and risk factors for sleep apnea, including a high BMI, family history of OSA, and observations of the bed partner [26].

Nocturnal/Diurnal Variation of Symptoms

Nocturnal worsening of asthma symptoms is well-described and should be considered in the management of patients' symptoms and control of the inflammatory process. Nocturnal asthma is relatively common with 30–70% of asthmatics reporting nocturnal worsening of symptoms at least one time per month [27]. There is a well-described circadian pattern of lung function with optimal pulmonary function occurring at approximately 4 pm and the poorest lung function occurring 12 hours later around 4 am[30]. This normal circadian variation in lung function ranges from a 5 to 8 percent variation from best to worst lung function over this circadian period. Asthmatics have a significantly greater variation in their circadian function over a 24-hour period with variations of 15 to 50% [28]. Several neurohormonal observations have been identified which may provide a potential explanation of the effect of chronobiology on lung function.

It has been well observed that cholinergic (vagal) tone is increased at night, this increase in parasympathetic tone is likely a contributor to some of the circadian changes in airway function. There is also a circadian variation in epinephrine release with corresponding variation in lung function [29, 30]. Additional neurohormonal changes which occur in a circadian pattern include hypothalamic and pituitary control of the cortisol levels [31]. Melatonin, a sleep-inducing hormone also has a proinflammatory effect which is enhanced in asthmatics and may contribute to worsening nocturnal asthma [32]. The circadian variability observations likely contribute to patterns of nighttime worsening of asthma in susceptible individuals.

Pediatric vs Adult Asthma

Asthma is a variable and heterogeneous disease and acts differently in children vs adults. Children have smaller airways and these smaller airways are more susceptible to symptom production with airway irritation and swelling. Asthma in childhood can be divided into two generalized groups, with the observation that many infants wheeze in the first few years of life but the majority of children will outgrow asthma by adulthood [33]. This group of children have intermittent symptoms, often in association with viral upper respiratory infections and tend to outgrow the episodes of wheezing as they get older [34]. The second group of wheezing children tend to have later onset of symptoms and those symptoms tend to be more persistent [35]. This cohort of childhood asthma tends to be characterized by atopy, a greater probability of a positive family history of asthma and allergies, and an increased risk for the asthma to continue as an adult [36].

The majority of adults with asthma were diagnosed as children and continue to have symptoms. Adults with new-onset asthma may represent a group of undiagnosed childhood asthma [37]. Another feature of adult-onset asthma is that it is twice as likely to occur in women, with the rate of onset being highest in the perimenopausal period [38]. Adult-onset asthma may also be associated with a greater rate of decline in lung function [39], with the severity of symptoms being associated with the degree of loss of pulmonary function [40]. Predisposing activities such as cigarette smoke and poor environmental exposures may also be contributing.

Diagnosis and Treatment of Asthma

The diagnosis of asthma utilizes a combination of patient symptoms, physical findings, and objective metrics of airflow. Treatment of asthma includes identifying and minimizing exposure to inciting events, prophylactic treatment to lessen airway responsiveness, and strategies to diminish airway inflammation. Both of these topics will be discussed in detail in subsequent chapters.

Summary

Asthma is a common and heterogeneous inflammatory disease that affects the airway and is not infrequently encountered in patients seeking medical care in the Otolaryngologist's clinic. Awareness of the disease presentation and triggers, risk factors associated with the variable presentation of the inflammation associated with asthma, and the variability of the inflammatory process should all be kept in mind when seeing patients with upper respiratory complaints.

References

1. Centers for Disease Control and Prevention. 2018. CDC – Asthma - Data and Surveillance - Asthma Surveillance Data. [online] Available at: http://www.cdc.gov/asthma/asthmadata.htm. Accessed 11 Jan 2021.
2. World Health Organization. https://www.who.int/features/factfiles/asthma/en/. Accessed 3rd Jan 2021.
3. Global Initiative for Asthma. Global strategy for asthma management and prevention https://www.ginasthma.org. Accessed 16th Dec 2020.
4. Bergeron C, Tulic M, Hamid Q. Airway remodeling in asthma: From benchside to clinical practice. Can Respir J. 2010;17(4):e85–93. https://doi.org/10.1155/2010/318029. https://www.ncbi.nlm.nih.gov/pmc/articles/PMC2933777/. Accessed 14th Dec 2020
5. Atsjournals.org. 2018. The economic burden of Asthma in the United States, 2008–2013 | Annals of the American Thoracic Society | Articles in Press. [online] Available at: https://www.atsjournals.org/doi/abs/10.1513/AnnalsATS.201703-259OC. Accessed 14th Jan 2021.
6. Toelle BG, Peat JK, Salome CM, et al. Toward a definition of asthma for epidemiology. Am Rev Respir Dis. 1992;146:633.
7. Enarson DA, Vedal S, Schulzer M, et al. Asthma, asthmalike symptoms, chronic bronchitis, and the degree of bronchial hyperresponsiveness in epidemiologic surveys. Am Rev Respir Dis. 1987;136:613.
8. Jenkins MA, Clarke JR, Carlin JB, et al. Validation of questionnaire and bronchial hyperresponsiveness against respiratory physician assessment in the diagnosis of asthma. Int J Epidemiol. 1996;25:609.
9. Worldwide variation in prevalence of symptoms of asthma, allergic rhinoconjunctivitis, and atopic eczema: ISAAC. The International Study of Asthma and Allergies in Childhood (ISAAC) Steering Committee. Lancet. 1998;351:1225.
10. Lai CK, Beasley R, Crane J, et al. Global variation in the prevalence and severity of asthma symptoms: phase three of the international study of asthma and allergies in childhood (ISAAC). Thorax. 2009;64:476.
11. Matricardi PM, Illi S, Grüber C, et al. Wheezing in childhood: incidence, longitudinal patterns and factors predicting persistence. Eur Respir J. 2008;32:585.
12. Bronnimann S, Burrows B. A prospective study of the natural history of asthma. Remission Relapse Rates Chest. 1986;90:480.
13. National Asthma Education and Prevention Program: Expert panel report III: Guidelines for the diagnosis and management of asthma. Bethesda, MD: National Heart, Lung, and Blood Institute. 2007. (NIH publication no. 08–4051) www.nhlbi.nih.gov/guidelines/asthma/asthgdln.htm. Accessed 3rd Dec 2020.
14. Castillo JR, Peters SP, Busse WW. Asthma exacerbations: pathogenesis, prevention, and treatment. J Allergy Clin Immunol Pract. 2017;5:918.
15. Leynaert B, Bousquet J, Neukirch C, et al. Perennial rhinitis: an independent risk factor for asthma in nonatopic subjects: results from the European Community respiratory health survey. J Allergy Clin Immunol. 1999;104:301.
16. Arbes SJ Jr, Gergen PJ, Vaughn B, Zeldin DC. Asthma cases attributable to atopy: results from the third National Health and nutrition examination survey. J Allergy Clin Immunol. 2007;120:1139.
17. Ploeger HE, Takken T, de Greef MH, Timmons BW. The effects of acute and chronic exercise on inflammatory markers in children and adults with a chronic inflammatory disease: a systematic review. Exerc Immunol Rev. 2009;15:6.
18. Nicholson PJ, Cullinan P, Taylor AJ, et al. Evidence based guidelines for the prevention, identification, and management of occupational asthma. Occup Environ Med. 2005;62:290.
19. Chipps BE, Haselkorn T, Paknis B, et al. More than a decade follow-up in patients with severe or difficult-to-treat asthma: the epidemiology and natural history of asthma: outcomes and treatment regimens (TENOR) II. J Allergy Clin Immunol. 2018;141:1590.
20. Mansfield LE, Hameister HH, Spaulding HS, et al. The role of the vague nerve in airway narrowing caused by intraesophageal hydrochloric acid provocation and esophageal distention. Ann Allergy. 1981;47:431.
21. Vincent D, Cohen-Jonathan AM, Leport J, et al. Gastro-oesophageal reflux prevalence and relationship with bronchial reactivity in asthma. Eur Respir J. 1997;10:2255.
22. Sant'Ambrogio FB, Sant'Ambrogio G, Chung K. Effects of HCl-pepsin laryngeal instillations on upper airway patency-maintaining mechanisms. J Appl Physiol. 1985;1998(84):1299.
23. Anderson SD, Daviskas E. The mechanism of exercise-induced asthma is .... J Allergy Clin Immunol. 2000;106:453.
24. Gilbert IA, McFadden ER Jr. Airway cooling and rewarming. The second reaction sequence in exercise-induced asthma. J Clin Invest. 1992;90:699.
25. Teodorescu M, Broytman O, Curran-Everett D, et al. Obstructive sleep apnea risk, asthma burden, and lower airway inflammation in adults in the severe asthma research program (SARP) II. J Allergy Clin Immunol Pract. 2015;3:566.
26. Kasasbeh A, Kasasbeh E, Krishnaswamy G. Potential mechanisms connecting asthma, esophageal reflux,

and obesity/sleep apnea complex--a hypothetical review. Sleep Med Rev. 2007;11:47.
27. Horner CC, Dula C, Bacharier LB, et al. Daily global stress is associated with nocturnal asthma awakenings in school-age children. J Allergy Clin Immunol. 2016;138:1196.
28. Hetzel MR, Clark TJ. Comparison of normal and asthmatic circadian rhythms in peak expiratory flow rate. Thorax. 1980;35:732.
29. Sutherland ER. Nocturnal asthma. J Allergy Clin Immunol. 2005;116:1179.
30. Barnes P, FitzGerald G, Brown M, Dollery C. Nocturnal asthma and changes in circulating epinephrine, histamine, and cortisol. N Engl J Med. 1980;303:263.
31. Sutherland ER, Ellison MC, Kraft M, Martin RJ. Altered pituitary-adrenal interaction in nocturnal asthma. J Allergy Clin Immunol. 2003;112:52.
32. Sutherland ER, Ellison MC, Kraft M, Martin RJ. Elevated serum melatonin is associated with the nocturnal worsening of asthma. J Allergy Clin Immunol. 2003;112:513.
33. Guilbert T, Krawiec M. Natural history of asthma. Pediatr Clin N Am. 2003;50:523.
34. Ernst P, Cai B, Blais L, Suissa S. The early course of newly diagnosed asthma. Am J Med. 2002;112:44.
35. Bisgaard H, Bønnelykke K. Long-term studies of the natural history of asthma in childhood. J Allergy Clin Immunol. 2010;126:187.
36. Morgan WJ, Stern DA, Sherrill DL, et al. Outcome of asthma and wheezing in the first 6 years of life: follow-up through adolescence. Am J Respir Crit Care Med. 2005;172:1253.
37. Stern DA, Morgan WJ, Halonen M, et al. Wheezing and bronchial hyper-responsiveness in early childhood as predictors of newly diagnosed asthma in early adulthood: a longitudinal birth-cohort study. Lancet. 2008;372:1058.
38. Triebner K, Johannessen A, Puggini L, et al. Menopause as a predictor of new-onset asthma: a longitudinal northern European population study. J Allergy Clin Immunol. 2016;137:50.
39. Lange P, Parner J, Vestbo J, et al. A 15-year follow-up study of ventilatory function in adults with asthma. N Engl J Med. 1998;339:1194.
40. Kelly WJ, Hudson I, Raven J, et al. Childhood asthma and adult lung function. Am Rev Respir Dis. 1988;138:26.

23 Pathology, Pathogenesis and Pathophysiology of Asthma

Rebecca J. Kamil, Venkataramana K. Sidhaye, and Murugappan Ramanathan Jr

Lung Anatomy and Physiology

Lung Function and Development

The main function of the lungs is to obtain oxygen from the environment to supply to cells for cellular respiration and then eliminate the carbon dioxide created by cells [36]. Critical functions of the respiratory system involve acid-base homeostasis, pulmonary defense against particles and microorganisms, and metabolism. In utero, the conducting airways (e.g., trachea, bronchi, and bronchioles) develop first and are followed by the formation and growth of the gas exchange portion (e.g., acini) of the lungs ([31], no. StatPearls [Internet]). The acini, or functional lung unit, involves a large surface area with a thin air-blood barrier where oxygen and carbon dioxide gas exchange take place. This unit includes alveolar ducts, sacs, and alveoli. Critical to this function is surfactant, a combination of lipids and proteins secreted into the alveolar space, which decreases surface tension to facilitate lung inflation and decrease the work of breathing ([70], pp. 427–444).

Lung Anatomy

Gross Anatomy

The lungs are connected to the heart through the pulmonary circulation ([34], p. Chap. 3). The upper airway connects to the trachea which enters the thorax and bifurcates into right and left mainstem bronchi. The right bronchus then further divides into upper, middle, and inferior lobar bronchi and supplies their respective right lung lobes. Left bronchus divides into superior and inferior lobar bronchi and supplies their respective left lung lobes. These bronchi then further divide into smaller bronchi and then bronchioles which end at the alveolar sac and the site of gas exchange.

R. J. Kamil
Department of Otolaryngology-Head and Neck Surgery, Johns Hopkins University School of Medicine, Baltimore, MD, USA
e-mail: rkamil1@jhmi.edu

V. K. Sidhaye
Division of Pulmonary Medicine, Johns Hopkins University School of Medicine, Baltimore, MD, USA
e-mail: Vsidhay1@jhmi.edu

M. Ramanathan Jr (✉)
Division of Rhinology and Endoscopic Skull Base Surgery, Department of Otolaryngology-HNS, Johns Hopkins University School of Medicine, Baltimore, MD, USA
e-mail: mramana3@jhmi.edu

C. Damask et al. (eds.), *Allergy in Otolaryngology Practice*,
https://doi.org/10.1007/978-3-031-93455-1_23

Histology

The lungs are covered in pleura which is a double-layered serous membrane ([31], no. StatPearls [Internet]). There are 300 million alveoli in an average 70-kilogram (kg) adult which equates to 80 square meters of surface area. Ciliated pseudostratified columnar respiratory epithelium lines the conducting portion of the airway. Ciliated cells are needed to moisturize the air and remove any irritants and microorganisms. This action is known as the mucociliary escalator. Goblet cells contain mucin granules and become less frequent in the smaller airways. There are also basal, brush, and neuroendocrine cells present which possess specialized functions.

Lung Physiology

In order for air to enter the lungs for gas exchange to take place, there must be a pressure gradient between the outside world and alveoli [37]. For this to occur, alveolar pressure must fall below atmospheric pressure through expansion of lungs by downward movement of diaphragm and contraction of intercostal muscles. When alveolar pressure is greater than atmospheric pressure to the point it can overcome the resistance to airflow of conducting airways, exhalation occurs.

Lung Volumes

The standardization of lung volumes and size is related to patient's height, weight, age, and gender [38]. There are four standard lung volumes and four standard lung capacities. These standardized volumes are measured during pulmonary function tests and spirometry, which are used to diagnose and follow asthma as well as many other pulmonary diseases.

(i) **Tidal volume (TV).**
Tidal volume (TV) is the volume of air entering or leaving the mouth with each breath. For a 70-kg adult, the average tidal volume is 500 mL during quiet breathing.

(ii) **Expiratory Reserve Volume (ERV).**
Expiratory reserve volume (ERV) is the volume of gas exhaled from the lungs during maximal forced expiration that starts at the end of the normal tidal expiration. It is also the difference of FRC and RV. In a 70-kg adult, the average ERV is 1500 mL.

(iii) **Inspiratory Reserve Volume (IRV).**
Inspiratory reserve volume (IRV) is the volume of gas inhaled into the lungs during a maximal forced inspiration starting at the end of a normal tidal inspiration. For a 70 kg adult, the average IRV is 2500 mL.

(iv) **Residual Volume (RV).**
Residual volume (RV) is the gas volume in the lungs after a maximal forced exhalation. This residual volume prevents lungs from collapsing. For a 70-kg adult, the average residual volume is 1500 mL.

(v) **Functional Residual Capacity (FRC).**
Functional residual capacity (FRC) is the volume of gas that is left in the lungs at the end of normal tidal expiration. This is comprised of the addition of RV and ERV. In a 70 kg adult, the average FRC is 3000 mL.

(vi) **Inspiratory Capacity (IC).**
Inspiratory capacity (IC) is the volume of gas inhaled during maximal inspiratory effort that begins at the end of normal tidal expiration. This is comprised of the addition of TV and IRV. In a 70 kg adult, the average IC is 3000 mL.

(vii) **Vital Capacity (VC).**
Vital capacity (VC) is the volume of gas exhaled from lungs during maximal forced expiration after maximal forced inspiration. The VC is RV subtracted from TLC. In a 70 kg adult, the average VC is 4500 mL.

(viii) **Total Lung Capacity (TLC).**
Total lung capacity (TLC) is the volume of gas left in the lungs after maximal inspiratory effort. The TLC is compromised of the addition of TV, RV, IRV, and ERV. In a 70 kg adult, the average TLC is 6000 mL.

Lung Volumes in Asthma

Asthma is an obstructive process that leads to increased resistance to airflow [38]. In this process, the RV, FRC, TV, and TLC are increased, while VC and ERV are decreased.

Asthma

Development of Asthma

Definition

Asthma is a heterogenous disease characterized by chronic airway inflammation that is generally associated with bronchial hyperresponsiveness [65]. Symptoms include wheezing, cough, and shortness of breath in conjunction with variable airflow obstruction. There are many clinical phenotypes that have been characterized including allergic asthma, non-allergic asthma, adult-onset asthma, and asthma associated with obesity. Allergic asthma often starts in childhood and is associated with atopic disease (e.g., eczema, food allergy, and allergic rhinitis). Sputum often contains eosinophils and symptoms are generally steroid-responsive.

Epidemiology

Asthma is a very common respiratory illness that affects up to 18% of the worldwide population [65]. In the United States, an estimated 7.7% of adults and 8.4% of children suffer from asthma [14]. There is an association between asthma and chronic rhinitis with up to 80% of individuals with asthma having some form of chronic rhinitis ([8], pp. 8–160). Conversely, up to 40% of people with chronic rhinitis have asthma. In this way, chronic rhinitis is risk factor for development of asthma and asthma history and symptoms should be elicited when treating patients with chronic rhinitis ([71], pp. 21–25; [15], pp. S781–6; [23], pp. 419–425).

Genetics

There is a genetic component to the development of asthma and children of asthmatics are at increased risk of developing the disease. It is estimated that children with no family history have a 5% risk of developing asthma, while children with two parents with asthma have a 50% risk ([74], p. 10.3402/ecrj.v2.24643. eCollection 2015). It is also estimated that nearly half of the cases of asthma in the United States are attributable to atopy, which also has a well-understood genetic component ([2], pp. 1139–1145). A Swedish study showed that family history of atopy had a 3- to four-fold increase of developing asthma compared to adults with no family history ([47], pp. 3–10).

Environment

There are numerous non-allergic factors that may also contribute to development and severity of asthma. These include viral respiratory infections ([28], pp. 1225–1229), chronic stress ([12], pp. 1014–1020), and obesity ([6], pp. 661–666). Other environmental factors include smoke exposure ([17], pp. 218–224), air pollution ([75], pp. 387–398), socioeconomic status ([12], pp. 1014–1020), and geographic location ([27], pp. 33–63).

Pathophysiology of Asthma

The lower airway is comprised of the trachea which stems into two mainstem bronchus and then into smaller bronchioles ([33], pp. 6–10). The respiratory epithelium is ciliated pseudostratified with a layer of smooth muscle beneath. Contraction of this smooth muscle characterizes the obstructive symptoms seen in asthma. Muscle contraction is influenced by many factors including neuroregulation by the parasympathetic system and inflammation. Inflammation is thought to be key to the development of asthma. With patients suffering from atopic asthma, there is a dominant T-helper cell 2 (TH2) response that leads to secretion of cytokines including IL-4, IL-5, and IL-13, which then recruit and activate eosinophils and mast cells. Several cells including lymphocytes and eosinophils migrate to the airway epithelium and promote an inflammatory response ([30], pp. 335–344). Degranulation of mast cells leads to histamine and leukotriene release which then leads to edema, hypertrophy of the smooth muscle, mucus hypersecretion, and basement membrane thickening. All of these factors then contribute to irreversible fibrosis over time. Moreover, an increase in specific IgE may occur locally at the site of respiratory epithelium in asthmatics, even in absence of systemic sensitization on testing ([73], pp. 213–218).

Physiologic Characteristics of Asthma

Diagnosis

The clinical presentation of asthma includes symptoms of chronic cough, expiratory wheezing, shortness of breath, and tight chest sensation [65]. These symptoms can be triggered by viral infection, exercise, cold, and stress. Common comorbid illnesses include: allergic rhinitis ([66], pp. S70–3; [32], pp. 1065–1076), GERD ([59], pp. 60–63), and eczema ([79], pp. 568–576). Co-existing COPD can complicate diagnosis and treatment of asthma ([54], pp. 1163–1165). Wheezing is common in childhood and can occur in up to 50% of children under age 6 ([22], pp. S115–6). Those children suffering from more severe episodes and who have co-morbid atopic diseases are more likely to develop asthma ([3], pp. 604–610). Asthma can develop early in life or can present well into adulthood. As people age, allergic disease tends to lessen in severity and inflammation related to asthma in older adults has been found to be more neutrophil, rather than eosinophil, driven ([13], pp. 901–909).

When eliciting history from asthma patients, it is important to be aware of possible irritants that can lead to worsening asthma symptoms including smoking, chemical irritants, and certain medications (e.g., NSAIDs, aspirin) ([1], pp. 370–378). Physical exam can be normal or there may be cough or expiratory wheezing on lung auscultation. It is important to look for other stigmata of allergic disease including eczema, allergic shiners and salute, and enlarged, boggy inferior turbinates on exam ([21], pp. S28–31).

Peak Expiratory Flow

Pulmonary function testing is the gold standard to diagnose and follow the treatment of asthma ([58], pp. 667–84, ix). Peak expiratory flow rate (PEFR) is airflow during the first 1–2 seconds of forceful exhalation ([57], pp. 39–53). PEFR is often used to monitor asthma severity by using a peak expiratory flow monitor at home or in the office. These are inexpensive devices that can be used to monitor asthma severity over time and determine the efficacy of treatments. For asthmatics with severe symptoms, it is recommended patients take measurements 2–3 times a day.

Spirometry

Spirometry involves the measurement of two volumes including the forced expiratory volume in 1 second (FEV1) and forced vital capacity (FVC), which measures the difference between maximum inhalation and exhalation in terms of lung volume ([57], pp. 39–53). In asthma, the FEV1/FVC ratio is decreased because obstructive processes decrease FEV1. These pulmonary function tests are performed in the office or by technician in a laboratory setting. This gives more information about location, severity, and type of disease process compared to PEFR. To diagnose asthma, this test is performed before and after bronchodilator application or bronchial provocation (e.g., methacholine or exercise). It is important to note that spirometry requires a conscious and cooperative participant and can be difficult to perform in small children ([77], pp. 379–388).

Treatment and Management of Asthma

The treatment of asthma involves multiple inhaled and oral medications [11]. Inhaled short-acting beta-$_2$-agonists, or rescue inhalers, are given to all patients with asthma to be used as

Table 23.1 —Treatment of asthma. Information is adapted from the National Health of Heart, Lung, and Blood Institute Guidelines for the Diagnosis and Management of Asthma [11]

Medication	Mechanism of action	Generic examples
Beta-$_2$-agonist[a] Short-acting Long-acting	Relaxation of smooth muscle which leads to bronchodilation	Albuterol Salmeterol Formoterol
Inhaled corticosteroids Low-dose Medium-dose High-dose	Inhibits phospholipase A2 and in effect, the arachidonic acid pathway	Fluticasone Mometasone Budesonide Ciclesonide Flunisolide
Oral corticosteroids	Inhibits phospholipase A2 and in effect, the arachidonic acid pathway	Methylprednisolone Prednisolone Prednisone
Leukotriene receptor antagonist	Prevents binding of leukotrienes to receptors	Montelukast Zafirlukast
5-lipoxygenase inhibitors	Prevents leukotriene synthesis	Zileuton
Cromolyn	Mast cell stabilizer	Cromolyn
Methylxanthines	Phosphodiesterase inhibition and adenosine receptor antagonism	Theophylline
Immunomodulators	Anti-IgE monoclonal antibody	Omalizumab

[a]There are several combination inhalers that include both corticosteroid and beta-2-agonist

needed. Asthma is an inflammatory disorder so inhaled low-dose corticosteroids are the first-line treatment. As severity increases, inhaled medium and high-dose corticosteroids, long-acting beta-$_2$-agonist, cromolyn, leukotriene receptor antagonist, theophylline, and oral corticosteroids are all treatment options. See Table 23.1 for details regarding their mechanisms of action and common examples. It is recommended that physicians should consider immunotherapy for patients with persistent, allergic asthma. There is strong evidence for the positive effects of immunotherapy in asthmatics with allergies to dust mites, animal dander, and pollen ([52], pp. 251–256; [25], pp. 943–948) and these effects are greater in children than adults [11].

The 2012 National Health of Heart, Lung, and Blood Institute Guidelines for the Diagnosis and Management of Asthma gives guidance on assessing the severity of asthma. According to symptoms, lung function, and frequency of rescue inhaler use, clinicians can determine status of asthma control and gives strategies for improvement. As otolaryngologists, history of inhaled corticosteroids becomes important when diagnosing and treating fungal laryngitis in a patient with hoarseness. It should be noted that inhalers used with a spacer can decrease the deposition of steroid onto the laryngeal mucosa and can help reduce symptoms if patients are unable to stop medication [69].

Long-term Consequences of Asthma

There are many long-term consequences of asthma. In children, poorly controlled asthma has negative effects on cardiovascular fitness and is associated with higher levels of obesity and learning disabilities ([55], pp. 511–523). While in adults, there is greater risk of depression, poor concentration, as well as upper and lower airway infections. There is airway remodeling in long-term asthma and effects are seen on the airway epithelium, smooth muscle, mucus glands, and extracellular matrix ([7], pp. 56–62). This remodeling is associated with a progressive decrease in lung function, but more research is needed to further characterize the mechanisms behind this decline ([60], pp. 477–86; quiz 487; [20], pp. 551–569).

Asthma and Otolaryngology

Unified Airway Theory

The unified airway theory describes the upper and lower airways as a single functional unit ([33], pp. 6–10). It describes that diseases affecting the upper airway, including inflammatory allergic rhinitis and chronic rhinosinusitis, affect inflammation occurring in the lower airway. The upper and lower airways share common histological features including ciliated epithelium, lamina propria, glands, and goblet cells ([40], pp. 499–508, [41], p. 44). For this reason, it is critical for otolaryngologists to have an understanding of asthma and the relationship it has to common diseases encountered in an otolaryngology clinic ([49], p. https://doi.org/10.3390/medsci7040053).

Asthma and Chronic Rhinosinusitis

There has long been noted an association between asthma and chronic rhinosinusitis (CRS) ([68], pp. 44–47; [56], pp. S22–209). CRS has been shown to contribute to the respiratory symptoms of asthma, decreased quality of life, and poorer control of asthma ([72], pp. 553–556; [49], p. https://doi.org/10.3390/medsci7040053). For patients with asthma, concurrent CRS symptoms are over three times as likely compared to those without asthma ([26], pp. 91–98), and asthma is a predictor of negative quality of life ([19], pp. 1314–1321). Presence of CRS is associated with more severe course of asthma, particularly in patients with nasal polyps ([44], pp. 1781–1788). Moreover, there is a significant association between asthma severity and abnormalities on CT sinus imaging ([50], pp. 52–58). The mechanism behind this association is not clearly understood, but both diseases have multifactorial etiologies with eosinophilia and airway remodeling as common features ([63], pp. 877–882).

Importantly, medical and surgical treatment for CRS is associated with improved asthma control and there is growing evidence that treatment for one condition can improve the other ([18], pp. 261–265; [64], pp. 68–74). There are new biologic therapies that have shown efficacy in treating nasal polyposis with co-morbid asthma ([9], pp. 181–187). Dupilumab, which is a monoclonal antibody against IL-4, omalizumab, which is an anti-IgE monoclonal antibody, and mepolizumab, which is an anti-IL-5 monoclonal antibody, all have been FDA approved for use in CRSwNP, as well as in asthma.

Asthma and Inhalant Allergy

Asthma, like allergic rhinitis, is more prevalent in the developed world ([76], pp. 204–2458–12–204; [51], pp. S18–20). In a study investigating bronchial hyper-responsiveness in children, 25% of children aged 8–10 with inhalant sensitivities on skin prick testing developed asthma ([62], pp. 65–74). This could be driven by a prolonged Th2 response initiated by inhalant allergies that leads to inflammation of airways ([24], pp. B12–7; [29], pp. S36–9). Adult patients with allergic rhinitis are 8 times more likely to develop asthma than those without allergic rhinitis ([39], pp. 301–304). However, it should be noted that patients with non-atopic rhinitis also had a significantly increased risk of asthma so rhinitis alone appears to be a risk factor. It has been found that perennial allergies are more likely to be associated with asthma than seasonal allergies ([43], pp. 1048–1052). There is evidence that treatment of allergic rhinitis with intranasal steroids ([46], pp. 569–579), oral antihistamines ([61], pp. 1161–1167), and leukotriene receptor antagonists ([4], pp. 307–313) may also improve asthma control ([78], pp. 108–352).

With co-morbid allergic disease, immunotherapy should be considered to help control asthma symptoms. Immunotherapy is a disease-modifying treatment and can be administered subcutaneously (SCIT) or sublingually (SLIT) ([42], pp. S55–9; [67], pp. S51–4). These two options are equally efficacious ([42], pp. S55–9). A large review found that immunotherapy improved asthma in terms of symptoms, medication use, and bronchial hyperresponsiveness ([16], pp. S1–55). For young patients, immunotherapy has been shown to decrease the development of asthma in long-term studies ([52], pp. 251–256; [25], pp. 943–948). Grass tablet immunotherapy reduced asthma symptoms in children 16 years old and younger in a placebo-controlled trial ([10], pp. 167–173.e7). In all patients, SLIT for grass allergy was shown to decrease the need for inhaled corticosteroid dose after only 1 year of treatment ([53], pp. 55–56). In another study, SLIT for grass allergy and inhaled steroids were found to be equally efficacious in treating asthma symptoms ([48], pp. 69–75). SLIT also had the additional benefit of improving nasal eosinophilia and bronchial hyperresponsiveness over the 5-year study. The current evidence shows immunotherapy can prevent children from developing asthma and can decrease asthma medication use and symptoms. In this way, immunotherapy could be a method to prevent the long-term consequences of asthma and viewed as a potential cost-mitigating strategy.

Asthma and Allergy Testing

Many patients undergoing allergy testing have co-morbid asthma. It is critical to elicit asthma medication regimen and recent rescue inhaler use. Anaphylaxis is a dreaded complication of allergy testing and immunotherapy, and active asthma has been identified as a major risk factor ([35], pp. S60–5). In a 2014 study, 46% of patients who experienced a major reaction had active asthma at the time of testing ([45], pp. 660–677). In a long-term study examining fatalities in SCIT and allergy skin testing, 15 of 17 deaths were in asthmatic patients who were not optimally controlled ([5], pp. 1129–1136). Extra watchfulness is warranted when providing care to an asthmatic patient in this setting.

Conclusions

It is critical to have a basic understanding of asthma when treating allergy and atopic disease. This chapter reviewed basic pulmonology and pulmonary function tests. It discussed the diagnosis and treatment of asthma. It also detailed the unified airway theory and importance of treating co-morbid rhinologic conditions to improve the control of asthma. It is always important to be mindful of asthma symptoms when conducting allergy testing and providing immunotherapy in clinic in order to avoid life-threatening anaphylaxis.

References

1. Al-Alawi M, Hassan T, Chotirmall SH. Advances in the diagnosis and management of asthma in older adults. 2014;127:370–8. https://doi.org/10.1016/j.amjmed.2013.12.013.
2. Arbes SJ Jr, Gergen PJ, Vaughn B, Zeldin DC. Asthma cases attributable to atopy: results from the third national health and nutrition examination survey. 2007;120:1139–45.
3. Bacharier LB, Phillips BR, Bloomberg GR, et al. Severe intermittent wheezing in preschool children: a distinct phenotype. 2007;119:604–10.
4. Baena-Cagnani CE, Berger WE, DuBuske LM, et al. Comparative effects of desloratadine versus montelukast on asthma symptoms and use of beta 2-agonists in patients with seasonal allergic rhinitis and asthma. 2003;130:307–13. https://doi.org/10.1159/000070218.
5. Bernstein DI, Wanner M, Borish L, et al. Twelve-year survey of fatal reactions to allergen injections and skin testing: 1990-2001. 2004;113:1129–36. https://doi.org/10.1016/j.aci.2004.02.006.
6. Beuther DA, Sutherland ER. Overweight, obesity, and incident asthma: a meta-analysis of prospective epidemiologic studies. 2007;175:661–6. https://doi.org/10.1164/rccm.200611-1717OC. [pii]
7. Boulet LP. Airway remodeling in asthma: update on mechanisms and therapeutic approaches. 2018;24:56–62. https://doi.org/10.1097/MCP.0000000000000441.
8. Bousquet J, Khaltaev N, Cruz AA, et al. Allergic rhinitis and its impact on asthma (ARIA) 2008 update (in collaboration with the World Health Organization, GA(2)LEN and AllerGen). 2008:8–160. https://doi.org/10.1111/j.1398-9995.2007.01620.x.
9. Brooks GD. Updated evaluation of dupilumab in the treatment of asthma: patient selection and reported outcomes. 2020;16:181–7. https://doi.org/10.2147/TCRM.S192392.

10. Bufe A, Eberle P, Franke-Beckmann E, et al. Safety and efficacy in children of an SQ-standardized grass allergen tablet for sublingual immunotherapy. 2009;123:167–173.e7. https://doi.org/10.1016/j.jaci.2008.10.044.
11. Busse W NIH Guidelines for the diagnosis and management of asthma. https://www.nhlbi.nih.gov/sites/default/files/media/docs/12-5075.pdf. 2020.
12. Chen E, Hanson MD, Paterson LQ, et al. Socioeconomic status and inflammatory processes in childhood asthma: the role of psychological stress. 2006;117:1014–20.
13. Chotirmall SH, Watts M, Branagan P, et al. Diagnosis and management of asthma in older adults. 2009;57:901–9. https://doi.org/10.1111/j.1532-5415.2009.02216.x.
14. Control C for D. 2018 Asthma Data. 2018. https://www.cdc.gov/asthma/most_recent_national_asthma_data.htm. Accessed 21 Apr 2020.
15. Corren J. Allergic rhinitis and asthma: how important is the link? 1997;99:S781–6.
16. Cox L, Nelson H, Lockey R, et al. Allergen immunotherapy: a practice parameter third update. 2011;127:S1–55. https://doi.org/10.1016/j.jaci.2010.09.034.
17. Cunningham J, O'Connor GT, Dockery DW, Speizer FE. Environmental tobacco smoke, wheezing, and asthma in children in 24 communities. 1996;153:218–24. https://doi.org/10.1164/ajrccm.153.1.8542119.
18. Dunlop G, Scadding GK, Lund VJ. The effect of endoscopic sinus surgery on asthma: management of patients with chronic rhinosinusitis, nasal polyposis, and asthma. 1999;13:261–5. https://doi.org/10.2500/105065899782102809.
19. Ek A, Middelveld RJ, Bertilsson H, et al. Chronic rhinosinusitis in asthma is a negative predictor of quality of life: results from the Swedish GA(2)LEN survey. 2013;68:1314–21. https://doi.org/10.1111/all.12222.
20. Fehrenbach H, Wagner C, Wegmann M. Airway remodeling in asthma: what really matters. 2017;367:551–69. https://doi.org/10.1007/s00441-016-2566-8.
21. Franzese CB. AAOA allergy primer: history and physical examination. 2014:S28–31. https://doi.org/10.1002/alr.21390.
22. Graham LM (2006) Preschool wheeze prognosis: how do we predict outcome? S115-S116.
23. Guerra S, Sherrill DL, Martinez FD, Barbee RA. Rhinitis as an independent risk factor for adult-onset asthma. 2002;109:419–25.
24. Holt PG, Macaubas C, Stumbles PA, Sly PD. The role of allergy in the development of asthma. 1999;402:B12–7. https://doi.org/10.1038/35037009.
25. Jacobsen L, Niggemann B, Dreborg S, et al. Specific immunotherapy has long-term preventive effect of seasonal and perennial asthma: 10-year follow-up on the PAT study. 2007;62:943–8.
26. Jarvis D, Newson R, Lotvall J, et al. Asthma in adults and its association with chronic rhinosinusitis: the GA2LEN survey in Europe. 2012;67:91–8. https://doi.org/10.1111/j.1398-9995.2011.02709.x.
27. Jie Y, Isa ZM, Jie X, et al. Urban vs rural factors that affect adult asthma. 2013;226:33–63. https://doi.org/10.1007/978-1-4614-6898-1_2.
28. Johnston SL, Pattemore PK, Sanderson G, et al. Community study of role of viral infections in exacerbations of asthma in 9–11 year old children. 1995;310:1225–9. https://doi.org/10.1136/bmj.310.6989.1225.
29. Jones CA, Holt PG. Immunopathology of allergy and asthma in childhood. 2000;162:S36–9. https://doi.org/10.1164/ajrccm.162.supplement_1.maic-10.
30. Kay AB. Inflammatory cells in bronchial asthma. 1989;26:335–44. https://doi.org/10.3109/02770908909073275.
31. Khan Y, Lynch D. Histology. Lung. 2019;
32. Krouse JH. Asthma management for the otolaryngologist. 2017;50:1065–76.
33. Krouse JH, Krouse HJ. Asthma, rhinitis, and the unified airway. 2013;31:6–10.
34. Kurt MD, Foreman KB, Albertine. Lungs. McGraw-Hill Companies; 2011.
35. Leatherman BD. Anaphylaxis in the allergy practice. 2014:S60–5. https://doi.org/10.1002/alr.21392.
36. Levitzky MG. Function and structure of the respiratory system. New York: McGraw-Hill; 2013.
37. Levitzky MG. Mechanics of breathing. New York: McGraw-Hill; 2013.
38. Levitzky MG. Diffusion of gases and interpretation of pulmonary function tests. New York: McGraw-Hill; 2013.
39. Leynaert B, Bousquet J, Neukirch C, et al. Perennial rhinitis: An independent risk factor for asthma in nonatopic subjects: results from the European community respiratory health survey. 1999;104:301–4.
40. Licari A, Caimmi S, Bosa L, et al. Rhinosinusitis and asthma: a very long engagement. 2014;27:499–508.
41. Licari A, Castagnoli R, Denicolo CF, et al. The nose and the lung: United Airway Disease? 2017;5:44. https://doi.org/10.3389/fped.2017.00044.
42. Lin SY. Sublingual immunotherapy: current concepts for the U.S. practitioner. 2014:S55–9. https://doi.org/10.1002/alr.21388.
43. Linneberg A, Henrik Nielsen N, Frolund L, et al. The link between allergic rhinitis and allergic asthma: a prospective population-based study. The Copenhagen Allergy Study. 2002;57:1048–52.
44. Liou A, Grubb JR, Schechtman KB, Hamilos DL. Causative and contributive factors to asthma severity and patterns of medication use in patients seeking specialized asthma care. 2003;124:1781–8.
45. Lockey RF, Benedict LM, Turkeltaub PC, Bukantz SC. Fatalities from immunotherapy (IT) and skin testing (ST). 1987;79:660–77.
46. Lohia S, Schlosser RJ, Soler ZM. Impact of intranasal corticosteroids on asthma outcomes in allergic rhinitis: a meta-analysis. 2013;68:569–79. https://doi.org/10.1111/all.12124.

47. Lundback B. Epidemiology of rhinitis and asthma. 1998; 3–10.
48. Marogna M, Spadolini I, Massolo A, et al. Long-term comparison of sublingual immunotherapy vs inhaled budesonide in patients with mild persistent asthma due to grass pollen. 2009;102:69–75. https://doi.org/10.1016/S1081-1206(10)60111-1.
49. Massoth L, Anderson C, McKinney KA. Asthma and chronic Rhinosinusitis: diagnosis and medical management. 2019;7 https://doi.org/10.3390/medsci7040053.
50. Matsuno O, Ono E, Takenaka R, et al. Asthma and sinusitis: association and implication. 2008;147:52–8. https://doi.org/10.1159/000128659.
51. Mims JW. Epidemiology of allergic rhinitis. 2014:S18–20. https://doi.org/10.1002/alr.21385.
52. Moller C, Dreborg S, Ferdousi HA, et al. Pollen immunotherapy reduces the development of asthma in children with seasonal rhinoconjunctivitis (the PAT-study). 2002;109:251–6.
53. Mosbech H. Tolerability and efficacy of house dust mite AIT. 2011:55–6. https://doi.org/10.1111/j.1398-9995.2011.02641.x.
54. Nyenhuis SM, Schwantes EA, Evans MD, Mathur SK. Airway neutrophil inflammatory phenotype in older subjects with asthma. 2010;125:1163–5. https://doi.org/10.1016/j.jaci.2010.02.015.
55. O'Byrne PM, Pedersen S, Schatz M, et al. The poorly explored impact of uncontrolled asthma. 2013;143:511–23.
56. Orlandi RR, Kingdom TT, Hwang PH, et al. International consensus statement on allergy and rhinology: Rhinosinusitis. 2016:S22–209. https://doi.org/10.1002/alr.21695.
57. Parker MJ. Interpreting spirometry: the basics. 2014;47:39–53. https://doi.org/10.1016/j.otc.2013.10.002.
58. Parker MJ. Asthma. 2011;44:667–84, ix. https://doi.org/10.1016/j.otc.2011.04.001.
59. Parsons JP, Mastronarde JG. Gastroesophageal reflux disease and asthma. 2010;16:60–3. https://doi.org/10.1097/MCP.0b013e328332ca2f.
60. Pascual RM, Peters SP. Airway remodeling contributes to the progressive loss of lung function in asthma: an overview. 2005;116:477–86; quiz 487.
61. Pasquali M, Baiardini I, Rogkakou A, et al. Levocetirizine in persistent allergic rhinitis and asthma: effects on symptoms, quality of life and inflammatory parameters. 2006;36:1161–7.
62. Peat JK, Salome CM, Woolcock AJ. Longitudinal changes in atopy during a 4-year period: relation to bronchial hyperresponsiveness and respiratory symptoms in a population sample of Australian schoolchildren. 1990;85:65–74. https://doi.org/10.1016/0091-6749(90)90223-q. [pii]
63. Ponikau JU, Sherris DA, Kephart GM, et al. Features of airway remodeling and eosinophilic inflammation in chronic rhinosinusitis: is the histopathology similar to asthma? 2003;112:877–82. https://doi.org/10.1016/j.jaci.2003.08.009.
64. Ragab S, Scadding GK, Lund VJ, Saleh H. Treatment of chronic rhinosinusitis and its effects on asthma. 2006;28:68–74. https://doi.org/10.1183/09031936.06.00043305. [pii]
65. Reddel H, Boulet L-P. Global Initiative for Asthma (GINA). 2020. https://ginasthma.org/gina-reports/.
66. Reisacher WR. Asthma and the otolaryngologist. 2014:S70–3. https://doi.org/10.1002/alr.21386.
67. Roche AM, Wise SK. Subcutaneous immunotherapy. 2014:S51–4. https://doi.org/10.1002/alr.21382.
68. Rosati MG, Peters AT. Relationships among allergic rhinitis, asthma, and chronic rhinosinusitis. 2016;30:44–7. https://doi.org/10.2500/ajra.2016.30.4252.
69. Rosen C, Simpson CB. Nonsurgical treatment of voice disorders. Berlin, Germany: Springer; 2008.
70. Schittny JC. Development of the lung. 2017;367:427–44. https://doi.org/10.1007/s00441-016-2545-0.
71. Settipane RJ, Hagy GW, Settipane GA. Long-term risk factors for developing asthma and allergic rhinitis: a 23-year follow-up study of college students. 1994;15:21–5. https://doi.org/10.2500/108854194778816634.
72. Slavin RG. The upper and lower airways: the epidemiological and pathophysiological connection. 2008;29:553–6. https://doi.org/10.2500/aap.2008.29.3169.
73. Takhar P, Corrigan CJ, Smurthwaite L, et al. Class switch recombination to IgE in the bronchial mucosa of atopic and nonatopic patients with asthma. 2007;119:213–8.
74. Thomsen SF. Genetics of asthma: an introduction for the clinician. eCollection. 2015;2 https://doi.org/10.3402/ecrj.v2.24643.
75. Thurston GD, Balmes JR, Garcia E, et al. Outdoor air pollution and new-onset airway disease. An Official American Thoracic Soc Workshop Report. 2020;17:387–98. https://doi.org/10.1513/AnnalsATS.202001-046ST.
76. To T, Stanojevic S, Moores G, et al. Global asthma prevalence in adults: findings from the cross-sectional world health survey. 2012;12:204-2458-12-204. https://doi.org/10.1186/1471-2458-12-204.
77. van den Wijngaart LS, Roukema J, Merkus PJ. Respiratory disease and respiratory physiology: putting lung function into perspective: paediatric asthma. 2015;20:379–88. https://doi.org/10.1111/resp.12480.
78. Wise SK, Lin SY, Toskala E, et al. International consensus statement on allergy and rhinology: allergic rhinitis. 2018;8:108–352. https://doi.org/10.1002/alr.22073.
79. Zhang H, Kaushal A, Soto-Ramirez N, et al. Acquisition, remission, and persistence of eczema, asthma, and rhinitis in children. 2018;48:568–76. https://doi.org/10.1111/cea.13096.

Classification of Asthma

24

Kelsey Ige and Shyam Joshi

Introduction

Asthma can be classified by phenotype, endotype, histology, association with other conditions (e.g., allergic rhinitis or nasal polyps), severity, or disease control. At the time of diagnosis, asthma is often categorized by disease severity to determine the initial treatment regimen. As asthma is a dynamic disease, control is typically used to guide changes in therapy. This chapter will concentrate on asthma severity and control as these both play a critical role in directing treatment plans.

Comparison: Asthma Severity or Asthma Control

Asthma severity includes both the severity of the underlying disease as well as its response to treatment. Classically, severity is defined at the time of asthma diagnosis through clinical features, objective spirometry data, and response to therapy.

K. Ige
Department of Pediatrics, Allergy and Asthma Medical Group of the Bay Area, Brentwood, CA, USA

S. Joshi (✉)
Section of Allergy and Immunology, Oregon Health and Science University, Portland, OR, USA
e-mail: JoshiSh@ohsu.edu

Severity was originally considered a static feature, but it has now been shown to evolve over time [1]. Previous asthma severity guidelines did not consider this; however, more recent recommendations have proposed periodically evaluating severity throughout the disease course [2]. While it remains a routinely used feature in clinical practice, patient-reported symptoms often do not correlate with asthma severity [3]. It is also not particularly useful to predict which treatments will be effective [4].

Asthma control, on the other hand, refers to the control of both clinical symptoms and airway inflammation independent of current medication use. Effective asthma management depends on the ability to measure changes in a patient's condition and make appropriate treatment adjustments by emphasizing goal-oriented, individualized therapy [5].

Control may have a different meaning for patients and providers, and both could vary significantly from the guidelines put forth by regulatory authorities. Studies have consistently shown most patients and providers overestimate asthma control, often leading to the undertreatment of the disease. Consequently, only a small percentage of patients reach good asthma control [6].

Asthma severity and asthma control measure different features of the disease (Table 24.1). Both of these measures remain useful tools in the management of asthma. Patients can have mild

C. Damask et al. (eds.), *Allergy in Otolaryngology Practice*,
https://doi.org/10.1007/978-3-031-93455-1_24

Table 24.1 Comparing asthma severity and asthma control measures

	Asthma severity	Asthma control
Frequency of assessment	At diagnosis and periodically with changes in therapy	Every clinical encounter
Factors assessed	Symptoms Spirometry Response to therapy	Symptoms Spirometry Objective measures of airway inflammation
Validated questionnaires	None	ATAQ ACQ ACT
Risk factors	Socioeconomic factors Environmental exposures	Socioeconomic factors Environmental exposures Disease severity Medication adherence and adverse effects
Therapy	Minimum required medication to achieve good symptom control (Step Therapy)	Goal-oriented and individualized Evaluates symptoms on current therapeutic regimen Indicates therapeutic changes

disease but can be poorly controlled or can have severe asthma that is well controlled. Better asthma control is achieved by using severity indices to guide the effectiveness of controller treatment. Conversely, improved asthma control over time may reduce severity. This chapter will explore the definitions of these two measures and how they are both used for effective asthma care.

Asthma Severity

Severity is evaluated at the time of asthma diagnosis as well as periodically through the disease course. While various severity assessments exist, most incorporate a finite set of measures including frequency of daytime symptoms, nighttime awakenings, degree of therapy needed to maintain control, interference with normal activity, and spirometry (Table 24.2) [7]. As asthma is an inflammatory airway disease, measurement of airway inflammation would be the most sensible gauge of severity. However, direct measurement of inflammation with sputum eosinophils and bronchoalveolar lavage is not in the current guidelines due to the difficulty in routinely performing these maneuvers. Fractional exhalation of nitric oxide (FeNO) may indirectly measure airway inflammation, which may prove to be an important objective measurement for asthma severity determination in the future [8].

Severity of Asthma and Exacerbation Risk

Severe and life-threatening asthma exacerbations can happen with any severity of asthma. However, risk factors of an asthma exacerbation, or death, strongly correlate with more severe asthma including severe/persistent airflow obstruction reflected in spirometry, systemic steroid use, two or more ED encounters or hospitalizations for asthma in the past year, and any history of intubation or ICU admission (especially in the last five years) [9–14].

Tobacco smoke and second-hand smoke exposure is associated with poor lung function, decreased responsiveness to treatment, and increased emergency department or urgent care visits [12]. Conclusive data is lacking on the effects of vaping; however, studies have suggested vaping will have similar adverse outcomes on asthma as tobacco smoke [15]. Air pollution, allergen exposure, obesity, psychosocial stressors, and socioeconomic status have been associated with poor asthma control and severe exacerbations, especially in children [16].

The single best predictor of a future severe asthma exacerbation is a severe asthma exacerbation in the last year. Children with at least one severe asthma exacerbation in the last year have a 2–2.5 times increased risk of a severe asthma exacerbation in the subsequent year despite using controller medications [17].

Table 24.2 NHLBI guidelines for measuring asthma severity

Components of Severity		Intermittent			Persistent: Mild			Persistent: Moderate			Persistent: Severe		
		Ages 0–4 years	Ages 5–11 years	Ages ≥12 years	Ages 0–4 years	Ages 5–11 years	Ages ≥12 years	Ages 0–4 years	Ages 5–11 years	Ages ≥12 years	Ages 0–4 years	Ages 5–11 years	Ages ≥12 years
Impairment	Symptoms	≤2 days/week			>2 days/week but not daily			Daily			Throughout the day		
	Nighttime awakenings	0	≤2x/month		1–2x/month	3–4x/month		3–4x/month	>1x/week but not nightly		>1x/week	Often 7x/week	
	SABA* use for symptom control (not to prevent EIB*)	≤2 days/week			>2 days/week but not daily	>2 days/week but not daily and not more than once on any day		Daily			Several times per day		
	Interference with normal activity	None			Minor limitation			Some limitation			Extremely limited		
	Lung function		Normal FEV_1 between exacerbations	Normal FEV_1 between exacerbations									
	➔ FEV_1* (% predicted)	Not applicable	>80%	>80%	Not applicable	>80%	>80%	Not applicable	60–80%	60–80%	Not applicable	<60%	<60%
	➔ FEV_1/FVC*		>85%	Normal†		>80%	Normal†		75–80%	Reduced 5%†		<75%	Reduced >5%†
Risk	Asthma exacerbations requiring oral systemic corticosteroids‡	0–1/year			≥2 exacerb. in 6 months, or wheezing ≥4x per year lasting >1 day AND risk factors for persistent asthma	≥2/year							
						Generally, more frequent and intense events indicate greater severity. →								
							Generally, more frequent and intense events indicate greater severity. →						
		*Consider severity and interval since last asthma exacerbation. Frequency and severity may fluctuate over time for patients in any severity category. Relative annual risk of exacerbations may be related to FEV_1.**											

* **Abbreviations:** EIB, exercise-induced bronchospasm; FEV_1, forced expiratory volume in 1 second; FVC, forced vital capacity; ICS, inhaled corticosteroid; SABA, short-acting beta$_2$-agonist.

† Normal FEV_1/FVC by age: 8–19 years, 85%; 20–39 years, 80%; 40–59 years, 75%; 60–80 years, 70%.

‡ Data are insufficient to link frequencies of exacerbations with different levels of asthma severity. Generally, more frequent and intense exacerbations (e.g., requiring urgent care, hospital or intensive care admission, and/or oral corticosteroids) indicate greater underlying disease severity. For treatment purposes, patients with ≥2 exacerbations may be considered to have persistent asthma, even in the absence of impairment levels consistent with persistent asthma.

Adopted from the National Asthma Education and Prevention Program Expert Panel Report-3 (NAEPP EPR-3). www.nhlbi.nih.gov/guidelines/asthma

Classifying Asthma Severity

Severity Classification Based on Impairment and Risk

The most widely used guideline in the United States is the National Heart, Lung, and Blood Institute (NHLBI) report based on the recommendations from National Asthma Education and Prevention Program Expert Panel Report-3 (NAEPP EPR-3) (Table 24.2) [18]. This age-based classification system separates patients into 1 of 4 categories. Overall, asthma severity is graded based on the most compromised variable within each group, including assessments on impairment and exacerbation risk. For example, in an adult patient with normal spirometry, minimal daytime symptoms, nighttime awakenings of >1 time per week, and no history of exacerbations requiring systemic corticosteroids, they would be categorized as moderate, persistent asthma due to their nocturnal symptoms.

The factors associated with progressive respiratory decline related to asthma are poorly understood, but measurement of lung function is a useful tool to indicate future risk of progressive impairment [19]. This is typically performed at diagnosis, 3–6 months after a change in treatment, and periodically while on maintenance therapy. The NAEPP ERP-3 recommends the use of spirometry instead of peak expiratory flow measures in the evaluation of asthma due to the latter's diurnal variability and poor reproducibility [18]. In adults, spirometry, specifically FEV_1 and FEV_1/FVC, are reliable metrics of asthma severity and are integrated into the classification system. FEV_1 values are not as reliable in children as the values can often be normal, regardless of their asthma severity [20]. Spirometry is not typically performed in children younger than 4 years of age due to their inability to perform the maneuvers required.

Severity Classification Based on Treatment Requirements

Severity can also be measured by the level of treatment required to control symptoms and exacerbations. This method is adopted by the Global Initiative for Asthma (GINA) (Table 24.3) [2]. This classification system can be particularly helpful in categorizing patients with more severe, episodic exacerbations requiring higher-intensity maintenance therapy, which would not be accurately classified using the NHLBI guidelines. For example, a patient with 1 severe exacerbation per year would be considered to have intermittent asthma based on the NHLBI criteria. However, if they are requiring maintenance use of a medium-dose combination inhaled corticosteroid and long-acting $beta_2$-agonist, then they would be classified with severe asthma per GINA guidelines. This would clearly change how the provider risk stratifies the patient and may change management considerations such as frequency of follow-up.

Other Severity Guidelines

In addition to the NHLBI and GINA guidelines, several other organizations have proposed classification systems including the World Health

Table 24.3 Global initiative for asthma guidelines on asthma severity. (Adopted from GINA Full Report 2020)

	Mild asthma	Moderate asthma	Severe asthma
Medication requirement for asthma control	As-needed rescue medication alone Low-dose ICS LTRA Chromones	Low-dose ICS-LABA Medium-dose ICS	Medium- or high-dose ICS-LABA ICS-LABA-LAMA Biologic therapy[a] OCS

[a]Anti-IgE, anti-IL5/5R, anti-TSLP or anti-IL4R monoclonal antibodies

ICS inhaled corticosteroid, *LTRA* leukotriene receptor antagonists, *LABA* long-acting $beta_2$-agonist, *LAMA* long-acting muscarinic antagonist, *OCS* oral corticosteroids, *TSLP* thymic stromal lymphopoietin

Organization (WHO) and American Thoracic Society (ATS) [21, 22]. These use similar metrics as those discussed earlier in this chapter.

Asthma Control

An alternate method to classify asthma is determining the level of control. This differs from asthma severity classification in that it is independent of current medication use, although many of the same metrics are used [1]. While severity is generally determined at the time of diagnosis and periodically evaluated throughout the disease course, control should be evaluated at every clinical encounter for asthma, both for scheduled and acute care visits. Many factors may play a role in poorly controlled asthma, which will be discussed later in this chapter, including poor medication adherence, frequent allergen exposure, and non-asthmatic respiratory symptoms [23].

Important measures of asthma control include frequency and intensity of asthma symptoms, nighttime awakenings, burden on normal activities (exercise, work, school, and recreation), rescue medication use, and validated questionnaires [5]. A thorough assessment of the patient includes input from family and/or caregivers as their observed symptoms can differ from the patient's reported symptoms and often more accurately represents the patient's asthma control. Acute healthcare use including urgent care and emergency room visits as well as hospitalizations correlates with the level of asthma control [24–26].

Objective measures (spirometry, FeNO, sputum eosinophils, and hyperresponsiveness studies) should be used when possible, as patient-reported symptoms do not always accurately reflect the degree of airway inflammation [5]. If these measures are in direct disconnect to the patient's reported symptoms, the provider must use their clinical judgment to evaluate asthma control.

The most frequently used guideline is from the NHLBI, which is based on the NAEPP EPR-3 recommendations (Table 24.4) [18]. It incorporates the patient's or caregiver's recall of asthma events over the previous 2–4 weeks as well as lung function measurements to assess impair-

Table 24.4 NHLBI guidelines for measuring asthma control

Components of Control		Well Controlled			Not Well Controlled			Very Poorly Controlled		
		Ages 0–4 years	Ages 5–11 years	Ages ≥12 years	Ages 0–4 years	Ages 5–11 years	Ages ≥12 years	Ages 0–4 years	Ages 5–11 years	Ages ≥12 years
Impairment	Symptoms	≤2 days/week	≤2 days/week but not more than once on each day	≤2 days/week	>2 days/week	>2 days/week or multiple times on ≤2 days/week	>2 days/week	Throughout the day		
	Nighttime awakenings	≤1x/month		≤2x/month	>1x/month	≥2x/month	1–3x/week	>1x/week	≥2x/week	≥4x/week
	Interference with normal activity	None			Some limitation			Extremely limited		
	SABA* use for symptom control (not to prevent EIB*)	≤2 days/week			>2 days/week			Several times per day		
	Lung function ➔ FEV_1* (*% predicted*) or peak flow (*% personal best*)	Not applicable	>80%	>80%	Not applicable	60–80%	60–80%	Not applicable	<60%	<60%
	➔ FEV_1/FVC*		>80%	Not applicable		75–80%	Not applicable		<75%	Not applicable
	Validated questionnaires† ➔ ATAQ* ➔ ACQ* ➔ ACT*	Not applicable	Not applicable	0 ≤0.75‡ ≥20	Not applicable	Not applicable	1–2 ≥1.5 16–19	Not applicable	Not applicable	3–4 Not applicable ≤15
Risk	Asthma exacerbations requiring oral systemic corticosteroids§	0–1/year			2–3/year	≥2/year		>3/year	≥2/year	
		Consider severity and interval since last asthma exacerbation.								
	Reduction in lung growth/Progressive loss of lung function	Not applicable	Evaluation requires long-term follow-up care.		Not applicable	Evaluation requires long-term follow-up care.		Not applicable	Evaluation requires long-term follow-up care.	
	Treatment-related adverse effects	*Medication side effects can vary in intensity from none to very troublesome and worrisome. The level of intensity does not correlate to specific levels of control but should be considered in the overall assessment of risk.*								

* **Abbreviations:** ACQ, Asthma Control Questionnaire®; ACT, Asthma Control Test™; ATAQ, Asthma Therapy Assessment Questionnaire®; EIB, exercise-induced bronchospasm; FVC, forced vital capacity; FEV_1, forced expiratory volume in 1 second; SABA, short-acting $beta_2$-agonist.

† Minimal important difference: 1.0 for the ATAQ; 0.5 for the ACQ; not determined for the ACT.

‡ ACQ values of 0.76–1.4 are indeterminate regarding well-controlled asthma.

§ Data are insufficient to link frequencies of exacerbations with different levels of asthma control. Generally, more frequent and intense exacerbations (e.g., requiring urgent care, hospital or intensive care admission, and/or oral corticosteroids) indicate poorer asthma control.

Adopted from the National Asthma Education and Prevention Program Expert Panel Report-3 (NAEPP EPR-3). www.nhlbi.nih.gov/guidelines/asthma

ment. In addition, a longitudinal review of asthma exacerbations over the past year requiring systemic therapy is an important feature. This guideline separates patients into three main asthma categories: Well Controlled, Not Well Controlled, and Very Poorly Controlled. Adjustments to the patient's management plan are considered based on asthma control measurements and discussed in another chapter.

Factors affecting asthma control include disease severity, poor medication adherence (due to side effects, inhaler technique, and cost of medications), repeated exposure to allergic triggers, respiratory infections, and non-asthmatic respiratory conditions [23]. These are further discussed in another chapter.

Limitations in Categorization Methods for Asthma Severity and Control

While multiple iterations of asthma severity and control guidelines have been published over the past 3 decades, there remain concerns regarding their utilization. Recent evidence suggests many primary care providers as well as asthma specialists are unclear on how to implement these guidelines in clinical practice [27]. Only 66% of allergists and pulmonologists assess asthma control with most patient visits. This implies the guidelines are underutilized and potentially this leads to suboptimal management decisions.

As discussed earlier in this chapter, a major limitation to these guidelines is the absence of directly evaluating airway inflammation due to difficulty in routinely performing the necessary techniques [23]. While sputum eosinophils and bronchoalveolar lavage have shown promise in guiding therapy, they are not easily attainable in the clinic setting and lack large randomized, controlled trials to support their routine use. Instead, guidelines utilize spirometry and patient-reported symptoms, which do not always directly correlate with airway inflammation. Peripheral biomarkers are being investigated to provide objective measurements of airway inflammation, but they are not currently validated to assist in evaluating asthma severity or control.

Finally, many factors (both related to and independent of the patient's asthma) can affect assessments using these guidelines. This could lead to undertreatment or overtreatment of asthma. When comparing women and men, women report more symptoms and typically rely more on short-acting beta-agonist therapy despite a similar level of airway inflammation [28]. This leads to a higher severity diagnosis and categorization of poor control, which could lead to an inappropriate increase in therapy. In addition, a similar situation frequently arises in patients with respiratory complaints not associated with their underlying asthma such as vocal cord dysfunction. Per guidelines, daily respiratory symptoms would indicate a step up in therapy; however, this would be misplaced as no clear increase in underlying airway inflammation or hyperresponsiveness would be present.

Utilization of questionnaires and symptom recall will continue to limit the usefulness and applicability of asthma severity. A combination of symptom evaluation and direct objective measurements of airway inflammation would provide the most useful and robust tool to determine severity and control.

Conclusions

Severity and control remain useful, yet limited, tools to categorize asthma. Asthma severity is typically assessed at diagnosis and periodically evaluated throughout the disease course. It is helpful in predicting the risk of exacerbations and plays a significant role in guiding management. Symptoms, spirometry, and medication requirements to maintain adequate control are all important factors in determining severity.

Symptom control remains a critical principle of chronic disease management, and routine assessments are recommended to guide individualized therapy. Asthma control, in contrast to asthma severity, is independent of current medication use and is calculated by clinical symptoms, limitations to daily life, and lung function measurements. Asthma control assessment should be performed at every patient encounter and is a key factor in long-term asthma management.

References

1. Cockcroft DW, Swystun VA. Asthma control versus asthma severity. J Allergy Clin Immunol. 1996;98(6):1016–8.
2. Global Initiative for Asthma. Global strategy for the diagnosis and prevention. Global Initiative for Asthma (updated 2020) 2020. Last accessed October 2020.
3. Ng TP. Validity of symptom and clinical measures of asthma severity for primary outpatient assessment of adult asthma. Br J Gen Pract. 2000;50(450):7–12.
4. Kwok MY, Walsh-Kelly CM, Gorelick MH, Grabowski L, Kelly KJ. National Asthma Education and prevention program severity classification as a measure of disease burden in children with acute asthma. Pediatrics. 2006;117:S71–7.
5. Joint Task Force on Practice Parameters, American Academy of Allergy, Asthma and Immunology; American College of Allergy, Asthma and Immunology and Joint Council of Allergy, Asthma and Immunology. Attaining optimal asthma control: a practice parameter. J Allergy Clin Immunol. 2005;116(5):S3–11. https://doi.org/10.1016/j.jaci.2005.08.017. Erratum in: J Allergy Clin Immunol. 2006 Feb;117(2):262
6. Gustafsson PM, Watson L, Davis KJ, Rabe KF. Poor asthma control in children: evidence from epidemiological surveys and implications for clinical practice. Int J Clin Pract. 2006;60:321–34.
7. Guidelines for the diagnosis and management of asthma. National Heart, Lung, and Blood Institute. National Asthma Education Program. Expert panel report. J Allergy Clin Immunol. 1991;88:425–534.
8. Diamant Z, Vijverberg S, Alving K, Bakirtas A, Bjermer L, Custovic A, Dahlen SE, Gaga M, Gerth van Wijk R, Giacco SD, Hamelmann E, Heaney LG, Heffler E, Kalayci Ö, Kostikas K, Lutter R, Olin AC, Sergejeva S, Simpson A, Sterk PJ, Tufvesson E, Agache I, Seys SF. Toward clinically applicable biomarkers for asthma: an EAACI position paper. Allergy. 2019;74(10):1835–51. https://doi.org/10.1111/all.13806.
9. Kitch BT, Paltiel AD, Kuntz KM, Dockery DW, Schouten JP, Weiss ST, Fuhlbrigge AL. A single measure of FEV_1 is associated with risk of asthma attacks in long-term follow-up. Chest. 2004;126(6):1875–82. https://doi.org/10.1378/chest.126.6.1875.
10. Adams RJ, Smith BJ, Ruffin RE. Factors associated with hospital admissions and repeat emergency department visits for adults with asthma. Thorax. 2000;55(7):566–73. https://doi.org/10.1136/thorax.55.7.566.
11. Belessis Y, Dixon S, Thomsen A, Duffy B, Rawlinson W, Henry R, Morton J. Risk factors for an intensive care unit admission in children with asthma. Pediatr Pulmonol. 2004;37(3):201–9. https://doi.org/10.1002/ppul.10443.
12. Eisner MD, Katz PP, Yelin EH, Shiboski SC, Blanc PD. Risk factors for hospitalization among adults with asthma: the influence of sociodemographic factors and asthma severity. Respir Res. 2001;2(1):53–60. https://doi.org/10.1186/rr37.
13. Lieu TA, Quesenberry CP, Sorel ME, Mendoza GR, Leong AB. Computer-based models to identify high-risk children with asthma. Am J Respir Crit Care Med. 1998;157(4 Pt 1):1173–80. https://doi.org/10.1164/ajrccm.157.4.9708124.
14. Cowie RL, Underwood MF, Revitt SG, Field SK. Predicting emergency department utilization in adults with asthma: a cohort study. J Asthma. 2001;38(2):179–84. https://doi.org/10.1081/jas-100000037.
15. Clapp PW, Peden DB, Jaspers I. E-cigarettes, vaping-related pulmonary illnesses, and asthma: a perspective from inhalation toxicologists. J Allergy Clin Immunol. 2020;145(1):97–9. https://doi.org/10.1016/j.jaci.2019.11.001. Epub 2019 Nov 9
16. Tomisa G, Horváth A, Szalai Z, Müller V, Tamási L. Prevalence and impact of risk factors for poor asthma outcomes in a large, specialist-managed patient cohort: a real-life study. J Asthma Allergy. 2019;23(12):297–307. https://doi.org/10.2147/JAA.S211246.
17. Puranik S, Forno E, Bush A, Celedon JC. Predicting severe asthma exacerbations in children. Am J Respir Crit Care. 2017;195(7):854–9. https://doi.org/10.1164/rccm.201606-1213PP.
18. 2020 Focused Updates to the Asthma Management Guidelines: A Report from the National Asthma Education and Prevention Program Coordinating Committee Expert Panel Working Group. J Allergy Clin Immunol. 2020;146(6):1217–1270.
19. O'Byrne P, Fabbri LM, Pavord ID, Papi A, Petruzzelli S, Lange P. Asthma progression and mortality: the role of inhaled corticosteroids. Eur Respir J. 2019;54(1):1900491. https://doi.org/10.1183/13993003.00491-2019.
20. Bacharier LB, Strunk RC, Mauger D, White D, Lemanske RF Jr, Sorkness CA. Classifying asthma severity in children: mismatch between symptoms, medication use, and lung function. Am J Respir Crit Care Med. 2004;170(4):426–32. https://doi.org/10.1164/rccm.200308-1178OC.
21. Bousquet J, Mantzouranis E, Cruz A, Aït-Khaled N, Baena-Cagnani CE, Bleecker ER, et al. Uniform definition of asthma severity. Control. And exacerbations: document presented for the world health organization consultation on severe asthma. J Allergy Clin Immunol. 2010;126(5):926–38.

22. Proceedings of the ATS workshop on refractory asthma: current understanding. Recommendations. And unanswered questions. Am Thorac Soc Am J Respir Crit Care Med. 2000;162(6):2341–51.
23. Colice GL. Categorizing asthma severity: an overview of national guidelines. Clin Med Res. 2004;2(3):155–63. https://doi.org/10.3121/cmr.2.3.155.
24. Vollmer WM, Markson LE, O'Connor E, Sanocki LL, Fitterman L, Berger M, et al. Association of asthma control with health care utilization and quality of life. Am J Respir Crit Care Med. 1999;160:1647–52.
25. Vollmer WM, Markson LE, O'Connor E, Frazier EA, Berger M, Buist AS. Association of asthma control with health care utilization: a prospective evaluation. Am J Respir Crit Care Med. 2002;165:195–9.
26. Van Ganse E, Laforest L, Pietri G, et al. Persistent asthma: disease control, resource utilization and direct costs. Eur Respir J. 2002;20:260–7.
27. Cloutier MM, Akinbami LJ, Salo PM, Schatz M, Simoneau T, Wilkerson JC, Diette G, Elward KS, Fuhlbrigge A, Mazurek JM, Feinstein L, Williams S, Zeldin DC. Use of National Asthma Guidelines by allergists and pulmonologists: a National Survey. J Allergy Clin Immunol Pract. 2020;S2213–2198(20):30377–9. https://doi.org/10.1016/j.jaip.2020.04.026. Epub ahead of print
28. Osborne ML, Vollmer WM, Linton KL, Buist AS. Characteristics of patients with asthma within a large HMO: a comparison by age and gender. Am J Respir Crit Care Med. 1998;157(1):123–8. https://doi.org/10.1164/ajrccm.157.1.9612063.

Therapy of Asthma

25

Alicia A. Alvarez and Jeffrey M. Chambliss

Introduction

Therapy options continue to evolve as asthma is further understood as a heterogenous disorder. Up to 80% of children and greater than 50% of adults with asthma are thought to have an allergic component [1]. Further understanding of the cellular mechanisms involved in asthma has led to the development of new therapies, including targeting specific pathways. These biologic therapies will be covered elsewhere. The focus of the following chapter is evidence for environmental interventions for inhalant allergens, pharmacologic treatment options for asthma, and finally immunotherapy and bronchial thermoplasty.

Cellular Mechanisms of Allergy in Asthma

Exposure to inhalant allergens has been linked to increased airway hyper-responsiveness and loss of asthma control [2]. It has been estimated that the prevalence of asthma is six times higher in patients with allergic rhinitis [3]. In addition, atopy and allergic sensitization are associated with an increased risk of developing asthma [4]. From a mechanistic standpoint, initial exposure to an allergen may lead to sensitization by the production of specific immunoglobulin E (IgE) antibodies. This is thought to be primarily mediated by type 2 helper T cells (Th2) and the production of interleukin-4 during B-cell activation.

With subsequent exposure to an allergen in a sensitized individual, both an acute and late-phase hypersensitivity reaction can occur. Initially, the allergen cross-links specific IgE antibodies bound to mast cells resulting in degranulation of preformed inflammatory mediators. The release of histamine, prostaglandin D2, and cysteinyl leukotrienes then leads to bronchoconstriction, mucous secretion, increased vascular permeability, and airway edema [5]. Simultaneously, macrophages and dendritic cells present the allergen to CD4+ T-helper cells that drive the production and recruitment of eosinophils and neutrophils. This leads to the late allergic response which typically begins three or more hours after allergen exposure and can persist for several weeks, manifesting as increased airway hyper-responsiveness and decreased forced expiratory volume in one second (FEV1) [6]. Thunderstorm asthma serves as a unique example of the early allergic response in asthma. In this phenomenon, initial dry updrafts

A. A. Alvarez
Sarasota Memorial Health Care System, FL, Sarasota, USA
e-mail: Alicia-Alvarez@smh.com

J. M. Chambliss (✉)
UT Southwestern Medical Center, Dallas, TX, USA
e-mail: Jeffrey.Chambliss@UTSouthwestern.edu

C. Damask et al. (eds.), *Allergy in Otolaryngology Practice*,
https://doi.org/10.1007/978-3-031-93455-1_25

carry whole pollen particles up to the cloud base where the increased humidity allows for higher concentration of pollen particles. The pollen grains rupture by osmotic shock, likely enhanced by the strong electric fields, and pollen fragments are then brought back down to ground level by cold down drafts. These small fragments can penetrate deeper into the lung than their whole granule predecessors. This can provoke severe asthma symptoms in sensitized patients with known asthma or allergic rhinitis in the first 30 minutes of a storm [7, 8]. While the triggers for asthma can be diverse, the focus of treatment involves prevention of allergic exposures and decreasing the effect of mediators involved in asthma inflammation.

Evidence for Allergen Mitigation Strategies

Evaluation of various allergen mitigation strategies has shown mixed results regarding clinical asthma outcomes. These strategies have generally focused on perennial allergens such as house dust mite, cockroach, rodents, mold, and furred pets. While allergen avoidance was previously recommended for all patients with asthma, there seems to be improved efficacy in using multicomponent techniques in patients with known sensitization, with interventions tailored to their specific allergens [9–12].

House Dust Mite

House dust mites are microscopic arthropods that feed on organic material including human skin cells, bacteria, and fungi. They live in upholstered material such as mattresses, bedding, and carpet and require a relative humidity above 50% to survive. Fecal pellets contain allergenic components that range in size from 20 to 40 micrometers. This size allows particles to become airborne when disturbed but will settle in 20–30 minutes. Acaricidal agents (dust mite insecticides) have not been shown to provide significant additional benefits when used with other physical barriers and are not recommended due to concerns for use of toxic chemicals in the home [9, 13, 14]. Washing fabrics with detergents in hot water is a safe and effective method to reduce house dust mite levels in bed linens [15, 16]. Pillow and mattress encasements have been shown to reduce dust mite levels, but this reduction was not sustained after 12 months of use [17]. Despite reducing allergen levels, the effect of these mitigation strategies on clinical outcomes has been variable. While large meta-analyses have shown no benefit in asthma symptom scores or FEV1 [18], individual studies have found an associated decrease in inhaled corticosteroid dosing in children [19] and decreased ER visits without impact on oral corticosteroid use [20].

Household Pests

Both mouse and cockroach pest control as interventions have shown mixed results in improving clinical asthma outcomes. There are a variety of cockroach allergens found in feces in addition to the pro-inflammatory chitin found in their exoskeleton [10]. While cockroach sensitization can be particularly problematic for patients with asthma living in inner cities and in crowded housing situations, rodents are found in urban and rural areas. Mouse and rat allergens are found in both fur and urine [21]. These particles are small enough to remain airborne for up to an hour and can easily travel throughout buildings by this route. Elevated mouse allergen levels can often be found at homes, as well as schools and office buildings [21]. Pest management for rodents and cockroaches primarily focuses on patient education to minimize food sources such as dirty dishes, garbage, and accessible stored dry goods such as grains and seeds. Rodent management also includes sealing cracks and holes that serve as entry points. Traps and pesticides can also be added.

Single interventions with professionally placed cockroach bait traps previously showed reduction in cockroach numbers, decreased asthma symptoms, and unscheduled healthcare utilization. This was more pronounced in homes of sensitized participants [22]. Another study focused on professional extermination of both rodents and cockroaches, in conjunction with mattress and pillow encasings and bedroom high-efficiency particulate air (HEPA) purifiers in the homes of asthmatic children that were predominantly sensitized to cockroach. This showed a reduction in cockroach allergen levels and daytime symptoms, but no significant change in mouse allergen levels, nighttime symptoms, or emergency department visits [23]. There is limited data on single mouse-focused mitigation strategies, but instead this is often included in multicomponent interventions which will be further discussed below. However, in one evaluation of rodent-focused pest management, there was no difference in asthma symptoms whether participants received pest management education and professional extermination or education alone [24].

Common Pets

Cats and dogs have a variety of allergens that can be found predominantly in hair and saliva. The length of pet hair does not impact the amount of allergen shed. These allergen particles are small in size and are easily airborne for hours. They can settle on clothing and travel to various locations. Cat allergen has been found in buses, workplaces, schools, and even homes of non-cat owners [25]. Pet removal may be considered in sensitized patients. A small study showed that cat removal reduced rates of inhaled corticosteroid use and bronchial hypersensitivity. However, the benefits of these pets, such as companionship, should be considered against health risks from exposure. Alternatively, it is recommended that pets be kept outside of the home or at a minimum outside of the bedroom. Washing pets may reduce the quantity of allergen shed, but this only lasts a few days and may not be a realistic option for pet owners [26, 27].

Carpet

Carpets serve as a reservoir for most allergens, yet carpet removal has not been studied as a single intervention. It has been included in multicomponent interventions with a reduction in allergen levels, but with an unclear impact on clinical outcomes [28]. Quantity of recovered allergen has been correlated with the square footage of carpet within the home, regardless of the style of fabric used [29]. Vacuuming carpet and upholstery have had mixed results in reducing allergen levels [25]. Cleaning with high-efficiency vacuums at least once per week for 12 months showed a reduction in cat allergen in homes that did not contain a cat. There was also a reduction in dog allergens on mattresses, but no significant change in dog and dust mite levels in carpet. There was no reduction in cat allergen levels in the homes of cat owners. However, participants who used high-efficiency vacuums showed a reduction in bronchodilator use and improvements in peak flow measurements [30]. Unfortunately, the act of vacuuming can agitate allergen particles causing them to become airborne [31]. Additionally, the design of many vacuum filtration systems is imperfect and can cause leaking of allergens into the ambient air. Central vacuum cleaning systems and double-walled vacuum bags, but not high-efficiency vacuums, reduced leakage of allergens from the vacuum itself [25].

Air Filters

Although HEPA filters were invented in the 1940s, the role of air purifiers in respiratory disease remains unclear. In theory, mechanical air filters can trap airborne allergen particles from the ambient air. This would be most effective for small particles that remain airborne for prolonged periods such as cat and dog allergens. However, the movement of air generated by the filter may disturb previously settled allergens and reintroduce them into the ambient air. Air filtration has been shown to produce modest reductions in cat, dust mite, and cockroach allergen levels, but has been less effective in reducing ragweed, Alternaria species levels or concentrations of allergens in floor dust. While meta-analyses have not shown a consistent improvement in clinical asthma outcomes, some individual studies have shown reduction in nighttime symptoms, bronchial hyperresponsiveness, and medication requirements [32, 33]. There has been some success in reducing tobacco smoke, mold, and cat allergen by adding filters to forced air household ventilation systems in air quality modeling system analysis, but its impact on clinical outcomes remains yet to be elucidated [34].

Multicomponent Mitigation Strategies

Overall, the evidence for environmental allergen avoidance measures is often contradictory and difficult to compare across studies [28]. The most benefit is seen in multicomponent interventions that are personalized to a patient's specific allergic sensitization. A large, randomized controlled trial in asthmatic inner-city children evaluated a yearlong intervention involving education on mitigation strategies and tobacco cessation for parents, bi-monthly home visits, impermeable mattress encasements, HEPA-filtered vacuum and air purifiers, and professional exterminator services. Children in the intervention arm showed lower cat, dust mite, and cockroach allergen levels and a decrease in symptoms that lasted over a year after completion of the intervention [11]. However, these large-scale multicomponent interventions can be difficult to implement due to cost, time commitment, health literacy, and fluctuating home environments [28].

Pharmacotherapy

The goal of medical management of asthma is to minimize symptoms and exacerbations while maintaining normal lung function and quality of life. Pharmacotherapy needs are dependent on the patient's asthma control and are titrated accordingly. Asthma control encompasses both current symptoms and the risk of future exacerbations. Assessment of current symptoms should include frequency of short-acting beta agonist (SABA) use, day and nighttime symptoms, and limitations on physical exertion. Ideally, patients with controlled asthma should have symptoms twice a week or less, with no limitations on exercise, work, or school, and no nighttime symptoms or early morning awakenings due to asthma.

There are multiple validated questionnaires such as the Asthma Control Test [35] that can provide an objective way to track symptoms over time. Factors that increase the risk of future exacerbations and poor asthma outcomes are detailed in Table 25.1 and focus on history of exacerbations, current lung function, and comorbid conditions [36]. While asthma severity can be determined based on frequency of symptoms, it may be difficult to assess if asthma is not well controlled [12]. A simpler method is to diagnose this retrospectively based on the level of therapy needed to maintain control as noted in Table 25.2.

Table 25.1 Risk factors for future exacerbations [36]

History
Frequent asthma symptoms
Previous ICU care or intubation for uncontrolled asthma
1 or more exacerbations within the last year
Medications
Frequent SABA use
Goal for controlled asthma: Twice a week or less
ICS not prescribed
Poor compliance
Incorrect inhaler technique
Comorbid conditions
Chronic rhinosinusitis
Obesity
Gastroesophageal reflux
Anxiety/depression
Pregnancy
Environmental exposures
Tobacco smoke
Allergens, if sensitized
Air pollution
Lung function
Decreased FEV1 or peak flow
High reversibility
Other
Socioeconomic barriers
Eosinophilia (sputum or blood)

Table 25.2 Pharmacotherapy by asthma severity [36]

Severity *Step*	Associated symptoms	Age 0–5	Age 6–11	Age 12+
Mild intermittent *Step 1*	Young children: Infrequent wheezing related to viral infection with rare interval symptoms Older children and adults: Symptoms less than twice a month	Maintenance:		
		Not needed	Not needed Consider: Daily low-dose ICS or as needed low-dose ICS taken when SABA is used	As needed low-dose ICS-formoterol Consider: Low-dose ICS whenever SABA is used
		Rescue:		
		As needed SABA	As needed SABA	As needed low-dose ICS-formoterol Consider: SABA alone
Mild persistent *Step 2*	Younger children: Wheezing episodes requiring SABA 3 or more times a year Older children and adults: Symptoms more than twice a month but less than daily	Maintenance:		
		Low-dose ICS Consider: Daily LTRA or short courses of ICS at the onset of viral illness	Low-dose ICS Consider: Adding LTRA or using as needed low-dose ICS taken when SABA is used	Daily low-dose ICS or as needed low-dose ICS-formoterol Consider: Adding LTRA or using low-dose ICS whenever SABA is used
		Rescue:		
		As needed SABA	As needed SABA	As needed low-dose ICS-formoterol Consider: SABA alone
Moderate persistent *Step 3*	Younger children: Symptoms not well controlled on low-dose ICS Older children and adults: Symptoms most days; weekly or more nighttime symptoms	Maintenance:		
		Double "low-dose" ICS Consider: Adding daily LTRA	Low-dose ICS-LABA or medium-dose ICS Consider: Low-dose ICS with LTRA	Low-dose ICS-LABA Consider: Medium-dose ICS or low-dose ICS with LTRA
		Rescue:		
		As needed SABA	As needed SABA	As needed low-dose ICS-formoterol if used as a maintenance Consider: As needed SABA
Severe persistent *step 4*	Younger children: Symptoms not well controlled on doubling of low-dose ICS Older children and adults: Symptoms most days, weekly or more nighttime symptoms or low lung function	Maintenance:		
		Double "low-dose" ICS and specialist referral Consider: Adding daily LTRA	Medium-dose ICS-LABA and specialist referral Consider: High-dose ICS-LABA or addition of tiotropium or LTRA	Medium-dose ICS-LABA Consider: High-dose ICS, addition of tiotropium or addition of LTRA
		Rescue:		
		As needed SABA	As needed SABA	As needed low-dose ICS-formoterol if used as a maintenance Consider: As needed SABA

(continued)

Table 25.1 (continued)

Severity *Step*	Associated symptoms	Age 0–5	Age 6–11	Age 12+
Severe persistent *Step 5*	Younger children: Not well controlled on previous step therapy Older children and adults: Symptoms most days, weekly or more nighttime symptoms or low lung function		Specialist referral and consideration of biologic therapy Consider addition of low-dose oral corticosteroids	Maintenance: High-dose ICS-LABA with add-on therapies (tiotropium, biologic) and specialist referral Consider: Addition of low-dose oral corticosteroids Rescue: As needed low-dose ICS-formoterol if used as a maintenance Consider: As needed SABA

LABA long-acting beta-agonist, *SABA* short-acting beta-agonist, *ICS* inhaled corticosteroid, *LTRA* leukotriene receptor antagonist

Inhaled corticosteroids are the backbone of asthma pharmacotherapy and the dose is often escalated with increasing severity of asthma. This is commonly described as a series of steps that providers can titrate up or down. See Table 25.2 for further details. Initial symptoms should guide which step to start a patient's therapy. Once symptoms are well controlled for at least three months, the provider can consider stopping some of the add-on medications or decreasing the ICS dose by 25–50%. This may not always be possible and should be a joint decision with the patient and provider. If therapy is stepped down, this is generally done outside of winter viral season and the patient's worst allergy season. If symptoms are not controlled despite appropriate initial therapies, pharmacotherapy should step up accordingly while considering add-on therapies and specialist referral. Additional recommendations on managing difficult-to-control asthma are detailed later in this chapter. Asthma control may vary throughout the year and medications should be re-evaluated regularly.

Formoterol is a unique long acting beta-agonist (LABA) as it has rapid onset of action within 3 minutes and reaches peak plasma concentrations in 10–15 minutes, unlike other LABAs that can take 30 minutes or more to reach peak effect [37, 38]. Several studies have demonstrated the safety of using ICS-formoterol as both a maintenance and rescue inhaler [39, 40] and its efficacy in reducing the risk of asthma exacerbation, primarily in intermittent or mild persistent asthma. Using ICS-formoterol as needed can provide rapid relief of bronchoconstriction and intermittent doses of corticosteroid when patients have worsening symptoms and increased underlying inflammation. Logistically, using ICS-formoterol as both a maintenance and rescue inhaler can simplify medication regimens and help improve compliance in patients with sporadic symptoms. Budesonide-formoterol was shown to be safe up to 12 puffs daily (72 mcg formoterol, 5 mcg delivered) [36]. However, due to insufficient data this method can be considered but is not yet recommended in patients less than 12 years of age. Daily ICS with rescue SABA or ICS taken with SABA as needed is recommended in lieu of this [36]. Furthermore, SABA alone or a short course of ICS + SABA can be used to treat wheezing with viral illnesses in children younger than 5 years of age. SABA as needed is the preferred rescue inhaler in patients whose maintenance regimen consists of medium or high doses of ICS or for treatment of exercise-induced asthma.

There is a wide variety of add-on therapies available in asthma which should be considered in patients at step 2 and higher. Leukotriene receptor antagonists (LTRA) are not preferred as a single maintenance treatment as ICS has been shown to be more effective in children and adults. However, they present an alternative for patients that are unable to tolerate or otherwise refuse ICS therapy. The addition of LTRA may help to reduce the dose of ICS needed to maintain asthma control.

Long-acting anti-muscarinic (LAMA) medications can be particularly helpful in patients with a component of chronic obstructive pulmonary disease (COPD). However, LAMA therapy should always be in conjunction with ICS as older patients with asthma-COPD overlap syndrome have been shown to have fewer hospitalizations on combination therapy [41].

A brief course of oral corticosteroids can be considered in patients with uncontrolled asthma to provide rapid control while simultaneously initiating ICS therapy. Daily oral corticosteroids should be reserved for patients with severe asthma refractory to standard-of-care treatment. Ideally, this can be used as a bridge to specialist evaluation and potential biologic therapy. If a patient requires prolonged high-dose steroids, additional medications for prophylaxis against gastrointestinal ulcers and pneumocystis pneumonia should be considered.

Difficult to Control Asthma

Medication noncompliance and poor inhaler technique are common causes of difficult to control asthma [42]. It has been estimated that approximately one-third of patients are not using their inhalers correctly and this has been associated with uncontrolled asthma [43]. Unfortunately, poor inhaler technique has been a persistent issue since the introduction of metered-dose inhalers in the 1960s [44]. Major errors in technique are related to poor coordination, insufficient depth or speed of inhalation and incomplete breath hold. Patient satisfaction with ease of use and effectiveness of asthma inhalers has been associated with improved adherence to medication regimens [45]. Multiple inhalers requiring different operating techniques and dosing regimens may further contribute to poor adherence. Proper education regarding use of inhalers, whether metered dose or dry powder inhalers, is an integral part of asthma management.

A number of comorbidities have been associated with decreased responsiveness to ICS such as concurrent tobacco use and obesity [12]. Smoking cessation [46] and weight reduction [47] have been shown to improve asthma symptoms. Uncontrolled rhinosinusitis can contribute to lower airway inflammation and its management has been shown to decrease asthma symptoms and ER visits, as well. Concomitant allergic bronchopulmonary aspergillosis is a rare non-invasive fungal infection that causes persistent inflammation of the airways and uncontrolled asthma symptoms. Many patients require prolonged treatment with oral corticosteroids and antifungal medications to prevent progression to pulmonary fibrosis [48]. In contrast, gastroesophageal reflux and obstructive sleep apnea can cause nocturnal symptoms that can masquerade as uncontrolled asthma. Treatment of these conditions has been associated with improved quality of life and decreased risk of exacerbations [12].

Immunotherapy

Allergen immunotherapy (AIT) for allergic asthma is an effective treatment and has been endorsed by multiple national and international guidelines for appropriate patients [49, 50]. AIT for aeroallergens can be delivered subcutaneously (subcutaneous immunotherapy, SCIT) or sublingually (sublingual immunotherapy, SLIT). Although via different routes, both forms involve administration of aeroallergen(s) to a sensitized individual with the goal of desensitization or achieving a state of tolerance to the allergens. When appropriate doses of allergens are administered over a period of time immunologic changes involving development of T and B cell tolerance leads to long-lasting improvements in asthma symptoms and quality of life [51]. SCIT has historically been more common, although SLIT has been increasingly utilized in the last several decades.

Appropriate patient selection is important prior to starting AIT. While also used for allergic rhinoconjunctivitis, AIT for allergic asthma involves identifying patients with evidence of sensitization to aeroallergens and worsening of symptoms with exposure to those allergens [52]. Sensitization can be determined by positive skin prick testing or demonstration of positive serum-specific IgE to aeroallergens. AIT can be considered in patients with mild or moderate persistent asthma and the patient's asthma should be well controlled prior to initiation of therapy [12]. AIT can also be considered in children with allergic rhinitis, at risk of developing asthma as a method of preventing asthma, as well as improving rhinitis symptoms [53]. Some factors to consider prior to starting AIT include the time commitment and patient access to care, along with the risk for reactions. Recommendations are commonly for AIT to be administered for 3 to 5 years to result in prolonged symptom improvement, even after stopping immunotherapy [50]. In the United States, multiple aeroallergens are often used to treat polysensitized patients whereas in Europe it is more common to treat with single allergens [54]. Reactions to AIT can range from mild, local erythema and itching, to severe systemic responses, including anaphylaxis. While overall uncommon anaphylaxis is more likely to occur with SCIT compared to SLIT, whereas symptoms with SLIT are more often oropharyngeal or gastrointestinal. Injection immunotherapy should be administered in a setting where prompt recognition and treatment of allergic reactions can be accomplished [52]. Similarly, patients should be observed for thirty minutes after an injection is given for signs of adverse reaction, as most systemic reactions occur within this time [55].

While dosing schedules can vary, SCIT is administered once or more a week during updosing with maintenance injections given every 2–4 weeks [49]. Systemic reviews in adult and pediatric patients have found that SCIT for allergic asthma improves symptom scores, reduces long-term control medication requirements, and improves bronchial hyper-reactivity [56–58]. SLIT doses are often administered daily, as the effective cumulative dose for SLIT appears to be higher than for SCIT [49]. While initiation or updosing of SLIT therapy should occur in an observed setting, daily dosing is often completed at home. There are several FDA-approved SLIT tablet products in the United States (house dust mite, ragweed, and grass) for the treatment of allergic rhinitis, but not asthma. SLIT similarly has been found to improve asthma symptoms and decrease use of long-term control medications [57]. However, direct comparisons of effectiveness for SCIT versus SLIT are limited.

Bronchial Thermoplasty

Bronchial thermoplasty (BT) is a technique of reducing smooth muscle mass in the airways through application of controlled thermal energy delivered during bronchoscopy [59]. It has been studied in adults and is approved in the United States and Europe. Trials have shown mild improvement in quality of life without improvement in airway hyperresponsiveness [60]. BT has not been studied in patients with low lung function or with frequent exacerbations, and its role in asthma therapy overall needs further investigation [59].

Conclusion

Asthma therapy is tied to understanding an individual patient's asthma triggers, condition, and ideally underlying mechanisms driving disease. Effective management of asthma requires frequent assessment of symptom control and appropriate titration of medications. Pharmacotherapy, primarily with ICS and SABA or LABA as detailed above, remains key to managing asthma. Environmental interventions may have a role for improving asthma management as non-pharmacologic options. In patients with asthma driven by allergic sensitization, immunotherapy offers the possibility of improved symptom control and enduring benefits even after therapy is completed.

References

1. Johansson SG, Hourihane JO, Bousquet J, Bruijnzeel-Koomen C, Dreborg S, Haahtela T, et al. A revised nomenclature for allergy. An EAACI position statement from the EAACI nomenclature task force. Allergy. 2001;56(9):813–24.
2. Holt PG, Macaubas C, Stumbles PA, Sly PD. The role of allergy in the development of asthma. Nature. 1999;402(6760 Suppl):B12–7.
3. Leynaert B, Neukirch C, Kony S, Guenegou A, Bousquet J, Aubier M, et al. Association between asthma and rhinitis according to atopic sensitization in a population-based study. J Allergy Clin Immunol. 2004;113(1):86–93.
4. Lee E, Lee SH, Kim YH, Cho HJ, Yoon J, Yang SI, et al. Association of atopy phenotypes with new development of asthma and bronchial hyperresponsiveness in school-aged children. Ann Allergy Asthma Immunol. 2017;118(5):542–50 e1.
5. Castillo JR, Peters SP, Busse WW. Asthma exacerbations: pathogenesis, Prevention, and treatment. J Allergy Clin Immunol Pract. 2017;5(4):918–27.
6. Diamant Z, Gauvreau GM, Cockcroft DW, Boulet LP, Sterk PJ, de Jongh FH, et al. Inhaled allergen bronchoprovocation tests. J Allergy Clin Immunol. 2013;132(5):1045–55 e6.
7. D'Amato G, Annesi Maesano I, Molino A, Vitale C, D'Amato M. Thunderstorm-related asthma attacks. J Allergy Clin Immunol. 2017;139(6):1786–7.
8. D'Amato G, Vitale C, D'Amato M, Cecchi L, Liccardi G, Molino A, et al. Thunderstorm-related asthma: what happens and why. Clin Exp Allergy. 2016;46(3):390–6.
9. Portnoy J, Miller JD, Williams PB, Chew GL, Miller JD, Zaitoun F, et al. Environmental assessment and exposure control of dust mites: a practice parameter. Ann Allergy Asthma Immunol. 2013;111(6):465–507.
10. Portnoy J, Chew GL, Phipatanakul W, Williams PB, Grimes C, Kennedy K, et al. Environmental assessment and exposure reduction of cockroaches: a practice parameter. J Allergy Clin Immunol. 2013;132(4):802–8 e1–25.
11. Morgan WJ, Crain EF, Gruchalla RS, O'Connor GT, Kattan M, Evans R 3rd, et al. Results of a home-based environmental intervention among urban children with asthma. N Engl J Med. 2004;351(11):1068–80.
12. National Asthma E, Prevention P. Expert panel report 3 (EPR-3): guidelines for the diagnosis and Management of Asthma-Summary Report 2007. J Allergy Clin Immunol. 2007;120(5 Suppl):S94–138.
13. El-Ghitany EM, Abd El-Salam MM. Environmental intervention for house dust mite control in childhood bronchial asthma. Environ Health Prev Med. 2012;17(5):377–84.
14. Bahir A, Goldberg A, Mekori YA, Confino-Cohen R, Morag H, Rosen Y, et al. Continuous avoidance measures with or without acaricide in dust mite-allergic asthmatic children. Ann Allergy Asthma Immunol. 1997;78(5):506–12.
15. Vyszenski-Moher DL, Arlian LG, Neal JS. Effects of laundry detergents on Dermatophagoides farinae, Dermatophagoides pteronyssinus, and Euroglyphus maynei. Ann Allergy Asthma Immunol. 2002;88(6):578–83.
16. McDonald LG, Tovey E. The role of water temperature and laundry procedures in reducing house dust mite populations and allergen content of bedding. J Allergy Clin Immunol. 1992;90(4 Pt 1):599–608.
17. Woodcock A, Forster L, Matthews E, Martin J, Letley L, Vickers M, et al. Control of exposure to mite allergen and allergen-impermeable bed covers for adults with asthma. N Engl J Med. 2003;349(3):225–36.
18. Gotzsche PC, Johansen HK. House dust mite control measures for asthma: systematic review. Allergy. 2008;63(6):646–59.
19. Halken S, Host A, Niklassen U, Hansen LG, Nielsen F, Pedersen S, et al. Effect of mattress and pillow encasings on children with asthma and house dust mite allergy. J Allergy Clin Immunol. 2003;111(1):169–76.
20. Murray CS, Foden P, Sumner H, Shepley E, Custovic A, Simpson A. Preventing severe Asthma exacerbations in children. A randomized trial of mite-impermeable bedcovers. Am J Respir Crit Care Med. 2017;196(2):150–8.
21. Phipatanakul W, Matsui E, Portnoy J, Williams PB, Barnes C, Kennedy K, et al. Environmental assessment and exposure reduction of rodents: a practice parameter. Ann Allergy Asthma Immunol. 2012;109(6):375–87.
22. Rabito FA, Carlson JC, He H, Werthmann D, Schal C. A single intervention for cockroach control reduces cockroach exposure and asthma morbidity in children. J Allergy Clin Immunol. 2017;140(2):565–70.
23. Eggleston PA. Methods and effectiveness of indoor environmental control. Ann Allergy Asthma Immunol. 2001;87(6 Suppl 3):44–7.
24. Matsui EC, Perzanowski M, Peng RD, Wise RA, Balcer-Whaley S, Newman M, et al. Effect of an integrated Pest management intervention on Asthma symptoms among mouse-sensitized children and adolescents with Asthma: a randomized clinical trial. JAMA. 2017;317(10):1027–36.
25. Portnoy J, Kennedy K, Sublett J, Phipatanakul W, Matsui E, Barnes C, et al. Environmental assessment and exposure control: a practice parameter--furry animals. Ann Allergy Asthma Immunol. 2012;108(4):223 e1–15.
26. Avner DB, Perzanowski MS, Platts-Mills TA, Woodfolk JA. Evaluation of different techniques for washing cats: quantitation of allergen removed from the cat and the effect on airborne Fel d 1. J Allergy Clin Immunol. 1997;100(3):307–12.
27. Hodson T, Custovic A, Simpson A, Chapman M, Woodcock A, Green R. Washing the dog reduces dog allergen levels, but the dog needs to be washed twice a week. J Allergy Clin Immunol. 1999;103(4):581–5.

28. Leas BF, D'Anci KE, Apter AJ, Bryant-Stephens T, Lynch MP, Kaczmarek JL, et al. Effectiveness of indoor allergen reduction in asthma management: a systematic review. J Allergy Clin Immunol. 2018;141(5):1854–69.
29. Lewis RD, Breysse PN. Carpet properties that affect the retention of cat allergen. Ann Allergy Asthma Immunol. 2000;84(1):31–6.
30. Popplewell EJ, Innes VA, Lloyd-Hughes S, Jenkins EL, Khdir K, Bryant TN, et al. The effect of high-efficiency and standard vacuum-cleaners on mite, cat and dog allergen levels and clinical progress. Pediatr Allergy Immunol. 2000;11(3):142–8.
31. Lewis RD, Ong KH, Emo B, Kennedy J, Kesavan J, Elliot M. Resuspension of house dust and allergens during walking and vacuum cleaning. J Occup Environ Hyg. 2018;15(3):235–45.
32. Sublett JL, Seltzer J, Burkhead R, Williams PB, Wedner HJ, Phipatanakul W, et al. Air filters and air cleaners: rostrum by the American Academy of Allergy, Asthma & Immunology indoor allergen committee. J Allergy Clin Immunol. 2010;125(1):32–8.
33. McDonald E, Cook D, Newman T, Griffith L, Cox G, Guyatt G. Effect of air filtration systems on asthma: a systematic review of randomized trials. Chest. 2002;122(5):1535–42.
34. Brown KW, Minegishi T, Allen JG, McCarthy JF, Spengler JD, MacIntosh DL. Reducing patients' exposures to asthma and allergy triggers in their homes: an evaluation of effectiveness of grades of forced air ventilation filters. J Asthma. 2014;51(6):585–94.
35. Nathan RA, Sorkness CA, Kosinski M, Schatz M, Li JT, Marcus P, et al. Development of the asthma control test: a survey for assessing asthma control. J Allergy Clin Immunol. 2004;113(1):59–65.
36. Global Initiative for Asthma. Global strategy for Asthma management and prevention. 2020. Available from: www.ginasthma.org.
37. Goldsmith DR, Keating GM. Budesonide/formoterol: a review of its use in asthma. Drugs. 2004;64(14):1597–618.
38. van Noord JA, Smeets JJ, Raaijmakers JA, Bommer AM, Maesen FP. Salmeterol versus formoterol in patients with moderately severe asthma: onset and duration of action. Eur Respir J. 1996;9(8):1684–8.
39. Rabe KF, Atienza T, Magyar P, Larsson P, Jorup C, Lalloo UG. Effect of budesonide in combination with formoterol for reliever therapy in asthma exacerbations: a randomised controlled, double-blind study. Lancet. 2006;368(9537):744–53.
40. O'Byrne PM, Barnes PJ, Rodriguez-Roisin R, Runnerstrom E, Sandstrom T, Svensson K, et al. Low dose inhaled budesonide and formoterol in mild persistent asthma: the OPTIMA randomized trial. Am J Respir Crit Care Med. 2001;164(8 Pt 1):1392–7.
41. Kendzerska T, Aaron SD, To T, Licskai C, Stanbrook M, Vozoris NT, et al. Effectiveness and safety of inhaled corticosteroids in older individuals with chronic obstructive pulmonary disease and/or Asthma. A population study. Ann Am Thorac Soc. 2019;16(10):1252–62.
42. Baddar S, Jayakrishnan B, Al-Rawas OA. Asthma control: importance of compliance and inhaler technique assessments. J Asthma. 2014;51(4):429–34.
43. Price DB, Roman-Rodriguez M, McQueen RB, Bosnic-Anticevich S, Carter V, Gruffydd-Jones K, et al. Inhaler errors in the CRITIKAL study: type, frequency, and association with Asthma outcomes. J Allergy Clin Immunol Pract. 2017;5(4):1071–81 e9.
44. Sanchis J, Gich I, Pedersen S. Aerosol drug management improvement T. Systematic review of errors in inhaler use: has patient technique improved over time? Chest. 2016;150(2):394–406.
45. Price D, Harrow B, Small M, Pike J, Higgins V. Establishing the relationship of inhaler satisfaction, treatment adherence, and patient outcomes: a prospective, real-world, cross-sectional survey of US adult asthma patients and physicians. World Allergy Organ J. 2015;8(1):26.
46. Perret JL, Bonevski B, McDonald CF, Abramson MJ. Smoking cessation strategies for patients with asthma: improving patient outcomes. J Asthma Allergy. 2016;9:117–28.
47. Porsbjerg C, Menzies-Gow A. Co-morbidities in severe asthma: clinical impact and management. Respirology. 2017;22(4):651–61.
48. Greenberger PA, Bush RK, Demain JG, Luong A, Slavin RG, Knutsen AP. Allergic bronchopulmonary aspergillosis. J Allergy Clin Immunol Pract. 2014;2(6):703–8.
49. Burks AW, Calderon MA, Casale T, Cox L, Demoly P, Jutel M, et al. Update on allergy immunotherapy: American Academy of Allergy, Asthma & Immunology/European academy of allergy and clinical immunology/PRACTALL consensus report. J Allergy Clin Immunol. 2013;131(5):1288–96 e3.
50. Jutel M, Agache I, Bonini S, Burks AW, Calderon M, Canonica W, et al. International consensus on allergy immunotherapy. J Allergy Clin Immunol. 2015;136(3):556–68.
51. Jutel M, Agache I, Bonini S, Burks AW, Calderon M, Canonica W, et al. International consensus on allergen immunotherapy II: mechanisms, standardization, and pharmacoeconomics. J Allergy Clin Immunol. 2016;137(2):358–68.
52. Cox L, Nelson H, Lockey R, Calabria C, Chacko T, Finegold I, et al. Allergen immunotherapy: a practice parameter third update. J Allergy Clin Immunol. 2011;127(1 Suppl):S1–55.
53. Muraro A, Roberts G, Halken S, Agache I, Angier E, Fernandez-Rivas M, et al. EAACI guidelines on allergen immunotherapy: executive statement. Allergy. 2018;73(4):739–43.
54. Mahler V, Esch RE, Kleine-Tebbe J, Lavery WJ, Plunkett G, Vieths S, et al. Understanding differences in allergen immunotherapy products and practices in North America and Europe. J Allergy Clin Immunol. 2019;143(3):813–28.

55. Epstein TG, Liss GM, Murphy-Berendts K, Bernstein DI. Immediate and delayed-onset systemic reactions after subcutaneous immunotherapy injections: ACAAI/AAAAI surveillance study of subcutaneous immunotherapy: year 2. Ann Allergy Asthma Immunol. 2011;107(5):426–31 e1.
56. Abramson MJ, Puy RM, Weiner JM. Injection allergen immunotherapy for asthma. Cochrane Database Syst Rev. 2010;(8):CD001186.
57. Lin SY, Azar A, Suarez-Cuervo C, Diette GB, Brigham E, Rice J, et al. The role of immunotherapy in the treatment of Asthma. Rockville (MD): AHRQ Comparative Effectiveness Reviews; 2018.
58. Rice JL, Diette GB, Suarez-Cuervo C, Brigham EP, Lin SY, Ramanathan M Jr, et al. Allergen-specific immunotherapy in the treatment of pediatric Asthma: a systematic review. Pediatrics. 2018;141(5)
59. Wahidi MM, Kraft M. Bronchial thermoplasty for severe asthma. Am J Respir Crit Care Med. 2012;185(7):709–14.
60. Torrego A, Sola I, Munoz AM, Roque IFM, Yepes-Nunez JJ, Alonso-Coello P, et al. Bronchial thermoplasty for moderate or severe persistent asthma in adults. Cochrane Database Syst Rev. 2014;2014(3):CD009910.

Asthma Phenotypes

26

Sandhya Khurana and Farrukh Abbas

Introduction

Asthma is a heterogenous disease usually characterized by chronic airway inflammation [1]. Our understanding of the many different mechanisms in asthma (endotypes) that result in a variety of disease expression and characteristics (phenotypes) has evolved. This heterogeneity has been extensively studied at clinical, cellular, and molecular levels. Clinically, patients with asthma differ with regard to symptoms, age of onset, airflow limitation, bronchodilator reversibility, response to treatment, triggers, and long-term outcomes [2]. This chapter briefly reviews the immunologic pathways involved in the pathogenesis of asthma and therapeutic targets, as well as provides an overview of the different asthma phenotypes.

S. Khurana
Pulmonary and Critical Care Medicine, University of Rochester School of Medicine, Rochester, NY, USA
e-mail: Sandhya_Khurana@urmc.rochester.edu

F. Abbas (✉)
Department of Pulmonary and Critical Care Medicine, Virginia Commonwealth University Health System, Richmond, VA, USA

Immunologic Basis and Inflammatory Pathways in Asthma

Chronic inflammation in asthma is broadly divided into "type-2 high" and "type-2 low", mediated by type-1 and type-2 immune responses respectively (Fig. 26.1) [4, 5].

Type-2 High Asthma

Type-2 inflammation is present in majority of patients with severe asthma. It is defined as absolute blood eosinophils ≥150/μL, and/or Fractional exhaled nitric oxide (FeNO) ≥20 ppb, and or sputum eosinophils ≥2%, and /or asthma is clinically allergen-driven [1]. Type-2 immune responses are the main defense against helminthic and parasitic infections. These pathways are also involved in asthma, atopy, and other allergic inflammatory disorders. Asthma was previously considered primarily a T helper cell 2 (Th2) disease driving the adaptive immune response to allergen exposure through cytokines IL-4, IL-5, and IL-13, resulting in allergic and eosinophilic inflammation [6]. The discovery of type-2 innate lymphoid cells (ILC2) revealed that the innate immune pathways are also involved in the pathogenesis of asthma and result in eosinophilic inflammation [7, 8]. Therefore, we now use the

C. Damask et al. (eds.), *Allergy in Otolaryngology Practice*,
https://doi.org/10.1007/978-3-031-93455-1_26

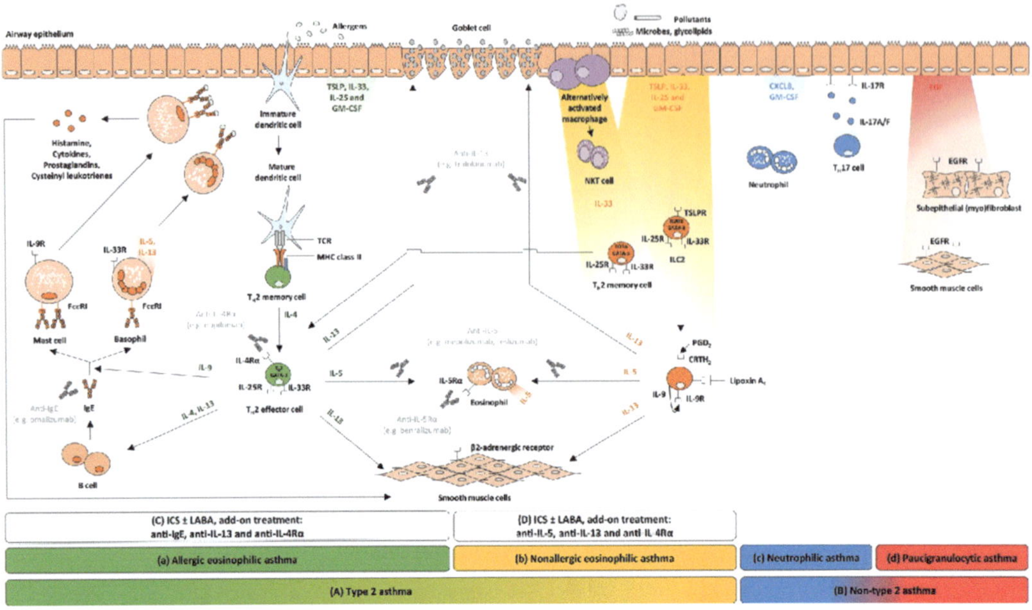

Fig. 26.1 Diagram showing type-2 and non-type-2 asthma pathways. Type-2 asthma can be allergic eosinophilic (**a**) or nonallergic eosinophilic (**b**). Non-type-2 asthma can be neutrophilic (**c**) or paucigranulocytic (**d**). (Reprinted by permission of the publisher (Taylor & Francis Ltd. http://www.tandfonline.com) [3])

term "type-2" inflammation that includes both Th2- and ILC2-related mechanisms. ILC2 are lineage-negative cells that lack markers for lymphocytes, dendritic cells, macrophages, or granulocytes [9, 10].

Type-2 immune responses can be mediated by allergic or non-allergic triggers. Th2 lymphocytes drive the allergic inflammatory response while ILC2s mediate non-allergic eosinophilic inflammation. Type-2 immune responses are initiated at the epithelial level in response to microbiome recognition, tissue destruction, or allergen exposure. Epithelial cytokines IL-25, IL-33, and TSLP, also known as "alarmins", are released by the epithelial cells and activate and mobilize dendritic cells, mast cells, basophils, and group 2 innate lymphoid cells (ILC2) [11, 12]. Once activated by TSLP, dendritic cells move to lymph nodes where they mediate maturation of naïve T cells to Th helper cells, e.g., Th2 cells [11]. Mature Th2 cells release cytokines IL-4, IL-5, IL-9, and IL-13. ILC2 also secrete cytokines IL-5 and IL-13 [13].

- IL-5 leads to tissue eosinophilia through a key role in differentiation, maturation, activation, and recruitment of eosinophils [11, 14, 15].
- IL-4 is involved in the differentiation of naïve T cells into Th2 CD4+ cells and mediates IgE class switching. IL-4 also mediates mucus secretion by airway epithelium and induces migration of eosinophils, monocytes, and basophils to the airway epithelium in response to allergen exposure [16–18].
- IL-9 has a role in allergic and eosinophilic asthma as it promotes Ig-E class switching, mucus secretion by epithelial cells, and mast cell hyperplasia [19–21].
- IL-13 is not only secreted by Th2 cells but also by ILC2 and mast cells. IL-13 has many similar properties as IL-4 and is involved in mucus secretion, chemotaxis of eosinophils, Ig-E class switching, and B-cell growth [22–24].

Type-2 high inflammation defines majority of the sub-phenotypes of asthma and therapeutic options have become available to target different steps of type-2 immune response. Monoclonal antibodies have shown efficacy in severe eosinophilic asthma and have important role as add-on therapy in patients with moderate to severe uncontrolled asthma and frequent exacerbations [25].

Eicosanoid Pathway-Mediated Type-2 Inflammation

Arachidonic acid is metabolized in the lipid layer of the cell membrane of eosinophils, mast cells, macrophages, and basophils [26]. This metabolism has two main pathways: the pathway involving the cyclooxygenase (COX) enzymes generates prostaglandins while the pathway involving 5-lipoxygenase enzyme generates cysteinyl leukotrienes (cyst-LT) [26]. Prostaglandin D2 (PGD2) is the major prostanoid released from mast cells and is involved in allergic asthma [27]. Higher levels of PGD2 have been found in asthmatic patients after allergen exposure [28, 29]. PGD2 causes tissue eosinophilia, bronchoconstriction, and it has been associated with asthma exacerbations and poor asthma control [30, 31]. Several trials have evaluated the efficacy of PGD2 receptor (DP2) antagonists and yielded mixed results [32–34]. Cysteinyl leukotrienes have been associated with bronchoconstriction, airway edema, increase vascular permeability, and mucus secretion [35, 36]. Inhibitor of 5-lipooxygenase (zileuton) and cyst-LT1 receptor (montelukast and zafirlukast) have shown efficacy in asthma, particularly in patients with aspirin-exacerbated respiratory disease (AERD) [37–39].

Type-2 Low Asthma

Type-2 low asthma is characterized by the absence of type-2 inflammatory markers. Type-2 low asthma may be more common in mild-to-moderate disease, with estimates of 64-73% [40, 41] Mechanisms of type-2 low asthma are not as well understood. Type-1 immune responses are mediated by Th1 & Th17 CD4 + T cells, type-3 innate lymphoid cells (ILC3), cytotoxic CD8 cells, and immunoglobin G (Ig G). Type-1 immune responses are involved in protection against fungi, viruses, bacteria, and protozoa. They can cause autoimmune diseases if directed against self-antigens [42]. The data supporting type-1 immune response as a mediator of asthma are not as robust as type-2 immune response. Th1 cells are characterized by interferon-gamma (IFNγ) production, which plays a role in viral infections and autoimmunity. Both Th1 and interferon-gamma are overexpressed in patients with asthma [43]. They may also be involved in severe and corticosteroid-resistant asthma [44, 45]. IL-17, mainly produced by CD4+ Th17 cells and other immune cells, is involved in airway neutrophilia and associated with airway hyperresponsiveness (AHR). [46, 47] Increased levels of IL-17 have been reported in bronchoalveolar lavage fluid (BALF), airway cells, and sputum of patients with asthma [48, 49]. Role of IL-17-producing ILC3 has been described in murine model in obesity-related asthma, airway smooth muscle dysfunction, and possibly in neutrophilic asthma [50, 51]. Neutrophils are involved in innate and cell-mediated inflammatory pathways in response to acute & chronic infections, smoking and environmental antigens [52]. Elevated airway epithelial neutrophils have been found in severe asthma and during asthma exacerbations [53–55]. The epithelial alarmins (TSLP, IL-25 and IL-33) released in response to tissue damage can drive type-2 inflammation but are also likely implicated in type-2 low inflammation as well particularly TSLP has been associated with steroid resistance of ILC-2 cells [56, 57]. Hence, anti-TSLP monoclonal antibody (tezepelumab) has shown efficacy in patients with type-2 high and type-2 low phenotypes [58].

Asthma Phenotyping Efforts

We have already briefly touched upon the immunologic basis of heterogeneity in asthma. Different approaches have been used over the years to classify asthma based on clinical, functional, molecular, and cellular phenotypes. Appreciation and understanding of asthma heterogeneity are critical to development and application of targeted effective therapies.

Inflammation in asthma has been broadly divided into eosinophilic and non-eosinophilic using sputum inflammometry. Normal sputum cell counts consist of about 2/3 macrophages and 1/3 neutrophils. Eosinophils are not usually seen in sputum of normal individuals but have been recognized as a major cell type in patients with asthma [59]. Eosinophilic asthma is characterized by elevated sputum eosinophils (>2%) [60] Eosinophilic asthma is associated with more frequent exacerbations and tends to be steroid responsive [61]. Non-eosinophilic asthma is characterized by the absence of sputum eosinophils. Sputum eosinophils of <1.9% on at least 2 occasions have been suggested as a threshold for defining non-eosinophilic asthma [52]. Non-eosinophilic asthma is further divided into neutrophilic, mixed granulocytic, and pauci-granulocytic [52]. Neutrophilic asthma is associated with reduced forced expiratory volume in 1 second (FEV-1) [62].

Mixed granulocytic inflammation, with increased eosinophils and neutrophils in the sputum, is associated with more refractory asthma, severe asthma exacerbations, poor lung function, and high health care utilization [52, 63]. Pauci-granulocytic asthma (PGA) patients have no evidence of increased sputum eosinophils or neutrophils. PGA is characterized by smooth muscle dysfunction independent of airway inflammation, can have fixed airway obstruction, and is frequently steroid insensitive [52, 64, 65].

There have been three major efforts to phenotype asthma using similar variables but different approaches: Severe Asthma Research Program (SARP), the Unbiased Biomarkers for the Prediction of Respiratory Disease Outcome (U-BIOPRED) program, and the Asthma Disease Endotyping for Personalized Therapeutics (ADEPT) study. The ADEPT study focused on molecular and genetic basis of asthma linking distinct endotypes to clinical phenotypes. These projects provide valuable insights into asthma phenotypes. We will be discussing SARP and U-BIOPRED.

Severe Asthma Research Program

In 2001, National Heart, Lung, and Blood Institute (NHLBI) funded the Severe Asthma Research Program (SARP) to generate a large cohort to better understand this heterogenous disease. One of the goals of SARP was to characterize patients with severe asthma and compare asthma across different severities. Moore and colleagues used data from SARP to define 5 different clusters of asthma phenotypes using 34 variables [66]. Cluster 1 included 15% of total population and had mild allergic asthma. This cluster was characterized by young patients, mostly females, who had early onset or atopic asthma and had normal lung function. Most of these patients were on two or less controller medications and reported minimal healthcare utilization. Cluster 2, the largest group, included 44% of the total population. This cluster also included patients with allergic asthma, early-onset, and atopy. This group had low-normal prebronchodilator FEV1 and bronchodilator reversal to normal FEV1. Cluster 2 required higher doses of ICS but similar health care utilization, symptoms, and rescue inhaler use as cluster 1. Cluster 3 included 8% of the cohort and was characterized by older age, mostly women, higher BMI, less atopy, daily asthma symptoms, mildly reduced pre-bronchodilator FEV1, less bronchodilator reversibility (BDR), higher systemic steroid use, more maintenance inhaler medications, and higher healthcare utilization.

Cluster 4 had individuals with early-onset atopic asthma but with longer duration, severely reduced FEV1 with reversibility to normal in only half the patients, daily symptoms, higher rescue inhaler use, more controller medications, higher need for systemic steroids, and higher health care utilization. Cluster 5 included individuals with later-onset asthma, less atopy, severely reduced lung function with less bronchodilator reversibility, daily symptoms, higher health care utilization, and higher systemic steroid use.

ADEPT and U-BIOPRED

ADPET and U-BIOPRED are independent asthma biomarkers study that were designed to better understand the disease and help devise personalized therapeutic plans [67, 68]. Loza and colleagues used ADPET and U-BIOPRED data to cluster clinically driven asthma phenotypes [69, 70]. Clinical phenotypes were created by using 9 variables from the ADEPT study which was used as training set and then U-BIOPRED data was used to validate ADEPT study-driven clinical phenotypes. Fuzzy partition-around-medoid (PAM) clustering was performed on 156 asthma patients from ADEPT study and determined four clinical phenotypes. Phenotype A1 had mild controlled early-onset asthma with normal lung function and low inflammation. 93% of patients in this group were not on ICS. This group had low sputum and blood eosinophils and lowest sputum neutrophils. Phenotype A2 had allergic and eosinophilic asthma of moderate severity with mild reversible airway obstruction. This group had the highest sputum and blood eosinophils, had highest atopy , and highest airway hyper-responsiveness (AHR) measured with methacholine concentration (provocative concentration (PC20)). Phenotype A3 contained non-eosinophilic asthmatics with less bronchodilator reversibility. This group contained patients of all asthma severity. They had lowest atopy, least sputum eosinophils, and highest sputum neutrophils of all the phenotypes identified. Phenotype A4 contained severe uncontrolled asthmatics with mixed inflammatory cells. This group had highest airway obstruction, highest BDR, and higher AHR. They had mixed eosinophilic/neutrophilic inflammation and low atopy. 12-month follow-up of these patients showed remarkable stability of these phenotypes with very low cross-over rate.

These clinical phenotypes were then validated using data from U-BIOPRED. Eighty-two patients were included in this analysis using similar inclusion criteria as ADEPT subjects. The same PAM clustering methodology generated four clinical phenotypes. These four clinical phenotypes demonstrated remarkably similar characteristics as ADEPT phenotypes (Table 26.1).

Table 26.1 The four clusters of clinical phenotypes in ADEPT and U-BIOPRED data

Phenotype	ADEPT	U-BIOPRED
Mild, controlled, low inflammation	A1	US1
Moderate, hyperreactive, eosinophilic	A2	US2
Mixed severity, non-eosinophilic, neutrophilic	A3	US3
Severe, uncontrolled, mixed granulocytic	A4	US4

Examples of Type-2 High Asthma Phenotypes

Early-Onset Allergic Asthma

Early-onset or childhood-onset asthma is a distinct phenotype characterized by atopy [71]. This type of asthma is linked to type-2 high allergic inflammation and relevant biomarkers (IL-4, IL-5, IL-13, and IgE) [11]. Patients with early-onset allergic asthma tend to have other comorbid allergic disorders such as allergic rhinitis and atopic dermatitis.

Late-Onset Eosinophilic Asthma

Late-onset eosinophilic asthma is characterized by eosinophilic inflammation, less reversible airway obstruction, and longer disease duration [72, 73]. Patients with this type of asthma have a more chronic course, tend to be non-atopic [74], have more rapid decline in lung function [75], and worse prognosis [76].

AERD

Aspirin-exacerbated respiratory disease (AERD) is a distinct asthma phenotype characterized by severe asthma, nasal polyposis, and acute respiratory symptoms upon exposure to nonsteroidal anti-inflammatory drugs (NSAIDS). [77] Arachidonic acid metabolites are involved in its pathogenesis. These patients usually have blood and tissue eosinophilia, and tend be corticosteroid dependent [78]. Nasal polyps are often difficult to manage and rapidly recur after surgical resection in these patients. Asthma in AERD is usually severe and difficult to control [79]. Careful history-taking is the key in identifying AERD. Atopy may be present in patients with AERD but it does not represent a true allergic disease [80].

Sensitizer-Induced Occupational Asthma

Occupational asthma is a distinct phenotype caused by workplace exposure and is different than work-exacerbated asthma, which is preexisting asthma exacerbated by work-related exposure [81]. Occupational asthma can be induced by sensitizers (sensitizer-induced occupational asthma) or by irritant (non-sensitizing occupational asthma). Sensitizers lead to an allergic immunologic response with IgE production and this type of asthma is often associated with allergic rhinitis [82]. It usually takes weeks to years to become sensitized to an allergen before the onset of asthma. Symptoms usually start at the onset of workday, and progress throughout the day and workweek, and typically resolve or improve on weekends and holidays.

Examples of Type-2 Low Asthma Phenotypes

Obesity-Associated Asthma

There is increasing evidence that asthma prevalence is higher in obese and overweight people [83, 84]. Obesity is considered a risk factor for new adult-onset asthma [85]. The risk of obese asthma phenotype is higher for women than men [85], and in nonatopic asthma than atopic asthma [86]. Patients with obesity-associated asthma have lower lung function [87, 88], lack airway eosinophilic inflammation, and have difficult to control asthma [88].

Smoking-Associated Asthma

Cigarette smoking can worsen asthma symptoms and disease control [89, 90]. Patients with asthma who smoke demonstrate a more rapid decline in lung function [91, 92], higher health care utilization, need for oral corticosteroids [92], and higher percentage of steroid-refractory asthma [93, 94]. Smoking can be a risk factor for new-onset asthma, and maternal smoking may lead to incident asthma in children [95–97].

Irritant-Induced Asthma

Irritant-induced asthma may be caused by workplace exposure to airway irritants, for example, cleaning products, ammonia, and organic dust [98]. Compared to sensitizer-induced asthma, there is no latency period as sensitization does not occur. The diagnosis of irritant-induced occupational asthma requires thorough history taking and monitoring of lung function during periods of exposure and no exposure [99, 100].

Paucigranulocytic Asthma

Patients with paucigranulocytic asthma tend to have stable disease, lower BMI [101], less AHR [102], less exacerbations, better lung function, and lower frequency of severe refractory asthma [65, 103].

Neutrophilic Asthma

Neutrophilic asthma phenotype is more prevalent in older patients [104]. Patients with neutrophilic asthma tend to have higher BMI [105], increased asthma duration, and fixed airflow limitation [106].

These asthma phenotypes may overlap as shown in Fig. 26.2.

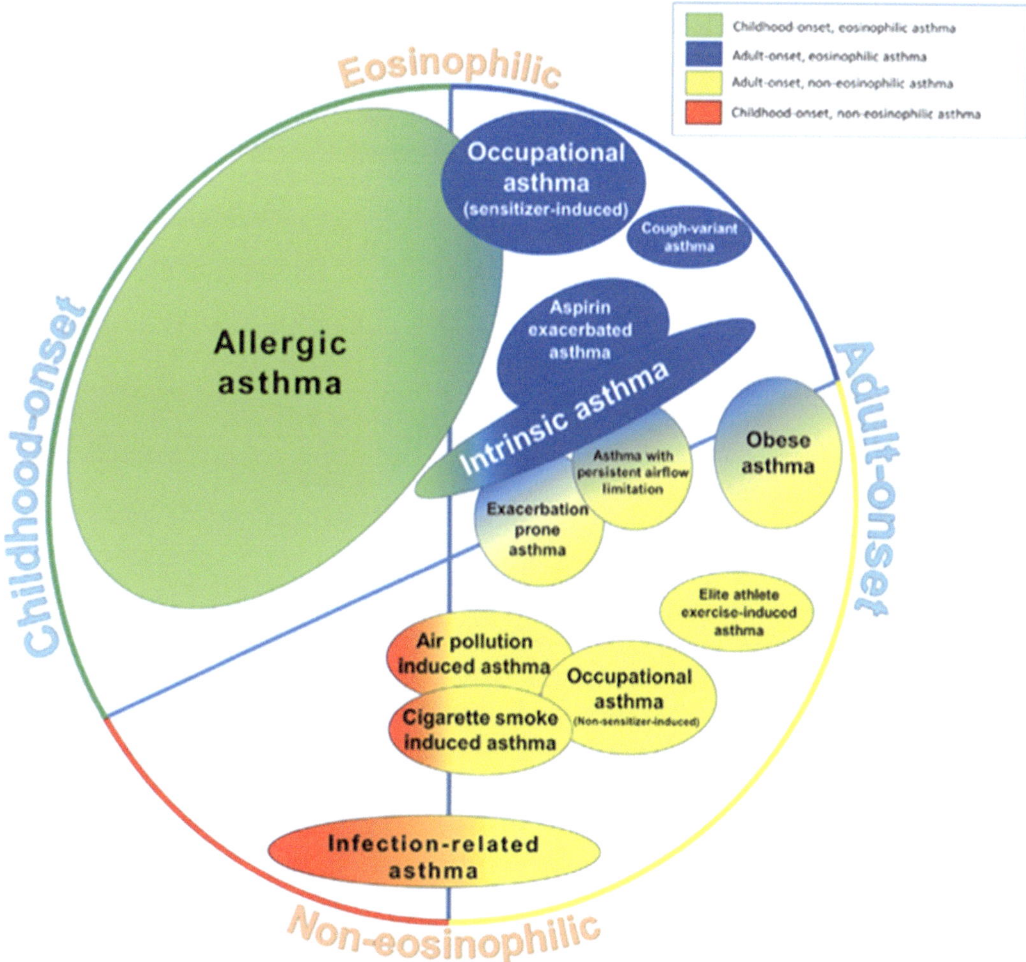

Fig. 26.2 Examples of common clinical asthma phenotypes across the spectrum of eosinophilic inflammation and age of onset. (Reprinted from [107], with permission of Elsevier)

Phenotypes Based on Biomarkers

Asthma phenotypes can also be defined based on markers of airway inflammation found in sputum, blood, exhaled air, and bronchial biopsy specimens [108, 109]. Some of these biomarkers are shown in Fig. 26.3. Eosinophilic and neutrophilic asthma, based on sputum, have been described in the above sections. Below, we discuss the role of other biomarkers.

Fractional Exhaled Nitric Oxide (FeNO)

FeNO is a marker of type-2 airway inflammation [111, 112]. Inhibitors of IL-4 and IL-13 are associated with lower FeNO level, suggesting a role in type-2 allergic eosinophilic asthma [63, 113]. Corticosteroids suppress FeNO level and are associated with clinical improvement [114]. Persistent elevation of FeNO despite adherence

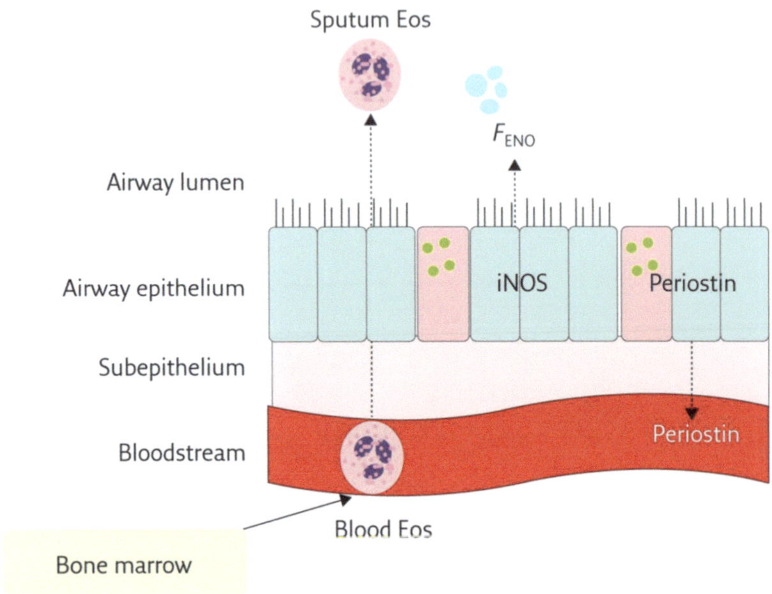

Fig. 26.3 Different biomarkers involved in type-2 asthma. *Eos* Eosinophil, *iNOS* inducible nitric oxide synthase. (Reproduced with permission of the © ERS 2020: [110] Published 25 September 2020)

with corticosteroid treatment is indicative of severe refractory asthma [115]. However, elevated FeNO levels are not a specific marker of eosinophilic inflammation and can be altered by many other conditions so should be used with caution [116].

Periostin

Periostin, an extracellular matrix protein, is a marker of type-2 inflammation and thought to reflect IL-13 activity [117]. Periostin has been used to successfully differentiate between T2-high and T2-low inflammation [118]. Periostin is not currently available for clinical use. It was being developed as a biomarker for anti-IL-13 antibody, lebrikizumab, which subsequently did not make it to clinical use after negative phase 3 clinical trials.

IgE

IgE is involved in atopic conditions including asthma, allergic rhinitis, and atopic dermatitis [119]. IgE can trigger mast cell-mediated acute-phase and late-phase bronchial constriction [120, 121]. Serum IgE levels correlate with asthma severity [120]. The production of antigen-specific IgE is mediated by class switching within B cells, induced by IL-4 and IL-13. Omalizumab is a monoclonal anti-IgE antibody approved as add-on therapy for moderate to severe allergic asthma. Dupilumab can also be effective in these patients.

Blood and Sputum Eosinophils

Eosinophilic inflammation in asthma can occur in both allergic and non-allergic phenotypes. Eosinophilic asthma can be defined by elevated eosinophils in blood, sputum, or airway biopsy specimens [122–124]. Sputum eosinophil threshold of ≥2% of the total white blood cell count [125, 126] has typically been used to identify eosinophilic asthma [63, 107, 127, 128]. Blood eosinophils have shown to have higher accuracy to predict sputum eosinophils when compared to serum periostin and FENO [129]. The clinical trials have demonstrated that peripheral blood eosinophils can be utilized to select patients and predict response to anti-IL5 therapies [130].

Currently Available Biologics and Future Directions

The biologic therapies currently available for clinical use as add-on therapy in moderate to severe uncontrolled asthma target IgE (omalizumab), IL-5 (mepolizumab, reslizumab), IL-5 receptor (benralizumab), IL-4 receptor alpha (dupilumab), and TSLP (tezepelumab). There are currently several clinical trials on biologics for severe asthma. Depemokimab is an ultra-long acting anti-IL-5 antibody with promising results in phase III trials as a twice-yearly biologic for type-2 high asthma [131]. Verekitug has similar dosing concept and targets TSLP, and is still undergoing phase II clinical trials [132]. Itepekimab/Tozorakimab (anti-IL33 antibodies) and Astegolimab (anti-IL-33 receptor ST2) could have a role in the future treatment of severe asthma [133–135]. [131 Lunsekimig (anti-IL13/anti-TSLP) is currently being investigated in phase II clinical trial for moderate to severe asthma [131].

Summary

Based on the type of inflammation, asthma is divided into type-2 high and type-2 low phenotypes. Type-2 high inflammation is mediated by Th2 helper and ILC2 cells. This type of asthma is characterized by eosinophilic infiltration of airways. Examples of type-2 high asthma include early-onset allergic, late-onset eosinophilic, sensitizer-induced occupational asthma, and aspirin-exacerbated respiratory disease (AERD). Biomarkers can assist with identification of asthma phenotypes as well as selection of appropriate treatments. Various biologic therapeutic options are available to treat patients with type-2 high moderate to severe uncontrolled asthma. Type-2 low asthma is mainly mediated by Th1 and Th17 cells. Examples of type-2 low asthma include obesity-associated, smoking-associated, irritant-induced occupational, paucigranulocytic, and neutrophilic asthma. Currently, there are no targeted therapies available for non-type-2 asthma.

References

1. Global Initiative for Asthma. Global Strategy for Asthma Management and Prevention, 2024. Updated May 2024. Available from: www.ginasthma.org
2. Szefler SJ, Martin RJ, King TS, Boushey HA, Cherniack RM, Chinchilli VM, et al. Significant variability in response to inhaled corticosteroids for persistent asthma. J Allergy Clin Immunol. 2002;109(3):410–8.
3. Godar M, Blanchetot C, de Haard H, Lambrecht BN, Brusselle G. Personalized medicine with biologics for severe type 2 asthma: current status and future prospects. mAbs. 2018;10(1):34–45. https://doi.org/10.1080/19420862.2017.1392425.
4. Licona-Limón P, Kim LK, Palm NW, Flavell RA. TH2, allergy and group 2 innate lymphoid cells. Nat Immunol. 2013;14(6):536.
5. Fahy JV. Identifying clinical phenotypes of asthma: steps in the right direction. Am J Respir Crit Care Med. 2010;181(4):296–7.
6. Mosmann TR, Cherwinski H, Bond MW, Giedlin MA, Coffman RL. Two types of murine helper T cell clone. I. Definition according to profiles of lymphokine activities and secreted proteins. J Immunol. 1986;136(7):2348–57.
7. Fort MM, Cheung J, Yen D, Li J, Zurawski SM, Lo S, et al. IL-25 induces IL-4, IL-5, and IL-13 and Th2-associated pathologies in vivo. Immunity. 2001;15(6):985–95.
8. Fallon PG, Ballantyne SJ, Mangan NE, Barlow JL, Dasvarma A, Hewett DR, et al. Identification of an interleukin (IL)-25–dependent cell population that provides IL-4, IL-5, and IL-13 at the onset of helminth expulsion. J Exp Med. 2006;203(4):1105–16.
9. Halim TY, Krauß RH, Sun AC, Takei F. Lung natural helper cells are a critical source of Th2 cell-type cytokines in protease allergen-induced airway inflammation. Immunity. 2012;36(3):451–63.
10. Liew FY, Girard J-P, Turnquist HR. Interleukin-33 in health and disease. Nat Rev Immunol. 2016;16(11):676.
11. Locksley RM. Asthma and allergic inflammation. Cell. 2010;140(6):777–83.
12. Angkasekwinai P, Park H, Wang Y-H, Wang Y-H, Chang SH, Corry DB, et al. Interleukin 25 promotes the initiation of proallergic type 2 responses. J Exp Med. 2007;204(7):1509–17.
13. Brusselle GG, Maes T, Bracke KR. Eosinophils in the spotlight: eosinophilic airway inflammation in nonallergic asthma. Nat Med. 2013;19(8):977–9.
14. Takatsu K. Interleukin-5 and IL-5 receptor in health and diseases. Proce Jpn Acad Ser B. 2011;87(8):463–85.
15. Fahy JV, Locksley RM. The airway epithelium as a regulator of Th2 responses in asthma. Am J Respir Crit Care Med. 2011;184(4):390–2.
16. Bochner BS, Luscinskas FW, Gimbrone MA Jr, Newman W, Sterbinsky SA, Derse-Anthony

CP, et al. Adhesion of human basophils, eosinophils, and neutrophils to interleukin 1-activated human vascular endothelial cells: contributions of endothelial cell adhesion molecules. J Exp Med. 1991;173(6):1553–7.
17. Masinovsky B, Urdal D, Gallatin WM. IL-4 acts synergistically with IL-1 beta to promote lymphocyte adhesion to microvascular endothelium by induction of vascular cell adhesion molecule-1. J Immunol. 1990;145(9):2886–95.
18. Brusselle G, Kips J, Tavernier J, Van der Heyden J, Cuvelier C, Pauwels R, et al. Attenuation of allergic airway inflammation in IL-4 deficient mice. Clin Exp Allergy. 1994;24(1):73–80.
19. Petit-Frere C, Dugas B, Braquet P, Mencia-Huerta J. Interleukin-9 potentiates the interleukin-4-induced IgE and IgG1 release from murine B lymphocytes. Immunology. 1993;79(1):146.
20. Dong Q, Louahed J, Vink A, Sullivan CD, Messler CJ, Zhou Y, et al. IL-9 induces chemokine expression in lung epithelial cells and baseline airway eosinophilia in transgenic mice. Eur J Immunol. 1999;29(7):2130–9.
21. Hültner L, Druez C, Moeller J, Uyttenhove C, Schmitt E, Rüde E, et al. Mast cell growth-enhancing activity (MEA) is structurally related and functionally identical to the novel mouse T cell growth factor P40/TCGFIII (interleukin 9). Eur J Immunol. 1990;20(6):1413–6.
22. Bochner BS, Klunk DA, Sterbinsky SA, Coffman RL, Schleimer RP. IL-13 selectively induces vascular cell adhesion molecule-1 expression in human endothelial cells. J Immunol. 1995;154(2):799–803.
23. Punnonen J, Aversa G, Cocks BG, McKenzie A, Menon S, Zurawski G, et al. Interleukin 13 induces interleukin 4-independent IgG4 and IgE synthesis and CD23 expression by human B cells. Proc Natl Acad Sci. 1993;90(8):3730–4.
24. Woodruff PG, Modrek B, Choy DF, Jia G, Abbas AR, Ellwanger A, et al. T-helper type 2–driven inflammation defines major subphenotypes of asthma. Am J Respir Crit Care Med. 2009;180(5):388–95.
25. Holguin F, Cardet JC, Chung KF, Diver S, Ferreira DS, Fitzpatrick A, et al. Management of severe asthma: a European respiratory society/american thoracic society guideline. Eur Respir J. 2020;55(1):1900588.
26. Laidlaw T, Boyce J. Cysteinyl leukotriene receptors, old and new; implications for asthma. Clin Exp Allergy. 2012;42(9):1313–20.
27. Fanning LB, Boyce JA. Lipid mediators and allergic diseases. Ann Allergy Asthma Immunol. 2013;111(3):155–62.
28. Liu MC, Hubbard WC, Proud D, Stealey BA, Galli SJ, Kagey-Sobotka A, et al. Immediate and late inflammatory responses to ragweed antigen challenge of the peripheral airways in allergic asthmatics: cellular, mediator, and permeability changes. Am Rev Respir Dis. 1991;144(1):51–8.
29. Murray M, Webb M, O'Callaghan C, Swarbrick A, Milner A. Respiratory status and allergy after bronchiolitis. Arch Dis Child. 1992;67(4):482–7.
30. Fajt ML, Gelhaus SL, Freeman B, Uvalle CE, Trudeau JB, Holguin F, et al. Prostaglandin D2 pathway upregulation: relation to asthma severity, control, and TH2 inflammation. J Allergy Clin Immunol. 2013;131(6):1504–12.e12.
31. Sampson SE, Sampson AP, Costello JF. Effect of inhaled prostaglandin D2 in normal and atopic subjects, and of pretreatment with leukotriene D4. Thorax. 1997;52(6):513–8.
32. Hall IP, Fowler AV, Gupta A, Tetzlaff K, Nivens MC, Sarno M, et al. Efficacy of BI 671800, an oral CRTH2 antagonist, in poorly controlled asthma as sole controller and in the presence of inhaled corticosteroid treatment. Pulm Pharmacol Ther. 2015;32:37–44.
33. Krug N, Gupta A, Badorrek P, Koenen R, Mueller M, Pivovarova A, et al. Efficacy of the oral chemoattractant receptor homologous molecule on TH2 cells antagonist BI 671800 in patients with seasonal allergic rhinitis. J Allergy Clin Immunol. 2014;133(2):414–9.e8.
34. Straumann A, Hoesli S, Bussmann C, Stuck M, Perkins M, Collins L, et al. Anti-eosinophil activity and clinical efficacy of the CRTH 2 antagonist OC 000459 in eosinophilic esophagitis. Allergy. 2013;68(3):375–85.
35. Mellor EA, Frank N, Soler D, Hodge MR, Lora JM, Austen KF, et al. Expression of the type 2 receptor for cysteinyl leukotrienes (CysLT2R) by human mast cells: functional distinction from CysLT1R. Proc Natl Acad Sci. 2003;100(20):11589–93.
36. Matsuda M, Tabuchi Y, Nishimura K, Nakamura Y, Sekioka T, Kadode M, et al. Increased expression of CysLT2 receptors in the lung of asthmatic mice and role in allergic responses. Prostaglandins Leukot Essent Fat Acids. 2018;131:24–31.
37. Dahlén S-E. Treatment of asthma with antileukotrienes: first line or last resort therapy? Eur J Pharmacol. 2006;533(1–3):40–56.
38. Fischer AR, Rosenberg MA, Lilly CM, Callery JC, Rubin P, Cohn J, et al. Direct evidence for a role of the mast cell in the nasal response to aspirin in aspirin-sensitive asthma. J Allergy Clin Immunol. 1994;94(6):1046–56.
39. Israel E, Fischer AR, Rosenberg MA, Lilly CM, Callery JC, Shapiro J, et al. The pivotal role of 5-lipoxygenase products in the reaction of aspirin-sensitive asthmatics to aspirin. Am Rev Respir Dis. 1993;148(6_pt_1):1447–51.
40. McGrath KW, Icitovic N, Boushey HA, Lazarus SC, Sutherland ER, Chinchilli VM, Fahy JV. Asthma Clinical Research Network of the National Heart L Blood I. A large subgroup of mild-to-moderate asthma is persistently noneosinophilic. Am J Respir Crit Care Med. 2012;185(6):612–619. https://doi.org/10.1164/rccm.201109-1640OC.
41. Lazarus SC, Krishnan JA, King TS, Lang JE, Blake KV, Covar R, Lugogo N, Wenzel S, Chinchilli VM,

Mauger DT, Dyer AM, et al. Blood Institute A. Mometasone or Tiotropium in Mild Asthma with a Low Sputum Eosinophil Level. N Engl J Med. 2019;380(21):2009–19. https://doi.org/10.1056/NEJMoa1814917.
42. Zhu J, Yamane H, Paul WE. Differentiation of effector CD4 T cell populations. Annu Rev Immunol. 2009;28:445–89.
43. Boniface S, Koscher V, Mamessier E, El Biaze M, Dupuy P, Lorec AM, et al. Assessment of T lymphocyte cytokine production in induced sputum from asthmatics: a flow cytometry study. Clin Exp Allergy. 2003;33(9):1238–43.
44. Raundhal M, Morse C, Khare A, Oriss TB, Milosevic J, Trudeau J, et al. High IFN-γ and low SLPI mark severe asthma in mice and humans. J Clin Invest. 2015;125(8):3037–50.
45. Chambers ES, Nanzer AM, Pfeffer PE, Richards DF, Timms PM, Martineau AR, et al. Distinct endotypes of steroid-resistant asthma characterized by IL-17Ahigh and IFN-γhigh immunophenotypes: potential benefits of calcitriol. J Allergy Clin Immunol. 2015;136(3):628–37.e4.
46. Miossec P, Kolls JK. Targeting IL-17 and TH 17 cells in chronic inflammation. Nat Rev Drug Discov. 2012;11(10):763–76.
47. Kudo M, Melton AC, Chen C, Engler MB, Huang KE, Ren X, et al. IL-17A produced by αβ T cells drives airway hyper-responsiveness in mice and enhances mouse and human airway smooth muscle contraction. Nat Med. 2012;18(4):547.
48. Molet S, Hamid Q, Davoineb F, Nutku E, Tahaa R, Pagé N, et al. IL-17 is increased in asthmatic airways and induces human bronchial fibroblasts to produce cytokines. J Allergy Clin Immunol. 2001;108(3):430–8.
49. Doe C, Bafadhel M, Siddiqui S, Desai D, Mistry V, Rugman P, et al. Expression of the T helper 17-associated cytokines IL-17A and IL-17F in asthma and COPD. Chest. 2010;138(5):1140–7.
50. Kim HY, Lee HJ, Chang Y-J, Pichavant M, Shore SA, Fitzgerald KA, et al. Interleukin-17–producing innate lymphoid cells and the NLRP3 inflammasome facilitate obesity-associated airway hyperreactivity. Nat Med. 2014;20(1):54–61.
51. Nagakumar P, Artusio L, Fainardi V, Fleming L, Bush A, Lloyd CM, et al. Role of airway ILC2 and ILC3 compared to Th2 and Th17 cells in paediatric severe therapy resistant asthma (STRA). C13 translational research in asthma. Am J Respir Crit Care Med. 2017;195:A4915-A.
52. Haldar P, Pavord ID. Noneosinophilic asthma: a distinct clinical and pathologic phenotype. J Allergy Clin Immunol. 2007;119(5):1043–52.
53. Fahy JV. Eosinophilic and neutrophilic inflammation in asthma: insights from clinical studies. Proc Am Thorac Soc. 2009;6(3):256–9.
54. Fahya JV, Kimb KW, Liub J, Bousheya HA. Prominent neutrophilic inflammation in sputum from subjects with asthma exacerbation. J Allergy Clin Immunol. 1995;95(4):843–52.
55. Nakagome K, Matsushita S, Nagata M. Neutrophilic inflammation in severe asthma. Int Arch Allergy Immunol. 2012;158(Suppl. 1):96–102.
56. Shikotra A, Choy DF, Ohri CM, Doran E, Butler C, Hargadon B, Shelley M, Abbas AR, Austin CD, Jackman J, Wu LC, et al. Increased expression of immunoreactive thymic stromal lymphopoietin in patients with severe asthma. J Allergy Clin Immunol. 2012;129(1):104–111–e101–109. https://doi.org/10.1016/j.jaci.2011.08.031.
57. Liu S, Verma M, Michalec L, Liu W, Sripada A, Rollins D, Good J, Ito Y, Chu H, Gorska MM, Martin RJ, Alam R. Steroid resistance of airway type 2 innate lymphoid cells from patients with severe asthma: The role of thymic stromal lymphopoietin. J Allergy Clin Immunol. 2018;141(1):257–268 e256. https://doi.org/10.1016/j.jaci.2017.03.032.
58. Menzies-Gow, A. et al. (2021) 'Tezepelumab in adults and adolescents with severe, uncontrolled asthma', New England Journal of Medicine, 384(19), pp. 1800–1809. https://doi.org./10.1056/nejmoa2034975.
59. Wenzel SE. Eosinophils in asthma—closing the loop or opening the door? N Engl J Med. 2009;360:1026.
60. Pizzichini E, Pizzichini MM, Efthimiadis A, Dolovich J, Hargreave FE. Measuring airway inflammation in asthma: eosinophils and eosinophilic cationic protein in induced sputum compared with peripheral blood. J Allergy Clin Immunol. 1997;99(4):539–44.
61. Green RH, Brightling CE, McKenna S, Hargadon B, Parker D, Bradding P, et al. Asthma exacerbations and sputum eosinophil counts: a randomised controlled trial. Lancet. 2002;360(9347):1715–21.
62. Woodruff PG, Fahy JV. A role for neutrophils in asthma? Am J Med. 2002;112(6):498–500.
63. Hastie AT, Moore WC, Meyers DA, Vestal PL, Li H, Peters SP, et al. Analyses of asthma severity phenotypes and inflammatory proteins in subjects stratified by sputum granulocytes. J Allergy Clin Immunol. 2010;125(5):1028–36.e13.
64. Schleich F, Sophie D, Renaud L. Biomarkers in the management of difficult asthma. Curr Top Med Chem. 2016;16(14):1561–73.
65. Tliba O, Panettieri RA Jr. Paucigranulocytic asthma: uncoupling of airway obstruction from inflammation. J Allergy Clin Immunol. 2019;143(4):1287–94.
66. Moore WC, Meyers DA, Wenzel SE, Teague WG, Li H, Li X, et al. Identification of asthma phenotypes using cluster analysis in the severe asthma research program. Am J Respir Crit Care Med. 2010;181(4):315–23.
67. Silkoff P, Strambu I, Laviolette M, Singh D, FitzGerald J, Lam S, et al. Asthma characteristics and biomarkers from the Airways Disease Endotyping for Personalized Therapeutics (ADEPT) longitudinal profiling study. Respir Res. 2015;16(1):142.

68. Shaw DE, Sousa AR, Fowler SJ, Fleming LJ, Roberts G, Corfield J, et al. Clinical and inflammatory characteristics of the European U-BIOPRED adult severe asthma cohort. Eur Respir J. 2015;46(5):1308–21.
69. Loza MJ, Adcock I, Auffray C, Chung KF, Djukanovic R, Sterk PJ, et al. Longitudinally stable, clinically defined clusters of patients with asthma independently identified in the ADEPT and U-BIOPRED asthma studies. Ann Am Thorac Soc. 2016;13(Supplement 1):S102–S3.
70. Loza MJ, Djukanovic R, Chung KF, Horowitz D, Ma K, Branigan P, et al. Validated and longitudinally stable asthma phenotypes based on cluster analysis of the ADEPT study. Respir Res. 2016;17(1):165.
71. Moore WC, Fitzpatrick AM, Li X, Hastie AT, Li H, Meyers DA, et al. Clinical heterogeneity in the severe asthma research program. Ann Am Thorac Soc. 2013;10 Suppl(Suppl):S118–24.
72. Wu W, Bleecker E, Moore W, Busse WW, Castro M, Chung KF, et al. Unsupervised phenotyping of severe asthma research program participants using expanded lung data. J Allergy Clin Immunol. 2014;133(5):1280–8.
73. Haldar P, Pavord ID, Shaw DE, Berry MA, Thomas M, Brightling CE, et al. Cluster analysis and clinical asthma phenotypes. Am J Respir Crit Care Med. 2008;178(3):218–24.
74. Amelink M, de Groot JC, de Nijs SB, Lutter R, Zwinderman AH, Sterk PJ, et al. Severe adult-onset asthma: a distinct phenotype. J Allergy Clin Immunol. 2013;132(2):336–41.
75. Amelink M, de Nijs SB, Berger M, Weersink EJ, ten Brinke A, Sterk PJ, et al. Non-atopic males with adult onset asthma are at risk of persistent airflow limitation. Clin Exp Allergy. 2012;42(5):769–74.
76. De Marco R, Locatelli F, Cerveri I, Bugiani M, Marinoni A, Giammanco G, et al. Incidence and remission of asthma: a retrospective study on the natural history of asthma in Italy. J Allergy Clin Immunol. 2002;110(2):228–35.
77. Laidlaw TM, Cahill KN. Current knowledge and management of hypersensitivity to aspirin and NSAIDs. J Allergy Clin Immunol Pract. 2017;5(3):537–45.
78. Carr TF, Kraft M. Management of severe asthma before referral to the severe asthma specialist. J Allergy Clin Immunol Pract. 2017;5(4):877–86.
79. Kim JE, Kountakis SE. The prevalence of Samter's triad in patients undergoing functional endoscopic sinus surgery. Ear Nose Throat J. 2007;86(7):396–9.
80. Nelson RK, Bush A, Stokes J, Nair P, Akuthota P. Eosinophilic asthma. J Allergy Clin Immunol Pract. 2020;8(2):465–73.
81. Tarlo SM, Lemiere C. Occupational asthma. N Engl J Med. 2014;370(7):640–9.
82. Ameille J, Hamelin K, Andujar P, Bensefa-Colas L, Bonneterre V, Dupas D, et al. Occupational asthma and occupational rhinitis: the united airways disease model revisited. Occup Environ Med. 2013;70(7):471–5.
83. Sideleva O, Black K, Dixon AE. Effects of obesity and weight loss on airway physiology and inflammation in asthma. Pulm Pharmacol Ther. 2013;26(4):455–8.
84. Amelink M, de Nijs SB, de Groot JC, van Tilburg PM, van Spiegel PI, Krouwels FH, et al. Three phenotypes of adult-onset asthma. Allergy. 2013;68(5):674–80.
85. Beuther DA, Sutherland ER. Overweight, obesity, and incident asthma: a meta-analysis of prospective epidemiologic studies. Am J Respir Crit Care Med. 2007;175(7):661–6.
86. Granell R, Henderson AJ, Evans DM, Smith GD, Ness AR, Lewis S, et al. Effects of BMI, fat mass, and lean mass on asthma in childhood: a Mendelian randomization study. PLoS Med. 2014;11(7):e1001669.
87. Van Veen I, Ten Brinke A, Sterk P, Rabe K, Bel E. Airway inflammation in obese and nonobese patients with difficult-to-treat asthma. Allergy. 2008;63(5):570–4.
88. Mosen DM, Schatz M, Magid DJ, Camargo CA Jr. The relationship between obesity and asthma severity and control in adults. J Allergy Clin Immunol. 2008;122(3):507–11.e6.
89. Thomson NC, Chaudhuri R, Heaney LG, Bucknall C, Niven RM, Brightling CE, et al. Clinical outcomes and inflammatory biomarkers in current smokers and exsmokers with severe asthma. J Allergy Clin Immunol. 2013;131(4):1008–16.
90. Dahms T, Bolin J, Slavin R. Passive smoking: effects on bronchial asthma. Chest. 1981;80(5):530–4.
91. Grol MH, Gerritsen J, Vonk JM, Schouten JP, Koeter GH, Rijcken B, et al. Risk factors for growth and decline of lung function in asthmatic individuals up to age 42 years: a 30-year follow-up study. Am J Respir Crit Care Med. 1999;160(6):1830–7.
92. Lazarus SC, Chinchilli VM, Rollings NJ, Boushey HA, Cherniack R, Craig TJ, et al. Smoking affects response to inhaled corticosteroids or leukotriene receptor antagonists in asthma. Am J Respir Crit Care Med. 2007;175(8):783–90.
93. Spears M, Cameron E, Chaudhuri R, Thomson NC. Challenges of treating asthma in people who smoke. Expert Rev Clin Immunol. 2010;6(2):257–68.
94. Westerhof GA, Vollema EM, Weersink EJ, Reinartz SM, de Nijs SB, Bel EH. Predictors for the development of progressive severity in new-onset adult asthma. J Allergy Clin Immunol. 2014;134(5):1051–6.e2.
95. Polosa R, Russo C, Caponnetto P, Bertino G, Sarvà M, Antic T, et al. Greater severity of new onset asthma in allergic subjects who smoke: a 10-year longitudinal study. Respir Res. 2011;12(1):16.
96. Polosa R, Knoke JD, Russo C, Piccillo G, Caponnetto P, Sarvà M, et al. Cigarette smoking is associated with a greater risk of incident asthma in allergic rhinitis. J Allergy Clin Immunol. 2008;121(6):1428–34.
97. Neuman Å, Hohmann C, Orsini N, Pershagen G, Eller E, Kjaer HF, et al. Maternal smoking in pregnancy and asthma in preschool children: a pooled

analysis of eight birth cohorts. Am J Respir Crit Care Med. 2012;186(10):1037–43.
98. Viegas S, Faísca VM, Dias H, Clérigo A, Carolino E, Viegas C. Occupational exposure to poultry dust and effects on the respiratory system in workers. J Toxic Environ Health A. 2013;76(4–5):230–9.
99. Bérubé D, Cartier A, L'Archevêque J, Ghezzo H, Malo J-L. Comparison of peak expiratory flow rate and FEV1 in assessing bronchomotor tone after challenges with occupational sensitizers. Chest. 1991;99(4):831–6.
100. Redlich CA, Tarlo SM, Hankinson JL, Townsend MC, Eschenbacher WL, Von Essen SG, et al. Official American Thoracic Society technical standards: spirometry in the occupational setting. Am J Respir Crit Care Med. 2014;189(8):983–93.
101. Moore WC, Hastie AT, Li X, Li H, Busse WW, Jarjour NN, et al. Sputum neutrophil counts are associated with more severe asthma phenotypes using cluster analysis. J Allergy Clin Immunol. 2014;133(6):1557–63.e5.
102. Brooks CR, van Dalen CJ, Zacharasiewicz A, Simpson JL, Harper JL, Le Gros G, et al. Absence of airway inflammation in a large proportion of adolescents with asthma. Respirology. 2016;21(3):460–6.
103. Ntontsi P, Loukides S, Bakakos P, Kostikas K, Papatheodorou G, Papathanassiou E, et al. Clinical, functional and inflammatory characteristics in patients with paucigranulocytic stable asthma: comparison with different sputum phenotypes. Allergy. 2017;72(11):1761–7.
104. Thomas RA, Green RH, Brightling CE, Birring SS, Parker D, Wardlaw AJ, et al. The influence of age on induced sputum differential cell counts in normal subjects. Chest. 2004;126(6):1811–4.
105. McGrath KW, Icitovic N, Boushey HA, Lazarus SC, Sutherland ER, Chinchilli VM, et al. A large subgroup of mild-to-moderate asthma is persistently noneosinophilic. Am J Respir Crit Care Med. 2012;185(6):612–9.
106. Little SA, MacLeod KJ, Chalmers GW, Love JG, McSharry C, Thomson NC. Association of forced expiratory volume with disease duration and sputum neutrophils in chronic asthma. Am J Med. 2002;112(6):446–52.
107. Hekking P-PW, Bel EH. Developing and Emerging clinical asthma phenotypes. J Allergy Clin Immunol Pract. 2014;2(6):671–80.
108. Wenzel SE. Asthma: defining of the persistent adult phenotypes. Lancet. 2006;368(9537):804–13.
109. Wenzel SE. Asthma phenotypes: the evolution from clinical to molecular approaches. Nat Med. 2012;18(5):716.
110. Breathe 16(2):200058. https://doi.org/10.1183/20734735.0058-2020.
111. Schleich FN, Seidel L, Sele J, Manise M, Quaedvlieg V, Michils A, et al. Exhaled nitric oxide thresholds associated with a sputum eosinophil count≥ 3% in a cohort of unselected patients with asthma. Thorax. 2010;65(12):1039–44.
112. Berry M, Shaw D, Green R, Brightling C, Wardlaw A, Pavord I. The use of exhaled nitric oxide concentration to identify eosinophilic airway inflammation: an observational study in adults with asthma. Clin Exp Allergy. 2005;35(9):1175–9.
113. Corren J, Lemanske RF Jr, Hanania NA, Korenblat PE, Parsey MV, Arron JR, et al. Lebrikizumab treatment in adults with asthma. N Engl J Med. 2011;365(12):1088–98.
114. Smith AD, Cowan JO, Brassett KP, Herbison GP, Taylor DR. Use of exhaled nitric oxide measurements to guide treatment in chronic asthma. N Engl J Med. 2005;352(21):2163–73.
115. Silkoff PE, Lent AM, Busacker AA, Katial RK, Balzar S, Strand M, et al. Exhaled nitric oxide identifies the persistent eosinophilic phenotype in severe refractory asthma. J Allergy Clin Immunol. 2005;116(6):1249–55.
116. Simpson JL, Scott R, Boyle MJ, Gibson PG. Inflammatory subtypes in asthma: assessment and identification using induced sputum. Respirology. 2006;11(1):54–61.
117. Jia G, Erickson RW, Choy DF, Mosesova S, Wu LC, Solberg OD, et al. Periostin is a systemic biomarker of eosinophilic airway inflammation in asthmatic patients. J Allergy Clin Immunol. 2012;130(3):647–54.e10.
118. Yates DH, Krishnan A, Chow S, Thomas PS. Non-invasive assessment of exhaled biomarkers in lung transplantation. J Breath Res. 2011;5(2):024001.
119. Postma DS, Bleecker ER, Amelung PJ, Holroyd KJ, Xu J, Panhuysen CI, et al. Genetic susceptibility to asthma—bronchial hyperresponsiveness coinherited with a major gene for atopy. N Engl J Med. 1995;333(14):894–900.
120. Oettgen HC, Geha RS. IgE regulation and roles in asthma pathogenesis. J Allergy Clin Immunol. 2001;107(3):429–41.
121. Howarth PH, Durham SR, Kay AB, Holgate ST. The relationship between mast cell-mediator release and bronchial reactivity in allergic asthma. J Allergy Clin Immunol. 1987;80(5):703–11.
122. Wenzel SE, Schwartz LB, Langmack EL, Halliday JL, Trudeau JB, Gibbs RL, et al. Evidence that severe asthma can be divided pathologically into two inflammatory subtypes with distinct physiologic and clinical characteristics. Am J Respir Crit Care Med. 1999;160(3):1001–8.
123. Hargreave FE. Quantitative sputum cell counts as a marker of airway inflammation in clinical practice. Curr Opin Allergy Clin Immunol. 2007;7(1):102–6.
124. Zhang XY, Simpson JL, Powell H, Yang IA, Upham JW, Reynolds PN, et al. Full blood count parameters for the detection of asthma inflammatory phenotypes. Clin Exp Allergy. 2014;44(9):1137–45.
125. Belda J, Leigh R, Parameswaran K, O'Byrne PM, Sears MR, Hargreave FE. Induced sputum cell counts in healthy adults. Am J Respir Crit Care Med. 2000;161(2):475–8.
126. Spanevello A, Confalonieri M, Sulotto F, Romano F, Balzano G, Migliori GB, et al. Induced spu-

tum cellularity: reference values and distribution in normal volunteers. Am J Respir Crit Care Med. 2000;162(3):1172–4.
127. Nair P, Pizzichini MM, Kjarsgaard M, Inman MD, Efthimiadis A, Pizzichini E, et al. Mepolizumab for prednisone-dependent asthma with sputum eosinophilia. N Engl J Med. 2009;360(10):985–93.
128. ten Brinke A, Zwinderman AH, Sterk PJ, Rabe KF, Bel EH. Factors associated with persistent airflow limitation in severe asthma. Am J Respir Crit Care Med. 2001;164(5):744–8.
129. Wagener AH, de Nijs SB, Lutter R, Sousa AR, Weersink EJ, Bel EH, et al. External validation of blood eosinophils, FENO and serum periostin as surrogates for sputum eosinophils in asthma. Thorax. 2015;70(2):115–20.
130. Katz LE, Gleich GJ, Hartley BF, Yancey SW, Ortega HG. Blood eosinophil count is a useful biomarker to identify patients with severe eosinophilic asthma. Ann Am Thorac Soc. 2014;11(4):531–6.
131. Jackson DJ, Wechsler ME, Jackson DJ, Bernstein D, Korn S, Pfeffer PE, Chen R, Saito J, de Luiz Martinez G, Dymek L, et al. Twice-yearly depemokimab in severe asthma with an eosinophilic phenotype. N. Engl. J. Med. 2024;391:2337–2349. https://doi.org/10.1056/NEJMoa2406673.
132. Seluk L, Davis AE, Rhoads S, Wechsler ME. Novel asthma treatments: Advancing beyond approved novel step-up therapies for asthma. Ann. Allergy Asthma Immunol. 2025;134:9–18. https://doi.org/10.1016/j.anai.2024.09.016
133. Rabe KF, Martinez FJ, Bhatt SP, Kawayama T, Cosio BG, Mroz RM, Boomsma MM, Goulaouic H, Nivens MC, Djandji M, et al. Aerify-1/2: Two phase 3, randomised, controlled trials of itepekimab in former smokers with moderate-to-severe copd. ERJ Open Res. 2024;10:00718–2023. https://doi.org/10.1183/23120541.00718-2023.
134. Corren J. Frontier-3: A randomized, phase 2a study to evaluate the efficacy and safety of tozorakimab (an anti-interleukin-33 monoclonal antibody) in early-onset asthma. Thorax. 2024 https://doi.org/10.1136/thorax-2024-BTSabstracts.96.
135. Kelsen SG, Agache IO, Soong W, Israel E, Chupp GL, Cheung DS, Theess W, Yang X, Staton TL, Choy DF, et al. Astegolimab (anti-st2) efficacy and safety in adults with severe asthma: A randomized clinical trial. J. Allergy Clin. Immunol. 2021;148:790–798. https://doi.org/10.1016/j.jaci.2021.03.044.

Part VI

Allergy and Related Conditions

Edited by Sarah K. Wise

Allergy and Sleep

27

Andrea F. Lewis and Brandon Shepherd

Introduction

The symptoms of allergic rhinitis (AR) greatly impact the quality of life for those who suffer from this inflammatory disease. AR can lead to significant fatigue and irritability which negatively affects school and work performance. Symptoms of nasal congestion and poor sleep quality are related to the decreased quality of life scores seen in the disease-specific quality of life tools, such as the Rhinoconjunctivitis Quality of Life Questionnaire. Sleep is one of the seven functional domains evaluated in this quality of life questionnaire [1]. The Allergic Rhinitis and its Impact on Asthma (ARIA) guidelines also use sleep disturbance as one of the troublesome symptoms to differentiate mild AR from moderate-severe AR as it is a debilitating problem for these patients [2] (Fig. 27.1).

In 2008, Craig et al. published a survey of 2355 patients showing that sleep impairment is very common in patients with AR, chronic rhinosinusitis (CRS), and nasal polyposis (NP) [3]. This study also showed that sleep disturbances have a significant negative impact on these patients' quality of life. The sleep symptoms correlated with the allergy season [3]. More recent studies have also shown the degree of sleep impairment to correlate to severity of allergic disease, which has also been associated with anxiety and depression [4].

Sleep disorders are very common in the general population. Insomnia affects up to 30% of adults [5]. Moderate hypersomnia, or the occurrence of episodes of sleepiness during daily life, affects 15% to 20% of people [6]. Estimates of obstructive sleep apnea (OSA) prevalence range from 9% to 38% with dramatic increases in prevalence in older populations [7]. With a nearly 20% estimated prevalence of atopic disease in the United States, there is opportunity for considerable overlap and comorbid disease burden of these chronic conditions [8]. This chapter reviews the relevant pathophysiology, diagnosis, and management of allergic disease as it relates to sleep.

A. F. Lewis (✉)
Department of Otolaryngology and Communicative Sciences, University of Mississippi Medical Center, Jackson, MS, USA
e-mail: aflewis@umc.edu; bashepherd@umc.edu

B. Shepherd
Mid-South Ear, Nose, Throat P.C., Jackson, MS, USA
e-mail: bshepherd@midsouthent.com

C. Damask et al. (eds.), *Allergy in Otolaryngology Practice*,
https://doi.org/10.1007/978-3-031-93455-1_27

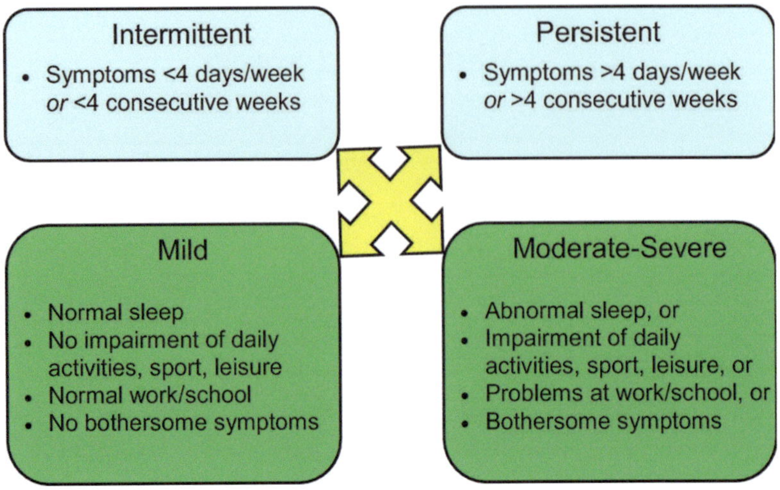

Fig. 27.1 ARIA guidelines for defining asthma severity. (Adapted from Bousquet [2])

Background: Sleep and Sleep-Disordered Breathing

Sleep is a reversible physiologic process involving a complex interplay of hormonal and neurophysiologic pathways between the central nervous system and multiple organ systems with benefits in neurocognitive functioning and overall health. These complex processes are also responsible for the division of sleep into many different stages which can be determined from signals on diagnostic tests such as the polysomnogram (PSG). Broadly, there is Rapid Eye Movement (REM) and non-REM (NREM) sleep. NREM sleep is further divided into three stages. Stages 1 and 2 are considered light stages of sleep with stage 3 sleep constituting deep restorative sleep. REM sleep is known for being particularly important as an almost complete paralysis of the body occurs during this stage, causing one to be particularly vulnerable to certain sleep disorders. REM sleep is also considered to be the period of restorative sleep when memory consolidation occurs. Various mechanisms exist by which this delicate framework can be disturbed.

One such disorder that can disrupt sleep is sleep-disordered breathing. Sleep-disordered breathing is a term which is used to describe a variety of obstructive respiratory-related events that can disrupt sleep, contributing to dysfunction in sleep-related quality of life. OSA occurs when repeated collapse of the airway leads to cessation of airflow and is considered the second most prevalent sleep disorder after insomnia.

OSA severity is described by the apnea-hypopnea index (AHI) which is the sum of apneas and hypopneas per hour. An apnea is defined by a cessation of airflow for at least 10 s. A hypopnea is defined by at least 30% reduction in the signal excursion that lasts at least 10 s. In order to be defined as a hypopnea, the event must also be associated with oxygen desaturation of 4% or greater, or a 3% or greater desaturation if the event is associated with an arousal. In children, no sleep-related respiratory events are expected, and thus an AHI of 1–5 is considered mild sleep apnea, 5–10 is considered moderate sleep apnea, and 10 or more is considered severe sleep apnea. In adults, an AHI of 5–15 is considered mild, 15–30 is considered moderate, and greater than 30 is considered severe sleep apnea [9]. The poor sleep quality seen in OSA exerts effects on various performance indices including reduced executive function.

Mechanism of obstruction in sleep apnea, as well as clinical presentation of OSA, vary among patients. The nose is rarely the sole site of obstruction but plays a significant role. The Starling Resistor model is widely used to describe the biomechanics of OSA with the nose regarded as a fixed inlet of air which can affect intraluminal pressures of the upper airway as a whole based on resistance [10]. Higher resistance to flow would thus lead to greater intraluminal pressures and collapse of the dynamic portion of the airway, predominantly involving the structures of the oropharynx—the palate, tongue base, lateral walls, and epiglottis. The pressure at which these structures collapse has been termed the critical pressure or P_{crit}. This pressure is unique to a patient based on anatomy, sleep position, neuromuscular tone, and other factors. Nasal resistance has been widely studied in OSA and sleep quality.

Pathophysiology of Allergic Rhinitis and Sleep Disturbance

There is a known association between AR and sleep-disordered breathing. Nasal congestion is frequently implicated in the pathogenesis of this association and is thought to be the main AR symptom causing sleep problems in rhinitis patients. In 1997, Young et al. did surveys and PSGs on over 900 people, demonstrating that those who reported nasal congestion due to allergy were 1.8 times more likely to have moderate to severe sleep-disordered breathing than were those without allergy-related nasal congestion [11]. Experimental induction of nasal obstruction in normal individuals has demonstrated disturbances on PSG including sleep fragmentation, increased apneas, and greater arousal index—corroborating the evidence that the nose is a significant contributor to sleep-disordered breathing and sleep disruption [12, 13]. In the Starling Resistor model for OSA, a collapsible tube (the pharynx) is mounted between a rigid upstream segment (the nasal cavity) and a rigid downstream segment (the trachea). This model shows how nasal congestion leads to increased upstream resistance contributing to obstruction of the airway. This also helps explain why approximately 15% of children have been shown to be at risk for persistent sleep-disordered breathing symptoms following adenoidectomy. In 81% of these cases, it is attributed to nasal pathologies [14]. Use of nasal steroids can significantly improve the symptoms in these patients, likely due to the adequate treatment of underlying nasal pathology [15].

There are many primary and secondary factors which promote sleep-related symptoms in atopic individuals with nasal congestion. Patients with OSA and AR with nasal congestion are more likely to snore, have excessive daytime somnolence, have chronic non-restorative sleep, and decreased quality of life scores compared to patients with OSA without nasal symptoms [16]. In addition to direct obstruction of nasal airflow, there are secondary effects of nasal congestion which may affect sleep quality. The increased nasal resistance elevates both respiratory and arousal events resulting in sleep fragmentation. Nasal receptors also appear to play a role in breathing as a whole. Higher minute ventilation, flow rate, and upper airway muscle tone are associated with effective nasal breathing [17–20]. Nasal congestion preferentially selects for mouth-breathing which promotes sleep-disordered breathing in patients regardless of OSA status by increasing upper airway collapsibility [21, 22]. Finally, the inflammatory cascade of allergic disease causes direct and indirect dysregulation of sleep, the details of which we will discuss in the following section.

Immune Mediators in Allergy and Sleep: Association with Circadian Rhythm

Aside from the proinflammatory effects of atopic disease and sleep disruption mediated through airway resistance and patient discomfort, systemic immunologic consequences appear to be implicated as well. Krouse et al. identified that inflammatory mediators in atopic patients (IL-1b, IL-4, and IL-10) are associated with decreased sleep latency (which suggests increased sleepiness), decreased REM latency, and shorter REM sleep periods [23, 24] (Table 27.1). This disruption in REM sleep can lead to difficulty with daytime functioning.

Conversely, quality of sleep is also implicated in promotion of atopy. Slow wave sleep and its

Table 27.1 Mediators generated in allergic rhinitis and associated with sleep changes

Mediator	Effect on sleep	Effect on nasal airway obstruction
Histamine	Involved in balance between wakefulness and slow-wave activity during sleep through H_1 receptors in the brain	Slight ↑
CysLT	↑ Slow-wave sleep	↑
IL-1	Effects probably mediated in part through ↑ PGD_2;↑ non-REM sleep; associated with ↓ latency to sleep onset; ↑ latency to REM and ↓ REM duration	
IL-4	Associated with ↓ latency to sleep onset; ↑ latency to REM and ↓ REM duration	
IL-10	Associated with ↓ latency to sleep onset; ↑ latency to REM and ↓ REM duration	
TNF-α	Probably mediated through ↑ PGD_2	
PGD_2	↑ REM, ↑ non-REM	↑
Bradykinin		↑
Substance P	↑ latency to REM, arousing effect	↑

From Ferguson [24] with permission
↑ Increase, ↓ decreased, *CysLT* cysteinyl leukotriene, *IL* interleukin, *TNF* tumor necrosis factor, *PGD_2* prostaglandin D_2, *REM* rapid eye movement

circadian, hormonal effectors play a role in immunological memory [25]. This phenomenon is well documented in the immunology literature and is considered part of consolidation or cellular-mediated memory formation. Aldosterone, growth hormone, and prolactin all have circadian releases which tend toward promotion of anti-inflammatory cytokines such as IL-12 [26]. High-quality slow wave sleep is, thus, thought to exert an inhibitory effect on the pro-inflammatory milieu by promoting Th1 differentiation of naïve CD4+ T cells. Thus, the anti-inflammatory effects of these hormones and cytokines can be adversely affected by poor sleep quality.

Subjectively, AR patients report diurnal exacerbation of nasal symptoms which coincide with nighttime sleep onset and awakening in the morning [27, 28] (Fig. 27.2). There is an increase in nasal reactivity in the morning hours—peaking at around 6 AM, underscored by a nighttime increase in circulating and mucosal inflammatory cells and cytokines which drive the timing and severity of these symptoms [29]. The increased nasal congestion in the early morning hours may further lead to an increased REM respiratory disturbance index (RDI) regardless of the overall AHI [30]. Further, circadian hormonal changes which also work against the atopic patient are managing nighttime symptoms including increased cholinergic and decreased corticosteroid and epinephrine tone [31]. Nasal congestion may be particularly susceptible to the effects of these hormonal changes.

Obstructive sleep apnea is also a known pro-inflammatory state. Fragmented sleep leads to poor circadian hormonal function and a shift toward the pro-inflammatory state. The adipokines, such as leptin, are elevated in OSA and have been identified as contributors to the inflammatory state and may concurrently worsen allergen-induced inflammation [32]. Thus, some of the morbidity of atopic diseases, such as asthma and AR, may be related to OSA. Treatment of OSA with CPAP has been shown to decrease the pro-inflammatory milieu and may be an important adjunctive treatment modality in some atopic patients [33].

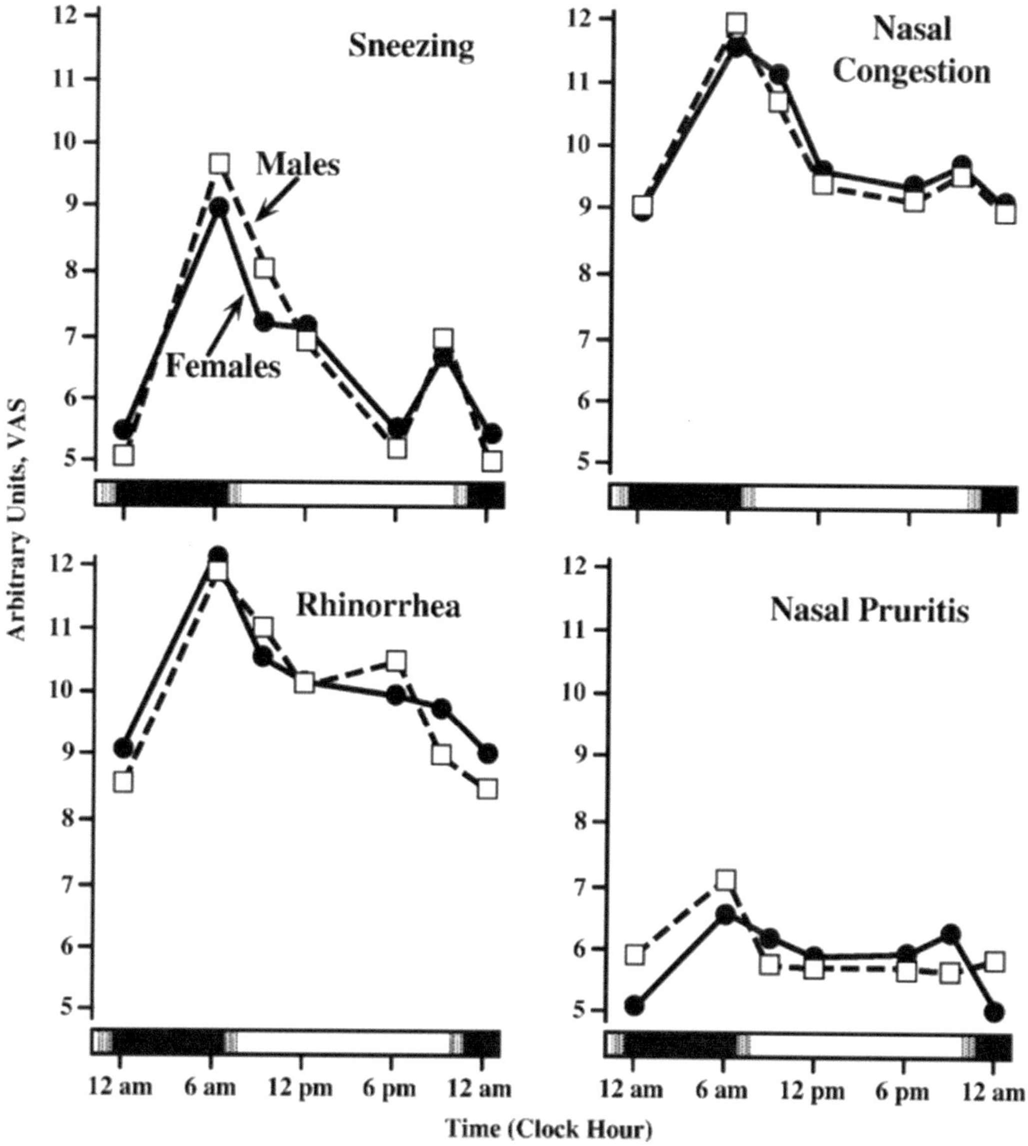

Fig. 27.2 Diurnal variation in AR symptoms—sneezing and nasal congestion, and rhinorrhea (runny nose), and pruritis (itchy nose) showing symptoms were greatest in the early morning. (From Smolensky et al. [77] with permission)

Perennial Versus Seasonal Allergy and Impact on Sleep

The pathophysiologic mechanisms of allergy symptoms predispose patients to also have worsened sleep quality and symptoms during seasonal exposure. Nasal congestion, nasal itching, rhinorrhea, sneezing, headache, and cough have been implicated in allergic symptoms which most frequently affect sleep [34]. McNichols et al. evaluated the effect of allergy on PSGs during and after ragweed exacerbation in seven patients and found that during the ragweed season, patients had longer and more frequent obstructive apneas in addition to an increase in nasal resistance [35]. Perennial allergy sufferers are thus expected to have concomitant sleep-related complaints. Several studies have associated perennial allergy with poor sleep, sleep-related quality of life, and productivity measures [34, 36]. One survey found that 68% of perennial allergy sufferers complained of sleep-related problems due to their allergy, compared with 48% of seasonal allergy sufferers [37]. The chronicity of perennial allergy can lead to a greater cumulative sleep deficit and predispose these patients to sleep-related complaints. Additionally, perennial allergens are more difficult to avoid, often being inhalational allergens within the home such as dust mites, molds, insects, and animal dander [2].

The Impact of Other Atopic Diseases on Sleep

Similar to AR, sleep disturbance is one of the associated symptoms of atopic dermatitis (AD) and is present in 47–80% of children and 33–87.1% of adults with AD [38]. Limited studies have been performed on AD and OSA; however, those which do exist have found poorer sleep efficiency and increased sleep disruption than controls [39–41]. The effects of pruritis and OSA have synergistic negative effects on sleep quality and quality of life, with pruritis negatively affecting sleep and poor sleep leading to pro-inflammatory cytokines. Circadian melatonin rhythm is dysregulated in AD patients and has been associated with the effects on sleep efficiency and sleep fragmentation [41, 42].

Sleep disturbance, including poor sleep quality, reduced sleep time, and changes in sleep architecture, is common in asthma and has been added to many asthma control questionnaires due to its importance [43–45]. Additionally, there is increased prevalence of OSA in asthmatics, along with worse clinical outcome, compared to controls [46]. Prevalence of OSA in severe asthma has been reported around 50% [47]. This is not surprising, given that some of the shared comorbidities of these two disease processes including obesity, inflammation, obstruction, and gastroesophageal reflux. When seen in combination, these effects are likely potentiated, leading to worse outcomes. This highlights the importance of appropriate suspicion for OSA and adequate treatment of both OSA and asthma to aid in adequate management of both disease processes. CPAP therapy has been shown to improve asthma-specific quality of life in this patient population [48]. Insomnia is also a known comorbid condition in asthmatics and may have independent adverse effects on asthma control [49].

Medical and Surgical Treatment of Allergy and its Impact on Sleep

Treatment of AR is most often aimed at adequate symptom control. One symptom which is often overlooked is sleep dysfunction and sleep-disordered breathing. CPAP is the first-line therapy for moderate and severe obstructive sleep apnea syndrome and has significant quality of life implications both in reduction of significant cardiovascular morbidity and improvement in sleep quality and daytime somnolence. However there is also morbidity from CPAP use, including nasal symptomatology, which may lead to poor compliance. Nasal symptoms such as rhinorrhea, nasal congestion, mucosal dryness, and nasal obstruction are present in as many as 15–45% of patients treated with CPAP [50]. These symptoms may have increased morbidity in patients with AR who use CPAP compared to those without [51]. Various conservative measures to reduce these adverse nasal effects of CPAP are routinely administered including nasal moisturization, humidification, changes in mask configuration, pressure ramps, routine education, and rigorous machine cleaning. These measures may improve the discomfort of use but likely represent a small contribution to overall compliance [52]. Despite the significant health-related improvements from CPAP use, there is a high rate of nonadherence with nearly 50% discontinuing use within the first 1–3 months [53] and an overall published rate of compliance of 40–85% [54, 55]. Nasal symptoms have been associated with as many as 42% of these dropouts [56].

Various medical, pharmacologic, psychiatric, and lifestyle factors have been found to impact sleep quality. In the following, we will review the mainstays of medical and surgical management of AR with particular attention to how they can improve sleep quality and CPAP compliance.

Topical Medications

Topical nasal medications represent the workhorse of nasal symptom treatment in AR. Inhaled nasal corticosteroids (INCS) are effective at reducing nasal symptom scores and improving quality of life and are superior to oral medications for symptom control [57]. There is also evidence that INCS use improves asthma control in patients with and without concurrent AR [58]. For this reason, INCS are widely used as first-line therapy for control of atopic disease.

INCS may improve quality of sleep as well as reduce disease severity in patients with OSA. As previously discussed, nasal symptoms are a significant factor related to poor CPAP compliance and INCS are used routinely to treat these symptoms. Additionally, AR may contribute to the development and severity of OSA in select patients. Various studies have evaluated the efficacy of INCS in OSA patients. In an unselected population of patients treated with INCS, there was no improvement in sleep measures or CPAP compliance at short term follow-up [59]. However, when comparing patients with OSA and AR to OSA without AR, INCS were able to improve sleep quality, Epworth Sleepiness Scale (ESS), and objective measures such as AHI, nasal airway resistance, and O2 saturation [60, 61]. These effects may be further potentiated with the addition of an antihistamine [62]. The fact remains that evidence in favor of INCS use for all patients with OSA on CPAP is lacking; however, for adults with concurrent AR, many will demonstrate improvement in sleep quality and objective sleep measures in addition to the improvement in nasal symptoms related to AR.

In children with OSA and AR, adenoidectomy or adenotonsillectomy has traditionally been pursued with excellent control of OSA in most cases. However, for those who wish to avoid or delay surgery, INCS reduces nasal symptoms, improves quality of life, shrinks adenoid tissue, and avoids the need for surgery in some cases [63, 64]. The long-term outcomes of such treatment are yet to be fully elucidated but INCS may be a safe and effective option.

Nasal decongestants are a routine rescue medication among those with nasal congestion or obstruction symptoms, owing to the powerful vasoconstriction of the nasal mucosa venous sinusoids and near immediate improvement of nasal airflow. However, medication overuse and rhinitis medicamentosa can become a problem in nasal symptoms sufferers including those with AR and nasal symptoms of OSA. Thus, routine education of these patients regarding the risks of daily nasal decongestant use is prudent. Fortunately, several studies have demonstrated that concurrent use of INCS with nasal decongestants can inhibit tachyphylaxis associated with frequent nasal decongestant use and reduce the incidence of rhinitis medicamentosa [65]. This is particularly helpful for the population of patients who suffer from both OSA and AR who, in addition to the benefits of INCS use, may have improvements in sleep architecture, AHI, and oxygen saturations with the use of nightly nasal decongestants [66]. This highlights the importance of nasal patency as both a risk factor and target for OSA treatment. Of note, patient selection is important as those without nasal obstruction symptoms are unlikely to benefit and, conversely, those who benefit may tolerate the reduced symptomatology yet still suffer from OSA and its deleterious health effects if nasal patency alone cannot provide cure.

Oral Medications

Systemic medications such as oral antihistamines, leukotriene receptor antagonists, and decongestants are routinely used in the treatment of AR and asthma. Although topical medications are more effective for symptom reduction, oral medications can be useful adjuncts for additional control or symptomatology. Additionally, access is widespread and patients will frequently attempt to treat their AR and insomnia symptoms with these medications without clinical instructions to do so.

The use of antihistamines has not been well studied with regard to improvement of sleep quality and CPAP compliance. This is likely due to sleep-related consequences that exist with these medications. Although they may assist with sleep onset, treatment of insomnia, and sleep quality in some, these symptoms are simply traded for daytime somnolence and negative effects on mood which have deleterious effects on quality of life [67]. These effects were originally thought to be present only in first-generation anti-histamines which cross the blood-brain barrier, but such effects are also present with the newer generation of medications. In clinical practice, balancing this class of medications can be challenging in patients with comorbid sleep-disordered breathing. There is a high ease of access of these medications to patients over the counter and many utilize them for their effectiveness as a sleep aid, unknowingly worsening their sleep quality and daytime sleepiness.

Oral leukotriene receptor antagonists such as montelukast have been widely used in the treatment of AR and asthma. Given the similar inflammatory cytokines in AR and OSA, a medication targeting the downregulation of these cytokines would be promising at improving OSA. In fact, several studies have found leukotriene antagonist therapy to be successful in children, correlating its use with or without INCS to a 55% (montelukast alone) to 70% (montelukast with INCS) reduction of AHI in pediatric patients with mild OSA, including patients who were refractory to adenotonsillectomy [68–71]. In the adult population, there is less evidence in favor of use. In one trial, unselected patients with mild sleep apnea were treated with montelukast plus INCS for 12 weeks and found to have no reduction of AHI despite subjective improvement in symptoms [72]. For those patients with concurrent OSA, asthma, and AR, the addition of montelukast therapy may provide some benefit in quality of life but must be weighed against the risk of the recently incurred a black box warning regarding serious mental health side effects.

Additional Therapies

Other pharmacologic and immunologic therapies exist for the treatment of allergic disease including subcutaneous or sublingual immunotherapy and biologics. To date, no studies have been undertaken to identify the implications of these treatments on sleep indices, although anecdotal evidence would suggest that effectiveness at improvement in nasal symptoms would lead to favorable responses with sleep as well. These treatments remain a mainstay of therapy for routine and refractory atopic disease and likely provide unreported benefit to the patients with comorbid OSA. Further investigation is needed.

As discussed, nasal patency contributes significantly to the disease burden of both OSA and AR. As such, surgical improvement of the nasal passages can be highly effective. Turbinate reduction, septoplasty, and functional septorhinoplasty have been utilized to increase nasal airflow, reduce nasal airway resistance, and reduce nasal obstruction in patients with both AR and OSA. Thus, there is opportunity for improvement of each disease process. However, OSA phenotype may affect outcome. The understanding of various phenotypes and endotypes in OSA pathophysiology is a burgeoning field, especially in the selection and response of various surgeries for OSA. Lack of delineation of OSA phenotypes and endotypes may have contributed to conflicting reports regarding the effectiveness of nasal surgery on reduction of AHI. In a meta-analysis by Ishii et al. of OSA patients with nasal obstruction undergoing nasal surgery, analysis of the pooled cohort of 320 patients demonstrated improvement in ESS and RDI but no improvement in AHI [73]. A similar study by Li et al. found no difference in AHI reduction in the surgical treatment of nasal obstruction in OSA compared to medical treatment in the main analysis but stratification by Friedman tongue position patients revealed significance in AHI reduction [74]. Additionally, 56% of patients had reduction of OSA disease severity by AHI and subjective improvement in symptoms with the non-responders correlating to unfavorable pharyngeal anatomy [75]. Thus, there are several important implications of these findings. First, as understanding of OSA phenotypes and endotypes evolves, targeted surgical interventions should become more effective for certain subsets of patients. Secondly, there is a robust body of literature demonstrating subjective improvement in sleep-related outcomes, especially in those patients who have concurrent nasal obstruction such as is common in patients with AR. This includes reduction of CPAP pressures [76] and improved CPAP compliance [77]. Finally, the AHI is but one measure of the complex and heterogeneous disease process of obstructive sleep apnea.

Conclusion

The disruption of sleep in patients with AR is multifactorial. The most common and well-known etiology of sleep impairment in AR is sleep-disordered breathing associated with nasal congestion, which is a complex process. Nasal congestion is also a factor in poor sleep quality even when it is not associated with OSA. Other lesser-known factors causing daytime sleepiness in the AR patient include the release of immune mediators which is tied to the circadian rhythm and can lead to decreased sleep efficiency. Medications and surgical treatments have been effective in reducing disease burden and symptoms and improving sleep quality and daytime function. Understanding these treatments and relationships is key to effectively improving the quality of life in patients suffering from AR.

Disclosure Statement The authors have nothing to disclose.

References

1. Juniper EF, Guyatt GH. Development and testing of a new measure of health status for clinical trials in rhinoconjunctivitis. Clin Exp Allergy. 1991;21(1):77–83.
2. Bousquet J, Van Cauwenberge P, Khaltaev N, Aria Workshop G, World Health Organization. Allergic rhinitis and its impact on asthma. J Allergy Clin Immunol. 2001;108(5 Suppl):S147–334.
3. Craig TJ, Ferguson BJ, Krouse JH. Sleep impairment in allergic rhinitis, rhinosinusitis, and nasal polyposis. Am J Otolaryngol. 2008;29(3):209–17.
4. Munoz-Cano R, Ribo P, Araujo G, Giralt E, Sanchez-Lopez J, Valero A. Severity of allergic rhinitis impacts sleep and anxiety: results from a large Spanish cohort. Clin Transl Allergy. 2018;8:23.
5. Leger D, Guilleminault C, Dreyfus JP, Delahaye C, Paillard M. Prevalence of insomnia in a survey of 12,778 adults in France. J Sleep Res. 2000;9(1):35–42.
6. Billiard M. Hypersomnias. In: Sleep: physiology, investigations, and medicine. 1st ed. New York: Springer; 2003. p. 333–6.
7. Senaratna CV, Perret JL, Lodge CJ, Lowe AJ, Campbell BE, Matheson MC, et al. Prevalence of obstructive sleep apnea in the general population: a systematic review. Sleep Med Rev. 2017;34:70–81.
8. National Institute of Allergy and Infectious Diseases. Airborne allergens: something in the air, NIH Publication No. 03–7045. Bethesda: National Institute of Allergy and Infectious Diseases; 2003.
9. Berry RB, Budhiraja R, Gottlieb DJ, Gozal D, Iber C, Kapur VK, et al. Rules for scoring respiratory events in sleep: update of the 2007 AASM manual for the scoring of sleep and associated events. Deliberations of the sleep apnea definitions task force of the American Academy of Sleep Medicine. J Clin Sleep Med. 2012;8(5):597–619.
10. Wellman A, Genta PR, Owens RL, Edwards BA, Sands SA, Loring SH, et al. Test of the Starling resistor model in the human upper airway during sleep. J Appl Physiol (1985). 2014;117(12):1478–85.
11. Young T, Finn L, Kim H. Nasal obstruction as a risk factor for sleep-disordered breathing. The University of Wisconsin Sleep and Respiratory Research Group. J Allergy Clin Immunol. 1997;99(2):S757–62.
12. Carskadon MA, Bearpark HM, Sharkey KM, Millman RP, Rosenberg C, Cavallo A, et al. Effects of menopause and nasal occlusion on breathing during sleep. Am J Respir Crit Care Med. 1997;155(1):205–10.
13. Millman RP, Acebo C, Rosenberg C, Carskadon MA. Sleep, breathing, and cephalometrics in older children and young adults. Part II – response to nasal occlusion. Chest. 1996;109(3):673–9.
14. Joshua B, Bahar G, Sulkes J, Shpitzer T, Raveh E. Adenoidectomy: long-term follow-up. Otolaryngol Head Neck Surg. 2006;135(4):576–80.
15. Yildirim YS, Senturk E, Eren SB, Dogan R, Tugrul S, Ozturan O. Efficacy of nasal corticosteroid in preventing regrowth after adenoidectomy. Auris Nasus Larynx. 2016;43(6):637–40.
16. Varendh M, Andersson M, Bjornsdottir E, Hrubos-Strom H, Johannisson A, Arnardottir ES, et al. Nocturnal nasal obstruction is frequent and reduces sleep quality in patients with obstructive sleep apnea. J Sleep Res. 2018;27(4):e12631.

17. White DP, Cadieux RJ, Lombard RM, Bixler EO, Kales A, Zwillich CW. The effects of nasal anesthesia on breathing during sleep. Am Rev Respir Dis. 1985;132(5):972–5.
18. McNicholas WT, Coffey M, Boyle T. Effects of nasal airflow on breathing during sleep in normal humans. Am Rev Respir Dis. 1993;147(3):620–3.
19. Douglas NJ, White DP, Weil JV, Zwillich CW. Effect of breathing route on ventilation and ventilatory drive. Respir Physiol. 1983;51(2):209–18.
20. Basner RC, Simon PM, Schwartzstein RM, Weinberger SE, Weiss JW. Breathing route influences upper airway muscle activity in awake normal adults. J Appl Physiol (1985). 1989;66(4):1766–71.
21. Wang W, Verin E, Series F. Influences of the breathing route on upper airway dynamics properties in normal awake subjects with constant mouth opening. Clin Sci (Lond). 2006;111(5):349–55.
22. Fitzpatrick MF, McLean H, Urton AM, Tan A, O'Donnell D, Driver HS. Effect of nasal or oral breathing route on upper airway resistance during sleep. Eur Respir J. 2003;22(5):827–32.
23. Krouse HJ, Davis JE, Krouse JH. Immune mediators in allergic rhinitis and sleep. Otolaryngol Head Neck Surg. 2002;126(6):607–13.
24. Ferguson BJ. Influences of allergic rhinitis on sleep. Otolaryngol Head Neck Surg. 2004;130(5):617–29.
25. Lange T, Born J, Westermann J. Sleep matters: CD4(+) T cell memory formation and the central nervous system. Trends Immunol. 2019;40(8):674–86.
26. Lange T, Dimitrov S, Fehm HL, Westermann J, Born J. Shift of monocyte function toward cellular immunity during sleep. Arch Intern Med. 2006;166(16):1695–700.
27. Reinberg A, Gervais P, Levi F, Smolensky M, Delcerro L, Ugolini C. Circadian and circannual rhythms of allergic rhinitis – an epidemiologic-study involving chronobiologic methods. J Allergy Clin Immunol. 1988;81(1):51–62.
28. Smolensky MH, Lemmer B, Reinberg AE. Chronobiology and chronotherapy of allergic rhinitis and bronchial asthma. Adv Drug Deliv Rev. 2007;59(9–10):852–82.
29. Aoyagi M, Watanabe H, Sekine K, Nishimuta T, Konno A, Shimojo N, et al. Circadian variation in nasal reactivity in children with allergic rhinitis: correlation with the activity of eosinophils and basophilic cells. Int Arch Allergy Immunol. 1999;120(Suppl 1):95–9.
30. Berson SR, Klimczak J, Prezio EA, Hu S, Abraham M. Clinical associations between allergies and rapid eye movement sleep disturbances. Int Forum Allergy Rhinol. 2018;8(7):817–24.
31. Greenberg H, Cohen RI. Nocturnal asthma. Curr Opin Pulm Med. 2012;18(1):57–62.
32. Wong CK, Cheung PF, Lam CW. Leptin-mediated cytokine release and migration of eosinophils: implications for immunopathophysiology of allergic inflammation. Eur J Immunol. 2007;37(8):2337–48.
33. Sanner BM, Kollhosser P, Buechner N, Zidek W, Tepel M. Influence of treatment on leptin levels in patients with obstructive sleep apnoea. Eur Respir J. 2004;23(4):601–4.
34. Romano M, James S, Farrington E, Perry R, Elliott L. The impact of perennial allergic rhinitis with/without allergic asthma on sleep, work and activity level. Allergy Asthma Clin Immunol. 2019;15:81.
35. McNicholas WT, Tarlo S, Cole P, Zamel N, Rutherford R, Griffin D, et al. Obstructive apneas during sleep in patients with seasonal allergic rhinitis. Am Rev Respir Dis. 1982;126(4):625–8.
36. Leger D, Bonnefoy B, Pigearias B, de La Giclais B, Chartier A. Poor sleep is highly associated with house dust mite allergic rhinitis in adults and children. Allergy Asthma Clin Immunol. 2017;13:36.
37. Blaiss MRT, Philpot E. A study to determine the impact of rhinitis on sufferers' sleep and daily routine. J Allergy Clin Immunol. 2005;115:S197.
38. Chang YS, Chiang BL. Sleep disorders and atopic dermatitis: a 2-way street? J Allergy Clin Immunol. 2018;142(4):1033–40.
39. Hon KL, Leung TF, Ma KC, Li AM, Wong Y, Yin JA, et al. Resting energy expenditure, oxygen consumption and carbon dioxide production during sleep in children with atopic dermatitis. J Dermatolog Treat. 2005;16(1):22–5.
40. Stores G, Burrows A, Crawford C. Physiological sleep disturbance in children with atopic dermatitis: a case control study. Pediatr Dermatol. 1998;15(4):264–8.
41. Chang YS, Chou YT, Lee JH, Lee PL, Dai YS, Sun C, et al. Atopic dermatitis, melatonin, and sleep disturbance. Pediatrics. 2014;134(2):e397–405.
42. Schwarz W, Birau N, Hornstein OP, Heubeck B, Schonberger A, Meyer C, et al. Alterations of melatonin secretion in atopic eczema. Acta Derm Venereol. 1988;68(3):224–9.
43. Teodorescu M, Consens FB, Bria WF, Coffey MJ, McMorris MS, Weatherwax KJ, et al. Correlates of daytime sleepiness in patients with asthma. Sleep Med. 2006;7(8):607–13.
44. Fitzpatrick MF, Engleman H, Whyte KF, Deary IJ, Shapiro CM, Douglas NJ. Morbidity in nocturnal asthma: sleep quality and daytime cognitive performance. Thorax. 1991;46(8):569–73.
45. Kales A, Beall GN, Bajor GF, Jacobson A, Kales JD. Sleep studies in asthmatic adults: relationship of attacks to sleep stage and time of night. J Allergy. 1968;41(3):164–73.
46. Davies SE, Bishopp A, Wharton S, Turner AM, Mansur AH. The association between asthma and obstructive sleep apnea (OSA): a systematic review. J Asthma. 2019;56(2):118–29.

47. Julien JY, Martin JG, Ernst P, Olivenstein R, Hamid Q, Lemiere C, et al. Prevalence of obstructive sleep apnea-hypopnea in severe versus moderate asthma. J Allergy Clin Immunol. 2009;124(2):371–6.
48. Davies SE, Bishopp A, Wharton S, Turner AM, Mansur AH. Does continuous positive airway pressure (CPAP) treatment of obstructive sleep apnoea (OSA) improve asthma-related clinical outcomes in patients with co-existing conditions? A systematic review. Respir Med. 2018;143:18–30.
49. Luyster FS, Strollo PJ Jr, Holguin F, Castro M, Dunican EM, Fahy J, et al. Association between insomnia and asthma burden in the severe asthma research program (SARP) III. Chest. 2016;150(6):1242–50.
50. Kreivi HR, Virkkula P, Lehto J, Brander P. Frequency of upper airway symptoms before and during continuous positive airway pressure treatment in patients with obstructive sleep apnea syndrome. Respiration. 2010;80(6):488–94.
51. Yang Q, Li H, Wu W, Huang X, Tu B, Ma Y, et al. Effect of continuous positive airway pressure on allergic rhinitis in patients with obstructive sleep apnea-hypopnea syndrome. Ther Clin Risk Manag. 2018;14:1507–13.
52. Ballard RD, Gay PC, Strollo PJ. Interventions to improve compliance in sleep apnea patients previously non-compliant with continuous positive airway pressure. J Clin Sleep Med. 2007;3(7):706–12.
53. Rosen CL, Auckley D, Benca R, Foldvary-Schaefer N, Iber C, Kapur V, et al. A multisite randomized trial of portable sleep studies and positive airway pressure autotitration versus laboratory-based polysomnography for the diagnosis and treatment of obstructive sleep apnea: the HomePAP study. Sleep. 2012;35(6):757–67.
54. Virk JS, Kotecha B. Otorhinolaryngological aspects of sleep-related breathing disorders. J Thorac Dis. 2016;8(2):213–23.
55. Donovan LM, Boeder S, Malhotra A, Patel SR. New developments in the use of positive airway pressure for obstructive sleep apnea. J Thorac Dis. 2015;7(8):1323–42.
56. Brander PE, Soirinsuo M, Lohela P. Nasopharyngeal symptoms in patients with obstructive sleep apnea syndrome. Effect of nasal CPAP treatment. Respiration. 1999;66(2):128–35.
57. Juel-Berg N, Darling P, Bolvig J, Foss-Skiftesvik MH, Halken S, Winther L, et al. Intranasal corticosteroids compared with oral antihistamines in allergic rhinitis: a systematic review and meta-analysis. Am J Rhinol Allergy. 2017;31(1):E19–28.
58. Lohia S, Schlosser RJ, Soler ZM. Impact of intranasal corticosteroids on asthma outcomes in allergic rhinitis: a meta-analysis. Allergy. 2013;68(5):569–79.
59. Charakorn N, Hirunwiwatkul P, Chirakalwasan N, Chaitusaney B, Prakassajjatham M. The effects of topical nasal steroids on continuous positive airway pressure compliance in patients with obstructive sleep apnea: a systematic review and meta-analysis. Sleep Breath. 2017;21(1):3–8.
60. Lavigne F, Petrof BJ, Johnson JR, Lavigne P, Binothman N, Kassissia GO, et al. Effect of topical corticosteroids on allergic airway inflammation and disease severity in obstructive sleep apnoea. Clin Exp Allergy. 2013;43(10):1124–33.
61. Kiely JL, Nolan P, McNicholas WT. Intranasal corticosteroid therapy for obstructive sleep apnoea in patients with co-existing rhinitis. Thorax. 2004;59(1):50–5.
62. Acar M, Cingi C, Sakallioglu O, San T, Fatih Yimenicioglu M, Bal C. The effects of mometasone furoate and desloratadine in obstructive sleep apnea syndrome patients with allergic rhinitis. Am J Rhinol Allergy. 2013;27(4):e113–6.
63. Zhang L, Mendoza-Sassi RA, Cesar JA, Chadha NK. Intranasal corticosteroids for nasal airway obstruction in children with moderate to severe adenoidal hypertrophy. Cochrane Database Syst Rev. 2008;2008(3):CD006286.
64. Sakarya EU, Bayar Muluk N, Sakalar EG, Senturk M, Aricigil M, Bafaqeeh SA, et al. Use of intranasal corticosteroids in adenotonsillar hypertrophy. J Laryngol Otol. 2017;131(5):384–90.
65. Baroody FM, Brown D, Gavanescu L, DeTineo M, Naclerio RM. Oxymetazoline adds to the effectiveness of fluticasone furoate in the treatment of perennial allergic rhinitis. J Allergy Clin Immunol. 2011;127(4):927–34.
66. An Y, Han D. The effects of nasal decongestion on obstructive sleep apnea: a detailed analysis. J Sleep Res. AmJOto. 2018;40:52–56
67. Ozdemir PG, Karadag AS, Selvi Y, Boysan M, Bilgili SG, Aydin A, et al. Assessment of the effects of antihistamine drugs on mood, sleep quality, sleepiness, and dream anxiety. Int J Psychiatry Clin Pract. 2014;18(3):161–8.
68. Tan HL, Gozal D, Kheirandish-Gozal L. Obstructive sleep apnea in children: a critical update. Nat Sci Sleep. 2013;5:109–23.
69. Kheirandish L, Goldbart AD, Gozal D. Intranasal steroids and oral leukotriene modifier therapy in residual sleep-disordered breathing after tonsillectomy and adenoidectomy in children. Pediatrics. 2006;117(1):e61–6.
70. Goldbart AD, Greenberg-Dotan S, Tal A. Montelukast for children with obstructive sleep apnea: a double-blind, placebo-controlled study. Pediatrics. 2012;130(3):e575–80.
71. Liming BJ, Ryan M, Mack D, Ahmad I, Camacho M. Montelukast and nasal corticosteroids to treat pediatric obstructive sleep apnea: a systematic review

and meta-analysis. Otolaryngol Head Neck Surg. 2019;160(4):594–602.
72. Smith DF, Sarber KM, Spiceland CP, Ishman SL, Augelli DM, Romaker AM. Effects of medical therapy on mild obstructive sleep apnea in adult patients. J Clin Sleep Med. 2019;15(7):979–83.
73. Ishii L, Roxbury C, Godoy A, Ishman S, Ishii M. Does nasal surgery improve OSA in patients with nasal obstruction and OSA? A Meta-analysis. Otolaryng Head Neck. 2015;153(3):326–33.
74. Li HY, Lee LA, Wang PC, Fang TJ, Chen NH. Can nasal surgery improve obstructive sleep apnea: subjective or objective? Am J Rhinol Allergy. 2009;23(6):E51–5.
75. Park CY, Hong JH, Lee JH, Lee KE, Cho HS, Lim SJ, et al. Clinical effect of surgical correction for nasal pathology on the treatment of obstructive sleep apnea syndrome. PLoS One. 2014;9(6):e98765.
76. Friedman M, Tanyeri H, Lim JW, Landsberg R, Vaidyanathan K, Caldarelli D. Effect of improved nasal breathing on obstructive sleep apnea. Otolaryng Head Neck. 2000;122(1):71–4.
77. Nakata S, Noda A, Yagi H, Yanagi E, Mimura T, Okada T, et al. Nasal resistance for determinant factor of nasal surgery in CPAP failure patients with obstructive sleep apnea syndrome. Rhinology. 2005;43(4):296–9.

28 Allergy and Ear Disease

Mallory J. Raymond, Matthew Ryan, and Sarah K. Wise

Introduction

Reports linking allergy and otologic conditions appear in the literature as early as the 1920s, with a clinical report of allergy linking Meniere's disease [1]. Over the last century, otologic manifestations of allergy have gained increasing attention with a plethora of work devoted to defining incidence and prevalence, clinical presentations, causal relationships, diagnostic criteria, and treatment algorithms. Otologic investigations have traditionally focused on the ear as three distinct anatomical subsites: the external ear, middle ear, and inner ear. This chapter reviews our current understanding of the link between allergy and pathology of these otologic subsites as well as evidence for causal relationships and current treatment modalities.

M. J. Raymond (✉)
Department of Otolaryngology-Head and Neck Surgery, Mayo Clinic, Jacksonville, FL, USA
e-mail: raymond.mallory@mayo.edu

M. Ryan
Department of Otolaryngology-Head and Neck Surgery, University of Texas Southwestern Medical Center, Dallas, TX, USA
e-mail: matthew.ryan@utsouthwestern.edu

S. K. Wise
Department of Otolaryngology, Emory University, Atlanta, GA, USA
e-mail: skmille@emory.edu

External Ear

Dermatoses

The external ear, like many other cutaneous sites, is susceptible to both irritant and allergic contact dermatoses. Often jointly referred to as eczematous otitis externa, these two entities commonly present with chronic external ear inflammation characterized by pruritis, erythema, and dry and scaling skin of the auricle or external auditory canal. Irritant contact dermatitis may result universally from exposure to noxious stimuli, like strong acids or alkalis, or from repeated exposure to relatively mild noxious stimuli in select susceptible individuals. Irritant dermatitis presents with well-defined lesions corresponding to the sites of exposure.

In contrast to irritant contact dermatitis, allergic contact dermatitis represents a delayed type IV hypersensitivity reaction, often resulting initially in vesicle formation followed by characteristic scaling [2]. Lesions are not necessarily limited to sites of exposure but can present more generalized, and an exposure sensitization phase is required [2]. Ear piercing has been linked with severe contact dermatitis and nickel sensitization in early case reports [3] and several large cohort studies [4, 5]. In the case of nickel allergy, diagnosis is often quite obvious as it presents as a dermatitis at the site of direct contact with a

C. Damask et al. (eds.), *Allergy in Otolaryngology Practice*,
https://doi.org/10.1007/978-3-031-93455-1_28

nickel-containing earring. Similarly, patients have demonstrated sensitivity to otic drop preparations, particularly those containing aminoglycosides, but also other antimicrobial agents and corticosteroids [6–8]. Diagnosis of these patients may remain elusive as they will often present with prolonged (3 months or more) pruritis and edema of the external auditory canal as well as otorrhea, causing the clinician to continue treatment for a suspected infectious otitis externa. Furthermore, patients have demonstrated contact allergy to hearing aid mold components including plastics, rubber, silicone, and most commonly methyl-methacrylate [9]. These patients may also present with external auditory canal pruritis, edema, erythema, otorrhea, and occlusive debris, making use of the hearing aid impossible. This may also be confused with an infectious otitis externa.

Because of the overlap in the presentation of these entities with infectious etiologies of otitis externa, diagnosis relies primarily on a thorough history, though in difficult-to-diagnose cases, allergy testing may be indicated. The gold standard for identification of an offending agent of allergic contact dermatitis is patch testing of any agents the individual has reported exposure to. The patches are applied to the back of the patient and left there for 2–3 days, after which time the site is examined for a reaction. In the case of nickel hypersensitivity, patch testing in patients who report a history of metal dermatitis has a sensitivity of 37% and a positive predictive value of 34.2%. The high specificity (85.2%) and negative predictive value (86.7%) make it reasonable to perform, but only in patients with a history of metal contact dermatitis in order to confirm sensitivity to the offending agent [5]. On the other hand, patch testing with otic drop preparations may reveal an allergy in 40–60% of patients with chronic otitis for greater than 3 months; therefore, it is also recommended to offer these patients testing [7]. Finally, patch testing for patients suspected to have an allergy to hearing aid molds may reveal a sensitivity in 27–56% of cases [9, 10]. Results of the testing must be considered in the context of the patient's history. It may be beneficial for the otolaryngologist to involve a dermatologic specialist in administration and review of patch testing.

The mainstay of treatment is avoidance of the offending allergen and providing single-compound topical steroid creams or ointments until patch testing results are available. Complex preparations should be avoided [9]. In the case of allergy to hearing aid molds, boiling the mold for 30 s, substituting the plastic in the mold for another, or plating the mold with a thin layer of gold may eliminate the problem [11]. In rare cases, patients have developed delayed type IV hypersensitivity reactions to cochlear implant components, resulting in implant extrusion. This requires the manufacturer to alter the coating material of future implants prior to reimplantation [12]. Expected prognosis for resolution of symptoms in all cases described is good once an offending agent has been identified. Allergen desensitization is almost never warranted or recommended because of the ability to avoid offending agents.

Dermatophytid

The external ear is also susceptible to dermatophytid reactions, classically described as noninfectious cutaneous eruptions secondary to allergy developed from a distant site of fungal infection [13]. The most common clinical presentation is that of a diffuse follicular or eczematoid rash over the trunk, extremities, or face, but it has also been reported to occur as a chronic otitis externa [14]. The essential criteria for diagnosis include: a proven dermatophyte infection; a distant cutaneous reaction free of fungal elements; and spontaneous resolution of the distant cutaneous reaction when the primary infection resolves [13]. It has also been suggested that diagnosis be confirmed with a positive allergy skin test of the isolated fungal elements to demonstrate an immediate type I IgE-mediated response [11]. The primary infection may be found in the nails, skin, or vagina and is most commonly due to the fungus, *Trichophyton* [15]. In cases of prolonged and refractory chronic otitis externa, clinicians should consider dermatophytid reaction and evaluate the patient for a distant site of fungal infection.

The treatment relies on the identification and treatment of the primary infection, though for this strategy, there is no data to advise the clinician on expected outcomes for the resolution of the chronic otitis externa. Desensitization with an allergenic extract of the most common fungal culprits (*Trichophyton, Oidiomycetes*, and *Epidermophyton*) has been performed in one study of 14 patients with chronic otitis externa and a suspicion for dermatophytid reaction [14]. In this series, a fungal source was identified in only four patients, but after 6 months of immunotherapy, 78.5% of patients had either symptom improvement or resolution. Though this rate of improvement is promising, the estimated prevalence of dermatophytid reaction is quite low. Clinicians should therefore rule out more common causes of chronic otitis externa prior to performing allergy skin testing, and immunotherapy should be considered only for very prolonged and refractory cases of chronic otitis externa of no known etiology or in patients who demonstrate fungal element sensitivity. The only evidence to date suggests following a six-month treatment course.

Middle Ear

Eustachian Tube Dysfunction

The eustachian tube functions as a corridor between the middle ear and nasopharynx and is in direct continuity with the upper airway. There are three basic functions in relation to the middle ear: pressure regulation, protection, and clearance of fluid or pathogens. Middle ear pressure is equalized with that of atmospheric pressure by active opening of the eustachian tube from contraction of the tensor veli palatini muscle during yawning or swallowing. The eustachian tube passively closes from lateral to medial allowing for middle ear clearance toward the nasopharynx and protection from nasopharyngeal reflux when at rest [16]. A dysfunctional eustachian tube can result from mechanical obstruction or a failure of effective opening secondary to inflamed mucosa or persistent negative pressure-generating habits such as sniffing or swallowing during nasal obstruction. Patients with eustachian tube dysfunction (ETD) may present with subjective complaints of ear fullness or pressure, autophony, otalgia, tinnitus, vertigo, clicking or popping sounds when swallowing, transient hearing loss, or difficulty with altitude change. ETD is typically diagnosed by clinical history of symptoms, but other findings may include the presence of a middle ear effusion, tympanic membrane retraction or perforation, cholesteatoma, or tympanometry indicating flat or negative middle ear pressure curves. It is important to note that an abnormal tympanogram is not a prerequisite for diagnosis of ETD, and many patients with ETD will have normal tympanograms.

A number of observations have been made linking ETD to allergic conditions, such as chronic rhinosinusitis [17, 18], allergic rhinitis [19, 20], and aspirin-exacerbated respiratory disease [21]. Theoretical causal mechanisms explaining this link include: (1) allergy-induced inflammation of the torus tubaris or eustachian tube mucosa, (2) allergy-induced nasal obstruction, or (3) reflux of allergic nasopharyngeal secretions into the eustachian tube. Studies focusing on the first theory utilized the 9-step inflation-deflation swallow test of eustachian tube function developed by Bluestone and Cantekin to establish this causal relationship [22]. Eustachian tube obstruction has since been demonstrated after intranasal challenge to pollen, histamine, and dust mite [23–25]. Studies relying on tympanometry suggest that nasal allergen challenge may mediate a direct positive correlation between intranasal resistance and negative middle ear pressure [26], and that intranasal allergy can both interfere with clearance of a middle ear effusion and worsen middle ear pressure when a history of effusion is present [27, 28]. While nasal resistance may correlate with ETD, little evidence points to nasal obstruction as a direct cause of ETD. In fact, nasal polyposis and nasal obstruction alone have not been significant predictors of eustachian tube dysfunction [29]. Finally, there is no definitive evidence in support of allergic reflux as a cause for ETD. Altogether, evidence strongly suggests that allergic rhinitis leads to ETD by promoting both mechanical obstruction and failure of the mucociliary clearance mechanism.

While evidence of a causal relationship between allergic rhinitis and ETD is strong, there is little evidence supporting effective treatments for ETD as a lone entity. Treatment options commonly considered include observation, nonsurgical pressure equalization technique, decongestants, antihistamines, corticosteroids, and leukotriene inhibitors, but none of these have been demonstrated to have definitive clinical benefit [30]. Indeed, in the absence of extrinsic factors, topical medications are not recommended for ETD [31]. However, in the setting of suspected or confirmed allergic rhinitis, treatments for allergic rhinitis, including topical and systemic antihistamines as well as topical corticosteroids, should be offered, though there is little evidence to guide the clinician in counseling of anticipated improvement in ETD symptoms. In a retrospective review of 155 patients with ETD and allergy who underwent diagnostic inhalant and food allergy testing and subsequent immunotherapy with elimination diet, Derebery et al. showed a 70% rate of improvement in ear fullness [32]. All of these patients demonstrated reactivity to inhalant allergens and nearly all to at least one food. In patients with food allergies, a statistically significant correlation between diet adherence and allergy symptoms was reported, as well as a near statistically significant correlation with ear fullness. Therefore, in patients with ETD, clinicians should query patients for the presence of allergic symptoms and treat allergic rhinitis if diagnosed, reserving immunotherapy only for patients who continue to have both symptoms of allergy and ETD. Even with immunotherapy, prognosis for resolution of ETD symptoms is unknown.

Otitis Media with Effusion

Otitis media with effusion (OME) is a common pediatric condition characterized by middle ear inflammation with subsequent effusion and often leading to hearing loss. A relationship between middle ear effusion and the upper airway, allergy, infection, and ETD has long been a subject of epidemiologic study. The reported incidence of allergy among patients with OME has varied widely, from essentially no difference compared to controls [33, 34], to some degree of difference [35–38], to a near-universal association between allergy and OME with up to 90% of patients with OME exhibiting allergy [39–43]. Additionally, several cross-sectional studies and one recent systematic review and meta-analysis suggest that allergic rhinitis and allergy are independent risk factors for OME [44, 45]. These inconsistencies likely represent differences between highly selected populations and variability of allergy testing methodologies and sensitivities. The relationship between food allergy and OME has not been as widely addressed, and yet is as equally inconsistent. The reported incidence of food allergies in children with OME has ranged from 45% to 78% [46, 47], and one cohort study found no association between cow's milk allergy and OME [48].

Although the pathogenesis of otitis media is accepted to be multifactorial, the exact causal mechanisms linking allergy and otitis media remain controversial. Most evidence to date suggests a role for ETD in the development of OME, but some have focused on the theory of the middle ear as a "shock organ," or a site of targeted allergic reaction [16]. The middle ear has been shown to be capable of developing a local IgE-mediated inflammatory reaction [49–51] and may do so in a targeted fashion, irrespective of a systemic inflammatory reaction [52]. Other Th2 inflammatory patterns have been found in effusions of atopic patients compared to non-atopics, including eosinophil growth, mucus production, and mast cell presence [53–55]. Furthermore, the chemoattractant cytokine RANTES (regulated upon activation, normal T cell expressed and secreted), eosinophilic cationic protein (ECP), as well as, IL-4 and IL-5 were found to be higher in effusions from atopic children than non-atopics [54, 56–58]. Arguably the strongest evidence to date directly establishing the middle ear as an allergic target and linking it with the upper airway is the presence of similar cytokine expression patterns from biopsy of middle ear and nasopharyngeal specimens in atopic patients [59].

Diagnosis of OME should be made by otomicroscopy, pneumatic otoscopy, and/or tympanometry, and treatment, by placement of tympanostomy tubes or observation, directed at the duration of the effusion, presence of hearing loss, and concern for risk factors [60, 61]. Randomized placebo-controlled trials have shown that intranasal steroids do not improve OME outcomes [62–64]. While antihistamines and steroids, both systemic and intranasal, are indicated for a number of allergic conditions, two Cochrane reviews have demonstrated the statistical ineffectiveness of antihistamines, decongestants, antihistamine/decongestant combinations, and intranasal steroids in resolution of OME [65, 66]. Although there may be a role for the use of decongestants for short-term improvement in ETD prior to flying or scuba diving or for intranasal steroids in resolving ETD [67], these medications should not be reflexively given in the hopes of improving OME. Leukotriene antagonists have been studied in three randomized controlled trials with mixed benefits and are not recommended for the treatment of OME alone [68–70].

Finally, there is limited data to guide clinicians in offering immunotherapy for the treatment of OME, however one non-randomized clinical trial demonstrated a significant improvement in OME after targeted subcutaneous immunotherapy [43]. Patients included had chronic OME or suppurative otitis media and underwent allergy skin testing with 11 inhalants and four molds. All patients were found to be atopic and over a third had otitis as the sole symptom. A group of controls self-selected to avoid immunotherapy, while the others underwent directed immunotherapy for a mean of 4 years. After just 1 year of treatment, 85% of ears became effusion-free, compared to 0% of the controls. This study suggests that patients with refractory OME, even those without atopic symptoms, should be offered allergy evaluation. If patients are found to allergic, they may be considered for immunotherapy. Clinicians should be cautioned however in offering immunotherapy without weighing the potential for spontaneous resolution of the effusion, cost and time effectiveness of immunotherapy compared to replacement of tympanostomy tubes, and lack of knowledge on hearing outcomes with immunotherapy. Further study is needed to address characterization of OME phenotypes and the role of allergens and sensitization in development of OME, and to better understand with randomized trials which patients may benefit from immunotherapy, prior to incorporating immunotherapy into a generalized treatment algorithm.

Eosinophilic Otitis Media

Eosinophilic otitis media (EOM) is a distinct middle ear entity first recognized in 1993 [71] and with diagnostic criteria established in 2011 [72]. It is characterized by OME or chronic otitis media with eosinophilic dominant effusion with two or more of the following minor criteria: an effusion which is highly viscous, resistant to conventional treatment, associated with bronchial asthma or nasal polyposis. It typically presents in middle age, more often in females (62%), and with a conductive hearing loss, which has potential to progress to a sensorineural hearing loss [72, 73]. It may also be associated with a history of aspirin intolerance [74]. Clinically, a mucinous yellow effusion may be seen, associated with varying degrees of edematous middle ear mucosa, but it is often missed because of its nonspecific nature [75]. EOM shares many clinical characteristics with eosinophilic granulomatosis with polyangiitis (EGPA) however patients with EGPA show elevated serum eosinophil levels as well as ANCA positivity [76].

Regarding pathophysiology, markers of active eosinophilic inflammation, ECP, and eosinophilic granule 2 (EG2)-positive cells, have been found in middle ear effusions [77]. Additionally, eosinophil chemoattractants, IL-5 and eotaxin, have been found in higher concentrations in middle ear effusion of EOM patients than controls [78, 79]. These findings combined with evidence of mRNA expression of RANTES and eotaxin signify active eosinophilic inflammation occurring in the middle ear [79, 80]. While the exact mechanism of eosinophilic inflammation has yet to be elucidated, it has been postulated that patulous eustachian tubes, seen in a cohort of asthmatics with EOM, may serve as a highway for antigen entry into the middle ear [81]. Potential antigenic agents responsible for inducing the eosinophilic inflammation could include bacteria, viruses, fungi, or any of their elements [82]. While this theory falls in line with historical postulations of the role of nasopharyngeal reflux contributing to ETD and ultimately middle ear disease, further evidence is needed.

Early diagnosis and treatment of EOM is critical due to the risk of progressive hearing loss. Diagnosis relies on the establishment of the clinical criteria discussed previously, both by history, physical exam, and sampling of the effusion. Initial treatment recommendations are for administration of topical (intratympanic injections) or systemic steroids after standard treatments of chronic otitis media, including antibiotic administration, myringotomy with placement of tympanostomy tube or tympanoplasty, have been performed [83]. Clinicians should work to optimize the treatment of concurrent bronchial asthma as this may improve EOM symptoms as well [84]. More recently, with the advances and success in treatment of bronchial asthma using targeted monoclonal antibodies, two studies have investigated concurrent treatment of EOM [85, 86]. Omalizumab was prospectively used for the treatment of eight patients with intractable EOM, and at 1 year, there was a significant improvement in symptom and clinical severity compared to controls [85]. Mepolizumab was also shown to significantly reduce objective severity scores and symptom severity after 3 months of treatment in seven out of nine patients [86]. Finally, one case study reports cessation of aural fullness and hearing loss and resolution of middle ear effusion in one patient with intractable EOM who was treated with benralizumab for just 2 months [74]. Thus, for patients with intractable EOM who have failed traditional treatments of EOM and transtympanic corticosteroids, it is reasonable to consider treatment with monoclonal antibodies. Currently, there is insufficient evidence to recommend which medication should be used. Additionally, there is no literature to date on the use of immunotherapy for EOM. Finally, in cases of severe EOM and profound hearing loss, cochlear implantation has been successfully performed and may be considered [87].

Inner Ear

Meniere's Disease

Meniere's disease (MD) is a chronic condition almost exclusively of adults, first described in 1861 by Prosper Meniere, and characterized by aural fullness, tinnitus, fluctuating sensorineural hearing loss, and episodic vertigo. MD is typically progressive with unpredictable fluctuations; vertiginous episodes increase in severity and frequency early in the disease course with a later decline but can also return after a long period of quiescence [88, 89]. Diagnosis remains clinically based and guidelines recommend categorizing cases as definite MD or probable MD based on the number of vertigo attacks, documented hearing loss, fluctuating aural symptoms, and exclusion of other causes [90].

MD has often been observed in association with allergic conditions. A survey of MD patients records a 41% rate of concurrent allergic rhinitis, estimated to be three times that of the general population [91], and a 58% rate of history of allergic symptoms [92]. Similar associations have been found in a self-reported questionnaire of allergic symptoms and migraine in MD and control patients [93]. Additionally, a higher prevalence of hearing loss and otoacoustic emission abnormalities has been observed in patients with allergic rhinitis [94]. MD has also been associated with heightened immunopathologic profiles. For example, higher rates of IgE hypersensitivity were observed in MD patients over controls and in a sample of neurotology clinic patients over the general population [95, 96]. MD patients have also been found to have higher levels of circulating immune complexes, interleukins, and autoantibodies than controls [97].

While the underlying pathophysiologic mechanism of MD remains uncertain, it has been associated with a dysregulation of inner ear fluid volume, coined "endolymphatic hydrops" [98]. Theories linking allergy to MD have centered on the role of the endolymphatic sac (ES) as a mediator in the development of hydrops and clinical symptoms [99]. First, the ES may be a "target organ" in the release of mediators caused by systemic inhalant or food allergy. Second, circulating immune complexes could infiltrate the ES through fenestrated vessels leading to local inflammation. Third, a dormant viral antigen sets the stage for the development of a later allergic reaction. Limited studies to date support any of these three causal mechanisms; however, electrocochleographic summation potential/action potential ratios have been shown to increase in response to inhalant and food allergen challenge in Meniere's patients [100–102], suggesting that allergy may worsen MD.

Diagnostic tests, including allergy testing, are not definitively recommended in the evaluation of MD, however certain aspects of a patient's MD history may incline the provider to pursue allergy testing. These include: a seasonal pattern to MD symptoms, other allergic symptoms such as rhinitis, bilateral symptoms, strong family history of allergy, history of childhood allergy, or history of developing symptoms immediately after antigenic exposure [103, 104]. Questions regarding a history of allergy may be used as screening tools for further evaluation, however, are not a mandatory part of the clinical evaluation of MD. If a history of allergy is suspected or strong, the suggested diagnostic methodology is allergy skin testing, and it should be primarily aimed at establishing a patient's reactivity to allergens, rather than correlating allergen dose exposure to MD symptom severity [104].

Even in the setting of concurrent allergies, the initial mainstay of treatment of MD remains dietary and lifestyle modifications, including salt, caffeine, and stress reduction [90]. However, if a diagnosis of allergy has been established, the clinician may consider concurrent immunotherapy as an adjunct for symptom management. MD patients undergoing immunotherapy and food elimination diets, both retrospectively and prospectively, have had statistically significant improvement in both the frequency and severity of tinnitus and vertigo compared to MD controls not receiving therapy [104, 105]. Physicians rated an overall group improvement of 68.5% of dizziness and 55.9% of tinnitus symptoms in those having undergone allergy treatment. While no randomized controlled trials have been performed to evaluate this further, it is not unreasonable, in patients who report a history of allergy and demonstrate sensitivity on testing, to include allergy control as part of a treatment plan [90]. In addition, oral agents with potential benefit include diuretics and betahistine. Betahistine is an H3 receptor antagonist and may lead to improvement in inner ear microcirculation [106]. There is mixed evidence of its effect on the control of vertigo [107, 108], but because of its relatively benign side effect profile, it may be given with little harm, and should be considered, especially for patients with concurrent allergies.

Conclusion

The outer, middle, and inner ear have strong links to allergy. The outer ear is subject to contact dermatitis and dermatophytid reactions. Primary management includes identification of the cause and removal of it. The middle ear is subject to OME, both secondary to ETD and as a primary site of allergic activity. While allergic rhinitis is associated with both ETD and OME, intranasal and systemic corticosteroids and antihistamines do not improve ETD and OME symptoms. However, in patients who demonstrate concurrent allergy, both by history and testing, immunotherapy may provide improvement in aural fullness and resolution of the effusion for some. Finally, MD, a condition of the inner ear, is associated with allergy, and similarly, immunotherapy may lead to reduced severity and frequency of tinnitus and vertigo in patients with concurrent allergy.

Condition	Presentation	Epidemiologic link to allergy	Pathophysiologic link to allergy	Diagnostic modalities	Treatment[a]	Outcomes of allergy treatment
Allergic contact dermatitis	Vesicles, scaling, pruritis, edema, otorrhea of contact site with external ear and/or canal	Direct relationship between contact and symptoms	Delayed type IV hypersensitivity reaction to allergen	(1) Clinical history; (2) Skin patch testing	(1) Removal of offending agent; (2) Single compound corticosteroid creams or ointments	Complete resolution expected
Dermatophytid reaction	Follicular or eczematoid rash over external ear	Secondary reaction after sensitization	Delayed type IV hypersensitivity reaction to dermatophyte	(1) Physical exam for distant dermatophyte infection; (2) Allergy skin test with isolated fungal element	(1) Treatment of primary fungal infection; (2) Allergen (*T.O.E* extract) immunotherapy	Potential 78% improvement rate, though otherwise limited evidence
Eustachian tube dysfunction	Ear fullness or pressure, autophony, otalgia, tinnitus, vertigo, clicking or popping sounds, transient hearing loss	Associated with allergic rhinitis, chronic rhinosinusitis, aspirin-exacerbated respiratory disease	Unknown, though strong evidence points to allergic rhinitis leading to ET mechanical obstruction and failure of mucociliary clearance	(1) Clinical history; (2) Physical exam; (3) Tympanometry; (4) Inhalant and food allergy testing	(1) Treat allergic rhinitis; (2) Inhalant and food immunotherapy for refractory ETD and allergic rhinitis	Potential 70% improvement rate in aural fullness, though evidence limited
Otitis media with effusion	Middle ear inflammation with effusion, possible conductive hearing loss, flat tympanogram	Associated with environmental allergies, allergic rhinitis, food allergies	Unknown, though some evidence points to ETD leading to OME and some to the middle ear as a "shock organ" or site of IgE-mediated hypersensitivity	(1) Otomicroscopy, pneumatic otoscopy; (2) Allergy testing	(1) AAO-HNS guidelines for OME; (2) Targeted immunotherapy	Potential for 85% resolution rate of middle ear effusion, though evidence limited
Eosinophilic otitis media	OME or chronic otitis media with eosinophilic dominant effusion and a viscous effusion, resistant to treatment	Associated with bronchial asthma, nasal polyposis, aspirin sensitivity	Unknown, though some evidence points patulous ET allowing antigen entry into middle ear and resulting in eosinophilic inflammation	(1) Clinical diagnostic criteria; (2) Eosinophil count in effusion	(1) PET and topical corticosteroids; (2) Transtympanic corticosteroid injection; (3) Monoclonal antibodies	Potential for 80–100% improvement in symptom and clinical severity, though evidence limited
Meniere's disease	Aural fullness, tinnitus, fluctuating sensorineural hearing loss, episodic vertigo	Associated with allergic rhinitis, history of allergy symptoms, heightened immunopathologic profiles	Unknown, though the endolymphatic sac may be a "target organ" for cytokine release or susceptible to circulating immune complexes or viral antigens	(1) Clinical history; (2) Allergy testing	(1) Salt, caffeine and stress reduction; (2) Diuretics and betahistine; (3) Directed immunotherapy	Potential for near 60% improvement rate in vertigo and tinnitus; uncertain benefit of betahistine; evidence limited

[a]Treatment for each condition includes historical and society-based guidelines for each condition as well as options in the setting of concurrent allergy

Financial Disclosures

- Raymond: None
- Ryan: None
- Wise: ALK-Abello (advisory board), OptiNose (advisory board), SinopSys Surgical (advisory board), NeurENT (consultant), Stryker (consultant)

References

1. Duke WW. Meniere's syndrome caused by allergy. JAMA. 1923;81:2179–81.
2. Fölster-Holst R, Sperl A, Albrecht T, Klimek L. Basis for the treatment of eczematous diseases in otorhinolaryngology. HNO. 2017 Oct;65(10):826–33.
3. Gaul JE. Development of allergic nickel dermatitis from earrings. JAMA. 1967;200(2):176–8.
4. McDonagh AJ, Wright AL, Cork MJ, Gawkrodger DJ. Nickel sensitivity: the influence of ear piercing and atopy. Br J Dermatol. 1992 Jan;126(1):16–8.
5. Dotterud LK, Falk ES. Metal allergy in north Norwegian schoolchildren and its relationship with ear piercing and atopy. Contact Derm. 1994 Nov;31(5):308–13.
6. Rasmussen PA. Otitis externa and allergic contact dermatitis. Acta Otolaryngol. 1974;77(5):344–7.
7. Fräki JE, Kalimo K, Tuohimaa P, Aantaa E. Contact allergy to various components of topical preparations for treatment of external otitis. Acta Otolaryngol. 1985;100(5–6):414–8.
8. Van Ginkel CJ, Bruintjes TD, Huizing EH. Allergy due to topical medications in chronic otitis externa and chronic otitis media. Clin Otolaryngol Allied Sci. 1995;20(4):326–8.
9. Sood S, Strachan DR, Tsikoudas A, Stables GI. Allergic otitis externa. Clin Otolaryngol Allied Sci. 2002;27(4):233–6. Review
10. Meding B, Ringdahl A. Allergic contact dermatitis from the earmolds of hearing aids. Ear Hear. 1992;13(2):122–4.
11. Derebery MJ, Berliner KI. Allergy and the contemporary otologist. Otolaryngol Clin N Am. 2003;36(5):989–1008. Review
12. Kunda LD, Stidham KR, Inserra MM, Roland PS, Franklin D, Roberson JB Jr. Silicone allergy: a new cause for cochlear implant extrusion and its management. Otol Neurotol. 2006;27(8):1078–82. Review
13. Burns T, Rook A. Rook's Textbook of Dermatology. Vol 8th ed. edited by Tony Burns ... [et al.]. Chichester: Wiley-Blackwell; 2010. http://search.ebscohost.com.proxy.library.emory.edu/login.aspx?direct=true&db=e000xna&AN=313118&site=ehost-live&scope=site. Accessed 7 Apr 2020.
14. Derebery J, Berliner KI. Foot and ear disease--the dermatophytid reaction in otology. Laryngoscope. 1996;106(2 Pt 1):181–6.
15. Becker GD. Treatment of chronic otitis externa with trichophyton, oidiomycetes, epidermophyton antigen. Otolaryngol Head Neck Surg (1979). 1980;88(3):293–4.
16. Bluestone CD. Eustachian tube function: physiology, pathophysiology, and role of allergy in pathogenesis of otitis media. J Allergy Clin Immunol. 1983;72(3):242–51.
17. Tangbumrungtham N, Patel VS, Thamboo A, Patel ZM, Nayak JV, Ma Y, Choby G, Hwang PH. The prevalence of Eustachian tube dysfunction symptoms in patients with chronic rhinosinusitis. Int Forum Allergy Rhinol. 2018;8(5):620–3.
18. Wu AW, Walgama ES, Higgins TS, Borrelli M, Vardanyan N, Hopp S, Shamsian A, Hopp ML. Eustachian tube quality of life and severity of disease in patients with chronic rhinosinusitis. Am J Rhinol Allergy. 2020;34(4):532–6.
19. Lazo-Sáenz JG, Galván-Aguilera AA, Martínez-Ordaz VA, Velasco-Rodríguez VM, Nieves-Rentería A, Rincón-Castañeda C. Eustachian tube dysfunction in allergic rhinitis. Otolaryngol Head Neck Surg. 2005;132(4):626–9.
20. Juszczak H, Aubin-Pouliot A, Sharon JD, Loftus PA. Sinonasal risk factors for eustachian tube dysfunction: cross-sectional findings from NHANES 2011-2012. Int Forum Allergy Rhinol. 2019 May;9(5):466–72.
21. Mullur J, Singer J, Roditi R, Cahill KN. Hearing loss and middle ear symptoms in aspirin-exacerbated respiratory disease. J Allergy Clin Immunol Pract. 2019;7(5):1671–1672.e3.
22. Bluestone CD, Cantekin EI. Current clinical methods indications and interpretation of Eustachian tube function tests. Ann Otol Rhinol Laryngol. 1981;90:556.
23. Friedman RA, Doyle WJ, Casselbrant ML, Bluestone C, Fireman P. Immunologic-mediated eustachian tube obstruction: a double-blind crossover study. J Allergy Clin Immunol. 1983;71(5):442–7.
24. Skoner DP, Doyle WJ, Chamovitz AH, Fireman P. Eustachian tube obstruction after intranasal challenge with house dust mite. Arch Otolaryngol Head Neck Surg. 1986;112(8):840–2.
25. Skoner DP, Doyle WJ, Fireman P. Eustachian tube obstruction (ETO) after histamine nasal provocation--a double-blind dose-response study. J Allergy Clin Immunol. 1987;79(1):27–31.
26. O'Connor RD, Ort H, Leong AB, Cook DA, Street D, Hamburger RN. Tympanometric changes following nasal antigen challenge in children with allergic rhinitis. Ann Allergy. 1984;53(6):468–71.
27. Mogi G, Chaen T, Tomonaga K. Influence of nasal allergic reactions on the clearance of middle ear effusion. Arch Otolaryngol Head Neck Surg. 1990;116(3):331–4.
28. Pelikan Z. The role of nasal allergy in chronic secretory otitis media. Ann Allergy Asthma Immunol. 2007 Nov;99(5):401–7.
29. Bakhshaee M, Ardakani HP, Ghazizadeh AH, Movahed R, Jarahi L, Rajati M. Middle ear function

in sinonasal polyposis. Eur Arch Otorrinolaringol. 2016;273(10):2911–6.
30. Norman G, Llewellyn A, Harden M, Coatesworth A, Kimberling D, Schilder A, McDaid C. Systematic review of the limited evidence base for treatments of Eustachian tube dysfunction: a health technology assessment. Clin Otolaryngol. 2014 Feb;39(1):6–21.
31. Tucci DL, McCoul ED, Rosenfeld RM, Tunkel DE, Batra PS, Chandrasekhar SS, Cordes SR, Eshraghi AA, Kaylie D, Lal D, Lee J, Setzen M, Sindwani R, Syms CA 3rd, Bishop C, Poe DS, Corrigan M, Lambie E. Clinical consensus statement: balloon dilation of the Eustachian tube. Otolaryngol Head Neck Surg. 2019;161(1):6–17.
32. Derebery MJ, Berliner KI. Allergic eustachian tube dysfunction: diagnosis and treatment. Am J Otol. 1997;18(2):160–5.
33. Caffarelli C, Savini E, Giordano S, Gianlupi G, Cavagni G. Atopy in children with otitis media with effusion. Clin Exp Allergy. 1998;28(5):591–6.
34. Yeo SG, Park DC, Eun YG, Cha CI. The role of allergic rhinitis in the development of otitis media with effusion: effect on eustachian tube function. Am J Otolaryngol. 2007;28(3):148–52.
35. Borge P. Atopy and secretory otitis media. Immunological studies and responses to topical corticosteroid therapy. J Laryngol Otol. 1983;97(2):117–29.
36. Tomonaga K, Kurono Y, Mogi G. The role of nasal allergy in otitis media with effusion. A clinical study. Acta Otolaryngol Suppl. 1988;458:41–7.
37. Corey JP, Adham RE, Abbass AH, Seligman I. The role of IgE-mediated hypersensitivity in otitis media with effusion. Am J Otolaryngol. 1994;15(2):138–44.
38. Chantzi FM, Kafetzis DA, Bairamis T, Avramidou C, Paleologou N, Grimani I, Apostolopoulos N, Papadopoulos NG. IgE sensitization, respiratory allergy symptoms, and heritability independently increase the risk of otitis media with effusion. Allergy. 2006;61(3):332–6.
39. McMahan JT, Calenoff E, Croft DJ, Barenholtz L, Weber LD. Chronic otitis media with effusion and allergy: modified RAST analysis of 119 cases. Otolaryngol Head Neck Surg. 1981;89(3 Pt 1):427–31.
40. Hurst DS. Allergy management of refractory serous otitis media. Otolaryngol Head Neck Surg. 1990;102(6):664–9.
41. Hurst DS. Association of otitis media with effusion and allergy as demonstrated by intradermal skin testing and eosinophil cationic protein levels in both middle ear effusions and mucosal biopsies. Laryngoscope. 1996;106(9 Pt 1):1128–37.
42. Alles R, Parikh A, Hawk L, Darby Y, Romero JN, Scadding G. The prevalence of atopic disorders in children with chronic otitis media with effusion. Pediatr Allergy Immunol. 2001;12(2):102–6. PubMed PMID: 11338283.
43. Hurst DS. Efficacy of allergy immunotherapy as a treatment for patients with chronic otitis media with effusion. Int J Pediatr Otorhinolaryngol. 2008;72(8):1215–23. https://doi.org/10.1016/j.ijporl.2008.04.013. Epub 2008 June 9.
44. Kreiner-Møller E, Chawes BL, Caye-Thomasen P, Bønnelykke K, Bisgaard H. Allergic rhinitis is associated with otitis media with effusion: a birth cohort study. Clin Exp Allergy. 2012;42(11):1615–20.
45. Cheng X, Sheng H, Ma R, Gao Z, Han Z, Chi F, Cong N, Wang J, Liu X, Luo X, Yu J, Ra Y. Allergic rhinitis and allergy are risk factors for otitis media with effusion: a meta-analysis. Allergol Immunopathol (Madr). 2017;45(1):25–32.
46. Nsouli TM, Nsouli SM, Linde RE, O'Mara F, Scanlon RT, Bellanti JA. Role of food allergy in serous otitis media. Ann Allergy. 1994;73(3):215–9.
47. Aydoğan B, Kiroğlu M, Altintas D, Yilmaz M, Yorgancilar E, Tuncer U. The role of food allergy in otitis media with effusion. Otolaryngol Head Neck Surg. 2004;130(6):747–50.
48. Juntti H, Tikkanen S, Kokkonen J, Alho OP, Niinimäki A. Cow's milk allergy is associated with recurrent otitis media during childhood. Acta Otolaryngol. 1999;119(8):867–73.
49. Bernstein JM, Ellis E, Li P. The role of IgE-mediated hypersensitivity in otitis media with effusion. Otolaryngol Head Neck Surg. 1981;89(5):874–8.
50. Bernstein JM, Lee J, Conboy K, Ellis E, Li P. The role of IgE mediated hypersensitivity in recurrent otitis media with effusion. Am J Otol. 1983;5(1):66–9.
51. Bernstein JM, Lee J, Conboy K, Ellis E, Li P. Further observations on the role of IgE-mediated hypersensitivity in recurrent otitis media with effusion. Otolaryngol Head Neck Surg. 1985;93(5):611–5.
52. Hurst DS, Weekley M, Ramanarayanan MP. Evidence of possible localized specific immunoglobulin E production in middle ear fluid as demonstrated by ELISA testing. Otolaryngol Head Neck Surg. 1999;121(3):224–30.
53. Hurst DS, Venge P. Evidence of eosinophil, neutrophil, and mast-cell mediators in the effusion of OME patients with and without atopy. Allergy. 2000;55(5):435–41.
54. Sobol SE, Taha R, Schloss MD, Mazer BD, Manoukian JJ, Tewfik TL, Hamid Q. T(H)2 cytokine expression in atopic children with otitis media with effusion. J Allergy Clin Immunol. 2002;110(1):125–30.
55. Tewfik TL, Mazer B. The links between allergy and otitis media with effusion. Curr Opin Otolaryngol Head Neck Surg. 2006;14(3):187–90.
56. Jang CH, Kim YH. Characterization of cytokines present in pediatric otitis media with effusion: comparison of allergy positive and negative. Int J Pediatr Otorhinolaryngol. 2002;66(1):37–40.
57. Jang CH, Kim YH. Demonstration of RANTES and eosinophilic cataionic protein in otitis media with effusion with allergy. Int J Pediatr Otorhinolaryngol. 2003;67(5):531–3.
58. Nguyen LH, Manoukian JJ, Sobol SE, Tewfik TL, Mazer BD, Schloss MD, Taha R, Hamid QA. Similar

allergic inflammation in the middle ear and the upper airway: evidence linking otitis media with effusion to the united airways concept. J Allergy Clin Immunol. 2004;114(5):1110–5.
59. Nguyen LH, Manoukian JJ, Tewfik TL, Sobol SE, Joubert P, Mazer BD, Schloss MD, Taha R, Hamid QA. Evidence of allergic inflammation in the middle ear and nasopharynx in atopic children with otitis media with effusion. J Otolaryngol. 2004;33(6):345–51.
60. Rosenfeld RM, Schwartz SR, Pynnonen MA, Tunkel DE, Hussey HM, Fichera JS, Grimes AM, Hackell JM, Harrison MF, Haskell H, Haynes DS, Kim TW, Lafreniere DC, LeBlanc K, Mackey WL, Netterville JL, Pipan ME, Raol NP, Schellhase KG. Clinical practice guideline: Tympanostomy tubes in children. Otolaryngol Head Neck Surg. 2013;149(1 Suppl):S1–35.
61. Rosenfeld RM, Shin JJ, Schwartz SR, Coggins R, Gagnon L, Hackell JM, Hoelting D, Hunter LL, Kummer AW, Payne SC, Poe DS, Veling M, Vila PM, Walsh SA, Corrigan MD. Clinical practice guideline: otitis media with effusion (update). Otolaryngol Head Neck Surg. 2016;154(1 Suppl):S1–S41.
62. Lildholdt T, Kortholm B. Beclomethasone nasal spray in the treatment of middle-ear effusion – a double-blind study. Int J Pediatr Otorhinolaryngol. 1982;4(2):133–7. PubMed PMID: 6752070
63. Shapiro GG, Bierman CW, Furukawa CT, Pierson WE, Berman R, Donaldson J, Rees T. Treatment of persistent eustachian tube dysfunction in children with aerosolized nasal dexamethasone phosphate versus placebo. Ann Allergy. 1982;49(2):81–5.
64. Williamson I, Benge S, Barton S, Petrou S, Letley L, Fasey N, Haggard M, Little P. Topical intranasal corticosteroids in 4-11 year old children with persistent bilateral otitis media with effusion in primary care: double blind randomised placebo controlled trial. BMJ. 2009;16(339):b4984.
65. Griffin G, Flynn CA. Antihistamines and/or decongestants for otitis media with effusion (OME) in children. Cochrane Database Syst Rev. 2011;(9):CD003423.
66. Simpson SA, Lewis R, van der Voort J, Butler CC. Oral or topical nasal steroids for hearing loss associated with otitis media with effusion in children. Cochrane Database Syst Rev. 2011;(5):CD001935.
67. Fireman P. Eustachian tube obstruction and allergy: a role in otitis media with effusion? J Allergy Clin Immunol. 1985;76(2 Pt 1):137–40.
68. Combs JT. The effect of montelukast sodium on the duration of effusion of otitis media. Clin Pediatr (Phila). 2004;43(6):529–33.
69. Schoem SR, Willard A, Combs JT. A prospective, randomized, placebo-controlled, double-blind study of montelukast's effect on persistent middle ear effusion. Ear Nose Throat J. 2010;89(9):434–7.
70. Ertugay CK, Cingi C, Yaz A, San T, Ulusoy S, Erdogmus N, Ertugay OC. Effect of combination of montelukast and levocetirizine on otitis media with effusion: a prospective, placebo-controlled trial. Acta Otolaryngol. 2013;133(12):1266–72.
71. Recent Advances in Otitis Media Treatment. Symposium proceedings. Minneapolis, Minnesota, October 1, 1993. Ann Otol Rhinol Laryngol Suppl. 1994;163:1–64.
72. Iino Y, Tomioka-Matsutani S, Matsubara A, Nakagawa T, Nonaka M. Diagnostic criteria of eosinophilic otitis media, a newly recognized middle ear disease. Auris Nasus Larynx. 2011;38(4):456–61.
73. Iino Y. Eosinophilic otitis media: a new middle ear disease entity. Curr Allergy Asthma Rep. 2008;8(6):525–30.
74. Chow K, Cosetti MK. Use of IL-5 inhibitor benralizumab as a novel therapy for eosinophilic otitis media: clinical capsule and review of literature. Otol Neurotol. 2020;41(2):e238–40.
75. Nagamine H, Iino Y, Kojima C, Miyazawa T, Iida T. Clinical characteristics of so called eosinophilic otitis media. Auris Nasus Larynx. 2002;29(1):19–28.
76. Fukuda A, Morita S, Nakamaru Y, Hoshino K, Fujiwara K, Homma A. Differentiation between eosinophilic otitis media and otitis media associated with eosinophilic granulomatosis with polyangiitis. Otol Neurotol. 2019;40(8):e796–802.
77. Iino Y, Nagamine H, Yabe T, Matsutani S. Eosinophils are activated in middle ear mucosa and middle ear effusion of patients with intractable otitis media associated with bronchial asthma. Clin Exp Allergy. 2001;31(7):1135–43.
78. Nonaka M, Fukumoto A, Ozu C, Mokuno E, Baba S, Pawankar R, Yagi T. IL-5 and eotaxin levels in middle ear effusion and blood from asthmatics with otitis media with effusion. Acta Otolaryngol. 2003;123(3):383–7.
79. Iino Y, Kakizaki K, Katano H, Saigusa H, Kanegasaki S. Eosinophil chemoattractants in the middle ear of patients with eosinophilic otitis media. Clin Exp Allergy. 2005;35(10):1370–6.
80. Iino Y. Role of IgE in eosinophilic otitis media. Allergol Int. 2010;59(3):233–8.
81. Kanazawa H, Yoshida N, Hara M, Hasegawa M, Matsuzawa S, Shinnabe A, et al. Risk factors for eosinophilic otitis media in patients with eosinophilic chronic rhinosinusitis. Int Adv Otol. 2013;9:353–8.
82. Kanazawa H, Yoshida N, Iino Y. New insights into eosinophilic otitis media. Curr Allergy Asthma Rep. 2015;15(12):76.
83. Iino Y, Nagamine H, Kakizaki K, Komiya T, Katano H, Saruya S, Kodera K. Effectiveness of instillation of triamcinolone acetonide into the middle ear for eosinophilic otitis media associated with bronchial asthma. Ann Allergy Asthma Immunol. 2006;97(6):761–6.
84. Tanaka Y, Nonaka M, Yamamura Y, Tagaya E, Pawankar R, Yoshihara T. Improvement of eosinophilic otitis media by optimized asthma

treatment. Allergy Asthma Immunol Res. 2013;5(3):175–8.
85. Iino Y, Hara M, Hasegawa M, Matsuzawa S, Shinnabe A, Kanazawa H, Yoshida N. Clinical efficacy of anti-IgE therapy for eosinophilic otitis media. Otol Neurotol. 2012;33(7):1218–24.
86. Iino Y, Takahashi E, Ida S, Kikuchi S. Clinical efficacy of anti-IL-5 monoclonal antibody mepolizumab in the treatment of eosinophilic otitis media. Auris Nasus Larynx. 2019;46(2):196–203.
87. Iwasaki S, Nagura M, Mizuta K. Cochlear implantation in a patient with eosinophilic otitis media. Eur Arch Otorrinolaringol. 2006;263(4):365–9.
88. Silverstein H, Smouha E, Jones R. Natural history vs. surgery for Menière's disease. Otolaryngol Head Neck Surg. 1989;100(1):6–16.
89. Havia M, Kentala E, Pyykkö I. Prevalence of Menière's disease in general population of southern Finland. Otolaryngol Head Neck Surg. 2005;133(5):762–8.
90. Basura GJ, Adams ME, Monfared A, Schwartz SR, Antonelli PJ, Burkard R, Bush ML, Bykowski J, Colandrea M, Derebery J, Kelly EA, Kerber KA, Koopman CF, Kuch AA, Marcolini E, McKinnon BJ, Ruckenstein MJ, Valenzuela CV, Vosooney A, Walsh SA, Nnacheta LC, Dhepyasuwan N, Buchanan EM. Clinical practice guideline: Ménière's disease executive summary. Otolaryngol Head Neck Surg. 2020;162(4):415–34.
91. Derebery MJ, Berliner KI. Prevalence of allergy in Meniere's disease. Otolaryngol Head Neck Surg. 2000;123(1 Pt 1):69–75.
92. Derebery MJ, Berliner KI. Characteristics, onset and progression in Meniere's disease. In: Lim DJ, editor. Proceedings of the 5th international symposium on Meniere's disease and inner ear homeostasis disorders. Los Angeles: House Ear Institute; 2005. p. 128–30.
93. Sen P, Georgalas C, Papesch M. Co-morbidity of migraine and Ménière's disease -- is allergy the link? J Laryngol Otol. 2005;119(6):455–60.
94. Singh S, Nagarkar AN, Bansal S, Vir D, Gupta AK. Audiological manifestations of allergic rhinitis. J Laryngol Otol. 2011;125(9):906–10.
95. Howard BK, Mabry RL, Meyerhoff WL, Mabry CS. Use of a screening RAST in a large neuro-otologic practice. Otolaryngol Head Neck Surg. 1997;117(6):653–9.
96. Keles E, Gödekmerdan A, Kalidağ T, Kaygusuz I, Yalçin S, Cengiz Alpay H, Aral M. Meniere's disease and allergy: allergens and cytokines. J Laryngol Otol. 2004;118(9):688–93.
97. Savastano M, Giacomelli L, Marioni G. Non-specific immunological determinations in Meniere's disease: any role in clinical practice? Eur Arch Otorrinolaringol. 2007;264(1):159.
98. Sajjadi H, Paparella MM. Meniere's disease. Lancet. 2008;372(9636):406–14.
99. Derebery MJ. Allergic and immunologic aspects of Meniere's disease. Otolaryngol Head Neck Surg. 1996;114(3):360–5.
100. Viscomi GJ, Bojrab DI. Use of electrocochleography to monitor antigenic challenge in Menière's disease. Otolaryngol Head Neck Surg. 1992;107(6 Pt 1):733–7.
101. Gibbs SR, Mabry RL, Roland PS, Shoup AG, Mabry CS. Electrocochleographic changes after intranasal allergen challenge: a possible diagnostic tool in patients with Meniere's disease. Otolaryngol Head Neck Surg. 1999;121(3):283–4.
102. Topuz B, Ogmen G, Ardiç FN, Kara CO. Provocation of endolymphatic hydrops with a prick test in Meniere's disease. Adv Ther. 2007;24(4):819–25.
103. Powers WH. Allergic factors in Meniere's disease. Trans Am Acad Ophthalmol Otolaryngol. 1973;77(1):ORL22-9.
104. Derebery MJ, Berliner KI. Allergy and its relation to Meniere's disease. Otolaryngol Clin N Am. 2010;43(5):1047–58.
105. Derebery MJ. Allergic management of Meniere's disease: an outcome study. Otolaryngol Head Neck Surg. 2000;122(2):174–82.
106. Dziadziola JK, Laurikainen EL, Rachel JD, Quirk WS. Betahistine increases vestibular blood flow. Otolaryngol Head Neck Surg. 1999;120(3):400–5.
107. Murdin L, Hussain K, Schilder AG. Betahistine for symptoms of vertigo. Cochrane Database Syst Rev 2016;(6):CD010696.
108. Adrion C, Fischer CS, Wagner J, Gürkov R, Mansmann U, Strupp M, BEMED Study Group. Efficacy and safety of betahistine treatment in patients with Meniere's disease: primary results of a long term, multicentre, double blind, randomised, placebo controlled, dose defining trial (BEMED trial). BMJ. 2016;21(352):h6816.

Allergy and Chronic Rhinosinusitis 29

Thomas S. Edwards, Samuel N. Helman, and John M. DelGaudio

Introduction

Much like allergic rhinitis (AR), chronic rhinosinusitis (CRS) is an inflammatory disorder of the nasal cavity and sinuses. CRS is defined as at least 12 weeks of sinonasal inflammation, characterized by nasal obstruction, mucoid anterior or posterior nasal drainage, facial pain, pressure, or fullness, and/or decreased sense of smell. These symptoms must be accompanied by objective findings of inflammation on imaging or nasal endoscopy (purulence, polyps, or edema) [1].

Epidemiology of Chronic Rhinosinusitis

CRS is estimated to have a prevalence of 10–15% [2, 3]. Population-based surveys do not typically differentiate between acute and chronic sinusitis making more accurate estimation difficult. The 2008 Global Allergy and Asthma European Network (GA^{2}LEN) questionnaire-based survey, using diagnostic criteria published in the European Position Paper on Rhinosinusitis and Nasal Polyps (EPOS), differentiated between acute and chronic rhinosinusitis based on patient-reported physician diagnosis. This work, likely the strongest estimate, reported the prevalence of CRS in Europe to be 10.9% [4, 5]. Best estimates of the prevalence of rhinosinusitis in the United States are approximately 12% [2]. In the 2012 US National Health Interview Survey, a patient-reported survey that did not differentiate between acute and chronic sinusitis, sinusitis was more common in women (14.5% vs 9.0%). The prevalence of sinusitis rises during young adult life, peaks in middle age, and falls in the elderly [6]. The estimated direct cost from this disease is $8.6 billion per year with the indirect cost estimated at $12.8 billion per year [2, 3].

Pathogenesis of Chronic Rhinosinusitis

The pathogenesis of CRS is not yet fully understood and likely to be multifactorial. It is believed that local mucosal abnormalities such as disrupted innate immunity, mucociliary dysfunction, immune hypersensitivity, and/or bacterial or fungal colonization in the presence of certain genetic, epigenetic, systemic, and/or environmental factors lead to the development of the disease [7]. Traditionally, CRS is categorized by phenotype: CRS without nasal polyps (CRSsNP) and CRS with nasal polyps (CRSwNP). Initial

T. S. Edwards · S. N. Helman · J. M. DelGaudio (✉)
Department of Otolaryngology, Emory University, Atlanta, GA, USA
e-mail: thomas.edwards@emory.edu; jdelgau@emory.edu

C. Damask et al. (eds.), *Allergy in Otolaryngology Practice*,
https://doi.org/10.1007/978-3-031-93455-1_29

research into the inflammatory profiles of CRSsNP and CRSwNP seemed to confirm a biologic basis for this system. The presence of neutrophils, interferon-γ (INF-γ), and transforming growth factor—beta1 (TGF-β1) in mucosal samples from patients with CRSsNP led to its characterization as a type 1 T helper cell (Th1) inflammatory process. The mucosa of patients with CRSwNP showed an abundance of eosinophils as well as elevated interleukin (IL)-5 and immunoglobulin-E (IgE) concentrations. This phenotype was thus described as having a type 2 T helper cell (Th2) polarization [8]. These inflammatory profiles, however, have significant geographic variability. While up to 80% of patients with CRSwNP in Europe and North America, a predominately white population, have a Th2 inflammatory profile, only 20% of patients with CRSwNP in China and Korea present with this inflammatory profile [9]. This variability has even been noted within diverse populations in the United States with one center reporting only 5% of patients with CRSsNP showing Th1 inflammation. Surprisingly, 37% of this CRSsNP population showed a Th2 inflammatory signature [10].

Recent studies suggest that subgroups within these broad phenotypic categories exist, frequently described as endotypes [11]. These subgroups are hypothesized to have different inflammatory and genetic signatures such as the presence or absence of IL-4, IL-5, IL-13, INF-γ, *Staphylococcus aureus* enterotoxin-specific IgE, and/or bitter taste receptor (T2R38). It is thought that these subgroups predict the likelihood of nasal polyps and associated diagnoses such as asthma and may correlate with treatment outcomes [12, 13]. These subgroups have yet to be clearly defined and may rather be a spectrum. Regardless, inflammation in general serves as a common thread for CRS.

The Role of Allergic Rhinitis in Chronic Rhinosinusitis

Proposed Mechanisms

Inhalant allergen exposure in patients with AR is also characterized as a Th2 inflammatory process. After initial exposure to an aeroallergen, antigen-presenting cells (APCs) process the allergen and activate Th2 ($CD4^+$) lymphocytes. These Th2 cells induce B-cells to differentiate into plasma cells and begin production of specific IgE (sIgE) to these allergens. These sIgE molecules bind to the surface of mast cells, priming them. Re-exposure to the allergen leads to early- and late-phase inflammatory responses [14, 15]. This Th2 immune profile has frequently raised the question of whether an association between AR and CRS, particularly CRSwNP, exists.

The hypothesized mechanism for this association revolves around the inflammatory response being both local and systemic on re-exposure to an aeroallergen. Locally, the response is driven by the direct activation of macrophages, mast cells, eosinophils, and B lymphocytes by aeroallergens to which the patient is sensitive. The systemic response is driven by the migration of activated Th2 lymphocytes to bone marrow. This leads to the release of inflammatory mediators that result in an increase in serum eosinophils [16]. Inflamed sinonasal tissue releases chemotactic signals such as eotaxin (C-C motif chemokine ligand 11) and increases expression of cell adhesion molecules such as vascular cell adhesion molecule 1 (VCAM1) recruiting serum eosinophils to these inflamed tissues [16].

Animal and Human Models

While several basic science studies utilizing both animal and human models seem to support the role of AR in CRS, clinical studies are inconclusive. In a mouse model sensitized to ovalalbumin and then exposed to both ovalbumin and *Streptococcus pneumoniae* simulating acute bacterial rhinosinusitis (ABRS) in the setting of AR, there was a threefold increase in the volume of the sinuses filled with neutrophil clusters and a twofold increase in the number of infiltrating neutrophils in sinus mucosa compared to non-allergic mice infected with *S. pneumoniae*. Nasal lavage from these allergic mice also showed heavier bacterial growth than controls suggesting a more severe infection [17].

In humans, it has been shown that aeroallergens do not enter unoperated sinuses spontaneously or with nose blowing [16, 18]. However, even without direct allergen uptake in unoperated sinuses, inflammatory changes are seen in the sinuses after nasal allergen challenge. Baroody et al. showed increased levels of histamine and eosinophils in lavage specimens from the ipsilateral maxillary sinus. Eosinophils were significantly more abundant than in subjects' serum. Interestingly, when these subjects were treated with loratadine there was an improvement in AR symptoms, but inflammatory markers from maxillary sinus lavage were unchanged. In the case of eosinophil cationic protein (ECP) there was actually an increase with loratadine [19]. Conversely, Keith et al. showed that while patients with CRSwNP and AR had elevated inflammatory markers (increased eosinophil and ECP levels) in nasal lavage at baseline, these markers did not increase significantly with exposure to allergens to which they were sensitive. Patients with only AR had significant increases in these markers on exposure to allergens to which they were sensitive. They hypothesized that the inflammatory environment may already be maximized in CRSwNP [20].

Conflicting Clinical Studies

Numerous clinical studies of the association between allergy and CRSsNP or CRSwNP have been undertaken. One of the largest studies to date of aeroallergen sensitivity in CRS by Tan et al. found 85.5% of patients with CRSwNP and 79.4% of patients with CRSsNP had reactivity to 1 or more allergens with skin prick testing (SPT). The authors compared this to the aeroallergen sensitivity rate of the general population as assessed by the National Health and Nutrition Examination Study III (NHANES III). This study showed 54.3% of 10,508 test subjects were sensitive to one or more allergens on SPT [21]. Another large study of aeroallergen sensitivity in CRS, however, found that aeroallergen sensitivity, assessed by in vitro testing, was equally prevalent in patients with CRSwNP (27.5%) and CRSsNP (32.3%) and was not associated with symptom scores. They concluded CRS was not influenced by aeroallergen sensitivity [22]. A comprehensive 2014 review of these studies and 22 others on the role of AR in CRS revealed widely contradictory findings. Seven of 18 studies showed no relationship between allergy and CRSwNP while 10 demonstrated a relationship. One study was equivocal. Of nine studies analyzing the role of AR in CRSsNP, four demonstrated a relationship between CRSsNP and allergy with five finding no relationship [23]. In a recent consensus statement, the overall evidence linking allergy to CRS is low (grade D) [15].

It is likely that the broad phenotypic categories of CRSsNP and CRSwNP obscure the association with allergy and that certain subtypes of CRS have an association with allergy while others do not. Allergic fungal rhinosinusitis (AFRS) is a widely described subtype of CRSwNP that is associated with allergy based upon published diagnostic criteria [24]. Newer subtypes of CRS such as central compartment atopic disease (CCAD) may also have an allergic etiology [25].

Allergy in Allergic Fungal Rhinosinusitis

AFRS is characterized by nasal polyps, eosinophilic mucin, characteristic radiographic findings, and type 1 hypersensitivity to fungi [24]. Wise et al. showed increased specific IgE (sIgE) to fungal species (specifically *Cladosporium* and *Aspergillus*) in sinus mucosa homogenates from patients with AFRS compared to tissue from patients with CRSsNP and control tissue. Interestingly, these AFRS patients also showed elevated levels of allergen-specific IgE (sIgE) to other perennial and seasonal aeroallergens (Timothy grass, red maple, cockroach, ragweed, and cocklebur) in addition to fungi [26]. A subset of patients with the classic phenotypic findings of AFRS lack a systemic type 1 hypersensitivity to fungi. Some of this subset have been found, however, to have fungal sIgE in their eosinophilic mucin and sinonasal tissue [27, 28]. This phenomenon, where no systemic evidence of sIgE to an allergen by traditional testing exists but sIgE to the allergen is found locally, has been described in AR by Powe et al. and termed local allergic rhinitis (LAR) or entopy [29].

Allergy in Central Compartment Atopic Disease

In 2014, White et al. demonstrated that polypoid edema of middle turbinate mucosa or polyps emanating from the middle turbinate (Fig. 29.1) was associated with positive skin or in-vitro testing for aeroallergens [30]. These results were supported by a larger retrospective study which showed that the degree of middle turbinate polypoid edema on nasal endoscopy (graded as focal, multifocal, diffuse, or polypoid) was associated with an increasing likelihood of AR [31]. Brunner et al. compared patients with isolated middle turbinate polyps to those with diffuse sinonasal polyposis, and found these to be two distinct entities, with the isolated middle turbinate polyp group having a significantly higher incidence of allergy (83 vs. 34%) and significantly lower Lund McKay scores (2.8 vs 14.9) [32].

DelGaudio et al. introduced the term "central compartment atopic disease" (CCAD) to describe patients with polyps of the central compartment, which includes the superior nasal septum, the middle turbinate (MT), and/or the superior turbinate (ST) [33]. It is hypothesized that these structures are involved because nasal airflow rises over the head of the inferior turbinate and travels between the nasal septum and middle and superior turbinates and then descends over the posterior aspect of the inferior turbinate to enter the nasopharynx [34]. Characteristic radiographic findings in CCAD include soft tissue thickening of the central nasal cavity, frequently bilaterally. Sinus involvement, if present, occurs in a medial to lateral progression as a result of sinus outflow tract obstruction. The roof and lateral walls of the ethmoid sinuses are typically spared in early obstructive sinus disease. In longer-standing disease, there can be near-complete or complete sinus opacification. It is thought that this pattern is related to either lateralization of the MT from central polypoid changes or from direct extension of the polypoid changes of the MT into the sinus outflow tracts leading to secondary obstruction of the sinuses [33]. The radiographic findings of cen-

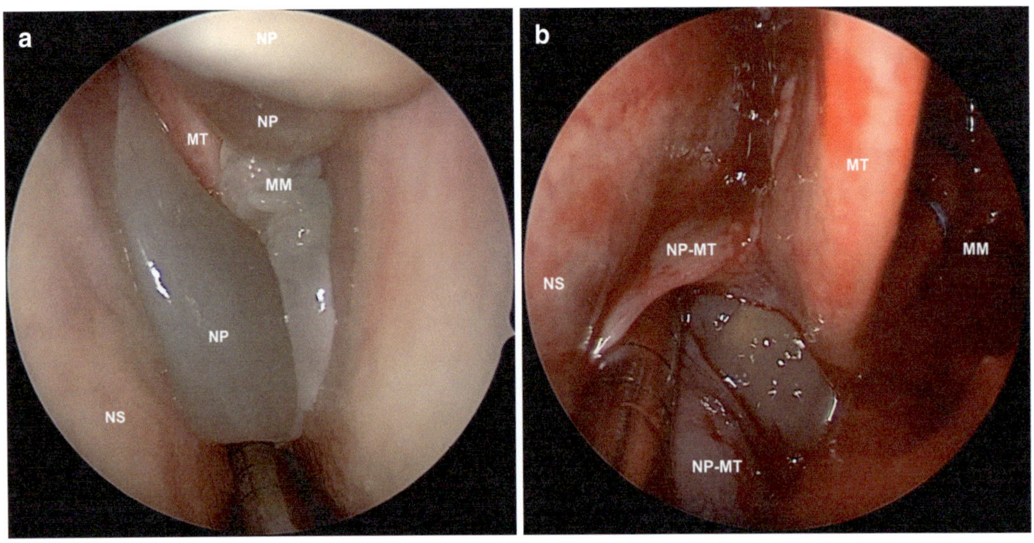

Fig. 29.1 Rigid nasal endoscopy of the left nasal cavity in a patient with central compartment atopic disease (CCAD). (**a**) Large nasal polyps (NP) emanating from between the nasal septum (NS) and middle turbinate (MT) and filling the middle meatus (MM). While possibly confused for traditional sinonasal polyps, (**b**) tracing the polyp (NP-MT) to its origin shows it arising from the MT. These findings, in combination with imaging (Fig. 29.2), are indicative of CCAD

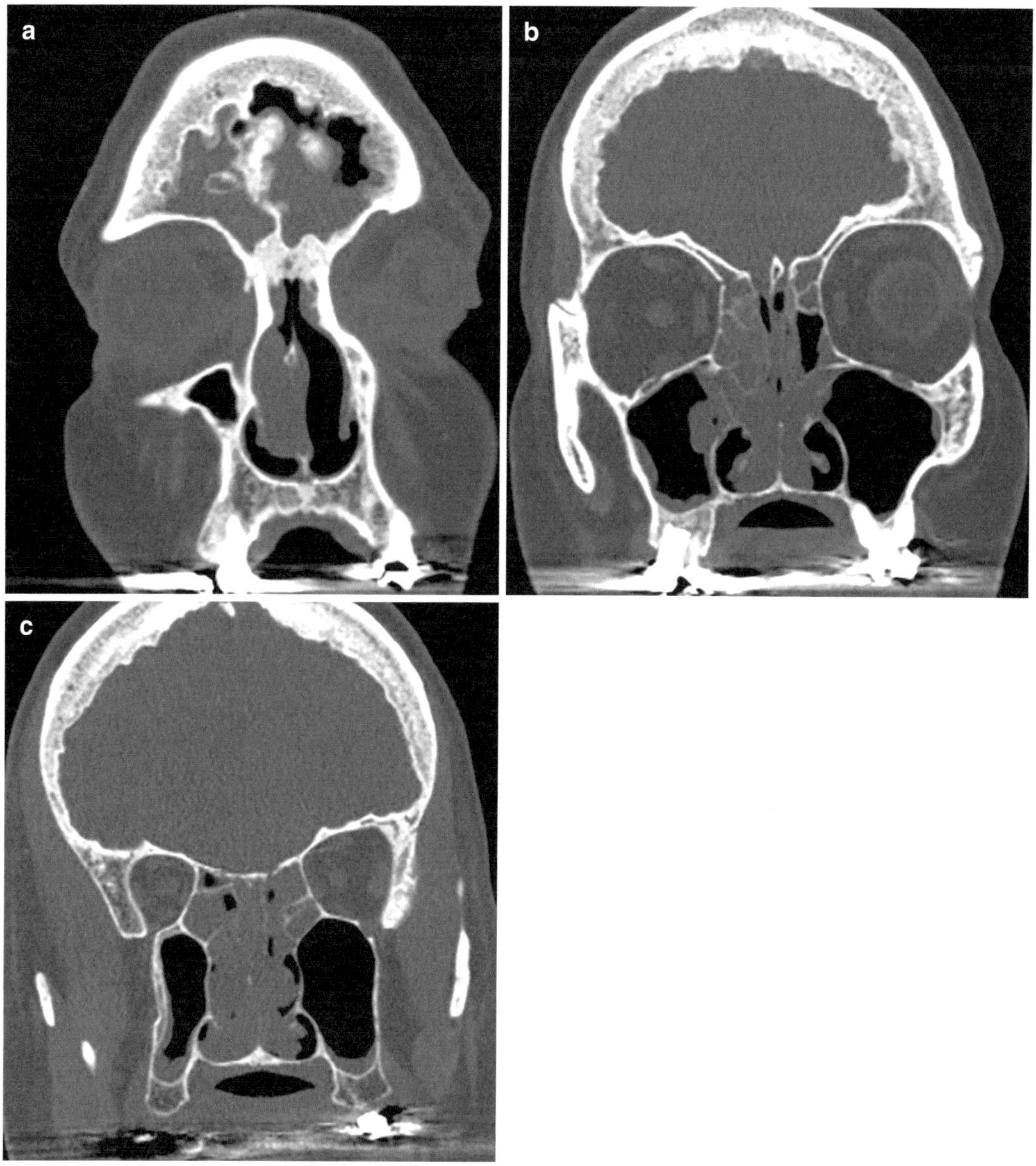

Fig. 29.2 Three-panel CT scan images of the sinuses in coronal view. Panel (**a**) shows the frontal sinuses and nasal cavity. Panel (**b**) displays the anterior ethmoid and maxillary sinuses. Panel (**c**) focuses on the posterior ethmoid and maxillary sinuses

tral nasal and sinus involvement (Fig. 29.2) predict atopy with 90.8% specificity [35].

Other Subtypes of Chronic Rhinosinusitis

While CCAD is a unique entity in itself, other subtypes of CRS such as aspirin-exacerbated respiratory disease (AERD, previously known as Samter's Triad), and respiratory epithelial adenomatoid hamartoma (REAH), frequently demonstrate similar imaging and endoscopy findings and increased rates of aeroallergen sensitivity. The pathophysiology of AERD is based on a non-IgE-mediated hypersensitivity to cyclooxygenase-1 (COX-1) inhibitors, such as acetylsalicylic acid (ASA) and other nonsteroidal anti-inflammatory drugs (NSAIDs). Alcohol sensitivity is a common symptom in patients with AERD and reported in 77% of patients [36–38]. Our group has found a prevalence of AR in 89.9% of patients with AERD treated in our practice from 2016 to 2019 with 81.9% demonstrating central compartment disease involvement [39]. Another retrospective analysis of patients with a pathologic diagnosis of REAH at our institution identified 26 patients between September 2006 and November 2019. Clinical AR was diagnosed in 18 of 19 patients with adequate allergy documentation. Allergy status was not documented in 7 patients. Concurrent sinonasal inflammatory disorders were frequently found including CRSwNP-NOS [6], CRSsNP [4], AERD [2], AFRS [1], CCAD [5], and IgG4-related sclerosing disease [40]. Although the evidence for allergy as an etiology for CRSwNP as a broad phenotypic group is low, there is strong evidence for the role of allergy in AFRS, growing evidence for its role in CCAD, and recent studies showing an increased incidence of allergy in AERD and REAH.

Diagnosis and Management

History

A detailed history can frequently identify features of both CRS and AR when they occur in unison. Thorough physical examination, however, is also required. As mentioned previously, CRS can only be diagnosed when sinonasal inflammation, characterized by nasal obstruction, mucoid anterior or posterior nasal drainage, facial pain, pressure, or fullness, and/or decreased sense of smell has been present for 12 weeks. A history evaluating for AR should include the type of allergic symptoms experienced (nasal congestion or obstruction, nasal pruritis, clear rhinorrhea, and sneezing), their timing (seasonality), and duration. Activities, exposures, or environments eliciting symptoms as well as medications or other measures that improve symptoms should be noted. Though outside of the scope of this chapter, the history and physical should also assess for symptoms of asthma due to the increased prevalence of asthma in both AR and CRSwNP [15, 41].

Evidence of Inflammation

Symptoms of CRS must be accompanied by objective findings of inflammation [1]. When CRS is suspected in conjunction with AR, inflammation of the central compartment is ideally assessed with nasal endoscopy. This allows for more precise assessment of the mucosa of the central compartment. It also may allow for the determination of where polyps are originating—from the turbinates or septum versus from within the sinuses themselves. Imaging is not recommended in the diagnosis of AR alone. However, when symptoms of CRS or central compartment mucosal abnormalities are present, imaging with computed tomography (CT) should also be obtained as inflammation of the sinuses is difficult to fully assess with nasal endoscopy.

Allergy Testing

When history and physical examination support a diagnosis of both CRS and AR, allergy testing is recommended in order to determine allergen sensitivity. In appropriately screened patients, skin testing is considered the gold standard. In patients deemed inappropriate for skin testing or those who decline skin testing, serum measurements of sIgE can be obtained. It is necessary for a strong correlation between patients' clinical history of allergic triggers and allergy testing results to be present. When a patient is sensitive to an allergen but denies symptoms with exposure, additional workup is not necessary. When the converse occurs, symptoms in the presence of a trigger but with negative systemic testing, additional evaluation can be considered to evaluate for LAR. Testing for LAR may consist of nasal provocation test, measurement of sIgE in nasal secretions/tissues, and/or basophil activation testing. Currently, these methods are most commonly used in research protocols and are not widely available commercially [15].

Other Diagnostics

A patient with AR and nasal polyposis may have various etiologies for their sinonasal disease and accurate diagnosis is key. Other diagnoses associated with the presence of nasal polyps, such as cystic fibrosis (CF) or inverted papilloma should be ruled out as these diagnoses may significantly alter the patient's management. Patients with a history of asthma, airway reactivity to aspirin or NSAIDs, and endoscopic evidence of nasal polyposis meet the criteria for AERD. The gold standard for the diagnosis of AERD is an aspirin challenge. In patients with AERD, aspirin challenge results in significant reaction including bronchospasm, urticaria, nasal congestion, rhinorrhea, and/or ocular pruritis. Aspirin challenge should only be undertaken in centers that specialize in this procedure and can provide appropriate resuscitative measures. Constant observation by qualified personnel is also mandatory [42].

Treatment of Allergen Sensitivity

The management of allergy-driven subtypes of CRS is similar to current therapies for CRSwNP though additional focus is placed on the management of aeroallergen sensitivity. In the case of AFRS and CCAD, medical management with intranasal and oral corticosteroids, antihistamines, and antibiotics is attempted. Antibiotics are given when endoscopy or CT demonstrates purulence or air-fluid levels. Frequently, medical management does not yield complete resolution of symptoms, with imaging obtained after medical therapy showing persistent sinonasal inflammation. In these patients, endoscopic sinus surgery is undertaken to remove obstructive sinonasal pathology and open the sinuses allowing for the application of topical therapies postoperatively. In patients with AFRS, there is a focus on removing all traces of fungal mucin in addition to widely opening the sinuses. In patients with CCAD, surgery of the central compartment is undertaken. In patients with early CCAD without involvement of the sinus this may be the full extent of surgery. In longer-standing disease, if sinus inflammation or opacification is present, the sinuses should be opened. Postoperatively, these patients are treated with topical corticosteroid irrigations and allergen immunotherapy (AIT).

There have been a limited number of studies of AIT in allergy-driven subtypes of CRS, and all studies were in AFRS. A review by Gan et al. found that AIT in AFRS potentially reduces mucosal inflammation and the need for topical and systemic corticosteroids. This evidence was of relatively low quality (level C), but AIT was determined to be an optional adjuvant therapy along with corticosteroids [43]. At the time of this writing, no studies have been completed to assess the role of AIT in CCAD. However, AIT has been widely and rigorously studied in patients with AR and been found to significantly reduce inflammation and symptoms on exposure to aeroallergens [15]. In light of these findings and in conjunction with those in AFRS, AIT may serve as an adjunct, particularly in the postoperative setting in patients with CCAD. Regardless, maintenance of therapies designed to limit inflammation is essential, as opening the affected sinuses could in theory expose previously allergen-naive mucosa to a greater burden of environmental allergens and lead to new or recurrent disease [33].

Adjuncts in AERD

In patients with AERD, the goals of surgical therapy are similar to those in AFRS with widely opened sinuses allowing for dispersion of topical corticosteroid irrigations post-operatively and conservative sculpting of the middle turbinates. In some instances, and particularly in recurrent AERD with central compartment involvement, a Draf 2b or Draf 3 procedure may be a helpful adjunct to clear the frontal sinus disease and central compartment polyps, including the polyp-bearing upper nasal septum. This provides improved access for topical therapy to this portion of the central compartment and the frontal sinuses. Additionally, due to the role of COX-1 inhibitor hypersensitivity, aspirin desensitization therapy may also be considered. Similar to aspirin challenge, aspirin desensitization should only be performed by experienced practitioners in an appropriate setting. Due to the resources required, aspirin challenge and desensitization are frequently performed at the same encounter. In addition, dietary salicylate avoidance and leukotriene-modifying medications may also be utilized [36, 38].

Monoclonal Antibody Therapies

In June 2019, dupilumab became the first monoclonal antibody (mAb) therapy approved for the treatment of CRSwNP. With several more mAb therapies under development, the study of these therapies in allergy-driven subtypes of CRSwNP is already beginning. Dupilumab blocks the IL-4 receptor α, which is bound by the two Th2 cytokines, IL-4 and IL-13. In a phase III randomized, double-blind, placebo-controlled trial (RDBPCT), dupilumab led to improvement in subjects' Lund-Mackay score by up to 7.44 and 22-item Sino-Nasal Outcome Test (SNOT-22) score by up to 21.12 after 24 weeks of treatment as compared to subjects taking a placebo [44]. With the Minimal Clinically Important Difference (MCID) of the SNOT-22 at 8.9 [45], treatment with dupliumab led to clinically significant improvements in symptoms in this population.

Omalizumab, an anti-IgE antibody, has been approved for the treatment of refractory allergen-exacerbated asthma and chronic urticaria. A small RDBPCT of omalizumab in 24 subjects with asthma and a diagnosis of CRSwNP by Gevaert et al. has been completed. This study included patients with both positive (n = 13) and negative (n = 11) allergy skin testing. Supporting the argument that AR is involved in the pathophysiology of CRSwNP, only patients with positive allergen sensitivity had significant improvements in Lund-Mackay score and polyp size [46]. These studies highlight a fundamental challenge of biologics, however. In the case of dupilumab, post-treatment SNOT-22 scores of 18.58 to 23.89 would still stratify patients into moderate CRS with 95% of patients responding that their quality of life is impacted [47]. While biologic therapies produce clinically significant results, surgical intervention and traditional medical management cannot be abandoned.

Example Case

A 71-year-old woman presented for evaluation of chronic nasal obstruction. She endorsed associated anosmia, thick nasal drainage, facial pressure, and hyponasal voice. She described these symptoms as existing for much of her life. She reported prior treatment for sinusitis with corticosteroid nasal spray and occasional oral corticosteroids which partially improved her symptoms. Since moving to the southeastern US, she noted worsening of her symptoms. A CT scan of her sinuses had been obtained about 6 years prior. She was told this did not show sinus disease at that time. She also endorsed symptoms of sneezing and thin rhinorrhea throughout the year but worse in the spring. She had been diagnosed with AR previously and had used oral antihistamines on-and-off for several years but not recently. She had allergy testing several times in the past and reported being most allergic to trees. She had undergone allergen immunotherapy 6 years previously but did not feel it was beneficial. She did not have any history of asthma or aspirin sensitivity. She had no history of sinus or nasal surgery. Her SNOT-22 score was 57.

Rigid nasal endoscopy showed large, obstructive polyps bilaterally, Fig. 29.1a. Initially, based on these findings, this appeared consistent with CRSwNP-NOS. However, a non-contrast CT scan of the sinuses was obtained which showed diffuse polypoid tissue throughout the nasal cavity and asymmetric, right worse than left, mucosal thickening of the medial aspect of the maxillary sinuses with peripheral clearing, Fig. 29.2. Allergy testing was performed using the modified quantitative testing (MQT) method [48]. She was sensitive to numerous perennial and seasonal allergens, Table 29.1. Based on endoscopy and imaging findings, she was diag-

Table 29.1 Modified quantitative allergy testing result for the patient in Figs. 29.1, 29.2, and 29.3

Panel A					**Panel C**				
Site: Right upper forearm					**Site: Left upper forearm**				
	P	**#5**	**#2**	**EP**		**P**	**#5**	**#2**	**EP**
1. Histamine (+ control)	7	–	–	**–**	1. Bahia	7	4	–	**4**
2. Mite, D.P.	13	–	–	**6**	2. English plantain	0	–	7	**3**
3. Mite, D.F.	13	–	–	**6**	3. Lamb's quarters	0	–	7	**3**
4. Alternaria	0	–	7	**3**	4. Birch	5	4	–	**4**
5. Aspergillus	6	6	–	**4**	5. White ash	5	4	–	**4**
6. Cat	5	4	–	**4**	6. E. Cottonwood	0	–	4	**NEG**
7. Dog	0	–	5	**NEG**	7. American elm	5	4	–	**4**
8. Glycerin (– control)	0	–	–	**–**	8. Red maple	0	–	8	**3**
Panel B					**Panel D**				
Site: Right lower forearm					**Site: Left lower forearm**				
	P	**#5**	**#2**	**EP**		**P**	**#5**	**#2**	**EP**
1. Cockroach	6	4	–	**4**	1. Cladosporium	0	–	5	**NEG**
2. Bermuda grass	5	4	–	**4**	2. B. Sorokiniana	0	–	7	**3**
3. Timothy grass	6	5	–	**4**	3. Penicillium	0	–	5	**NEG**
4. Oak, White	5	5	–	**4**	4. Mouse	0	–	5	**NEG**
5. Pecan, pollen	0	–	6	**NEG**	5. Histamine (+ Conf ctrl)	0	–	–	**–**
6. Red cedar	0	–	5	**NEG**	6. Mixed feathers	0	–	5	**NEG**
7. Short ragweed	0	–	5	**NEG**	7. Epicoccum	0	–	5	**NEG**
8. Rough pigweed	0	–	6	**NEG**					

Allergy skin testing endpoints (EP) by this method range from 0 (negative; NEG) to 6 (maximum positive reactivity)

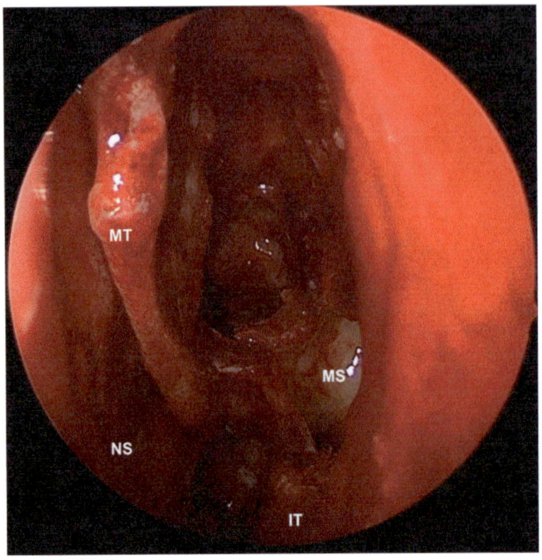

Fig. 29.3 Rigid nasal endoscopy of the left nasal cavity of the patient in Figs. 29.1 and 29.2 at the conclusion of surgery illustrating a sculpted middle turbinate (MT) and widely patent maxillary sinus (MS) with no evidence of gross mucosal inflammation. *NS* nasal septum, *IT* inferior turbinate

nosed with CCAD. As she had previously failed medical management, functional endoscopic sinus surgery was recommended which she elected to pursue.

Intraoperatively, the polyps were traced to their origin and were noted to be emanating from the middle turbinate, Fig. 29.1b, confirming CCAD. The polyps were removed and the polypoid middle turbinates were sculpted but largely preserved. Due to the inflammation noted on preoperative imaging, the sinuses were opened, Fig. 29.3. After surgical intervention, she was started on high-volume topical budesonide irrigations as well as AIT to reduce sinonasal inflammation. Her symptoms improved significantly with a SNOT-22 score of 5 at 2 months post-operatively. Long-term follow-up results are pending.

Conclusion

This chapter explores the relationship between AR and CRS. It is evident that while CRS broadly may not be associated with AR there are certain CRS subtypes where allergy is prominent. Chronic inflammation underpins all forms of CRS. Allergy-mediated inflammation may be the driving force for the development of AFRS and CCAD. Additionally, allergy may be a mitigating factory in AERD and even REAH. Additional study is needed to further clarify the specific subtypes of CRS and their association with allergy.

Financial Disclosures

- Edwards: None.
- Helman: None.
- DelGaudio: Medtronic (consultant), ProDex (consultant), IntersectENT (stockholder).

References

1. Orlandi RR, Kingdom TT, Hwang PH, Smith TL, Alt JA, Baroody FM, et al. International consensus statement on allergy and rhinology: rhinosinusitis. Int Forum Allergy Rhinol. 2016;6(Suppl 1):S22–209.
2. DeConde AS, Soler ZM. Chronic rhinosinusitis: epidemiology and burden of disease. Am J Rhinol Allergy. 2016;30(2):134–9.
3. Bhattacharyya N, Villeneuve S, Joish VN, Amand C, Mannent L, Amin N, et al. Cost burden and resource utilization in patients with chronic rhinosinusitis and nasal polyps. Laryngoscope. 2019;
4. Fokkens WJ, Lund VJ, Mullol J, Bachert C, Alobid I, Baroody F, et al. EPOS 2012: European position paper on rhinosinusitis and nasal polyps 2012. A summary for otorhinolaryngologists. Rhinology. 2012;50(1):1–12.
5. Hastan D, Fokkens WJ, Bachert C, Newson RB, Bislimovska J, Bockelbrink A, et al. Chronic rhinosinusitis in Europe–an underestimated disease. A GA(2)LEN study. Allergy. 2011;66(9):1216–23.
6. Blackwell DL, Lucas JW, Clarke TC. Summary health statistics for U.S. adults: national health interview survey, 2012. Vital Health Stat. 2014;10(260):1–161.
7. Flint PW, Haughey BH, Lund V, Niparko JK, Robbins KT, Thomas JR, et al. Cummings otolaryngology–head & neck surgery. 6th ed. Philadelphia: Elsevier/Saunders; 2015.
8. Van Zele T, Claeys S, Gevaert P, Van Maele G, Holtappels G, Van Cauwenberge P, et al. Differentiation of chronic sinus diseases by measurement of inflammatory mediators. Allergy. 2006;61(11):1280–9.
9. Zhang Y, Gevaert E, Lou H, Wang X, Zhang L, Bachert C, et al. Chronic rhinosinusitis in Asia. J Allergy Clin Immunol. 2017;140(5):1230–9.
10. Tan BK, Klingler AI, Poposki JA, Stevens WW, Peters AT, Suh LA, et al. Heterogeneous inflammatory patterns in chronic rhinosinusitis without nasal polyps in Chicago, Illinois. J Allergy Clin Immunol. 2017;139(2):699–703 e7.

11. Tomassen P, Vandeplas G, Van Zele T, Cardell LO, Arebro J, Olze H, et al. Inflammatory endotypes of chronic rhinosinusitis based on cluster analysis of biomarkers. J Allergy Clin Immunol. 2016;137(5):1449–56 e4.
12. Gurrola J 2nd, Borish L. Chronic rhinosinusitis: endotypes, biomarkers, and treatment response. J Allergy Clin Immunol. 2017;140(6):1499–508.
13. Wang X, Zhang N, Bo M, Holtappels G, Zheng M, Lou H, et al. Diversity of TH cytokine profiles in patients with chronic rhinosinusitis: a multicenter study in Europe, Asia, and Oceania. J Allergy Clin Immunol. 2016;138(5):1344–53.
14. Rosenwasser LJ. Current understanding of the pathophysiology of allergic rhinitis. Immunol Allergy Clin N Am. 2011;31(3):433–9.
15. Wise SK, Lin SY, Toskala E, Orlandi RR, Akdis CA, Alt JA, et al. International consensus statement on allergy and rhinology: allergic rhinitis. Int Forum Allergy Rhinol. 2018;8(2):108–352.
16. Kennedy JL, Borish L. Chronic sinusitis pathophysiology: the role of allergy. Am J Rhinol Allergy. 2013;27(5):367–71.
17. Blair C, Nelson M, Thompson K, Boonlayangoor S, Haney L, Gabr U, et al. Allergic inflammation enhances bacterial sinusitis in mice. J Allergy Clin Immunol. 2001;108(3):424–9.
18. Adkins TN, Goodgold HM, Hendershott L, Slavin RG. Does inhaled pollen enter the sinus cavities? Ann Allergy Asthma Immunol. 1998;81(2):181–4.
19. Baroody FM, Mucha SM, Detineo M, Naclerio RM. Nasal challenge with allergen leads to maxillary sinus inflammation. J Allergy Clin Immunol. 2008;121(5):1126–32 e7.
20. Keith PK, Conway M, Evans S, Wong DA, Jordana G, Pengelly D, et al. Nasal polyps: effects of seasonal allergen exposure. J Allergy Clin Immunol. 1994;93(3):567–74.
21. Tan BK, Zirkle W, Chandra RK, Lin D, Conley DB, Peters AT, et al. Atopic profile of patients failing medical therapy for chronic rhinosinusitis. Int Forum Allergy Rhinol. 2011;1(2):88–94.
22. Robinson S, Douglas R, Wormald PJ. The relationship between atopy and chronic rhinosinusitis. Am J Rhinol. 2006;20(6):625–8.
23. Wilson KF, McMains KC, Orlandi RR. The association between allergy and chronic rhinosinusitis with and without nasal polyps: an evidence-based review with recommendations. Int Forum Allergy Rhinol. 2014;4(2):93–103.
24. Bent JP 3rd, Kuhn FA. Diagnosis of allergic fungal sinusitis. Otolaryngol Head Neck Surg. 1994;111(5):580–8.
25. Marcus S, Roland LT, DelGaudio JM, Wise SK. The relationship between allergy and chronic rhinosinusitis. Laryngoscope Investig Otolaryngol. 2019;4(1):13–7.
26. Wise SK, Ahn CN, Lathers DM, Mulligan RM, Schlosser RJ. Antigen-specific IgE in sinus mucosa of allergic fungal rhinosinusitis patients. Am J Rhinol. 2008;22(5):451–6.
27. Collins M, Nair S, Smith W, Kette F, Gillis D, Wormald PJ. Role of local immunoglobulin E production in the pathophysiology of noninvasive fungal sinusitis. Laryngoscope. 2004;114(7):1242–6.
28. Wise SK, Ahn CN, Schlosser RJ. Localized immunoglobulin E expression in allergic rhinitis and nasal polyposis. Curr Opin Otolaryngol Head Neck Surg. 2009;17(3):216–22.
29. Powe DG, Jagger C, Kleinjan A, Carney AS, Jenkins D, Jones NS. 'Entopy': localized mucosal allergic disease in the absence of systemic responses for atopy. Clin Exp Allergy. 2003;33(10):1374–9.
30. White LJ, Rotella MR, DelGaudio JM. Polypoid changes of the middle turbinate as an indicator of atopic disease. Int Forum Allergy Rhinol. 2014;4(5):376–80.
31. Hamizan AW, Christensen JM, Ebenzer J, Oakley G, Tattersall J, Sacks R, et al. Middle turbinate edema as a diagnostic marker of inhalant allergy. Int Forum Allergy Rhinol. 2017;7(1):37–42.
32. Brunner JP, Jawad BA, McCoul ED. Polypoid change of the middle turbinate and paranasal sinus polyposis are distinct entities. Otolaryngol Head Neck Surg. 2017;157(3):519–23.
33. DelGaudio JM, Loftus PA, Hamizan AW, Harvey RJ, Wise SK. Central compartment atopic disease. Am J Rhinol Allergy. 2017;31(4):228–34.
34. Zhao K, Jiang J. What is normal nasal airflow? A computational study of 22 healthy adults. Int Forum Allergy Rhinol. 2014;4(6):435–46.
35. Hamizan AW, Loftus PA, Alvarado R, Ho J, Kalish L, Sacks R, et al. Allergic phenotype of chronic rhinosinusitis based on radiologic pattern of disease. Laryngoscope. 2018;128(9):2015–21.
36. White AA, Stevenson DD. Aspirin-exacerbated respiratory disease. N Engl J Med. 2018;379(11):1060–70.
37. Ta V, White AA. Survey-defined patient experiences with aspirin-exacerbated respiratory disease. J Allergy Clin Immunol Pract. 2015;3(5):711–8.
38. Levy JM, Rudmik L, Peters AT, Wise SK, Rotenberg BW, Smith TL. Contemporary management of chronic rhinosinusitis with nasal polyposis in aspirin-exacerbated respiratory disease: an evidence-based review with recommendations. Int Forum Allergy Rhinol. 2016;6(12):1273–83.
39. DelGaudio JM, Levy JM, Wise SK. Central compartment involvement in aspirin-exacerbated respiratory disease: the role of allergy and previous sinus surgery. Int Forum Allergy Rhinol. 2019;9(9):1017–22.
40. Schertzer JS, Levy JM, Wise SK, Magliocca KR, DelGaudio JM. Is respiratory epithelial adenomatoid hamartoma related to central compartment atopic disease? Am J Rhinol Allergy. 2020;1945892420914212
41. Marcus S, Schertzer J, Roland LT, Wise SK, Levy JM, DelGaudio JM. Central compartment atopic disease: prevalence of allergy and asthma compared with other subtypes of chronic rhinosinusitis with nasal polyps. Int Forum Allergy Rhinol. 2019;
42. Macy E, Bernstein JA, Castells MC, Gawchik SM, Lee TH, Settipane RA, et al. Aspirin challenge and

desensitization for aspirin-exacerbated respiratory disease: a practice paper. Ann Allergy Asthma Immunol. 2007;98(2):172–4.
43. Gan EC, Thamboo A, Rudmik L, Hwang PH, Ferguson BJ, Javer AR. Medical management of allergic fungal rhinosinusitis following endoscopic sinus surgery: an evidence-based review and recommendations. Int Forum Allergy Rhinol. 2014;4(9):702–15.
44. Bachert C, Han JK, Desrosiers M, Hellings PW, Amin N, Lee SE, et al. Efficacy and safety of dupilumab in patients with severe chronic rhinosinusitis with nasal polyps (LIBERTY NP SINUS-24 and LIBERTY NP SINUS-52): results from two multicentre, randomised, double-blind, placebo-controlled, parallel-group phase 3 trials. Lancet. 2019;394(10209):1638–50.
45. Hopkins C, Gillett S, Slack R, Lund VJ, Browne JP. Psychometric validity of the 22-item sinonasal outcome test. Clin Otolaryngol. 2009;34(5):447–54.
46. Gevaert P, Calus L, Van Zele T, Blomme K, De Ruyck N, Bauters W, et al. Omalizumab is effective in allergic and nonallergic patients with nasal polyps and asthma. J Allergy Clin Immunol. 2013;131(1):110–6 e1.
47. Toma S, Hopkins C. Stratification of SNOT-22 scores into mild, moderate or severe and relationship with other subjective instruments. Rhinology. 2016;54(2):129–33.
48. Marple BF, Mabry RL. Quantitative skin testing for allergy : IDT and MQT. New York: Thieme Medical Publishers; 2006. xiv, 113 p.

Aspirin-Exacerbated Respiratory Disease

30

Mark Arnold and Joshua M. Levy

Introduction

Aspirin-exacerbated respiratory disease (AERD), NSAID-exacerbated respiratory disease, or Samter's triad, is a progressive inflammatory disease defined clinically by a triad of asthma, chronic rhinosinusitis with nasal polyposis (CRSwNP), and sensitivity to aspirin and other COX-1 inhibiting nonsteroidal anti-inflammatory drugs (NSAID). These patients have a characteristic anaphylactoid reaction following aspirin or NSAID ingestion, with systemic symptoms involving multiple organ systems, including the upper and lower airways. This reaction may be tested as part of an aspirin provocation challenge, currently considered the gold standard in diagnosis. However, in clinical practice, aspirin provocation challenges are not consistently performed, potentially resulting in under-diagnosis. With a unique patient population, diagnostic workup, and complementary medical and surgical treatment options, this disease remains challenging to control. However, the increased recognition and prudent use of emerging therapies, such as aspirin desensitization and biologic therapies, offer hope for improved patient outcomes and disease control.

Prevalence

With substantial reliance on self-reported symptoms and a lack of in vitro testing, the prevalence of AERD is difficult to determine. Furthermore, aspirin provocation challenge is not routinely performed in prevalence studies [1]. However, AERD is thought to affect 8–26% of patients with CRSwNP [2]. In one study, 80 patients with nasal polyposis were recruited prospectively for oral aspirin challenge, and 48% subsequently had a positive test. Yet two-thirds of these patients denied any history of NSAID hypersensitivity and were felt to be "aspirin tolerant" prior to the positive test [2]. This group of patients, who do not identify aspirin sensitivity prior to a formal challenge likely, represent a significant population that are under-diagnosed and under-treated. In a 2017 study, Cahill et al. developed an informatics algorithm to identify patients meeting criteria for suspected AERD with asthma, nasal polyps, and reactions to NSAIDs. 12% of these patients lacked a diagnosis of AERD and had not been referred for formal diagnostic testing with

M. Arnold
Department of Otolaryngology at Upstate Medical University, Syracuse, NY, USA
e-mail: arnoldm@upstate.edu

J. M. Levy (✉)
Department of Otolaryngology-Head and Neck Surgery, Emory University School of Medicine, Atlanta, GA, USA
e-mail: joshua.levy2@emory.edu

C. Damask et al. (eds.), *Allergy in Otolaryngology Practice*,
https://doi.org/10.1007/978-3-031-93455-1_30

aspirin provocation [3]. This group of patients were also less likely to have been seen by an allergist or immunologist [3].

The median age of onset of AERD is around 30 years [4]. It is also suspected that the prevalence and severity of AERD is higher among women. The underlying mechanism for this unexpected finding is felt to be secondary to elevated expression of COX-1 in men [2]. Patients with asthma also have higher rates of AERD, likely from a shared underlying pathophysiology. In a recent meta-analysis, 7.2% of asthmatics had AERD [5]. Moreover, this prevalence doubles to 14.9% in patients with severe asthma [5].

AERD represents a notable healthcare burden in the United States, with an annual expenditure estimated to be over 4.5 billion dollars [2]. This group represents over two million people living in the United States [2]. Under-diagnosis and inadequate treatment outcomes lead to the high healthcare expenditures associated with this chronic disease.

Pathophysiology

Role of Arachidonic Acid Metabolism

The characteristic symptomatology of aspirin ingestion followed by bronchospasm, rhinitis, and urticaria is well described, yet the underlying pathophysiology of AERD is relatively unknown. However, arachidonic acid has been felt to be the key mediator of the disease [6]. Arachidonic acid serves as the building block of both pro-inflammatory leukotrienes and anti-inflammatory prostaglandins. Under physiologic conditions, these powerful inflammatory mediators are kept in careful balance. However, this metabolism is characteristically dysregulated in AERD (Fig. 30.1). At baseline, decreased levels of both COX-2 and prostaglandin (PG) E2 synthase result in partial shunting of arachidonic acid away from PG pathways with an associated reliance on COX-1 to maintain their production. The result is decreased baseline levels of anti-inflammatory PGE2, and an abundance of pro-inflammatory cysteinyl leukotrienes. Should patients take a COX-1 inhibitor, the arachidonic acid pathway is further shunted toward pro-inflammatory leukotrienes, resulting in acute symptoms.

In a 1991 study, urinary leukotriene levels were compared between asthmatics with and without comorbid aspirin intolerance. Christie et al. found that levels of urinary leukotriene E4 (uLTE4) had a sixfold increase in AERD versus aspirin-tolerant asthma [6]. Furthermore, they found a fourfold increase in uLTE4 following aspirin ingestion.

Mast Cell Activation

In addition to the role of dysregulated arachidonic acid metabolism, mast cell activation has also been implicated in the pathophysiology of AERD. In 2019, Cahill et al. evaluated markers of mast cell activation in AERD subjects undergoing aspirin provocation challenge. Of 39 subjects, half demonstrated mast cell activation, with a corresponding 10% rise in serum tryptase. This elevation in serum tryptase inversely correlated with FEV_1, associating mast cell activation to bronchoconstriction caused by released mediators including PGD_2.

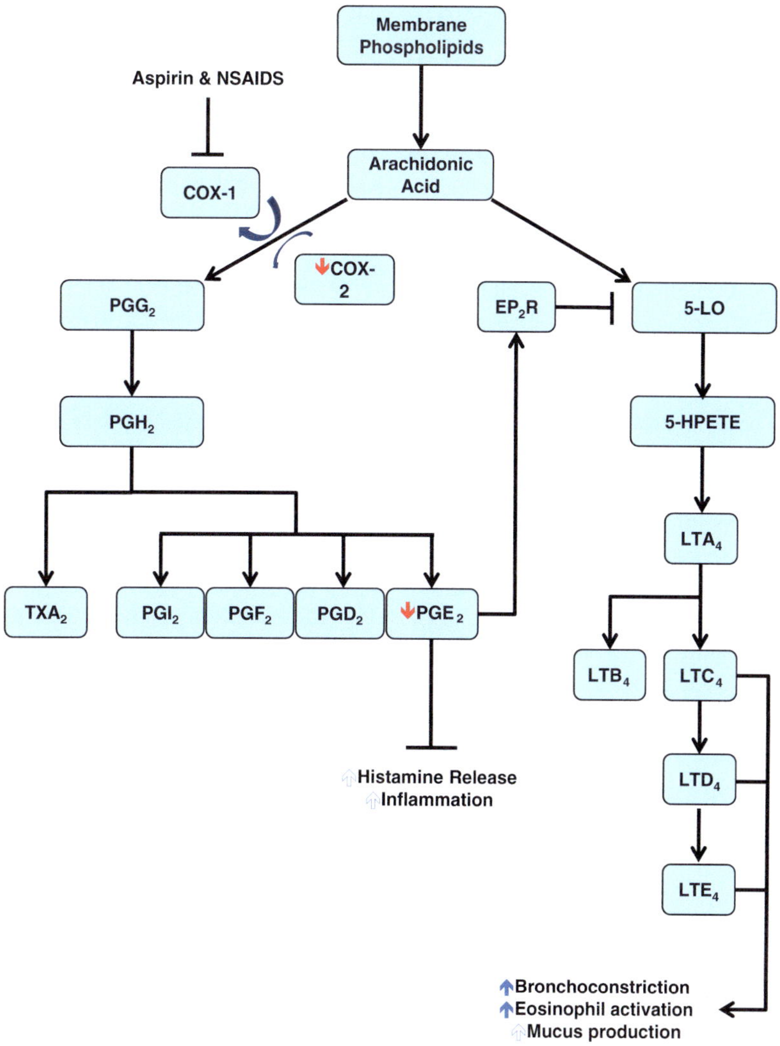

Fig. 30.1 Arachidonic acid pathway in AERD. In patients with AERD, there is decreased baseline expression of COX-2 and PGE_2 (red arrows). With aspirin and other NSAID ingestion, there is inhibition of COX-1, resulting in further decreased levels of PGE_2, histamine release, and disinhibition of the lipoxygenase pathway. This results in bronchoconstriction and mucus hypersecretion (blue arrows). COX denotes cyclooxygenase [1, 2], 5-HPETE 5-hydroperoxyeicosatetraenoic acid, 5-LO 5-lipoxygenase, LT leukotriene (A_4, B_4, C_4, D_4, and E_4), NSAID nonsteroidal anti-inflammatory drug, PG prostaglandin (D_2, E_2, F_2, G_2, H_2, I_2), EP_2R prostaglandin E_2 receptor, and TXA_2 thromboxane A_2

Diagnosis

Clinical Presentation

While AERD may have a "classic" triad of asthma, nasal polyps, and aspirin sensitivity, the presentation varies. Typically, symptoms are non-specific [1]. Upper airway involvement includes congestion, rhinorrhea, sneezing, and evidence of nasal polyps on nasal examination, while lower airway symptoms present with laryngospasm, cough, or wheezing. In addition, patients may have other symptoms of systemic inflammation. Gastrointestinal involvement includes abdominal pain and nausea, and cutaneous manifestations may occur with flushing and urticaria [1]. These symptoms may be present at baseline, but characteristically flare with certain triggers including aspirin, NSAIDS, or alcohol.

Nearly all patients with AERD present with nasal polyposis (Fig. 30.2) [2, 7]. Patients with AERD may be initially misdiagnosed as AFRS, as tenacious eosinophilic mucin is associated with both conditions.

Despite the anaphylactoid attacks characteristic of AERD, this disease is not caused by classic IgE-mediated atopic reactions. Interestingly, patients often display a progression of symptoms, akin to an "allergic march" [8]. Although concomitant IgE-mediated disease is found in up to two-thirds of patients with AERD, a classic type I IgE-mediated hypersensitivity reaction is not thought to be causative of the acute symptom flares in AERD [2].

If there is suspicion for AERD, it is paramount that the history includes sensitivity to aspirin and NSAIDS. However, 15% of AERD patients are unable to identify if they are sensitive to these medications [4]. Furthermore, in patients with CRSwNP and asthma, AERD should not be ruled out if they take aspirin. In a cohort of 163, seven patients (4.2%) were found to tolerate a low dose of 81 mg of aspirin prior to a formal positive aspirin provocation challenge [9]. The underlying pathophysiology may be due to a threshold dose necessary for a clinical reaction [10]. Given this potential diagnostic dilemma with aspirin provocation challenge, it is reasonable to consider a history of two symptomatic reactions to NSAIDs sufficient to make a clinical diagnosis [7].

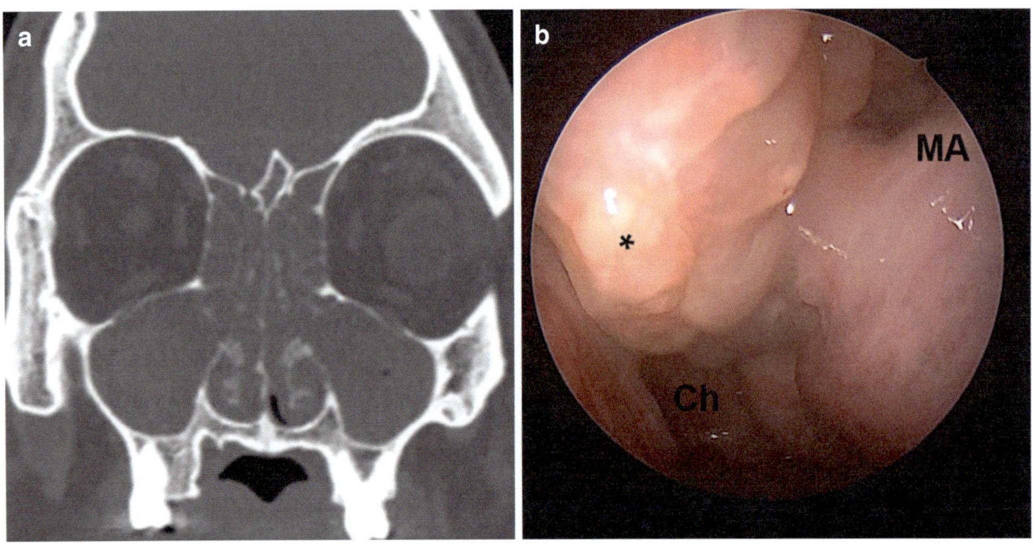

Fig. 30.2 Nasal polyps in AERD. Diffuse sinonasal inflammation with obstructive nasal polyps (*) and eosinophilic mucin is often found in AERD. (**a**) Characteristic coronal CT and (**b**) nasal endoscopic findings in the left nare following postoperative disease recurrence. *Ch* Choana, *MA* Maxillary antrostomy

Aspirin Provocation Challenge

The aspirin provocation challenge defines the diagnosis of AERD. While monitoring for anaphylaxis, the challenge is considered positive if FEV_1 decreases by over 15%. Historically, the challenge was performed in the ICU setting, but this is no longer necessary. Furthermore, the test can be immediately followed with aspirin desensitization. Patients should not be offered the test if FEV_1 is less than 75%, or if they have a history of a severe reaction or anaphylaxis to aspirin.

While the aspirin provocation challenge is the gold standard, unfortunately it is not widely utilized. In a survey of the American Academy of Allergy, Asthma & Immunology (AAAAI), 37.5% of respondents did not offer aspirin challenge [11]. Furthermore, 28.2% did not refer patients suspected to have AERD to a provider who would offer the test. Furthermore, a recent analysis of a national insurance claims database found that among patients with AERD, there exist significant geographic disparities in areas that offer aspirin desensitization. Of 5628 patients meeting clinical criteria for AERD between 2009 and 2015, only 7% underwent diagnostic aspirin challenge [8]. Furthermore, desensitization occurred in limited geographic areas in the United States, contributing to the low overall rates of desensitization.

Smoking Cessation and Alcohol Sensitivity

Interestingly, smoking cessation may precede the onset of symptoms associated with AERD. In a cohort study of 114 patients, smoking cessation was associated with an increased odds ratio of 4.63 for the development of AERD symptoms versus patients with aspirin-tolerant asthma [12]. Smoking is felt to be pro-inflammatory, resulting in increase in COX-2 expression that potentially compensates for the decreased baseline expression characteristic of AERD.

Conversely, patients with AERD often demonstrate alcohol sensitivity. The mechanism is largely unknown, but up to 75% of patients with AERD demonstrate upper airway symptoms (rhinorrhea, sneezing, nasal congestion) with alcohol ingestion [13]. Furthermore, these reactions were not specific to a type nor an amount of alcohol ingested [13]. However, these findings can be non-specific, as up to 30% of patients with aspirin-tolerant asthma also have a similar sensitivity to alcohol. Curiously, patients can tolerate more alcohol after aspirin desensitization [14]. This finding is clinically relevant, and may be a motivating factor for some to pursue desensitization to improve their ability to socialize in certain settings.

Treatment

The treatment of AERD is multi-disciplinary and depends on patient factors including the severity of the disease. At varying points throughout their treatment, patients with AERD may require coordinated care from a pulmonologist, allergist, and an otolaryngologist.

Avoidance

In patients with nasal polyps and asthma, any history of reaction to aspirin or other NSAIDs should prompt avoidance of all NSAIDs, especially those with inhibition of COX-1 activity [15]. However, baseline symptoms of AERD tend to be progressive independent of NSAID ingestion. Dietary non-acetylated salicylates may represent an underappreciated exposure. The first randomized trials by Sommer et al. evaluated the efficacy of a low salicylate diet for the control of respiratory and sinonasal symptoms in AERD, with the hypothesis that dietary sources of COX-inhibiting salicylates, such as leafy greens and dried fruits, among many others, may contribute to chronic symptoms in AERD [16, 17]. They reported improvement in mean SNOT-22 and objective Lund-Kennedy endoscopic scores. Additional study is needed to explore these early findings.

Medical Management: Topical and Oral Therapies

Recommended first-line therapies for AERD are the same as for nasal polyps and/or asthma without aspirin sensitivity. Primary asthma therapies include inhaled corticosteroids and beta-agonists [18]. Primary CRSwNP therapies include topical nasal saline and intranasal corticosteroids. While not specific to AERD, topical corticosteroids as a maintenance therapy have been well studied in CRSwNP, and are recommended before or after sinus surgery [19]. Multiple preparations are available and are equally effective, including fluticasone propionate, mometasone, and budesonide [19]. Systemic corticosteroids may also be used as needed for either condition. Leukotriene modifying drugs (LTMDs) represent a cogent option in the treatment of AERD as they inhibit the cysteinyl leukotriene mediators and/or receptors that drive this disease. Two currently available drugs montelukast and zileuton, and randomized trials have demonstrated that both result in improved sinonasal symptoms [20, 21]. As an added benefit, premedication with LTMDs improves safety during aspirin provocation challenge without leading to false-negative results [22]. However, there are also known side effects. Montelukast carries a risk of mental health side effects, including complete suicide [23]. Zileuton, on the other hand, has a risk of self-limited hepatotoxicity that requires liver function monitoring during therapy [24].

Medical Management: Aspirin Desensitization

Aspirin desensitization is the only disease-specific therapy currently offered for AERD. This procedure immediately follows a diagnostic challenge and requires daily administration of oral aspirin to maintain a desensitized state. New exposures after missing aspirin for as few as 1–2 days may lead to a life-threatening reaction [25]. Unlike desensitization for a classic, type-I IgE-mediated hypersensitivity reaction, the mechanism for aspirin desensitization is currently unknown [26].

The benefits of aspirin desensitization have been demonstrated in several randomized, double-blinded, placebo-controlled studies [27–31]. In 2013, Comert and colleagues followed 40 patients with AERD who were desensitized and maintained on 300 mg a day of aspirin. They found utilization of systemic corticosteroids, incidence of sinusitis, and endoscopic sinus surgery was decreased at both 1 and 3 years versus patients without desensitization [27]. A randomized controlled trial in 2015 followed 34 patients, with the randomized group undergoing aspirin desensitization followed by 625 mg twice daily [28]. Compared to placebo, symptom scores and medication needs in the aspirin group were significantly lower at 6 months. Also, objective measure of pulmonary function, forced expiratory volume in 1 s (FEV_1), was higher in the aspirin group. Interestingly, serum levels of IL-10, TGF-β, and IFN-γ did not vary between treatment arms, suggesting either the involvement of other inflammatory cytokines or local variation of these inflammatory mediators.

In 2013, Fruth and colleagues evaluated the efficacy of 100 mg low-dose daily aspirin as maintenance therapy following desensitization [29]. After surgery, 70 individuals were randomized to 100 mg a day or placebo. Although there was a high dropout rate of the 31 individuals, the patients in the aspirin group showed decreased polyp scores on nasal endoscopy, increased quality of life scores, and a reduction in CRS-related symptoms. Desensitization therapy is also cost-effective. In an analysis of reimbursements of a large Midwestern healthcare plan, desensitization cost $6768 per quality-adjusted life year, or just $18.54 per additional symptom-free day [32].

There are multiple aspirin desensitization protocols that exist, and these vary depending on the region and clinician experience. Usually, these protocols can be initiated immediately following aspirin provocation challenge. Protocols are now more expedient, with several completing in just 24–48 hours. In addition, protocols exist utilizing triggering drugs beyond aspirin. For example, in

Europe, intranasal ketorolac often initiates the challenge, followed by oral aspirin [33, 34]. Several recommended protocols for diagnostic aspirin challenge and desensitization are currently used in clinical practice [35].

The widely used protocol by White and colleagues at the Scripps Clinic in San Diego begins with a first morning of 30-min escalating doses of nasal ketorolac to induce local reactions and desensitization of the entire respiratory tract. Following this are two doses of 60 mg of aspirin at 90-min intervals. Desensitization is achieved the first day, but doses of 150 and 325 mg of aspirin are given the second day to prove protocol completion [25]. Another protocol, developed by Chen et al. at UT Southwestern in 2015, offers even earlier time to desensitization [36]. They successfully treated 56 of 57 patients with hourly dose-escalation. During the morning, escalating doses of aspirin are given each hour (40.5, 81, 120, 162, and finally 325 mg). The afternoon is then reserved for treating any reactions generated during the morning session. The following day, additional doses of 325 mg can be given. Nine of the 57 patients finished the protocol in a single day, as their challenges were negative, while the rest completed on the second day.

In general, the refractory period after aspirin ingestion is 48–72 h. Therefore, brief interruptions in aspirin therapy <48 h are generally tolerated without the need for repeated desensitization. However, if the interruption is ≥48 h, repeat desensitization is recommended [25].

The daily maintenance dose of aspirin varies, but is typically up to 650 mg taken twice daily [30]. In a 2007 study, 137 patients took either 650 mg or 325 mg twice daily, and after 1 month changed their dose based on symptom control and maintained this dosing for 1 year [30]. They found that both dosages were equally efficacious and had similar adverse events, with the most common, at 10%, being dyspepsia. The authors recommended starting at the higher 650 mg twice daily dosing, with consideration of de-escalation to 325 mg twice daily for those with improved symptoms. Additional study is needed to define daily dosage protocols for AERD.

While benefits of maintenance aspirin therapy have been reported, the duration and overall safety of lifelong therapy remains a concern to both clinicians and patients. In 2018, Walters et al. surveyed 92 patients with AERD an average of 15 years following desensitization and daily aspirin therapy [31]. Among this group, 38% reported stopping aspirin therapy. The reasons for discontinuation were split between adverse reactions, lack of clinical benefit, and to allow other surgical procedures. While most adverse reactions were minor, three patients in this group required urgent or emergent evaluation due to gastrointestinal or bleeding side effects associated with aspirin therapy. The other 62% remained on aspirin treatment; with the majority (85%) of patients felt that aspirin desensitization improved their overall quality of life.

Historically, aspirin desensitization was often performed in the ICU. However, the use of premedication increases the safety and utilization of desensitization protocols in the ambulatory setting. Premedication blunts the severity of a diagnostic reaction by pre-emptively treating with leukotriene inhibitors, oral corticosteroids, and other medications [37]. In addition, a full airway and crash cart system is mandatory, with supplies including epinephrine, antihistamines, and an intubation kit. Incentive spirometry is also a necessity to monitor FEV_1 closely. In a review of 210 patients, 90% had naso-ocluar reactions, while 43% had lower airway reactions, all of which were treated with topical and oral medications without complications [38]. In a review of 1400 patients undergoing diagnostic aspirin challenge, three had systemic hypotensive reactions requiring epinephrine [25].

Despite the benefits of aspirin desensitization, not all patients are eligible. Chronic aspirin use is contraindicated in pregnancy, unstable asthma, anticoagulant use, comorbid gastric ulcers, eosinophilic esophagitis, and patients under the age of 14 due to concern for Reye syndrome [1]. Compliance may also be problematic, as patients may discontinue therapy due to dyspepsia, bleeding, or for planned surgeries.

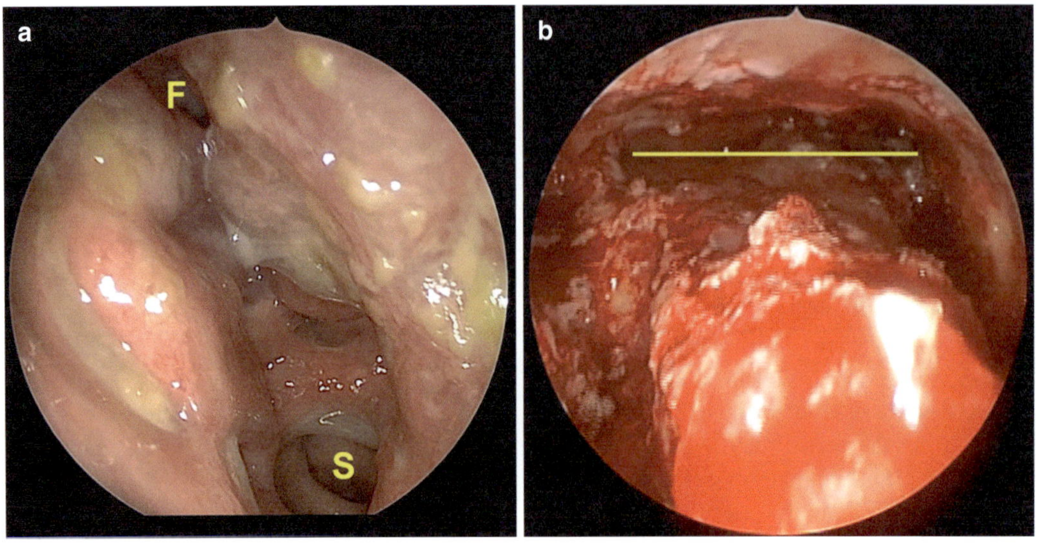

Fig. 30.3 Surgical approach for the management of nasal polyposis in AERD. Extent of surgery for the control of CRSwNP is determined by surgeon preference and patient factors. However, given the high likelihood of disease recurrence is it recommended to consider a "full house" endoscopic sinus surgery with bilateral maxillary antrostomies, sphenoethmoidectomies, and frontal sinusotomies as primary procedures, as well as a Modified Endoscopic Lothrop Procedure for disease recurrence. (**a**) Right post-operative full house cavity with evidence of polypoid inflammation and mucostasis. (**b**) Postoperative Lothrop procedure with frontal neo-ostium (line). *F* Frontal ostium, *S* Sphenoid ostium

Surgical Management: Endoscopic Sinus Surgery

Endoscopic sinus surgery is an important adjunct to appropriate medical therapy for the control of CRSwNP in AERD (Fig. 30.3). Often, treatment requires a strong multi-disciplinary connection between the allergist and surgeon. To reduce the risk of bleeding, aspirin desensitization is recommended to begin shortly after ESS. To avoid the need for repeated desensitization among patients already on daily aspirin, protocols have been developed to decrease daily aspirin prior to surgery.

In a recent study, Jerschow et al. elucidated the synergetic relationship between aspirin desensitization and ESS [39]. In this observational trial, 28 patients with known AERD and prior desensitization underwent elective ESS followed by repeated desensitization 3–4 weeks after surgery. There was a significant decrease in the reaction severity to aspirin after ESS in all patients, with 43% having no clinical reaction to the challenge at all. After ESS, there was also an increase in lipoxin A4, a marker of less severe asthma. Furthermore, urinary leukotriene E4 (uLTE4) and prostaglandin D2 metabolite (PGDM), biomarkers of AERD, also decreased after ESS. These results suggest that the sinonasal polyp load is directly linked to the systemic reaction to aspirin, and a reduction in polyps facilitates a safer aspirin provocation challenge. These findings were subsequently replicated by Huang et al. [40]. These findings highlight the need for a coordinated multi-disciplinary treatment team. The most appropriate timing for a diagnostic aspirin challenge relative to ESS remains unsettled and decided on a local basis [41].

Patients with AERD often have sinonasal disease with a polyp burden that is more severe than other patients with CRSwNP [42, 43]. With extensive disease that is often recalcitrant, it is felt that these patients merit a primary comprehensive ESS to facilitate delivery of topical therapies. While primary Lothrop procedures are not recommended at this time, it remains a topic of debate and regional variation in practice. Morrissey and colleagues followed 31 patients with AERD who had undergone a complete ESS with maxillary antrostomies, sphenoethmoidectomies, and an endoscopic modified Lothrop procedure (EMLP) [44]. Despite this approach, over an average follow-up of 36 months, 58% had polyp recurrence and 22.5% went on to have a revision EMLP. This high revision rate highlights the need to maximize adjunctive medical therapies.

Emerging Therapies: Ifetroban and Role of Biologics

AERD remains a difficult-to-treat disease. However, as insight into the underlying pathophysiology of the disease continues to grow, researchers are seeking out alternative medical therapies. In 2012, Laidlaw et al. examined the polyps of patients with AERD and found a higher proportion of platelet-bound leukocytes [45]. These adherent platelets contributed to more than half of the total LTC_4 synthase activity, and therefore uLTE4. By binding platelets, these leukocytes are hyperproducing leukotrienes, leading to tissue inflammation. Therefore, the PGH2 and thromboxane A2 receptor on platelets could represent novel therapeutic targets. Currently, a phase 2 trial is underway to assess the safety and efficacy of oral Ifetroban, a thromboxane receptor antagonist in patients with AERD.

Over the past few years, humanized monoclonal antibody (i.e., biologic) therapies have begun to play an increasing role in the management of CRSwNP. These drugs act by targeting specific immune cells or inflammatory pathways to modify the course of the disease while maintaining a minimal side effect profile. Many of these biologics began as therapies for other type-2-mediated inflammatory diseases, such as asthma and atopic dermatitis. However, biologics like omalizumab, an anti-IgE antibody, were found to have additional benefits in treating nasal polyps in those patients with concurrent CRSwNP [46].

In a recent clinical trial, dupilumab was shown to reduce polyp size, sinus opacification, and improve symptoms in 143 patients with CRSwNP [47]. The results of this trial led to recent FDA approval for CRSwNP in June of 2019. Dupilumab acts by binding and antagonizing the IL-4α receptor, resulting in reductions of both IL-4 and IL-13. The result is a reduction in the local Th2 pro-inflammatory biomarkers seen in CRSwNP [48].

With the emerging role that biologics play in both CRS and asthma, naturally, AERD investigators are eager to explore these drugs as a treatment for AERD. From a nested analysis of the phase 2 dupilumab study, Laidlaw et al. analyzed a subset of 19 patients with AERD, among the larger cohort of 60 patients [47, 49]. They confirmed that patients with AERD had a more severe disease than the other aspirin tolerant patients with CRSwNP with poorer sense of smell, greater sinus opacification, and poorer baseline lung function. They also found that dupilumab significantly improved CRSwNP disease outcomes in patients with AERD, in addition to improving their asthma control and lung function.

Although there is emerging evidence of the added benefit of biologics in patients with CRSwNP, further studies are necessary. Current trials have yet to examine the specific role of biologics after ESS [46–48, 50, 51]. Instead, ESS was evaluated as an outcome measure between the two randomized treatment arms. Certainly, with the clear benefit of aspirin desensitization after ESS in patients with AERD, the additional role for biologics within this treatment algorithm remains unclear.

Conclusion

With diverse treatment options for an often-recalcitrant disease, it is important for the clinician to formulate a step-wise approach with individualized modifications as necessary. Patients with AERD should be initiated on appropriate medical management with saline irrigations, topical steroids, and possible courses of oral steroids. Should symptoms persist, a comprehensive sinus surgery is warranted with opening of all affected paranasal sinuses. Primary EMLP has been advocated by some, but the true necessity of this is still being evaluated. However, should patients fail an initial full-house ESS, a revision with EMLP may be considered. Postoperative aspirin desensitization may also be offered, especially if the patient has undergone revision sinus surgery. Biologic therapies may also be considered. Dietary modification by reducing dietary salicylic acid intake to 10–20 mg and antileukotrienes are additional considerations for the management of AERD.

References

1. White AA, Stevenson DD. Aspirin-exacerbated respiratory disease. N Engl J Med. 2018;379(11):1060–70.
2. Nabavi M, Esmaeilzadeh H, Arshi S, Bemanian MH, Fallahpour M, Bahrami A, et al. Aspirin hypersensitivity in patients with chronic rhinosinusitis and nasal polyposis: frequency and contributing factors. Am J Rhinol Allergy. 2014;28(3):239–43.
3. Cahill KN, Johns CB, Cui J, Wickner P, Bates DW, Laidlaw TM, et al. Automated identification of an aspirin-exacerbated respiratory disease cohort. J Allergy Clin Immunol. 2017;139(3):819–25.e6.
4. Szczeklik A, Nizankowska E, Duplaga M. Natural history of aspirin-induced asthma. AIANE Investigators. European Network on Aspirin-Induced Asthma. Eur Respir J. 2000;16(3):432–6.
5. Rajan JP, Wineinger NE, Stevenson DD, White AA. Prevalence of aspirin-exacerbated respiratory disease among asthmatic patients: a meta-analysis of the literature. J Allergy Clin Immunol. 2015;135(3):676–81.e1.
6. Christie PE, Tagari P, Ford-Hutchinson AW, Charlesson S, Chee P, Arm JP, et al. Urinary leukotriene E4 concentrations increase after aspirin challenge in aspirin-sensitive asthmatic subjects. Am Rev Respir Dis. 1991;143(5 Pt I):1025–9.
7. Berges-Gimeno MP, Simon RA, Stevenson DD. The natural history and clinical characteristics of aspirin-exacerbated respiratory disease. Ann Allergy Asthma Immunol. 2002;89(5):474–8.
8. Roland LT, Nagy C, Wang H, Moore R, Cahill KN, Laidlaw TM, et al. Treatment practices for aspirin-exacerbated respiratory disease: analysis of a national insurance claims database. Int Forum Allergy Rhinol. 2019;10(2):3–6.
9. Lee-Sarwar K, Johns C, Laidlaw TM, Cahill KN. Tolerance of daily low-dose aspirin does not preclude aspirin-exacerbated respiratory disease. J Allergy Clin Immunol Pract. 2015;3(3):449–51.
10. Hope AP, Woessner KA, Simon RA, Stevenson DD. Rational approach to aspirin dosing during oral challenges and desensitization of patients with aspirin-exacerbated respiratory disease. J Allergy Clin Immunol. 2009;123(2):406–10.
11. Waldram JD, White AA. A survey of aspirin desensitization practices among allergists and fellows in training in the United States. J Allergy Clin Immunol. 2015;135(2):AB113.
12. Hayashi H, Fukutomi Y, Mitsui C, Nakatani E, Watai K, Kamide Y, et al. Smoking cessation as a possible risk factor for the development of aspirin-exacerbated respiratory disease in smokers. J Allergy Clin Immunol Pract. 2018;6(1):116–25.e3.
13. Carlos Cardet J, White AA, Barrett NA, Feldweg AM, Wickner PG, Savage J, et al. Alcohol-induced respiratory symptoms are common in patients with aspirin exacerbated respiratory disease. J Allergy Clin Immunol Pract. 2014;2:208–13.e2.
14. Glicksman JT, Parasher AK, Doghramji L, Brauer D, Waldram J, Walters K, et al. Alcohol-induced respiratory symptoms improve after aspirin desensitization in patients with aspirin-exacerbated respiratory disease. Int Forum Allergy Rhinol. 2018;8(10):1093–7.
15. Kowalski ML, Makowska JS, Blanca M, Bavbek S, Bochenek G, Bousquet J, et al. Hypersensitivity to nonsteroidal anti-inflammatory drugs (NSAIDs) – classification, diagnosis and management: review of the EAACI/ENDA and GA2LEN/HANNA. Allergy. 2011;66:818–29.
16. Sommer DD, Rotenberg BW, Sowerby LJ, Lee JM, Janjua A, Witterick IJ, et al. A novel treatment adjunct for aspirin exacerbated respiratory disease: the low-salicylate diet: a multicenter randomized control crossover trial. Int Forum Allergy Rhinol. 2016;6(4):385–91.
17. Sommer DD, Hoffbauer S, Au M, Sowerby LJ, Gupta MK, Nayan S. Treatment of aspirin exacerbated respiratory disease with a low salicylate diet: a pilot crossover study. Otolaryngol Head Neck Surg (United States). 2015;152(1):42–7.
18. Global Initiative for Asthma. Global strategy for asthma management and prevention; 2019. Available from: www.ginasthma.org
19. Orlandi RR, Kingdom TT, Hwang PH, Smith TL, Alt JA, Baroody FM, et al. International consensus statement on allergy and rhinology: rhinosinusitis. Int Forum Allergy Rhinol. 2016;6:S22–209.
20. Schäper C, Noga O, Koch B, Ewert R, Felix SB, Gläser S, et al. Anti-inflammatory properties of montelukast, a leukotriene receptor antagonist in patients with asthma and nasal polyposis. J Investig Allergol Clin Immunol. 2011;21(1):51–8.
21. Dahlén B, Nizankowska E, Szczeklik A, Zetterström O, Bochenek G, Kumlin M, et al. Benefits from adding the 5-lipoxygenase inhibitor zileuton to conventional therapy in aspirin-intolerant asthmatics. Am J Respir Crit Care Med. 1998;157(4 PART I):1187–94.

22. White AA, Stevenson DD, Simon RA. The blocking effect of essential controller medications during aspirin challenges in patients with aspirin-exacerbated respiratory disease. Ann Allergy Asthma Immunol. 2005;95(4):330–5.
23. FDA requires boxed warning about serious mental health side effects for asthma and allergy drug montelukast (Singulair); advises restricting use for allergic rhinitis Risks may include suicidal thoughts or actions 3-4-2020 FDA Drug Safety Communication.
24. Zileuton. LiverTox: clinical and research information on drug-induced liver injury. Bethesda: National Institute of Diabetes and Digestive and Kidney Diseases; 2012.
25. Lee RU, Stevenson DD. Aspirin-exacerbated respiratory disease: evaluation and management. Allergy Asthma Immunol Res. 2010;3:3–10.
26. Widal F, Abraimi P, Lermoyex J. Anaphylaxie et idiosyncrasie. LA PRESSE MEDICALE 30: 189–193, 1922
27. Comert S, Celebioglu E, Yucel T, Erdogan T, Karakaya G, Onerci M, et al. Aspirin 300 mg/day is effective for treating aspirin-exacerbated respiratory disease. Allergy Eur J Allergy Clin Immunol. 2013;68(11):1443–51.
28. Esmaeilzadeh H, Nabavi M, Aryan Z, Arshi S, Bemanian MH, Fallahpour M, et al. Aspirin desensitization for patients with aspirin-exacerbated respiratory disease: a randomized double-blind placebo-controlled trial. Clin Immunol. 2015;160(2):349–57.
29. Fruth K, Pogorzelski B, Schmidtmann I, Springer J, Fennan N, Fraessdorf N, et al. Low-dose aspirin desensitization in individuals with aspirin-exacerbated respiratory disease. Allergy Eur J Allergy Clin Immunol. 2013;68(5):659–65.
30. Lee JY, Simon RA, Stevenson DD. Selection of aspirin dosages for aspirin desensitization treatment in patients with aspirin-exacerbated respiratory disease. J Allergy Clin Immunol. 2007;119(1):157–64.
31. Walters KM, Waldram JD, Woessner KM, White AA. Long-term clinical outcomes of aspirin desensitization with continuous daily aspirin therapy in aspirin-exacerbated respiratory disease. Am J Rhinol Allergy. 2018;32(4):280–6.
32. Shaker M, Lobb A, Jenkins P, O'Rourke D, Takemoto SK, Sheth S, et al. An economic analysis of aspirin desensitization in aspirin-exacerbated respiratory disease. J Allergy Clin Immunol. 2008;121(1):81–7.
33. Sanchez-Jareño M, Barranco P, Lluch-Bernal M, López-Carrasco V, Quirce S. Nasal challenge with ketorolac: utility and safety in clinical practice. J Allergy Clin Immunol. 2019;143(2):AB283.
34. Lee R, Woessner K, Simon R, Stevenson D. Intranasal ketorolac for desensitization in patients with aspirin exacerbated respiratory disease. J Allergy Clin Immunol. 2008;121(2):S73.
35. Woessner KM, White AA. Evidence-based approach to aspirin desensitization in aspirin-exacerbated respiratory disease. J Allergy Clin Immunol. 2014;133(1):286–7.e1–9. https://doi.org/10.1016/j.jaci.2013.11.016. PMID: 24369807.
36. Chen JR, Buchmiller BL, Khan DA. An hourly dose-escalation desensitization protocol for aspirin-exacerbated respiratory disease. J Allergy Clin Immunol Pract. 2015;3(6):926–31.e1.
37. White AA, Bosso JV, Stevenson DD. The clinical dilemma of "silent desensitization" in aspirin-exacerbated respiratory disease. Allergy Asthma Proc. 2013;34(4):378–82.
38. Williams AN, Simon RA, Woessner KM, Stevenson DD. The relationship between historical aspirin-induced asthma and severity of asthma induced during oral aspirin challenges. J Allergy Clin Immunol. 2007;120(2):273–7.
39. Jerschow E, Edin ML, Chi Y, Hurst B, Abuzeid WM, Akbar NA, et al. Sinus surgery is associated with a decrease in aspirin-induced reaction severity in patients with aspirin exacerbated respiratory disease. J Allergy Clin Immunol Pract. 2019;7(5):1580–8.
40. Huang GX, Palumbo ML, Cahill KN, Laidlaw TM. Nasal sinus surgery improves lower airway reactivity during aspirin desensitization for AERD. J Allergy Clin Immunol [Internet]. 2019;143(2):AB283. Available from: https://doi.org/10.1016/j.jaci.2018.12.866.
41. Mathur SK. Sinus surgery effects on diagnosis and management of patients with AERD. J Allergy Clin Immunol Pract [Internet]. 2019;7(5):1589–90. Available from: https://doi.org/10.1016/j.jaip.2019.03.029.
42. Amar YG, Frenkiel S, Sobol SE. Outcome analysis of endoscopic sinus surgery for chronic sinusitis in patients having Samter's triad. J Otolaryngol. 2000;29(1):7–12.
43. Young J, Frenkiel S, Tewfik MA, Mouadeb DA. Long-term outcome analysis of endoscopic sinus surgery for chronic sinusitis. Am J Rhinol. 2007;21(6):743–7.
44. Morrissey DK, Bassiouni A, Psaltis AJ, Naidoo Y, Wormald PJ. Outcomes of modified endoscopic Lothrop in aspirin-exacerbated respiratory disease with nasal polyposis. Int Forum Allergy Rhinol. 2016;6(8):820–5.
45. Laidlaw TM, Kidder MS, Bhattacharyya N, Xing W, Shen S, Milne GL, et al. Cysteinyl leukotriene overproduction in aspirin-exacerbated respiratory disease is driven by platelet-adherent leukocytes. Blood. 2012;119(16):3790–8.
46. Gevaert P, Calus L, Van Zele T, Blomme K, De Ruyck N, Bauters W, et al. Omalizumab is effective in allergic and nonallergic patients with nasal polyps and asthma. J Allergy Clin Immunol. 2013;131(1):110–6.e1.
47. Bachert C, Han JK, Desrosiers M, Hellings PW, Amin N, Lee SE, et al. Efficacy and safety of dupilumab in patients with severe chronic rhinosinusitis with nasal polyps (LIBERTY NP SINUS-24 and LIBERTY NP SINUS-52): results from two multicentre, randomised, double-blind, placebo-controlled, parallel-group phase 3 trials. Lancet. 2019;394(10209):1638–50.
48. Jonstam K, Swanson BN, Mannent LP, Cardell LO, Tian N, Wang Y, et al. Dupilumab reduces local type 2 pro-inflammatory biomarkers in chronic rhinosinusitis with nasal polyposis. Allergy Eur J Allergy Clin Immunol. 2019;74(4):743–52.

49. Laidlaw TM, Mullol J, Fan C, Zhang D, Amin N, Khan A, et al. Dupilumab improves nasal polyp burden and asthma control in patients with CRSwNP and AERD. J Allergy Clin Immunol Pract. 2019;7(7):2462–5.e1.
50. Gevaert P, Van Bruaene N, Cattaert T, Van Steen K, Van Zele T, Acke F, et al. Mepolizumab, a humanized anti-IL-5 mAb, as a treatment option for severe nasal polyposis. J Allergy Clin Immunol. 2011;128(5):989–95.e1-8.
51. Bachert C, Sousa AR, Lund VJ, Scadding GK, Gevaert P, Nasser S, et al. Reduced need for surgery in severe nasal polyposis with mepolizumab: randomized trial. J Allergy Clin Immunol. 2017;140(4):1024–31.e14.

Local Respiratory Allergy

31

Ibon Eguiluz-Gracia, Almudena Testera-Montes, and Carmen Rondón

Introduction

Chronic rhinitis and asthma are inflammatory conditions of the respiratory mucosa affecting >30% and >4% of the adult Western population, respectively [1, 2]. Chronic rhinitis has been classically divided into the allergic rhinitis (AR) and the non-allergic rhinitis (NAR) phenotypes [1, 3]. AR patients are defined by the positivity of skin prick test (SPT) and/or serum allergen-specific (s)IgE in association with corresponding symptoms [4]. Conversely, the negativity of both classical markers of atopy identifies NAR individuals [5]. Nevertheless, accumulating data indicate the existence of a new allergic phenotype of rhinitis in non-atopic patients who display nasal-specific reactivity to aeroallergens. This phenotype has been termed local allergic rhinitis (LAR) [6], and the diagnosis requires the implementation of the nasal allergen challenge (NAC) in the clinic [7]. To further complicate the field, recent evidence suggests that nasal reactivity to aeroallergens with and without positive SPT can coexist in the same patient [8]. This phenotype is called dual allergic rhinitis (DAR). Conversely, asthma phenotypes are divided into those with eosinophilic infiltrate and those without eosinophilic infiltrate [9]. Eosinophilic asthma represents >80% of the total cases of the disease and was historically divided between allergic asthma (AA) and eosinophilic non-allergic asthma, based on the presence of atopy [9]. Nevertheless, recent data demonstrates that non-atopic patients with eosinophilic asthma can display positive responses to the bronchial allergen challenge (BAC) [10]. This new phenotype has been called local allergic asthma (LAA) and illustrates how atopy and allergy represent two different phenomena. Overall these data identify local respiratory allergy (LRA) as a relevant pathological mechanism driving chronic airway disease in both atopic and non-atopic patients. In this chapter, we will review the clinical phenotype, pathophysiology, epidemiology, and natural evolution of LRA. Treatment options will be also addressed with a focus on the beneficial effect of allergen immunotherapy (AIT) for LRA.

I. Eguiluz-Gracia · A. Testera-Montes · C. Rondón (✉)
Allergy Unit, Hospital Regional Universitario de Málaga. IBIMA-Plataforma BIONAND. RICORS Inflammatory Diseases, Málaga, Spain

C. Damask et al. (eds.), *Allergy in Otolaryngology Practice*,
https://doi.org/10.1007/978-3-031-93455-1_31

Clinical Phenotypes

The diagnosis of AR and AA requires the positivity of at least one of the two classical markers of atopy in a patient with a clinical history suggestive of allergy [4]. In case of discrepancies between the results of SPT/serum sIgE and symptoms pattern, an allergen challenge can help investigate a potential allergic etiology [7]. By definition, AR and AA patients test positive to the challenge, whereas NAR and non-allergic asthma (NAA) individuals display negative results [11]. Interestingly, up to one-fourth of non-atopic rhinitis patients display positive NAC responses, thus fulfilling the criteria for LAR diagnosis [6, 12]. Therefore, a NAC is required to discriminate between LAR and NAR [13]. Several features help identify candidate subjects for a NAC among non-atopic rhinitis patients. As compared with NAR, LAR individuals are more frequently nonsmoker women with family history of atopy and an earlier rhinitis onset [6]. LAR individuals with asthma can also display positive BAC responses [10]. This finding expands the unified airway concept and identifies LAA as a new eosinophilic asthma phenotype [9]. Similar to LAR, LAA can only be diagnosed if a BAC is implemented in the clinical protocol. In LAA patients, the BAC induces an increase in airway hyperreactivity measurable by methacholine provocation [10].

Patients who react only to seasonal allergens on SPT but also suffer from perennial rhinitis are frequently found in the clinic. This scenario was classically explained by the cooperation of allergic and non-allergic mechanisms (mixed rhinitis, MR) [14]. Nevertheless, recent evidence suggests that a significant proportion of these subjects display positive NAC responses to both seasonal and perennial allergens [8]. The coexistence of "local" and "systemic" sensitization to different aeroallergens in the same individual has been termed DAR. As compared with MR individuals, DAR patients are younger and their nasal symptoms start more frequently with a seasonal pattern with further progression to perennial symptoms [8] (Fig. 31.1).

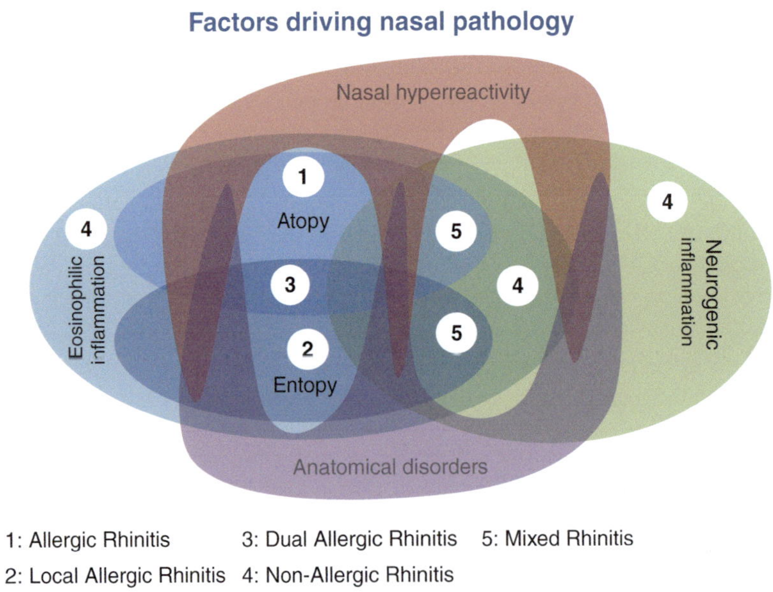

Fig. 31.1 Diagram of the different factors driving nasal pathology. The numbers indicate the distinct phenotypes of chronic rhinitis. Every phenotype can coexist or not with nasal hyperreactivity and/or anatomical disorders. The conjunction of factors affecting an individual will explain the specific features of chronic rhinitis in each patient

Immunological Mechanisms

Specific nasal and bronchial reactivity to aeroallergens is associated with eosinophilic inflammation, regardless of the atopic status for the corresponding allergen [15, 16]. Patients with AR, AA, LAR, LAA, MR, or DAR experience a progressive increase of eosinophil cationic protein (ECP) in the respiratory secretions [8, 17] during the 24 h following a positive NAC or BAC [18, 19]. Conversely, a negative challenge does not induce increase of nasal or bronchial ECP, even in atopic patients [8]. Monocytes also increase in the sputum of AA and LAA individuals after a positive BAC [10]. Moreover, a positive NAC in AR and LAR subjects induces an increase of nasal tryptase, peaking 15 min after allergen administration and rapidly returning to baseline values [15, 18]. Overall, these observations suggest that nasal reactivity to aeroallergens is associated with the classical phases of allergic inflammation (early and late), regardless of the atopic status [19, 20].

The involvement of sIgE in LRA has been more controversial, especially due to the relatively small proportion of LAR patients (20–40%) with detectable sIgE in the nasal secretions [17, 18, 21]. Moreover, sIgE has not been detected in the sputum of LAA individuals [10]. Nevertheless, the pooled analysis of LAR subjects demonstrated that nasal sIgE significantly increased during the 24 h following a positive NAC [18, 19]. In any case, in our opinion, it is not surprising that many LRA patients do not have detectable sIgE in the respiratory secretions, as these biological fluids drain in the lymphoid vessels, which in turn drain in the blood [15]. Conversely, a recent article using Merocel© sponges detected nasal sIgE in 91% of LAR individuals [22]. Merocel© sponges expand inside the nostril to perfectly adapt to the anatomy, and upon removal, they scratch a significant amount of mucosal cells.

Interestingly, 50–66% of patients with LAR and DAR display positive basophil activation test (BAT) responses [8, 23–25]. Wortmannin experiments confirmed that the activation of peripheral basophils in these patients is mediated by sIgE [23]. These findings might indicate that most patients with LRA are sensitized to the allergens they test positive to in the challenge, yet their sIgE is not bound to skin mast cells, but to peripheral basophils. To explain this observation, we hypothesize that similar to atopic respiratory allergy [26, 27], in individuals with LRA, sIgE against aeroallergens is mostly produced at the mucosal level, following sequential class switch recombination of IgG_1+ B cells [28]. After sensitizing mucosal resident cells, sIgE would traffic to the bloodstream through the lymphoid vessels to sensitize circulating basophils initially [15]. After saturating FcεRI on peripheral basophils, sIgE would sensitize resident mast cells in the different tissues, including skin mast cells [20]. Only after the saturation of the whole receptor system, sIgE would be found at the free status in serum and other biological fluids [15]. The extremely high affinity of IgE (K_d:10^{-10}) for FcεRI determines this binding sequence to the receptors expressed in different tissues [29]. Therefore, the state of each biomarker would derive from the amount of sIgE synthetized by patients with the different allergic phenotypes of rhinitis and asthma (Fig. 31.2).

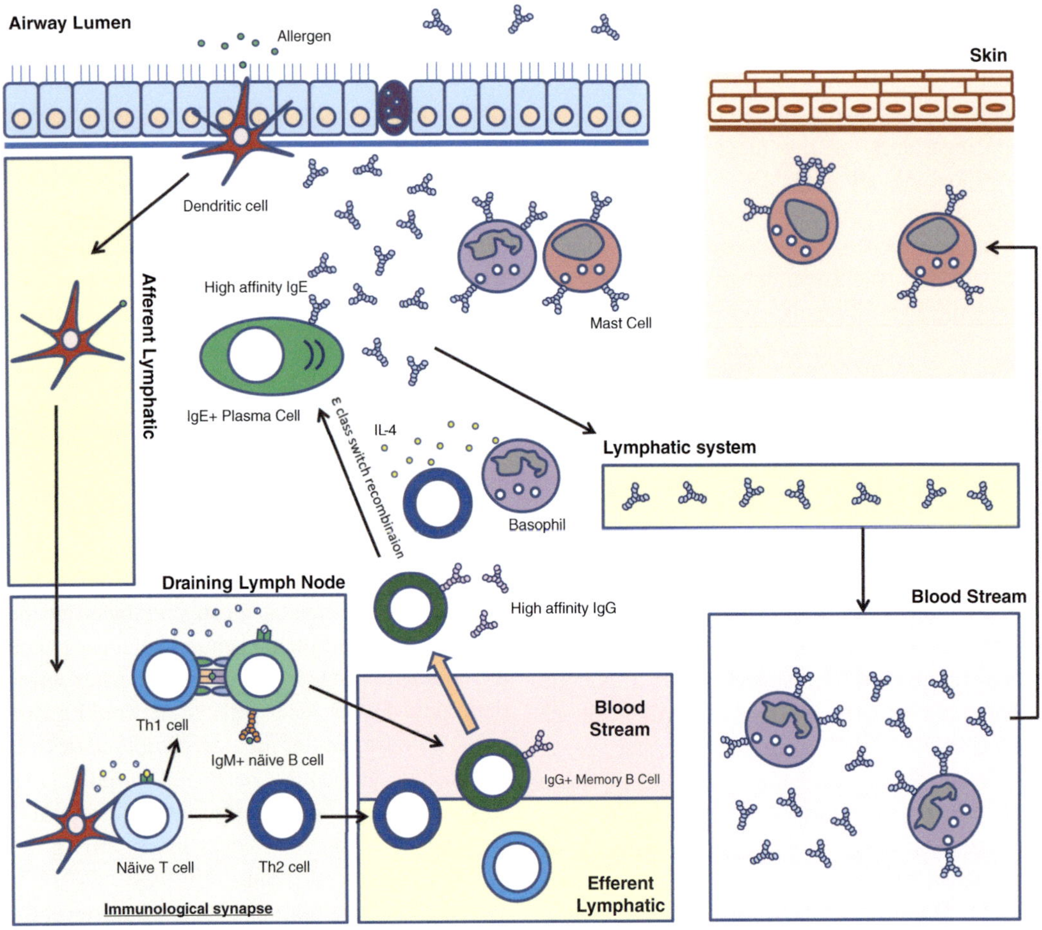

Fig. 31.2 In allergic diseases of the airways, allergen-specific (s)IgE is preferentially synthetized in the respiratory mucosa. Resident dendritic cells capture the allergens and transport them to secondary lymphoid tissues where the immunological synapse takes place. The generation of sIgE+ B cells is not functional at this level. On the other hand, significant amounts of sTh2, sTh1, and sIgG1+ B cells are produced in the germinal centers before trafficking to the bloodstream to extravasate at peripheral tissues, including the respiratory mucosa. Upon the effect of IL-4 (provided by allergen-activated sTh2 cells or basophils), sIgG1+ B cells undergo sequential class switch recombination to IgE to give rise to plasma cells producing increased amounts of high-affinity sIgE. Thereafter, sIgE binds to FcεRI expressed on resident mast cells and basophils (sensitization). After saturating the mucosal receptor system, the remaining sIgE molecules traffic through the lymphoid vessels to the bloodstream where they sensitize circulating basophils first. After saturating peripheral basophils, sIgE is distributed to all peripheral tissues where it sensitizes resident mast cells, including skin mast cells. Only after the saturation of the whole receptor system of the organism, sIgE can be found at the free state in serum and other biological fluids

Epidemiology

Clinical and epidemiological studies show that LRA is a common entity affecting patients of different ages and ethnic and geographical background [17, 30–35]. Within LRA spectrum, LAR is the condition that has been defined in a more detailed way. LAR is an underdiagnosed entity, especially due to the scarce implementation of the NAC [7, 36]. A recent systematic review of 46 studies concluded that the prevalence of LAR among non-atopic adults with rhinitis was 26.5% [12]. Nevertheless, a population study is still lacking. Published literature identifies significant differences in LAR prevalence among distinct geographical areas (Table 31.1). This fact proba-

Table 31.1 Epidemiological studies in local allergic rhinitis

Author	Year	Country	Study groups	Age	Allergens	Positive NAC response n (%)
Carney et al. [37]	2002	UK	21 IR (perennial)	Adults	Dp/Df, epithelia, grass	13/21 (61.9%)
Wedback et al. [38]	2005	Sweden	15 IR (seasonal)	Adults	Grass birch, timothy	7/15 (46.7%)
Rondón et al. [17]	2007	Spain	50 IR (perennial)	Adults	Dp	27/50 (54%)
Rondón et al. [39]	2008	Spain	32 IR (seasonal)	Adults	Grass, olive	21/32 (65.6%)
Cruz Niesvaara [31]	2012	Spain	30 IR (perennial)	Adults	Dp	19/30 (63.3%)
Rondón et al. [30]	2012	Spain	158 IR (seasonal & perennial)	Adults	Dp, alternaria, pollens, epithelia	110/158 (69.6%)
Fuiano et al. [40]	2012	Italy	36 NAR (perennial)	4–18	Alternaria	23/36 (64%)
Cheng et al. [32]	2013	China	147 IR (perennial)	Adults	Df	12/147 (8.1%)
Chang et al. [33]	2014	Korea	62 IR (perennial)	Adults	Dp	22/62 (35.5%)
Bozek et al. [41]	2015	Poland	131 IR (perennial)	Adults >65 years	Dp, pollens, molds, cat	46/131 (35.1%)
Klimek et al. [42]	2015	Germany	2 IR (perennial)	Adults	Alternaria	2 case report
Jang et al. [43]	2015	Korea	110 IR (perennial)	Adults	Dp	12/110 (10.9%)
Refaat et al. [44]	2015	Egypt	40 IR (perennial)	Adults	Dp	25/40 (62.5%)
Buntarickporpan et al. [45]	2015	Thailand	25 NAR (perennial)	8–18	Dp	2/54 (3.7%)
Blanca-López et al. [46]	2016	Spain	52 NAR (seasonal)	Adults	Phleum	28/52 (53.8%)
Duman et al. [47]	2016	Turkey	28 NAR (seasonal & perennial)	5–16	Dp, Df, grass	7/28 (25%)
Zicari et al. [48]	2016	Italy	18 NAR (perennial)	6–12	Dp, Df, lolium	12/18 (66.6%)
Prieto et al. [49]	2016	Spain	45 NAR (perennial)	10–20	Dp, Df, pollens, epithelia	30/45 (66%)
Krajewska-Wojtys et al. [50]	2016	Poland	121 NAR (seasonal)	12–18	Phleum, artemisia, birch	73/121 (60.3%)
Badran et al. [51]	2016	Egypt	273 NAR	Adults	Dp, Df, pollen	231/273 (84.6%)(total results with all allergens)

(continued)

Table 31.1 (continued)

Author	Year	Country	Study groups	Age	Allergens	Positive NAC response n (%)
Duman et al. [47]	2016	Turkey	28 NAR (seas/ perennial)	Adults	Dp, Df, grass mix	7/28 (25%) (total results with all allergens)
Jung et al. [52]	2017	Korea	81 NAR (perennial)	Adults	Df	6/81 (7.4%)
Venegas-Díaz et al. [53]	2017	Spain	80 NAR (seasonal & perennial)	Adults	Dp, salsola, cupressus	21/80 (26.25%)
Shin et al. [54]	2017	Korea	81 NAR (perennial)	Adults	Dp, Df	6/81 (7.4%)
Krajewska- Wojtys et al. [50]	2017	Poland	84 NAR (perennial)	Adults	Dp, alternaria, cat	21/84 (25%) (total with all allergens)
Ha et al. [55]	2017	Korea	64 NAR (perennial)	1–18	Dp	5/64 (7.8%)
Tao et al. [34]	2018	China	79 NAR (seasonal & perennial)	Adults	Pollen/Dp	15/79 (18.9%) local Ig E, no NAC
Tantilipikorn, et al. [56]	2019	Thailand	62 NAR (perennial)	Adults	Dp	15/62 (24.2%)
Meng Y et al. [22]	2019	China	73 NAR (seasonal)	Adults	Dp, Df	12/73 (16.4%)
Bozek et al. [57]	2019	Poland	621 NAR (perennial)	>5 years	Dp, Phleum, artemisia, birch, cat	360/621 (57.97%)
Duarte-Ferreira et al. [24]	2019	Portugal	20 NAR (perennial)	Adults	Dp,Df	17/20 (85%)
Tsilochristou et al. [58]	2019	Greece	24 NAR (seasonal & perennial)	Adults	Phleum, olea, alternaria, Dp	7/24 (29%) (total result with all allergens)
Ishida M et al. [35]	2020	Japan	50 NAR (seasonal & perennial)	Adults	Dp, Df, Jcp	5/21 (23.8%) Dp,Df 2/24 (14.3%) Jcp

IR Idiopathic rhinitis, *NAR* non-allergic rhinitis, *Dp* Dermatophagoides pteronyssinus, *Df* Dermatophagoides farinae, *NAC* nasal allergen challenge, *Jcp* Japanese cedar pollen bly derives from the distinct models of health care, the heterogeneity of referral criteria to specialized centers, or the lack of standardization of the NAC methodology [46]. Moreover, there might be a lower prevalence of LAR in Asian countries (0–25%) as compared to Western Europe (29.2–69.6%) [32, 34, 40, 43, 45, 47, 48, 50, 54, 58]. Regarding age, the prevalence in young adults seems higher than in the elderly population [41].

Natural History

After the identification of LAR, one of the biggest questions about the disease was whether LAR constituted an initial step in the development of AR [6, 59]. A preliminary study including 180 non-atopic rhinitis patients reported that 24% of the subjects developed systemic atopy over time, suggesting that LAR evolves frequently to AR [60]. However, this study did not differentiate between LAR and NAR patients. Subsequently, another retrospective study conducted in 42 LAR individuals showed a 40% conversion rate to AR. However, this study did not include a sufficiently large sample size or a control group [61]. The best quality information regarding the natural history of LAR was provided by a 10-year follow-up study of a cohort of 194 LAR patients and 130 healthy controls. This study showed that the conversion rate to systemic atopy was similar between LAR patients and the healthy population (<10% for both groups) [62]. This finding indicates that LAR is a differentiated rhinitis phenotype [63]. This study also identified that the proportion of LAR individuals suffering from asthma symptoms increased from 18.8% to 30.7% during the first 10 years after the disease is established. Moreover, conjunctivitis symptoms followed a similar trend. During the study period, a significant increase in rhinitis severity and the number of visits to the Emergency Room was also observed. Of note, this worsening occurred more quickly during the first 5 years after the disease is established with slower progression during the subsequent 5 years [63].

Diagnostic Testing

LAR should be considered in the differential diagnosis of patients with nasal symptoms suggestive of allergy but no evidence of systemic atopy [49, 59, 64]. The diagnostic approach should begin with a complete clinical history, including interrogation about asthma and conjunctivitis symptoms. Thereafter, a nasal exploration with anterior rhinoscopy and/or nasal endoscopy should be performed [7, 13, 65]. In case of history suggestive of AR but absent systemic sensitization, the nasal response to the allergen should be evaluated by a NAC. NAC is the gold standard to establish the allergic triggers of rhinitis and is needed for the confirmation of LAR diagnosis [6, 7, 66]. Before the application of the allergen, the existence of nasal hyperresponsiveness needs to be investigated by the performance of a saline challenge. Provided the saline challenge is negative, the administration of the allergen can be done with a micropipette or a nasal spray applied bilaterally. The use of standardized allergenic extracts is required to guarantee the reliability of the test [7, 66]. NAC monitoring should be conducted by evaluating both objective (nasal patency) and subjective (naso-ocular symptom score) parameters. Accepted methods to measure the nasal patency include acoustic rhinometry, active anterior rhinomanometry, and peak nasal inspiratory flow. NAC is considered positive when there is a clear change in objective and/or subjective parameters, or when there are moderate changes in both parameters simultaneously [7]. NAC is a safe and reproducible technique. A study by our group analyzing 11,499 procedures performed in children and adults with rhinitis and asthma demonstrated that adverse effects rarely occur [67]. Importantly, no severe effects (e.g., bronchospasm) were observed. International guidelines recommend testing only one allergen per session. However, our group described a protocol for multiple allergen provocation in the same session, which is a very convenient approach for the screening of LAR patients [68].

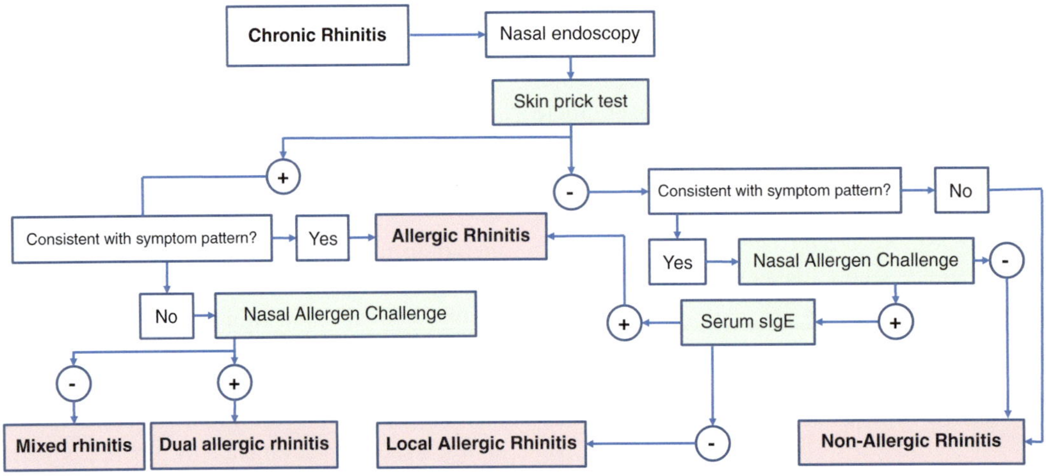

Fig. 31.3 Diagnostic algorithm for chronic non-infectious rhinitis: the green color indicates diagnostic tests; the red color indicates phenotypes of chronic rhinitis (diagnosis); *sIgE* allergen-specific IgE

The measurement of nasal sIgE has been also applied for the diagnosis of LAR, but the quantification of sIgE in the nasal secretions has demonstrated a low sensitivity and cannot be recommended for routine LAR diagnosis [15, 17, 21, 64]. Several samples have been used to measure nasal sIgE (secretions, scraping, brushing, etc.), but not all of them have been applied to LAR. Therefore, the quantification of nasal sIgE should be considered a research tool at this time [69, 70].

Conversely, the BAT is a more promising tool for the facilitation of LAR diagnosis. Published studies have demonstrated high specificity, yet the sensitivity is overall lower than that of the NAC (50–60%) [24, 25]. Unlike nasal sIgE, the BAT counts on a standardized methodology and defined cut-off points. Moreover, a previous NAC is not needed to increase the sensitivity of the test [8]. Nonetheless, BAT should be still considered a research tool until further validation.

An algorithm for LAR diagnosis in the clinic is presented in Fig. 31.3.

Therapeutic Strategies

The treatment of LRA (LAR and DAR with/without asthma) is complex and should follow *Allergic Rhinitis and its Impact of Asthma* (ARIA) recommendations [71] for atopic respiratory allergy: patient's education, allergen avoidance, pharmacologic treatment, and AIT.

Nasal and ocular symptoms in LAR and DAR patients can be controlled with allergen avoidance measures and pharmacotherapy (nasal corticosteroids and oral antihistamines) [62, 63]. However, these measures are not effective in many patients, as allergen avoidance is not always feasible and pharmacotherapy may induce bothersome side effects. Moreover, corticosteroids and antihistamines do not prevent disease progression.

On the other hand, severe and difficult-to-control rhinitis and asthma phenotypes constitute a worldwide health problem as they are responsible for >80% of the costs associated with chronic respiratory diseases [72, 73]. Some biological drugs can control the symptoms of eosinophilic asthma but do not represent a solution for the issue, because, similar to standard pharmacotherapy, they do not modify the natural course of the disease. Moreover, long-lasting treatment with costly symptomatic drugs, like biologicals, imposes a high economic burden to health systems.

Currently, AIT constitutes the only etiologic treatment available for airway allergy, targeting the underlying pathophysiology and possibly displaying a disease-modifying effect [74]. The identification of the allergen(s) triggering the symptoms is the first step in the stratification of rhinitis patients, thus ensuring that the correct allergen solution will be used for AIT [74] Despite its relevance, this issue is especially complex in LRA patients who, by definition, test negative in the SPT and serum sIgE.

Clinical Impact of Allergen Immunotherapy in Local Respiratory Allergy

AIT is an etiologic and cost-effective therapeutic intervention for airway allergy, controlling associated morbidity, inducing a long-lasting beneficial effect, and modifying the natural course of the disease. AIT modifies the Th2-biased response and induces and state of permanent immune-tolerance to the allergen which is associated with a sustained clinical effect after treatment discontinuation (long-term effect) [74–78].

The pathophysiological similarities between AR and LAR served as basis for the first grass pollen subcutaneous AIT (grass-SCIT) observational study conducted in LAR individuals in 2011 [79]. Five SCIT studies with commercialized and standardized allergen extracts have been conducted in LAR adult patients in the last decade: one open observational study [79] and four double-blind placebo-control clinical trials (RCT) [80–83]. Overall, these studies demonstrate that SCIT is an effective treatment for LAR adult patients. Other administration routes as sublingual, intranasal, epicutaneous, transcutaneous, intradermal, or intralymphatic have not been evaluated yet in patients with LRA.

In 2011 the first grass-SCIT observational real-life study included 20 patients with seasonal LAR to grass pollen [79]. Ten patients were treated with 6 months of preseasonal grass-SCIT and seasonal pharmacotherapy (rescue medication) during the pollen season and ten patients only with rescue medication. Grass-SCIT induced a significant improvement of symptoms and medications scores, number of medication-free days, and rhinitis severity. A 100% reduction of severe rhinitis cases and a 57% reduction of moderate rhinitis cases were observed. In addition, AIT increased the nasal tolerance to grass as measured by the NAC, and 30% of patients tested negative in the NAC after the treatment period. Serum allergen-specific IgG4 (sIgG4) also increased progressively in the treated group and the difference became significant after 12 months [79].

In 2016, a 2-year RCT of DP-SCIT vs placebo in 36 patients with perennial persistent moderate-to-severe LAR was published [80]. In this trial the clinical effect of SCIT was closely monitored, at baseline, and after 1, 3, 6, 12, 18, and 24 months of treatment. The results revealed an early and sustained clinical beneficial effect of DP-SCIT on symptoms, medication, and allergen tolerance outcomes, starting from the sixth month of therapy and progressively increasing to the end of the study. This improvement was apparent in combined symptom and medication scores (CSMS), individual symptoms and medication scores, number of medication-free days, and allergen concentration tolerated in the NAC [80]. At the end of the study, 67% of patients tolerated a concentration of Der p1 $\geq$ 10 times higher than that before SCIT initiation, and half of them tested negative in the NAC. Moreover, patients treated with DP-SCIT, displayed progressively increasing serum DP-sIgG4 titles from the beginning of the study period, showing significant differences from the first year of AIT [80]. These results were confirmed in the next RCTs [81–83].

The beneficial effect of AIT on multimorbidity (conjunctivitis and asthma) and also on health-related quality of life was first evidenced in the Phleum-SCIT vs placebo RCT [81]. The improvement of the quality of life was later confirmed in the Betula-SCIT vs placebo RCT [82]. The evaluation of health-related quality of life is a helpful tool to assess patients' self-perceived benefit and the cost-effectiveness of therapeutic interventions.

More recently, a 3-year RCT of Betula-SCIT vs placebo demonstrated for the first time a significant decrease of bronchial responsiveness to birch pollen in 5 out of 7 LAR-LAA patients who were treated with AIT [83].

The current knowledge about the immunologic effect of AIT in LRA is limited. However, all the studies carried out to date show that the clinical improvement induced by AIT is accompanied by a significant and progressive increase of serum sIgG4 levels and mucosal tolerance to the allergen [79–83]. These results suggest that sIgG4 is a useful response biomarker for AIT in LRA.

The potential long-term clinical effect of AIT after treatment discontinuation in LAR patients is currently under investigation. Preliminary data from PI17/01410 project indicate that AIT induces antibodies blocking sIgE (IgG4 and IgA) at the mucosal level [84] and 95% of LAR patients responding to AIT maintain the improvement at least during the 2 years following treatment discontinuation [85]. Overall, these data suggest that, similar to atopic respiratory allergy, AIT is able to modify the natural course of LRA.

Conclusion

LRA constitutes a diagnostic and therapeutic challenge for clinicians. The disease often starts during childhood and quickly progresses towards the clinical worsening and the association of comorbidities, most importantly LAA. The first five years of evolution constitute a window of opportunity to implement specific measures aiming to prevent disease progression and the association of comorbidities.

LAR diagnosis relies on the positivity of the NAC, whereas the BAT and nasal sIgE require further validation before their recommendation for clinical use. Thus, the implementation of the NAC in the diagnostic algorithms for rhinitis is a prerequisite for an early recognition of the condition and the prescription of specific therapies with disease-modifying potential. In this regard, AIT is the only existing etiological treatment for airway allergy, and it also seems to have the ability to control LAR symptoms while is being administered. Preliminary data, suggesting that AIT may induce a long-term clinical effect on LRA after therapy discontinuation, warrants further investigation.

References

1. Papadopoulos NG, Guibas GV. Rhinitis subtypes, endotypes, and definitions. Immunol Allergy Clin N Am. 2016;36(2):215–33.
2. Rondon C, et al. Nonallergic rhinitis and lower airway disease. Allergy. 2017;72(1):24–34.
3. Mullol J, Del Cuvillo A, Lockey RF. Rhinitis phenotypes. J Allergy Clin Immunol Pract. 2020;8(5):1492–503.
4. Greiner AN, et al. Allergic rhinitis. Lancet. 2011;378(9809):2112–22.
5. Hellings PW, et al. Non-allergic rhinitis: position paper of the European academy of allergy and clinical immunology. Allergy. 2017;72(11):1657–65.
6. Rondon C, et al. Local allergic rhinitis: concept, pathophysiology, and management. J Allergy Clin Immunol. 2012;129(6):1460–7.
7. Auge J, et al. EAACI position paper on the standardization of nasal allergen challenges. Allergy. 2018;73(8):1597–608.
8. Eguiluz-Gracia I, et al. Coexistence of nasal reactivity to allergens with and without IgE sensitization in patients with allergic rhinitis. Allergy. 2020;75:1689.
9. Holgate ST, et al. Asthma. Nat Rev Dis Primers. 2015;1:15025.
10. Campo P, et al. Bronchial asthma triggered by house dust mites in patients with local allergic rhinitis. Allergy. 2019;74(8):1502–10.
11. Pepper AN, Ledford DK. Nasal and ocular challenges. J Allergy Clin Immunol. 2018;141(5):1570–7.
12. Hamizan AW, et al. Positive allergen reaction in allergic and nonallergic rhinitis: a systematic review. Int Forum Allergy Rhinol. 2017;7(9):868–77.
13. Eguiluz-Gracia I, et al. How to diagnose and treat local allergic rhinitis: a challenge for clinicians. J Clin Med. 2019;8(7):1062.
14. Greiwe JC, Bernstein JA. Allergic and mixed rhinitis: diagnosis and natural evolution. J Clin Med. 2019;8(11):2019.
15. Rondon C, et al. IgE test in secretions of patients with respiratory allergy. Curr Allergy Asthma Rep. 2018;18(12):67.
16. Eguiluz-Gracia I, et al. Rapid recruitment of CD14(+) monocytes in experimentally induced allergic rhinitis in human subjects. J Allergy Clin Immunol. 2016;137(6):1872–1881 e12.
17. Rondon C, et al. Local IgE production and positive nasal provocation test in patients with persistent nonallergic rhinitis. J Allergy Clin Immunol. 2007;119(4):899–905.
18. Rondon C, et al. Nasal inflammatory mediators and specific IgE production after nasal challenge with grass pollen in local allergic rhinitis. J Allergy Clin Immunol. 2009;124(5):1005–11 e1.
19. Lopez S, et al. Immediate and dual response to nasal challenge with Dermatophagoides pteronyssinus in local allergic rhinitis. Clin Exp Allergy. 2010;40(7):1007–14.

20. Eguiluz-Gracia I, et al. Mucosal IgE immune responses in respiratory diseases. Curr Opin Pharmacol. 2019;46:100–7.
21. Campo P, et al. Direct intranasal application of the solid phase of ImmunoCAP(R) increases nasal specific immunoglobulin E detection in local allergic rhinitis patients. Int Forum Allergy Rhinol. 2018;8(1):15–9.
22. Meng Y, et al. Specific immunoglobulin E in nasal secretions for the diagnosis of local allergic rhinitis. Rhinology. 2019;57(4):313–20.
23. Gomez E, et al. Role of the basophil activation test in the diagnosis of local allergic rhinitis. J Allergy Clin Immunol. 2013;132(4):975–6 e1–5.
24. Duarte Ferreira R, et al. Contribution of in vivo and in vitro testing for the diagnosis of local allergic rhinitis. J Investig Allergol Clin Immunol. 2019;29(1):46–8.
25. Campo P, et al. Immunologic responses to the major allergen of Olea europaea in local and systemic allergic rhinitis subjects. Clin Exp Allergy. 2015;45(11):1703–12.
26. KleinJan A, et al. Local production and detection of (specific) IgE in nasal B-cells and plasma cells of allergic rhinitis patients. Eur Respir J. 2000;15(3):491–7.
27. Takhar P, et al. Allergen drives class switching to IgE in the nasal mucosa in allergic rhinitis. J Immunol. 2005;174(8):5024–32.
28. Wu YC, et al. Influence of seasonal exposure to grass pollen on local and peripheral blood IgE repertoires in patients with allergic rhinitis. J Allergy Clin Immunol. 2014;134(3):604–12.
29. Kinet JP. The high-affinity IgE receptor (Fc epsilon RI): from physiology to pathology. Annu Rev Immunol. 1999;17:931–72.
30. Rondon C, et al. Prevalence and clinical relevance of local allergic rhinitis. Allergy. 2012;67(10):1282–8.
31. Cruz Niesvaara D, Rondon C, Almeida Quintana L, Correa A, Castillo Sainz R, Melendez L, et al. Evidence of local allergic rhinitis in areas with high and permanent aeroallergens exposure. J Allergy Clin Immunol. 2012;129(2):AB111.
32. Cheng KJ, et al. Serum eosinophil cationic protein level in Chinese subjects with nonallergic and local allergic rhinitis and its relation to the severity of disease. Am J Rhinol Allergy. 2013;27(1):8–12.
33. Chang GU, et al. Nonspecific hyper-reactivity and localized allergy: cause of discrepancy between skin prick and nasal provocation test. Otolaryngol Head Neck Surg. 2014;150(2):194–200.
34. Tao XY, et al. Clinical characteristics and allergen sensitization patterns of patients with local allergic rhinitis in Southern China. Int Arch Allergy Immunol. 2018;175(1–2):107–13.
35. Ishida M, et al. Possibility of local allergic rhinitis in Japan. Am J Rhinol Allergy. 2020;34(1):26–34.
36. Rondon C, et al. More research is needed for local allergic rhinitis. Int Arch Allergy Immunol. 2015;167(2):99–100.
37. Carney AS, et al. Atypical nasal challenges in patients with idiopathic rhinitis: more evidence for the existence of allergy in the absence of atopy? Clin Exp Allergy. 2002;32(10):1436–40.
38. Wedback A, et al. Seasonal non-allergic rhinitis (SNAR)--a new disease entity? A clinical and immunological comparison between SNAR, seasonal allergic rhinitis and persistent non-allergic rhinitis. Rhinology. 2005;43(2):86–92.
39. Rondon C, et al. Seasonal idiopathic rhinitis with local inflammatory response and specific IgE in absence of systemic response. Allergy. 2008;63(10):1352–8.
40. Fuiano N, Fusilli S, Incorvaia C. A role for measurement of nasal IgE antibodies in diagnosis of Alternaria-induced rhinitis in children. Allergol Immunopathol (Madr). 2012;40(2):71–4.
41. Bozek A, et al. Local allergic rhinitis in elderly patients. Ann Allergy Asthma Immunol. 2015;114(3):199–202.
42. Klimek L, et al. Local allergic rhinitis to Alternaria alternata : evidence for local IgE production exclusively in the nasal mucosa. HNO. 2015;63(5):364–72.
43. Jang TY, Kim YH. Nasal provocation test is useful for discriminating allergic, nonallergic, and local allergic rhinitis. Am J Rhinol Allergy. 2015;29(4):e100–4.
44. Refaat MM, et al. Serum indolamine 2,3 dioxygenase as a marker in the evaluation of allergic rhinitis. Am J Rhinol Allergy. 2015;29(5):329–33.
45. Buntarickpornpan P, et al. The proportion of local allergic rhinitis to Dermatophagoides pteronyssinus in children. Pediatr Allergy Immunol. 2016;27(6):574–9.
46. Blanca-Lopez N, et al. Seasonal local allergic rhinitis in areas with high concentrations of grass pollen. J Investig Allergol Clin Immunol. 2016;26(2):83–91.
47. Duman H, et al. The relevance of nasal provocation testing in children with nonallergic rhinitis. Int Arch Allergy Immunol. 2016;170(2):115–21.
48. Zicari AM, et al. Local allergic rhinitis in children: novel diagnostic features and potential biomarkers. Am J Rhinol Allergy. 2016;30(5):329–34.
49. Papadopoulos NG, et al. Phenotypes and endotypes of rhinitis and their impact on management: a PRACTALL report. Allergy. 2015;70(5):474–94.
50. Krajewska-Wojtys A, et al. Local allergic rhinitis to pollens is underdiagnosed in young patients. Am J Rhinol Allergy. 2016;30(6):198–201.
51. Badran HS, et al. Identification and prevalence of allergic, nonallergic, and local allergic rhinitis patients in western area, Saudi Arabia. Ann Otol Rhinol Laryngol. 2016;125(8):634–43.
52. Jung CG, et al. Prevalence and clinical characteristics of local allergic rhinitis to house dust mites. Yonsei Med J. 2017;58(5):1047–50.
53. Venegas Díaz I. Estudio de base poblacional sobre prevalencia de rinitis alérgica local (RAL) en un área geográfica definida (Comarca de L'Alacantí). Universidad Miguel Hernández; 2017.
54. Shin YS, Jung CG, Park HS. Prevalence and clinical characteristics of local allergic rhinitis to house dust mites. Curr Opin Allergy Clin Immunol. 2018;18(1):10–5.
55. Ha EK, et al. Prevalence and clinical characteristics of local allergic rhinitis in children sensitized

to house dust mites. Int Arch Allergy Immunol. 2017;174(3–4):183–9.
56. Tantilipikorn P, et al. Prevalence of local allergic rhinitis to Dermatophagoides pteronyssinus in chronic rhinitis with negative skin prick test. Asian Pac J Allergy Immunol. 2021;39:111–6.
57. Bozek A, et al. The prevalence and characteristics of local allergic rhinitis in Poland. Rhinology. 2019;57(3):213–8.
58. Tsilochristou O, et al. Detection of local allergic rhinitis in children with chronic, difficult-to-treat, nonallergic rhinitis using multiple nasal provocation tests. Pediatr Allergy Immunol. 2019;30(3):296–304.
59. Campo P, et al. Local allergic rhinitis. Immunol Allergy Clin N Am. 2016;36(2):321–32.
60. Rondon C, et al. Evolution of patients with nonallergic rhinitis supports conversion to allergic rhinitis. J Allergy Clin Immunol. 2009;123(5):1098–102.
61. Sennekamp J, et al. Local allergic nasal reactions convert to classic systemic allergic reactions: a long-term follow-up. Int Arch Allergy Immunol. 2015;166(2):154–60.
62. Rondon C, et al. Local allergic rhinitis is an independent rhinitis phenotype: the results of a 10-year follow-up study. Allergy. 2018;73(2):470–8.
63. Rondon C, et al. Follow-up study in local allergic rhinitis shows a consistent entity not evolving to systemic allergic rhinitis. J Allergy Clin Immunol. 2014;133(4):1026–31.
64. Campo P, et al. Local IgE in non-allergic rhinitis. Clin Exp Allergy. 2015;45(5):872–81.
65. Fokkens WJ, et al. European position paper on rhinosinusitis and nasal polyps 2020. Rhinology. 2020;58(Suppl S29):1–464.
66. Dordal MT, et al. Allergen-specific nasal provocation testing: review by the rhinoconjunctivitis committee of the Spanish Society of Allergy and Clinical Immunology. J Investig Allergol Clin Immunol. 2011;21(1):1–12. quiz follow 12
67. Eguiluz-Gracia I, et al. Safety and reproducibility of nasal allergen challenge. Allergy. 2019;74(6):1125–34.
68. Rondon C, et al. Nasal allergen provocation test with multiple aeroallergens detects polysensitization in local allergic rhinitis. J Allergy Clin Immunol. 2011;128(6):1192–7.
69. De Schryver E, et al. Local immunoglobulin e in the nasal mucosa: clinical implications. Allergy Asthma Immunol Res. 2015;7(4):321–31.
70. Gelardi M, et al. Local allergic rhinitis: entopy or spontaneous response? World Allergy Organ J. 2016;9(1):39.
71. Bousquet J, et al. Next-generation Allergic Rhinitis and Its Impact on Asthma (ARIA) guidelines for allergic rhinitis based on Grading of Recommendations Assessment, Development and Evaluation (GRADE) and real-world evidence. J Allergy Clin Immunol. 2020;145(1):70–80 e3.
72. O'Neill S, et al. The cost of treating severe refractory asthma in the UK: an economic analysis from the British Thoracic Society Difficult Asthma Registry. Thorax. 2015;70(4):376–8.
73. Ferreira de Magalhaes M, et al. Cost of asthma in children: a nationwide, population-based, cost-of-illness study. Pediatr Allergy Immunol. 2017;28(7):683–91.
74. Roberts G, et al. A new framework for the interpretation of IgE sensitization tests. Allergy. 2016;71(11):1540–51.
75. Calderon MA, et al. Allergy immunotherapy across the life cycle to promote active and healthy ageing: from research to policies: an AIRWAYS Integrated Care Pathways (ICPs) programme item (action plan B3 of the European innovation partnership on active and healthy ageing) and the Global Alliance against Chronic Respiratory Diseases (GARD), a World Health Organization GARD research demonstration project. Clin Transl Allergy. 2016;6:41.
76. Jutel M, et al. Allergen-specific immunotherapy with recombinant grass pollen allergens. J Allergy Clin Immunol. 2005;116(3):608–13.
77. Durham SR, et al. Long-term clinical efficacy of grass-pollen immunotherapy. N Engl J Med. 1999;341(7):468–75.
78. Burks AW, et al. Update on allergy immunotherapy: American Academy of Allergy, Asthma & Immunology/European Academy of Allergy and Clinical Immunology/PRACTALL consensus report. J Allergy Clin Immunol. 2013;131(5):1288–96 e3.
79. Rondon C, et al. Local allergic rhinitis: allergen tolerance and immunologic changes after preseasonal immunotherapy with grass pollen. J Allergy Clin Immunol. 2011;127(4):1069–71.
80. Rondon C, et al. Efficacy and safety of D. pteronyssinus immunotherapy in local allergic rhinitis: a double-blind placebo-controlled clinical trial. Allergy. 2016;71(7):1057–61.
81. Rondon C, et al. Specific immunotherapy in local allergic rhinitis: a randomized, double-blind placebo-controlled trial with Phleum pratense subcutaneous allergen immunotherapy. Allergy. 2018;73(4):905–15.
82. Bozek A, Kolodziejczyk K, Jarzab J. Efficacy and safety of birch pollen immunotherapy for local allergic rhinitis. Ann Allergy Asthma Immunol. 2018;120(1):53–8.
83. Bozek A, et al. Different development forms of local allergic rhinitis towards birch. Biomed Res Int. 2020;2020:3408561.
84. Parkin R, Eguiluz-Gracia I, Jaen MT, Durham S, Mayorga L, Segovia CR, Shamji M. Nasal allergen neutralizing antibodies correlate closely with tolerated intranasal allergen challenge dose following grass pollen subcutaneous immunotherapy in patients with local allergic rhinitis. J Allergy Clin Immunol. 2020;145:AB184.
85. Eguiluz-Gracia I, Rondón C, Bogas G, Campo P, Gomez F, Barrionuevo E, Prieto A, Cardenas N, Molina A, Espino T, Mayorga C, Torres MJ. Long-term clinical effect of grass-allergen immunotherapy in local allergic rhinits and its capacity to modify the natural course of the disease. J Allergy Clin Immunol. 2019;143(2):AB305.

32 Drug Allergy

Merin Kuruvilla (Kalangara)

Introduction

Adverse drug reactions are a major clinical problem affecting up to 20% of hospitalized patients and 10% of the general population [1]. Drug allergic reactions account for about 10% of all adverse drug reactions, which are broadly categorized as type A or type B. Type A adverse drug reactions are mediated by recognized pharmacologic drug effects, that are generally dose-dependent and include side effects and overdose. Type B reactions account for less than 20% of adverse drug reactions and include drug hypersensitivities. While type B reactions were originally described as unpredictable and idiosyncratic with an immunologic basis, many of these features have been called into question.

For decades, the Gell and Coombs classification has served as the archetype for classifying drug allergy, and broadly categorizes reactions as (1) Type 1—immediate onset, IgE mediated; (2) Type 2—cytotoxic, IgG-mediated; (3) Type 3—serum sickness, immune complex-mediated; and (4) Type 4—delayed, T-cell-mediated. However, our knowledge of the different mechanisms whereby drugs cause hypersensitivity reactions has significantly advanced over the past decade, and many reaction types are not fully described by this classification. There has been a recent paradigm shift in drug allergy using phenotypes and endotypes to provide a more personalized approach to diagnosis and management (Fig. 32.1) [2]. The phenotypes focus on observable manifestations such as timing and symptoms of the reaction. These clinical presentations are mediated by various underlying mechanisms or endotypes. Some of these reactions are determined by genetic predisposition, and genotyping has recently become an important component of drug allergic evaluation.

M. Kuruvilla (Kalangara) (✉)
Division of Allergy/Immunology, Emory University School of Medicine, Atlanta, GA, USA

C. Damask et al. (eds.), *Allergy in Otolaryngology Practice*,
https://doi.org/10.1007/978-3-031-93455-1_32

	Phenotype	Endotype	Diagnostic evaluation
Immediate hypersensitivity	Pruritus, urticaria, angioedema, shortness of breath, GI distress, cardiovascular collapse	Type 1 hypersensitivity: Mast cell/basophil degranulation	Acute: tryptase, Urinary histamine and eicosanoids Follow up: SPT, IDT, specific IgE, BAT if indicated
	Fever, chills, rigors, nausea, pain, headache	Cytokine release: T-cells, monocytes, macrophages	Acute: IL-6
	Mixed constellation of above features	Mixed: Mast cell mediated and cytokine release	Acute: tryptase, IL-6 Follow up: SPT, IDT, specific IgE, BAT if indicated
Delayed hypersensitivity	Drug exanthem: Maculopapular pruritic eruption without blistering or mucosa involvement	CD4+/CD8+ T-cells, often underlying viral/bacterial infection	IDT if appropriate, DPT
	Fixed drug eruption: annular pigmented patches that recur at the same site with re-exposure	CD8+/memory effector T-cells	Patch test at site of eruption (high yield)
	AGEP: generalized small non-follicular pustules on an erythematous base	IL-8/CXCL8 production Neutrophilic infiltration	Patch testing (high yield)
	SJS/TEN: blistering of skin/mucosa due to keratinocyte necrosis	P-i reaction: CD8+ T-cell activation with Fas apoptosis and release of cytotoxic peptides	Genotype pre-screening if appropriate Patch test, IDT (low yield)
	DRESS: Fever, rash, eosinophilia, organ involvement	P-i reaction: CD4+ T-cell activation often with HHV reactivation	Genotype pre-screening if appropriate Patch testing (30-50%), IDT

Fig. 32.1 Drug allergy phenotypes and endotypes

Drug Allergy Phenotypes and Endotypes

Phenotypically, drug hypersensitivity reactions can be broadly classified as immediate versus delayed based on the interval between drug exposure and onset of reaction.

Phenotypes of Immediate Drug Hypersensitivity Reactions

Immediate reactions manifest within minutes to 6 h (most within 1 h) following drug exposure with a constellation of cutaneous, respiratory, gastrointestinal, and cardiovascular symptoms including pruritus, urticaria and angioedema, shortness of breath, desaturation, nausea, vomiting diarrhea, hypotension, and cardiovascular collapse. The diagnosis of anaphylaxis is based upon the acute development of symptoms in 2 or more organ systems, or isolated hypotension following exposure to an allergic trigger [1].

Drug-induced anaphylaxis is associated with more severe, potentially fatal, anaphylaxis compared to other triggers such as food. The incidence of drug-induced anaphylaxis has increased in the past few decades secondary to newly approved chemotherapy and biologics. In a review of electronic medical record data from approximately two million patients, there was a 1.1% prevalence of drug-induced anaphylaxis as recorded in the allergy module [3]. The main culprit in the United States continues to be antibiotics, specifically beta-lactams, while NSAIDs have been highlighted as a leading cause in recent studies out of Europe [4].

Endotypes of Immediate Drug Hypersensitivity Reactions

Type 1 immediate hypersensitivity involves mast cell and basophil activation. These reactions were originally confined to IgE-mediated mechanisms; however, their definition has now expanded to include mast cell/basophil activation through other mechanisms as outlined below. Immediate drug reactions may also be accounted for by complement activation, cytokine release, and enzyme inhibition.

IgE-Mediated A recent paradigm shift is the emergence of two distinct phenotypes of IgE-mediated drug allergy. The first represents traditional IgE-mediated allergy and develops after multiple drug exposures. However, IgE-mediated drug allergy may also manifest with the first dose, as with cetuximab. This occurs due to the presence of pre-existing IgE directed against a carbohydrate antigen galactose-α-1,3-galactose (alpha-gal), which is also present on cetuximab. Certain tick bites induce IgE formation to galactose-α-1,3-galactose, and patients who acquire this sensitization from tick bites subsequently react to cetuximab.

Direct Mast Cell Activation Mast cells may also be directly activated by medications that contain THIQ motifs via the MRGPRX2 receptor on their surface, as with vancomycin, fluoroquinolones, and neuromuscular blocking agents [5]. Other medications can cause direct non-immunologic mast cell activation through different receptor interactions (e.g. opioids) or direct membrane effect (e.g. iodinated contrast media).

Cytokine Release Cytokine storm reactions are triggered by the administration of chimeric, humanized, or human monoclonal antibodies and also certain chemotherapeutic agents. These manifest with atypical anaphylactic symptoms such as fever, chills, and malaise, followed by desaturation and hypotension. The mechanism involves activation of immune cells expressing IgG antibody receptors (FcγR) with the consequent release of inflammatory mediators such as IL-6 and TNF- α. Some of these reactions are mixed with an IgE-mediated component as well, and present additionally with hives and pruritus. Steroid premedication appears to protect from mild, but not severe, reactions.

COX-1 Inhibition Patients with aspirin/NSAID hypersensitivity can have various immediate reactions caused by mediators induced by COX-1 inhibition. NSAID-exacerbated respiratory disease (also known as aspirin-exacerbated respiratory disease or Samter's triad) is caused by aberrations in arachidonic acid metabolism, mediated by underlying decreased production of, or response to, prostaglandin E2 [6]. COX-1 inhibition exacerbates the baseline overproduction of cysteinyl leukotrienes and prostaglandin D2. NSAID hypersensitivity also manifests as urticaria/angioedema, the underlying mechanism being COX-1 inhibition-related loss of prostaglandin E2 production. Prostaglandin E2 stabilizes mast cells, and a decrease in production causes an acute increase in tryptase levels and cysteinyl leukotriene production [6].

Phenotypes of Delayed-Onset Hypersensitivity Reactions

Delayed reactions by definition develop 6 or more hours following drug exposure but usually take days to weeks to manifest [7]. They have heterogeneous manifestations ranging from mild exanthems to life-threatening systemic illnesses.

Drug Exanthems Delayed exanthems account for approximately 90% of delayed drug reactions [8], and complicate approximately 5% of antibiotic prescriptions [9]. These typically occur within a week of drug initiation but can be accelerated in patients who were previously sensitized. Cutaneous eruptions secondary to antibiotics may even develop up to 2 weeks following treatment discontinuation. These reactions present as erythematous and pruritic maculopapular rashes that spread in a centrifugal fashion from the torso to the extremities. Drug exanthems often develop in conjunction with underlying viral or bacterial infections. It is unclear whether exanthems are predominantly para-infectious events as opposed to pathogen stimulation of the immune system with a secondary drug reaction.

These reactions are typically benign and self-limited upon drug discontinuation. There is limited evidence showing that drug exanthems may even be "treated through" with close monitoring when the drug (such as an antibiotic) is still necessary [10]. However, there is no consensus definition on acceptable reaction severity for continued treatment.

Severe Cutaneous Adverse Reactions (SCAR)

SCAR may be life-threatening and includes Stevens–Johnson syndrome (SJS) and toxic epidermal necrolysis (TEN) and drug reaction with eosinophilia and systemic symptoms (DRESS). Acute generalized exanthematous pustulosis (AGEP) and multifocal fixed drug eruption are also classified as SCAR but these entities are in general not as severe or potentially fatal.

SJS and TEN are reported at 1 to 2 cases per million patients per year, and are medication-induced in approximately 70% of cases. Both involve massive keratinocyte apoptosis causing epidermal detachment. SJS primarily manifests with mucosal involvement (epidermal involvement less than 10% of body surface area) and TEN represents more severe cases with greater than 30% epidermal detachment. SJS/TEN has overall mortality of around 30% [11], and can be up to 90% in severe TEN [12]. Close to 90% of survivors will have residual sequelae, mostly scarring of the lids and ocular surface [13].

DRESS presents with fever, a generalized exanthem, lymphadenopathy, and facial edema with a latency period of 2 to 8 weeks. Laboratory studies demonstrate eosinophilia and atypical lymphocytosis. Internal organ involvement is frequent, most commonly with nephritis and hepatitis. The immunopathogenesis of DRESS also involves the reactivation of human herpes viruses (HHV), especially HHV-6, in up to two-thirds of cases around 2–3 weeks after symptom onset [14]. Viral reactivation has been associated with more severe and prolonged symptoms and systemic inflammation despite drug discontinuation.

Endotypes Underlying Delayed T-Cell-Mediated Reactions

Regardless of the precise clinical phenotype, delayed drug hypersensitivity is mostly T-cell-mediated. While a number of mechanistic models have been constructed in recent years, there are no in vivo studies to support the hypotheses. Overall, T-cell activation by drugs occurs in a mostly non-covalent and dose-dependent manner [15].

Hapten/Pro-hapten Model This theory states that drugs and their reactive metabolites act as haptens that are essentially incomplete antigens. Haptens are too small to be immunogenic on their own and require covalent attachment to a larger host carrier protein. This binding generates a new composite antigen that is presented by the HLA molecule and recognized by the T-cell receptor to elicit an immune response. Several drugs act as haptens, notably penicillins [15].

Pharmacological Interaction with Immune Receptors (p-i) Concept According to the p-i concept, a drug undergoes direct and non-covalent binding to HLA or T-cell receptor proteins to trigger a T-cell response. This bypasses the antigen-processing requirements by antigen-presenting cells. Activated T-cells expand and migrate into tissues and present clinically within a week of treatment initiation. The p-i concept has important clinical implications, and underscores the lack of utility for skin testing in delayed drug hypersensitivity [16]. In vitro T-cell analysis from patients indicates that p-i reactions are most frequently responsible for SCARs such as AGEP, DRESS, and SJS/TEN [17].

Altered Peptide Repertoire Model In this model, a drug binds non-covalently to the antigen-binding cleft of HLA. This alters the properties of bound peptides, leading to the presentation of novel ligands to T-cells that trigger an immune response [15].

Pharmacogenomics and Drug Allergy

Certain HLA class I types are strongly associated with increased risk of specific T-cell mediated reactions, and in these instances, HLA screening may be performed to rule out this propensity when clinically appropriate. This susceptibility is usually specific to discrete ancestries and for certain reaction types. Screening for HLA-B*57:01 and abacavir hypersensitivity syndrome, and HLA-B*15:02 and carbamazepine-induced SJS in Asian populations, are now implemented in routine clinical practice.

Diagnosis of Drug Allergy

Biomarkers of Acute, Immediate Drug Reactions

Tryptase Serum tryptase is a mast cell-specific protease and is the most ubiquitously used biomarker for drug anaphylaxis. Elevations can be detected within minutes of reaction onset and normalize within 24–48 h. Samples should ideally be drawn at 30 min to 2 h since this time frame corresponds with peak levels. Levels greater than 11.4 ng/ml indicate acute mast cell/basophil degranulation. Also, every individual has a baseline level of tryptase that is stable. An increase from the baseline tryptase value by 2 ng/ml + 1.2 × the baseline level during an acute drug reaction is also regarded as a meaningful rise [18].

Histamine While histamine is also released following mast cell activation, detectable levels in the serum are transient and rapidly cleared. Therefore, while serum histamine is limited as a biomarker, urine histamine, and its metabolites can be measured using a 24-h urine collection.

Arachidonic Acid Metabolites Leukotriene C4 and prostaglandin D2 are important mediators that are newly synthesized in response to immediate drug reactions. They are produced from mast cells as well as other inflammatory cells. The urinary metabolites leukotriene E4 and 9α,11β-prostaglandin F2 can be measured in 24-h urine collection. Despite the high specificity, a 24-h urine collection timed to symptom onset can be difficult resulting in low sensitivity.

Interleukin-6 (IL-6) IL-6 has been used as a biomarker for the detection of cytokine release reactions triggered by biological agents and chemotherapy [19], and can even guide management in terms of pre-medication for future desensitization. An isolated surge in the IL-6 level without accompanying increase in serum tryptase correlates with atypical clinical symptoms such as fever, chills, and pain.

Skin Testing

Skin testing is widely used for the evaluation of immediate drug reactions. However, it must be noted that skin testing lacks consistent predictive values for most antibiotics and other medications. There are no commercially available standardized extracts for skin testing other than penicillin (PRE-PEN; ALK-Abelló, Inc., Port Washington, NY), as will be discussed later. In general, positive skin tests are predictive of reactivity when non-irritant drug concentrations are used. However, negative tests are less useful due to unknown negative predictive values.

A negative skin test is often unreliable for excluding drug allergy in view of several factors. For instance, the native drug is often not responsible for the reaction but rather a drug metabolite. Also, many drugs skin testing reagents for most drugs are yet to be standardized. It is also generally agreed that skin testing should be deferred for at least 4–6 weeks following an acute reaction to minimize false positive as well as false negative reactions, although the evidence to support this is weak at best.

Skin Prick Testing (SPT) SPT is still used frequently for the evaluation of immediate IgE-mediated reactions, and compared with results of negative (saline) and positive (histamine) control testing. SPT must be interpreted cautiously with direct MC activators, and are unlikely to be high yield in pure cytokine storm reactions.

Intradermal Testing Intradermal testing appears to be more sensitive for drug exanthems as compared with patch testing [20], although some groups endorse direct oral challenge without antecedent skin tests for benign rashes [21]. Intradermal testing may be performed for DRESS when more than 6 months have elapsed since the index reaction. A recent prospective study even suggests safety of intradermal testing for SCAR within 6 months for reactors [22]. There is no standardized methodology nor consistent drug concentrations advised for intradermal testing. Guidelines issued by different societies have varying recommendations, making the comparison of results between centers impossible [9]. In general, a delayed positive intradermal testing is interpreted based on infiltration and erythema at the site within 24–48 h [20].

Patch Testing The approach to patch testing for drugs is fairly consistent in Europe, using test chambers incorporated with the medication compounded to its maximal non-irritating concentration and applied to the skin. Patch tests are read at 48 to 96 h and have established safety in the evaluation of SCAR [14]. Patch testing has variable sensitivity: 30–50% for DRESS and approximately 20% for SJS/TEN [14]. The incriminated drug also affects patch test sensitivity, for instance is higher with amoxicillin (approximately 44%) and lower with macrolides and cephalosporins (less than 5%).

Drug Provocation Testing (DPT)

DPT is the "gold standard" in the diagnosis of any drug hypersensitivity. It consists of the controlled administration of an incriminated drug to rule out sensitization, thus removing erroneous allergy labels. DPTs have been shown to be safe after risk stratification and using individualized protocols, when performed by experienced allergists. They may be performed as full dose or graded challenges, the latter at 30- to 60-min intervals. This is sufficient in ruling out immediate hypersensitivity to the culprit medication, and is also considered adequate for an established history of a benign exanthem [23]. Multi-day challenges are currently not recommended due to the theoretical risk of antibiotic resistance, the caveat being that even with a negative single-dose challenge, subsequent prolonged courses may trigger a reaction. However, a negative single-dose DPT appears to be reassuring for most benign delayed reactions [24].

On the other hand, DPT may be dangerous with a history of SCAR especially in the scenario of a recent reaction, and is obviously contraindicated in those with a positive skin test. There is still a lack of consensus regarding those who should be selected for DPT after negative IDT/patch testing in this setting.

Serum-Specific Drug IgE

Drug-specific IgE measurements are available only for a few medications and are of limited utility. The commercial IgE assay for penicillin has low sensitivity and correlates poorly with skin tests and drug challenges [25]. Drug-directed IgE has also been demonstrated with good specificity for quinolones, platins, and certain biologic agents [26]. Finally, the detection of alpha-gal specific IgE in the serum prior to treatment can be predictive of cetuximab hypersensitivity [27].

Basophil Activation Test (BAT)

BAT has been used to demonstrate IgE sensitization based on the upregulation of basophil activation markers CD63 and CD203 when incubated with the culprit drug [12]. BAT has been studied for various drugs such as antibiotics and neuromuscular blocking agents, and may also be useful in predicting reactions in sensitized patients.

Drug Desensitization

Drug desensitization enables the continued treatment of patients with immediate hypersensitivity reactions, and allows them to be maintained on first-line therapies while protecting from anaphylaxis. This involves the rapid incremental administration of doubling doses of the drug, and mostly uses a standard 12-step, three-bag protocol with the concentration in each bag increasing by a factor of ten. Desensitization induces a temporary state of tolerance that requires continuing drug exposure for maintenance. It was previously thought that desensitization would be efficacious only for IgE-mediated anaphylaxis. However, standard multistep protocols for desensitization also appear to be effective for immediate drug reactions that are not IgE mediated. Gradual reintroduction or a more prolonged drug desensitization over days may even have a role in non-severe delayed reactions such as benign exanthems, although the mechanism underlying efficacy in these cases is unknown [28]. Desensitization is contraindicated with a history of SCARs since even a minute exposure may trigger severe even fatal reactions.

The mechanism underlying mast cell unresponsiveness in desensitization is yet to be fully elucidated, but more than 90% of desensitizations are performed uneventfully or with only mild reactions. A few patients have moderate to severe breakthrough reactions, and there have been no fatalities. These procedures were initially undertaken in the critical care unit, but are now performed safely in the outpatient setting with adequate personnel support and resuscitation equipment readily accessible.

Penicillin Allergy

While approximately 10% of the United States population, or an estimated 20 million individuals, harbor penicillin allergy labels, these are proven erroneous in up to 98% of evaluations in recent cohorts [29]. Erroneous penicillin allergy labels have been recognized as a public health risk, and have been associated with a multitude of personal health and societal ramifications. Multiple studies have quantified the impact of these inaccurate allergy label levels, and individuals with penicillin allergy labels more frequently receive alternative broad-spectrum antibiotics and have longer durations of hospitalization, resulting in increased healthcare costs [30].

The substantial clinical and economic consequences of a penicillin allergy label have driven current guidelines encouraging routine penicillin allergy verification in all comers with this diagnosis. Blumenthal et al. used a time-driven activity-based costing model to estimate base penicillin allergy testing costs of $220, which was even lower at $84 with direct drug challenge only [31]. This is a fairly small investment when weighed against the clinical and economic consequences of alternative antibiotic use [30].

Evaluation of Penicillin Allergy Labels

Penicillin skin testing (PST) followed by DPT to confirm the absence of clinical reactivity has long been the traditional criterion standard for evaluation. Overall, IgE-mediated allergy directed against the beta-lactam core has decreased in recent years, while reactions directed against the side chains of bet-lactams are on the rise. Amoxicillin is thus preferred for DPT because it accounts for approximately 80% of prescribed penicillin and bears the antigenic determinants.

Penicillin Skin Testing In the United States, penicilloyl polylysine (the major determinant) and benzyl penicillin (a single minor determinant) are used for PST. However, PST ideally requires both major and multiple other minor determinants since patients with anaphylaxis may well be sensitized to the minor determinants but these are not commercially available [32]. A negative PST has a high predictive value, greater than 97% [33]. However, a caveat is that a positive PST does not necessarily predict challenge reactions. A recent study demonstrated that 60% of patients with a positive skin test were challenge-negative to the culprit penicillin [34]. Further, PST itself may be prohibited by time, personnel, and/or other resource constraints.

Direct Oral Amoxicillin Challenge There is a growing trend toward direct oral challenge without antecedent PST among low-risk patients without a history of anaphylaxis. The safety of this approach has been reproduced in several single-center studies and most recently in a multicenter cohort that support the efficacy of direct oral amoxicillin challenge in low-risk patients [21, 35–37]. With careful selection, the vast majority of direct PCN challenges in the literature have been negative. Less than 1 in 20 persons will have an acute reaction to direct drug challenge based on these studies. Further, several reactors in these studies developed subjective adverse reactions that were not thought to be truly anaphylactic.

A recent guideline has been published for outpatient non-allergist penicillin allergy evaluation based on DPT based on the validation of an optimal low-risk protocol for use in the allergy clinic in a multicenter study [38]. Stevenson et al. published a risk-stratified strategy for penicillin allergy de-labeling in the setting of non-allergist outpatient clinics, and a modified algorithm for beta-lactam use is presented in Fig. 32.2 for implementation in otolaryngology clinics. This simple risk-based strategy will provide a more efficient provision to de-label penicillin allergies, and translate into a meaningful public health intervention in the future.

Cross-Reactivity Among Beta-Lactams

All beta-lactams share an identical core beta-lactam ring but with different side chains. The beta-lactam ring does not appear to mediate cross-reactivity amongst beta-lactams. Once the beta-lactam ring structure breaks down, the penicilloyl group in penicillins are prone to become haptens. This is in contrast with cephalosporin degradation of the beta-lactam ring, the products of which do not undergo haptenation [39]. On the other hand, substantial evidence exists for side chain structural similarity as opposed to the shared beta-lactam ring being responsible for cross-reactivity in both immediate and delayed hypersensitivity [39].

The overall rate of cross-reactivity between penicillins and cephalosporins is no more than 2%. However, this increases significantly up to 35% in the scenario of identical side chains such as between aminopenicillins and aminocephalosporins (such as amoxicillin and cephalexin) [40]. This is in contrast to drugs such as cefazolin with unique side chains and negligible rates of clinical cross-reactivity with penicillin, and even other cephalosporins. Thus, the approach to cross-reactivity in this setting has become more nuanced.

Carbapenems and aztreonam have minimal rates of clinical cross-reactivity with penicillins at less than 1% and 0% respectively, with the only caveat that aztreonam and ceftazidime have similar side chains [40]. However, it must be noted that cross-reactivity rates were mostly studied in cohorts with benign cutaneous reactions. Caution must be exercised when prescribing alternative beta-lactams in patients with SCAR.

Beta-Lactam Allergy Pathways

The concept of drug allergy pathways was first developed at Massachusetts General Hospital, based on a risk-stratified and standardized approach to beta-lactam allergy labels to optimize their use [41]. This pathway employed a clinical decision support tool that was incorporated in the electronic medical record and implemented across their healthcare system. A similar methodology has been adopted subsequently by several other institutions within the United States. These pathways involve risk stratification based on historical reaction details and assessment of

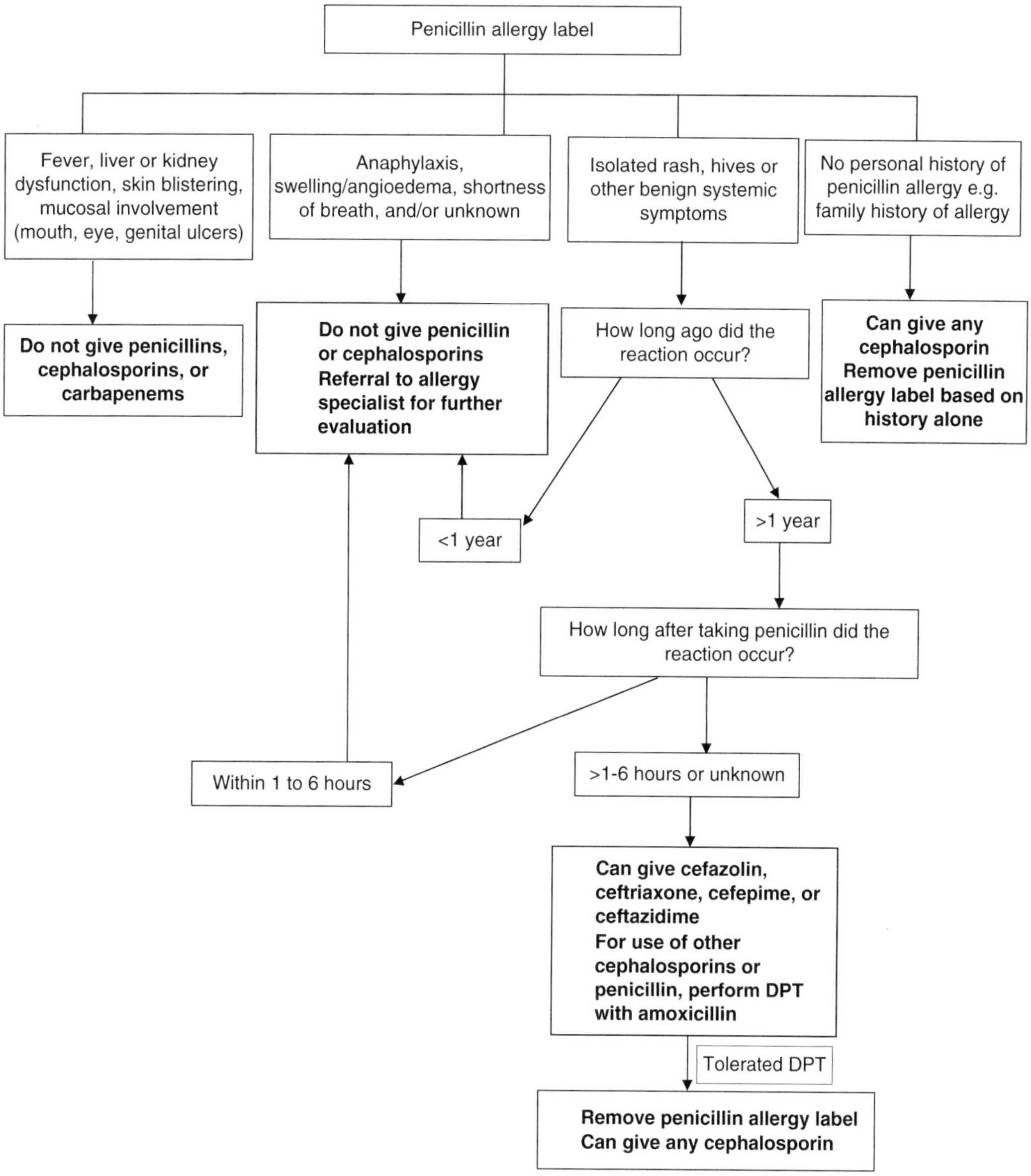

Fig. 32.2 Approach to penicillin allergy labels in non-allergist outpatient clinics

their clinical condition. Risk stratification is also contingent upon institutional factors, including the interview instrument, interviewer, and resources. Overall, erring on the side of caution to maintain safety while optimizing beta-lactam use is recommended. Drug allergy pathways have translated into promotion of antibiotic stewardship and other quality improvement metrics.

Summary

We anticipate drug allergy to increase in incidence and relevance with the continued discovery and approval of new and improved medications. However, there are numerous unmet needs in drug allergy evaluation specifically the lack of reliable diagnostic tests and the paucity of standardized testing reagents. Future studies should focus on these challenges, in particular the validation of diagnostic methods for most drug reactions.

References

1. Shaker MS, et al. Anaphylaxis-a 2020 practice parameter update, systematic review, and Grading of Recommendations, Assessment, Development and Evaluation (GRADE) analysis. J Allergy Clin Immunol. 2020;145(4):1082–123.
2. Jakubovic BD, et al. Drug hypersensitivity in the fast lane: what clinicians should know about phenotypes, endotypes, and biomarkers. Ann Allergy Asthma Immunol. 2020;124:566.
3. Dhopeshwarkar N, et al. Drug-induced anaphylaxis documented in electronic health records. J Allergy Clin Immunol Pract. 2019;7(1):103–11.
4. Jares EJ, et al. Drug-induced anaphylaxis, elicitors, risk factors, and management in Latin America. J Allergy Clin Immunol Pract. 2020;8(4):1403–1405 e1.
5. McNeil BD, et al. Identification of a mast-cell-specific receptor crucial for pseudo-allergic drug reactions. Nature. 2015;519(7542):237–41.
6. Laidlaw TM, Cahill KN. Current knowledge and management of hypersensitivity to aspirin and NSAIDs. J Allergy Clin Immunol Pract. 2017;5(3):537–45.
7. Dykewicz MS, Lam JK. Drug hypersensitivity reactions. Med Clin North Am. 2020;104(1):109–28.
8. Abrams EM, Khan DA. Diagnosing and managing drug allergy. CMAJ. 2018;190(17):E532–8.
9. Phillips EJ, et al. Controversies in drug allergy: testing for delayed reactions. J Allergy Clin Immunol. 2019;143(1):66–73.
10. Trautmann A, et al. "Treating through" decision and follow-up in antibiotic therapy-associated exanthemas. J Allergy Clin Immunol Pract. 2017;5(6):1650–6.
11. Wheatley LM, et al. Report from the National Institute of Allergy and Infectious Diseases workshop on drug allergy. J Allergy Clin Immunol. 2015;136(2):262–71 e2.
12. Muraro A, et al. Precision medicine in allergic disease-food allergy, drug allergy, and anaphylaxis-PRACTALL document of the European academy of allergy and clinical immunology and the American academy of allergy, asthma and immunology. Allergy. 2017;72(7):1006–21.
13. Schwartz RA, McDonough PH, Lee BW. Toxic epidermal necrolysis: part II. Prognosis, sequelae, diagnosis, differential diagnosis, prevention, and treatment. J Am Acad Dermatol. 2013;69(2):187 e1–16. quiz 203-4
14. Adler NR, et al. Recent advances in the understanding of severe cutaneous adverse reactions. Br J Dermatol. 2017;177(5):1234–47.
15. White KD, et al. Evolving models of the immunopathogenesis of T cell-mediated drug allergy: the role of host, pathogens, and drug response. J Allergy Clin Immunol. 2015;136(2):219–34. quiz 235
16. Pichler WJ, et al. Pharmacological interaction of drugs with immune receptors: the p-i concept. Allergol Int. 2006;55(1):17–25.
17. Adam J, et al. Avidity determines T-cell reactivity in abacavir hypersensitivity. Eur J Immunol. 2012;42(7):1706–16.
18. Schwartz LB, et al. Quantitation of histamine, tryptase, and chymase in dispersed human T and TC mast cells. J Immunol. 1987;138(8):2611–5.
19. Isabwe GAC, et al. Hypersensitivity reactions to therapeutic monoclonal antibodies: phenotypes and endotypes. J Allergy Clin Immunol. 2018;142(1):159–170 e2.
20. Barbaud A, et al. A multicentre study to determine the value and safety of drug patch tests for the three main classes of severe cutaneous adverse drug reactions. Br J Dermatol. 2013;168(3):555–62.
21. Mill C, et al. Assessing the diagnostic properties of a graded oral provocation challenge for the diagnosis of immediate and nonimmediate reactions to amoxicillin in children. JAMA Pediatr. 2016;170(6):e160033.
22. Trubiano JA, et al. The safety of antibiotic skin testing in severe T-cell-mediated hypersensitivity of immunocompetent and immunocompromised hosts. J Allergy Clin Immunol Pract. 2019;7(4):1341–1343 e1.
23. Lammintausta K, Kortekangas-Savolainen O. Oral challenge in patients with suspected cutaneous adverse drug reactions: findings in 784 patients during a 25-year-period. Acta Derm Venereol. 2005;85(6):491–6.
24. Waton J, et al. Drug re-challenges in cutaneous adverse drug reactions: information and effectiveness in the long-term management of patients. Allergy. 2011;66(7):941–7.
25. Macy E, Goldberg B, Poon KY. Use of commercial anti-penicillin IgE fluorometric enzyme immunoassays to diagnose penicillin allergy. Ann Allergy Asthma Immunol. 2010;105(2):136–41.
26. Aranda A, et al. In vitro evaluation of IgE-mediated hypersensitivity reactions to quinolones. Allergy. 2011;66(2):247–54.
27. Chung CH, et al. Cetuximab-induced anaphylaxis and IgE specific for galactose-alpha-1,3-galactose. N Engl J Med. 2008;358(11):1109–17.
28. Scherer K, et al. Desensitization in delayed drug hypersensitivity reactions – an EAACI position paper of the Drug Allergy Interest Group. Allergy. 2013;68(7):844–52.
29. Macy E, Ngor EW. Safely diagnosing clinically significant penicillin allergy using only penicilloyl-polylysine, penicillin, and oral amoxicillin. J Allergy Clin Immunol Pract. 2013;1(3):258–63.
30. Blumenthal KG, et al. High-cost, high-need patients: the impact of reported penicillin allergy. Am J Manag Care. 2020;26(4):154–61.

31. Blumenthal KG, et al. The cost of penicillin allergy evaluation. J Allergy Clin Immunol Pract. 2018;6(3):1019–1027 e2.
32. Voelker D, et al. Minor determinants of penicillin and amoxicillin are still key components of penicillin skin testing. J Allergy Clin Immunol Pract. 2020;8:1980.
33. Fox S, Park MA. Penicillin skin testing in the evaluation and management of penicillin allergy. Ann Allergy Asthma Immunol. 2011;106(1):1–7.
34. Tannert LK, et al. Positive skin test or specific IgE to penicillin does not reliably predict penicillin allergy. J Allergy Clin Immunol Pract. 2017;5(3):676–83.
35. Confino-Cohen R, et al. Oral challenge without skin testing safely excludes clinically significant delayed-onset penicillin hypersensitivity. J Allergy Clin Immunol Pract. 2017;5(3):669–75.
36. Iammatteo M, et al. Safety and outcomes of Oral graded challenges to amoxicillin without prior skin testing. J Allergy Clin Immunol Pract. 2019;7(1):236–43.
37. Tucker MH, et al. Amoxicillin challenge without penicillin skin testing in evaluation of penicillin allergy in a cohort of marine recruits. J Allergy Clin Immunol Pract. 2017;5(3):813–5.
38. Stevenson B, et al. Multicenter Australian study to determine criteria for low- and high-risk penicillin testing in outpatients. J Allergy Clin Immunol Pract. 2020;8(2):681–689 e3.
39. Zagursky RJ, Pichichero ME. Cross-reactivity in beta-lactam allergy. J Allergy Clin Immunol Pract. 2018;6(1):72–81 e1.
40. Castells M, Khan DA, Phillips EJ. Penicillin allergy. N Engl J Med. 2019;381(24):2338–51.
41. Blumenthal KG, et al. Addressing inpatient beta-lactam allergies: a multihospital implementation. J Allergy Clin Immunol Pract. 2017;5(3):616–625 e7.

Food Allergy

33

Christopher P. Parrish, Shyam Joshi, and J. Andrew Bird

Introduction

Immune-mediated reactions to food are common and significantly impair the quality of life of affected individuals. Recent estimates suggest 5.6 million US children [1] and more than 26 million US adults [2] may have a food allergy with even more individuals believing they are food allergic. Because of its prevalence in the population and its perception in the public, it is paramount for physicians who see allergic disease to be familiar with characteristic symptoms and to be comfortable with applying validated testing measures when indicated to ensure appropriate diagnosis. This chapter will review the basic definitions of food allergy, prevalence and epidemiology, pathophysiology, diagnosis, and appropriate management strategies with insight into future treatment options currently under investigation.

C. P. Parrish · J. A. Bird (✉)
Division of Allergy and Immunology, University of Texas Southwestern Medical Center, Dallas, TX, USA
e-mail: Christopher.Parrish@UTSouthwestern.edu; Drew.Bird@UTSouthwestern.edu

S. Joshi
Section of Allergy and Immunology, Oregon Health and Science University, Portland, OR, USA

Food Allergy Definitions

Any clinically evident sign or symptom that occurs upon food ingestion may be considered an adverse reaction to food [3]. Some reactions are the result of an immunologic response to food (allergy), while others are not (intolerance). The term food allergy most commonly refers to immediate hypersensitivity reactions mediated by food allergen binding to IgE antibodies on the surface of mast cells and basophils, resulting in cross-linking and release of histamine and other mediators. While contact or inhalation of allergen may trigger a reaction, the most typical encounter with food allergens is via ingestion. It is important to note that sensitization (the presence of IgE antibodies targeting foods) is necessary but not sufficient for diagnosis of IgE-mediated food allergy. As discussed below in more detail, clinical allergy is defined by the reproducible occurrence of symptoms upon ingestion. IgE-mediated reactions differ in pathophysiology and clinical presentation from non-IgE-mediated immunologic reactions. Examples of non-IgE-mediated reactions to foods include food protein-induced enterocolitis syndrome (FPIES), which is characterized by delayed (onset 1–4 h after ingestion), profuse, repetitive vomiting resulting in dehydration with associated pallor and lethargy. Eosinophilic esophagitis (EoE) and other eosinophilic gastrointestinal dis-

C. Damask et al. (eds.), *Allergy in Otolaryngology Practice*,
https://doi.org/10.1007/978-3-031-93455-1_33

eases (EGIDs) are thought to have a mixed pathophysiology with perhaps some involvement of IgE but mostly non-IgE-mediated mechanisms involving Th2 inflammation. Celiac disease is an example of an immunologic reaction to food that involves Th1 inflammation.

The term intolerance should be reserved for symptoms that occur with ingestion of food but are not the result of an immunologic reaction to the food [3]. Instead, they may be due to the inherent properties of the food and/or of the individual eating the food. Lactose intolerance, with gastrointestinal manifestations occurring after ingestion of lactose-containing foods such as milk, is an example of intolerance—in this case due to deficiency of lactase enzymes in the intestines of the affected individual. Scombroid poisoning is an example of intolerance in which the characteristics of the food (conversion of histidine to histamine in spoiled fish) lead to symptoms upon ingestion. The term "sensitivity" is not well-defined and is often used by laypersons to describe a non-specific intolerance of a food. Given potential confusion with sensitization (the presence of IgE antibodies to food), this term likely should be avoided.

For the remainder of this chapter, food allergy will be used to refer to IgE-mediated allergy to foods with immediate hypersensitivity reaction. Tolerance refers to the natural state in which a food may be eaten ad lib without symptoms of allergy even with periods of abstinence.

Prevalence and Epidemiology

Extensive data is available suggesting that food allergies are common, affecting up to 10% of the population [4]. Food allergy commonly begins in childhood, and most food allergies are outgrown. Only 15% of adult cases have their initial allergic reaction in adulthood [5]. Recent epidemiologic surveys suggest that ~8% of US children have a food allergy and more than 11% are perceived as food allergic [1]. Survey data in adults suggest that 1 in 10 US adults are food allergic (10.8%), whereas nearly 19% of adults believe they have a food allergy and only 1 in 20 have a physician-diagnosed food allergy [2]. It should be noted that self-reported food allergy rates are substantially higher than those confirmed with supervised oral food challenges (OFCs), implying that many individuals carry unconfirmed and possibly inaccurate diagnoses. Moreover, the precise prevalence remains unknown as individual studies lack a standardized definition of food allergy, concentrate on specific foods or manifestations, or focus on particular study populations.

The highest rates of food allergy are seen in western societies including Canada, several European nations, Australia, and the United States [6]. Countries with drastically lower rates include India, Thailand, and Iceland. Interestingly, in adults there are reports of higher sensitization rates in India compared to western countries (up to 27%); however, clinically relevant food allergy is rare at 1–2% [7]. The high variability between countries is likely due to diet exposure effects, genetic predisposing, microbiome diversity, and specific environmental exposures, although additional studies are needed to further explore this phenomenon.

The vast majority of food allergy reactions occur to a rather limited number of foods: peanut, tree nuts, fish, shellfish, egg, milk, wheat, soy, and seeds. However, nearly all foods have been reported in literature as culprits. Many studies have demonstrated a 1–2% relative increase in food allergy prevalence over the past 2–3 decades, especially in relation to peanut allergy [8]. The cause of this increase is not well understood, but several theories have been proposed including the delayed introduction of high-risk foods.

Importantly, most food allergies that develop in childhood are outgrown. A high rate of resolution is seen with allergies to milk (>50% by ages 5–10 years), egg (~50% by ages 2–9 years), wheat (50% by 7 years), and soy (45% by 6 years) [4]. Allergies to peanut, tree nuts, fish, and shellfish are more persistent. Approximately 20% of peanut-allergic children will develop natural tolerance by 4 years of age, and only approximately 10% of tree-nut-allergic children will develop tolerance [4]. The natural history of seed, fish, and shellfish allergies has not been closely studied, though shellfish allergy commonly develops in adulthood [2].

Race remains a controversial issue in terms of prevalence. While reports have shown higher rates of food allergy in black and Hispanic population, the underlying cause of this association has not been well studied [8]. Therefore, using this information for clinical decision-making should be done cautiously as many external factors including healthcare and socioeconomic disparities may play a significant role [9].

Pathophysiology of IgE-Mediated Food Allergy

IgE-mediated food allergy is the most common presentation of true immunologic-induced food reactivity. Its pathophysiology is important in understanding symptoms consistent with true disease and secondarily application of validated testing modalities to confirm clinical suspicion. Underlying the development of food allergy is a loss of oral tolerance, a physiologic state of systemic unresponsiveness to food antigens [10]. When oral tolerance fails to develop or is lost, food allergy develops. A number of factors have been shown or hypothesized to contribute to the loss of oral tolerance, though a unifying factor to explain most food allergy development is lacking. Failure of oral tolerance to develop and/or loss of tolerance has been observed in immune deficiency states (e.g., selective IgA deficiency, common variable immunodeficiency, and immunodysregulation polyendocrinopathy enteropathy X-linked (IPEX) syndrome). Other pre-disposing or contributing factors that have been hypothesized to contribute include proton pump inhibitor (PPI) use which may contribute to impaired digestion of proteins, genetic and environmental risk factors including male sex, African ancestry, Caesarean section delivery, IL10 and IL13 gene polymorphisms and a westernized low fiber diet [10].

Food allergens are typically proteins, with few exceptions. Conceptually any food may trigger a food-induced allergic reaction, but in clinical practice more than 90% of reactions are caused by 9 foods or food groups (cow's milk, hen's egg, peanut, tree nuts [e.g. almond, cashew, walnut, etc.], wheat, soy, finned fish, crustacean shellfish, and sesame seed) [1]. These common food allergens are water-soluble, 10–70 kilo-Dalton animal or plant glycoproteins that are resistant to heat, processing, and enzymatic digestion [11]. Less stable proteins found in fruits and vegetables may cross-react with pollen-homologous proteins leading to the sensation of oral itching known as pollen food allergy syndrome (PFAS) or oral allergy syndrome [12]. PFAS reactions are typically limited to the oropharynx, are transient, and are unlikely to induce anaphylaxis. Complex carbohydrates found in mammalian meat (galactose-alpha-1,3-galactose) have also been reported to produce delayed anaphylactic reactions [4].

Sensitization to food allergens may occur before ingestion has occurred. The dual allergen exposure hypothesis suggests that low-dose cutaneous exposure to allergen is sensitizing and facilitated by an impaired skin barrier and inflammation such as that seen in atopic dermatitis [4]. This hypothesis was developed by Gideon Lack and supported by his studies showing atopic infants are less likely to develop a peanut allergy if peanut is introduced into their diet before allergy has developed compared to high-risk infants who avoid peanut [13]. Cutaneous exposure to allergen induces thymic stromal lymphopoietin (TSLP) production, activation of basophils, production of type 2 T-helper-cell (Th2) cytokines, and accumulation of mast cells in the gut [10, 14].

In a non-allergic individual, food antigens are processed primarily through the gut-associated lymphoid tissue (GALT). CD103+ dendritic cells (DC) take up the antigen in the gut mucosa and CD11b + dermal dendritic cells and Langerhans cells in the skin migrate to regional lymph nodes where tolerance is induced, partly through induction of T regulatory cells (Treg) [4]. In allergic individuals, Th2 responses replace the Treg response driving IgE class switching and expansion of allergic effector cells (e.g., mast cells, basophils) via production of interleukin (IL) 4 and IL-13. Allergen-specific IgE binds to high-affinity surface IgE receptors (Fc epsilon RI) primarily on mast cells and basophils, and cross-linking of IgE on the cell surface leads to degranulation releasing inflammatory mediators including prostaglandins, histamine, leukotrienes, and platelet-activating factor, resulting in the characteristic allergic response [15].

Mast cell activation is the major cause of allergic inflammation, and mast cells are located primarily in mucosal tissues of the respiratory tract and gastrointestinal tract, and in the dermal layers of the skin [16]; therefore, symptoms of allergic reactivity are primarily characterized by objective symptoms in those systems. Basophils also play a role in human anaphylaxis, though their contribution to the pathology of anaphylaxis is less clear [17]. Within minutes to no more than 2 h of ingestion of allergen an allergic patient may develop anaphylaxis, a severe, life-threatening, systemic allergic response. Skin symptoms may include acute urticaria, angioedema, or diffuse pruritis. Gastrointestinal symptoms include acute vomiting, cramping abdominal pain, or diarrhea. Both upper and lower respiratory symptoms may develop including repetitive coughing, wheezing, laryngeal edema, repetitious sneezing, copious mucus production, and congestion. Cardiovascular symptoms such as hypotension or dysrhythmia may develop, though they are rare.

Relationship Between Food Allergy and Other Atopic Diseases

Early Introduction of Allergenic Foods and the "Atopic March"

As discussed above, food allergy prevalence has increased in recent decades. Delayed introduction of highly allergenic foods is thought to be a contributing factor to this rising prevalence. Previous guidelines in western societies recommended avoidance of allergenic foods for the first several years of life, [18] but recent studies have shifted the paradigm from avoidance to early introduction of allergenic foods to prevent food allergy [19]. An observational study noted tenfold higher rates of peanut allergy among Jewish children in the United Kingdom compared with those in Israel [20]. The Israeli children ate peanut-containing snack foods beginning around age 7 months with a median consumption of 7.1 g per month versus 0 g per month in the UK children. This observation led to a landmark prospective study comparing early introduction (beginning at age 4–11 months) and ongoing consumption of peanut (2 g peanut protein, 3 times per week) to strict avoidance from infancy to age 5 years in high-risk children [13]. The high-risk group was defined by severe eczema (frequent need for topical corticosteroids) and/or egg allergy. The relative reduction in peanut allergy prevalence at age 5 years for the consumption group was 86% compared to the avoidance group among those without sensitization at baseline and 70% among those with mild sensitization (peanut skin prick test wheal of 3–4 mm diameter). This drastic reduction led to changes in guideline recommendations for timing of peanut introduction around the world. Current guidelines from the NIAID recommend testing for peanut sensitization prior to introduction between 4 and 6 months of age in high-risk children (severe eczema and/or egg allergy) and introduction without testing for those with mild to moderate eczema at around age 6 months [21].

The dual allergen exposure hypothesis discussed above proposes an explanation for the effectiveness of early allergen introduction. Atopic dermatitis is often the earliest manifestation in what is commonly referred to as the "atopic march", with infantile eczema preceding IgE-mediated food allergy and later followed by wheezing/asthma and allergic rhinitis. According to the dual allergen exposure hypothesis, exposure to foods through the cutaneous route, especially in low doses via eczematous skin with Th2 predominant inflammation tends to lead to IgE sensitization and food allergy, while exposure via mouth leads to natural tolerance [19]. The goal of early introduction is to introduce the allergenic food by mouth prior to the development of allergy and to keep the food in the diet on a regular basis for the ongoing promotion of tolerance.

While expert guidelines and recommendations worldwide encourage early peanut introduction, there is less consensus relating to introduction of other common food allergens [22]. Multiple studies of early egg introduction have shown conflicting results likely related to varying baseline risk among the studied populations and variance in the allergenicity of the egg products used. Two trials of early introduction of heated egg protein resulted in significant benefit without sacrificing safety [23, 24]. Four other trials used raw egg protein, which is more allergenic than heated egg protein, with only one of the trials showing benefit of early introduction [25–28]. A major limiting factor in most of these studies was the presence of egg allergy upon study entry, suggesting that earlier introduction or use of the less allergenic heated form of egg protein may be preferable. British (https://www.bsaci.org/about/early-feeding-guidance) and Australian (https://www.allergy.org.au/patients/allergy-prevention/ascia-how-to-inroduce-solid-foods-to-babies) guidelines recommend early introduction of egg, while US guidelines do not directly recommend early egg introduction, though it is to be noted that there appears to be no benefit to delayed introduction of allergenic foods in any population. Data regarding the early introduction of other common food allergens is lacking. A single prospective cohort study reported lower rates of cow's milk allergy in infants who were fed cow's milk protein within the first 14 days of life versus between days 105 and 194 of life [29]. The EAT trial, which attempted introduction of 6 common food allergens at age 3 months in an unselected population, showed benefit for introduction of peanut and egg but did not show any benefit with early introduction of milk, sesame, fish, or wheat [23]. At this time the evidence is strongest for early introduction of peanut and possibly egg, especially in high-risk infants, and ongoing studies aim to further inform and optimize early introduction as a food allergy prevention strategy.

Food Allergy and Atopic Dermatitis

Atopic dermatitis (AD) is relatively common in the pediatric population with an incidence between 10% and 30% [30]. Its onset is typically in early infancy and often resolves by adolescence. Adult-onset AD is rare and only accounts for 9–14% of total cases. The pathophysiology of AD is complex and involves genetic factors (defective skin barrier and immune dysregulation) as well as environmental exposures (allergens, irritants, and microbes). Most known genetic mutations associated with AD involve skin barrier function with filaggrin (*FLG*), an epidermal structural protein, being the strongest known genetic risk factor. Interestingly, the odds ratio for *FLG* mutations and peanut allergy is even stronger than that for AD (5.3 vs. 3.1) [31]. This correlation provides a strong connection between skin barrier disturbances and the pathogenesis of food allergy. In addition, both AD and food allergy share similar immunologic abnormalities leading to Th2-high inflammatory processes as discussed earlier in this chapter.

More severe, earlier onset, and persistent forms of AD are associated with higher rates of both food sensitization and food allergy, which has been consistently illustrated in various populations. In the large Australia-based HealthNuts cohort, up to 50% of infants with moderate to severe AD during their first 3 months of life requiring topical corticosteroids use subsequently developed OFC-proven food allergy [32]. This relationship is not as convincing in patients with mild AD.

Food allergy sensitization in AD patients has classically been thought to occur through the gastrointestinal tract due to gut barrier dysfunction. However, more recent studies have demonstrated that sensitization can occur prior to first ingestion. Direct peanut oil application on inflamed skin and household peanut exposure have been shown to increase the risk of peanut allergy, suggesting food protein contact with inflamed skin may also be a common mechanism [33].

The role of foods as a trigger for AD flares is less well defined. Studies are conflicting with several revealing up to 30% of patients with moderate to severe AD may have a food trigger but other reports have substantially lower numbers [30]. While the common food allergens are the most frequently implicated foods in younger children, birch pollen-related foods have been described as potential triggers of AD in older children and adults. This phenomenon called pollen food allergy syndrome will be discussed in more detail in the following sections of this chapter.

As specific IgE tests are often positive to multiple food allergens in AD patients, testing should be restricted only to foods with a convincing history of an IgE-mediated allergy. It is not recommended to perform screening food-specific IgE panels on all patients presenting with moderate-to-severe AD before food introduction as this practice commonly results in misdiagnosis of food allergy and may lead to nutritional deficiencies secondary to unnecessary dietary avoidance [34, 35]. It is also important to note that removal of a food to which a child is sensitized may result in loss of tolerance and trigger an anaphylactic reaction with reintroduction [36, 37]. It is advisable to refer patients with moderate to severe AD that is inadequately responsive to standard topical therapies to an allergist comfortable in assessing food allergy and performing oral food challenges when necessary rather than performing an indiscriminate battery of food allergy tests and recommending dietary avoidance [30].

Food Allergy and Allergic Rhinitis

Reported food allergies are common in patients with allergic rhinitis with prevalence estimates ranging from 20% to 70% based on geographic location and are more often seen in adults compared to children [38]. The vast majority of these are consistent with pollen food allergy syndrome (PFAS), but classic IgE-mediated food allergy is also reportedly higher in this population.

PFAS is an overarching term for several described subtypes including birch-pollen, mugwort-celery-spice, and ragweed-melon syndromes. While considered a food allergy by the strict definition of the term, PFAS is clearly a different entity and often classified as class II food allergy. Prior aeroallergen sensitization can lead to immunologic recognition of cross-reactive proteins found in many common foods (Table 33.1). Upon exposure to these food allergens, most patients develop localized oral-pharyngeal pruritus. As the majority of these allergens are heat labile, the symptoms may only occur when eating raw foods while the patient may tolerate cooked or processed products. Systemic reactions can occur in up to 3% of cases including urticaria, dyspnea, and anaphylaxis. The diagnosis is often made clinically based on history alone, but specific IgE testing can be used in select situations.

Management of PFAS varies widely. For minor localized symptoms, conservative mea-

Table 33.1 Cross-reactivity between pollen and associated foods that are seen in pollen-food allergy syndrome [38]

	Cross-reactive triggers		
Pollens	Fruits	Vegetables/spices	Other
Alder	Apple, cherry, peach, pear	Celery, parsley	Almond, hazelnut
Birch/oak	Apple, apricot, cherry, kiwi, peach, pear, plum, tomato	Carrot, celery, coriander, cumin, green pepper, parsley	Almond, beans, hazelnut, lentils, peanut, soybean
Cedar			
Mugwort	Peach, lychee, mango, grape	Bell pepper, broccoli, cabbage, cauliflower, coriander, garlic, onion	Mustard seeds, sunflower seeds, peanut
Northern pasture grasses (e.g., Timothy, orchard)	Kiwi, melon, orange, tomato, watermelon	Swiss chard, white potato	Peanut
Ragweed	Banana, canteloupe, honeydew, watermelon	Cucumber, squash, zucchini	

sures are often recommended including removing the peel (if applicable) or heating the food through baking/microwaving to reduce allergenicity. In patients with a history of more severe or systemic symptoms, avoidance may be the only option. Prescription of an epinephrine autoinjector is left to the discretion of the provider and practices differ based on geographic location.

Furthermore, rhinitis can be a common symptom encountered during a classic IgE-mediated food reaction along with other systemic symptoms. The literature has not supported a clear correlation between the ingestion of foods with isolated, immune-mediated rhinitis as a result [39, 40]. Neurogenic activation of rhinorrhea can occur in some patients regardless of the food ingested, which is termed gustatory rhinitis. This is a unique and separate disease process and should be considered in patients presenting with singular rhinitis symptoms with food ingestion. In these circumstances, food-specific IgE testing (e.g., serum IgE testing or skin prick testing) is not indicated.

Food Allergy and Asthma

Asthma is a complex multifactorial disorder that is attributed to the interaction between genetic factors, environmental exposures (air pollution, pollens and other aeroallergen, and weather), and host factors (obesity, infections, and allergic sensitization). It is now recognized that asthma is not a singular disease but a group of heterogeneous phenotypes with varied etiologies, prognoses, and management considerations. It remains a major cause of morbidity and mortality globally with a prevalence of approximately 4–5%, although it is much higher in many western countries [41].

Early childhood asthma and wheezing is thought to share a similar pathophysiologic basis with food allergy, as both are important components of the atopic march. Approximately one-third of children with food allergy have asthma and 4–8% of children with asthma have food allergy [42]. The development of asthma by 4–5 years of age is twice as common in those with challenge-proven food allergy at 1 year of age, irrespective of whether the food allergy subsequently resolves. Those with multiple food allergies and coexistent eczema were almost 3 times as likely to develop asthma compared with those with no food allergies [43].

Respiratory symptoms including wheezing are common manifestations of food allergy with other systemic symptoms; however, it is rarely the only symptom. Patients with poorly controlled asthma are more likely to have a fatal allergic reaction to foods. Consequently, aggressive asthma control is vital in this specific patient population. There is no evidence that dietary elimination helps with asthma control [44]. Apart from avoiding documented IgE-mediated food allergens, avoiding specific foods is not recommended for the treatment of asthma [42].

Diagnosis

Patient History

Food allergy diagnosis relies heavily on the patient's clinical history, keeping in mind that validated testing modalities evaluate for the presence of food-specific IgE. In addition, the sensitivity and specificity of IgE testing, as with all tests, is heavily reliant on the pre-test probability of disease. With these factors in mind, it is important to consider the pathophysiology of IgE-mediated food allergy, and to focus on the history of the following relevant facts about IgE-mediated food allergy (Fig. 33.1).

1. *More than 90% of food-induced allergic reactions are caused by 9 major foods or food groups* [4].
   - Cow's milk, hen's egg, peanut, tree nuts (e.g., walnut, cashew, almond, etc.), wheat, soy protein, finned fish, crustacean shellfish, and sesame seed are responsible for the overwhelming majority of food-induced reactions. With this in mind, carefully consider the patient's diet within 2 h

1. **Did the reaction occur after eating a food containing milk, egg, wheat, soy, peanut, a tree nut, sesame seed, fish or shellfish?**
   - More than 90% of food-induced allergic reactions are caused by one of these foods.
2. **Does the patient have an aversion to the suspected food?**
   - Allergic patients, especially children, do not typically prefer the food that has caused an allergic reaction.
3. **How long after ingestion did the reaction occur?**
   - IgE-mediated food-induced allergic reactions typically occur within minutes to no more than 2 hours after ingestion.
4. **What organ systems were involved in the reaction?**
   - Symptoms of an allergic reaction are present in organ systems that contain mast cells (e.g. respiratory mucosa, skin, GI mucosa)
5. **Does the reaction occur reproducibly with ingestion?**
   - A food-induced allergic reaction will occur each time the food is ingested in sufficient quantity, often requiring a small amount of exposure to trigger a reaction.*
6. **How long has it been since the last reaction?**
   - Most food allergies are outgrown; however, peanut, tree nut, fish, shellfish and seed allergies tend to persist into adulthood.
7. **Are symptoms consistent with the above characteristics?**
   - Do not test for specific IgE to foods if the pathophysiology is not consistent with IgE-mediated food allergy even though many diseases may be attributed to an "allergy" in non-medical literature (e.g. fatigue, headaches, behavioral changes).

*Baked milk and baked egg products may be tolerated by most milk and egg-allergic individuals because heating alters protein conformation.

Fig. 33.1 Important questions to consider when evaluating a patient for food allergy

of the reaction in light of these common food allergens.

2. *Patients (especially children) may have an aversion to the suspected food.*
   - It is uncommon for a patient with a food allergy to have a taste preference for a food which triggers immediate reactivity. In young children this may present with a parent stating they have tried giving the child eggs, for example, but the child spits the food out of their mouth. In older children or adults who are peanut-allergic, the smell of peanut products is not typically appealing.
3. *IgE-mediated reactions usually occur within 20 min of ingestion and almost always within 2 h of ingestion* [45].
   - Ask for the temporal relation between the onset of symptoms and the time of last ingestion. If the patient states they developed symptoms hours later, especially if the following day, then it is very unlikely the symptoms are related to food allergy. The exception to this rule is with delayed anaphylaxis related to ingestion of mammalian meat (alpha-gal syndrome), when symptoms may appear as many as 6 h after ingestion [4].
4. *Mast cells are primarily located in the respiratory mucosa, GI mucosa, and skin* [16].
   - Cross-linked IgE bound to the high-affinity surface IgE receptors on mast cells and circulating basophils leads to degranulation. This results in the characteristic symptoms of IgE-mediated food allergy, and mast cell degranulation is the primary driver of allergic anaphylaxis. [16] Symptoms of IgE-mediated disease are characteristically present at the sites where mast cells are concentrated.
5. *A food-induced allergic reaction will occur each time the patient is exposed to the allergen in sufficient quantity; however, some factors, such as baking, may affect protein conformation and food matrices, such as wheat, may affect absorption* [45].
   - Food-induced allergic reactions are reproducible with repeat ingestion, especially if a standard serving size of the food has been ingested. The patient's history will suggest

characteristic symptoms each time the patient eats the food of concern rather than a history of tolerance on occasion with reactivity at other times. Heating alters milk and egg protein conformation, and the majority of milk and egg allergic individuals will tolerate these foods in a baked good while reacting to lesser cooked forms (e.g., yogurt, scrambled egg, etc.).

6. *Peanut, tree nut, fish, shellfish, and sesame seed allergies are persistent, while most other food allergies are outgrown with age* [46].
   - It is important to ask patients when they last had a reaction to the food of concern since the majority of patients will develop natural tolerance to cow's milk, hen's egg, wheat, soy, fruit, and vegetable allergies. If a patient has not had a reaction in more than 1–2 years, then it may be reasonable to consider additional testing or observed food challenges to see if natural tolerance has developed.
7. *Limit testing to scenarios in which patients are likely food-allergic based on the above facts.*
   - Patients may attribute a number of disease states to a food trigger without any physiologic basis to have underlying IgE specificity. Food allergy is not the underlying cause of chronic rhinitis, asthma, behavior or mood changes, headaches, chronic urticaria, chronic GI complaints, or fatigue.

Serum IgE Testing, Component Testing, and Skin Prick Testing

Serum IgE testing detects food-specific IgE antibodies in the serum. Sensitization to allergens is not equivalent to clinical reactivity, and panel testing for a non-specific array of food allergens commonly leads to misdiagnosis [34]. Several investigators have established 95% positive predictive value cut-offs associated with ImmunoCAP-specific IgE testing for cow's milk, hen's egg, and peanut test interpretation (Table 33.2) [57]. Other foods do not have similarly established interpretive capabilities. It is also important to note there are no tests which predict reaction severity, rather test results should be interpreted as the likelihood of reacting with ingestion of the food allergen.

Rather than using crude allergen extracts, component resolved diagnostics (CRD) measure IgE to individual allergens within the food [58]. CRD has proven more helpful in diagnosing pea-

Table 33.2 Predictive values of diagnostic tests used to diagnose food allergy [47]

Food	Serum food-IgE (kU/L)[a] ~95% Positive OFC	Serum food-IgE (kU/L)[a] ~50% Negative OFC[b]	SPT wheal (mm)[a] ~95% Positive OFC	SPT wheal (mm)[a] ~50% Negative OFC[b]
Cow's milk	≥15 [48]	≤2 [49]	≥8 [50]	
	≥5 if younger than 1 year [51]			
Egg white	≥7 [48]	≤2 [49]	≥7 [50]	≤3 [52]
	≥2 if younger than 2 years [53]			
Peanut	≥14 [48]	≤2 with and ≤ 5 without history of peanut reaction [54]	≥8 [50, 55]	≤3 [55]

A subset of patients with undetectable serum food-specific IgE antibody and negative SPT has been reported to have objective reactions confirmed by OFC [56]

OFC oral food challenge, *SPT* skin prick test

[a]Phadia ImmunoCAP; SPT with commercial food extracts

[b]Serum IgE levels, when applied to patients with a history supporting IgE-mediated food allergy, may assist in predicting when it would be prudent to consider an observed oral food challenge. In general, oral food challenges are considered for patients with a 50% or greater likelihood of passing a challenge

nut allergy than using the whole peanut extract, with IgE to Ara h 2 providing higher diagnostic accuracy than whole peanut-sIgE or peanut-sIgE to other peanut components [4]. CRD has also proven useful in the diagnosis of hazelnut allergy (specificity of testing improved when using component testing for Cor a 9 and 14) [59]. Results from studies measuring the usefulness of CRD testing for milk, egg, wheat, soy, and fruit allergies have not conclusively shown superiority in CRD testing over whole allergen testing [58].

Skin prick testing (SPT) is very sensitive with a negative predictive value greater than 90% [58]. A SPT wheal diameter 3 mm larger than the negative control is considered positive, and the larger the SPT wheal diameter, the more likely the result indicates a clinically meaningful allergic response. SPT is performed by using commercial extracts, though these extracts have not been standardized and may contain varying amounts of allergen [60, 61]. Fresh food testing (especially for fruits and vegetables) may be more accurate than when using commercial extracts [62, 63]. Several investigators have attempted to establish 95% PPVs for SPT wheal interpretation; however, values vary between patient populations, ages, and foods studied [58].

Oral Food Challenge

The diagnostic standard for food allergy is an ingestion challenge, with the highest degree of certainty present when both the patient and provider are blinded to administration of the challenge food or placebo, termed a double-blind, placebo-controlled food challenge (DBPCFC) [64]. The DBPCFC is typically performed in research studies, but it is uncommonly administered in clinical practice. An open oral food challenge (OFC), however, is commonly performed in an allergist's practice. This is typically done to assess for the development of tolerance since serum IgE testing and skin prick testing results may not clearly align with the patient's ingestion history.

The total amount of food administered should approximate a standard serving size, with a minimum cumulative challenge dose of at least 3500 mg of protein [64]. The serving is typically divided into 4–7 servings, starting with a small portion and gradually giving larger amounts every 20–30 min. The OFC is stopped when objective signs of an allergic reaction are observed. Subjective symptoms are not clearly indicative of an allergic reaction, and oftentimes visualization of the oropharynx via rhinolaryngoscopy may assist with differentiating objective angioedema versus a subjective globus sensation or vocal cord dysfunction that may be present in some individuals.

OFCs are considered safe. Fatalities have been reported, though these are extremely rare [64]. It is recommended that OFCs are performed in a monitored setting by providers experienced in the recognition and treatment of anaphylaxis with emergency medications readily available.

Unproven Diagnostic Approaches

Presently, the diagnostic tools available for food allergy are limited. Serum-specific IgE testing and SPT are useful only in IgE-mediated reactions, while OFCs may be time-consuming, fear-inducing, and not readily available for many patients [65]. Due to these factors, alternative diagnostic methods are often sought out by patients and caregivers with over 1 in 5 patients with self-reported food allergy undergoing unproven diagnostic testing [66]. This form of non-validated testing can lead to incorrect diagnoses, unnecessary food avoidance, and a significant decline in quality of life for patients and their families.

Atopy patch testing (APT) is a frequently used diagnostic modality in the diagnosis of delayed hypersensitivity reactions including contact dermatitis and drug allergy. APT is not recommended in the evaluation of IgE-mediated food allergy as it has shown low sensitivity, specificity, positive predictive value (PPV), and negative predictive value (NPV) in multiple studies [67]. APT has also been evaluated as a diagnostic tool for specific non-IgE-mediated food allergies such as eosinophilic esophagitis (EoE) and food protein-induced enterocolitis syndrome (FPIES). Its utility in these conditions remains unknown as conflicting results exist across multiple studies. Additional research is needed before a clear recommendation can be made.

The production of food-specific IgG is the body's natural response to ingested food, which is supported by the fact that 98% of children by the age of 2 develop cow's milk protein-specific IgG [68]. Many laboratories and clinicians that recommend testing for food-specific IgG claim that it is not helpful in diagnosing immediate-type reactions but is useful to diagnose the contribution of food in chronic diseases such as irritable bowel syndrome (IBS), chronic fatigue, migraines, and nonspecific joint pain. Reliable data is significantly lacking in the utility of this test with the majority of studies being of low quality [65]. While several studies have shown that food elimination based on food-specific IgG testing can lead to a decrease in reported symptoms, most of these lack control groups and have a high degree of bias. Despite this, large panel assays are available to providers and directly to patients with their use increasing over the past decade. Caution should be taken while interpreting these tests as more rigorous studies are needed before their use can be recommended.

Several other testing modalities have been evaluated and proven to be unhelpful in food allergy diagnosis. This includes provocation and neutralization testing, pulse testing, electrodermal testing, cytotoxic testing, and applied kinesiology testing [65].

Management of IgE-Mediated Food Allergy

The primary recommendations for management of IgE-mediated food allergy are allergen avoidance and emergency preparedness with education on the prompt treatment of systemic reactions with auto-injectable epinephrine [3]. Options for food allergy management are expanding, with a strong focus of research on interventional therapies aimed at mitigating reactions. One such interventional therapy, a peanut oral immunotherapy product has been FDA-approved and studies are ongoing assessing other therapies.

Food Allergen Avoidance

In general, consumption of allergenic food is necessary to trigger an allergic reaction, thus it follows logically that avoidance should be an effective strategy. However, accidental ingestion does occur despite avoidance efforts. For peanut allergy, accidental ingestion may occur in up to 50% of affected children over 2 years and in up to 75% over 10 years [69]. In order to minimize accidental ingestion and subsequent reactions, label reading and prevention of cross-contact are key [57].

The Food Allergy Labeling and Consumer Protection Act of 2004 (FALCPA) requires the listing of most common allergens (milk, egg, peanut, tree nuts, wheat, soy, fish, and crustacean shellfish) in plain English on the ingredient label for all packaged foods (except meat, poultry, specific egg products, and alcoholic beverages) sold in the United States. This requirement may be met by simply listing the allergen in the ingredient list, or through use of a separate "Contains" statement. Other common food allergens such as sesame seed, are not mandated to be listed on the label in the United States. Precautionary allergy labeling, with the use of phrases such as "may contain" or "processed in a facility with", is not mandated by FALCPA but is voluntarily provided by some manufacturers with the intent to warn of potential cross-contact. Excellent consumer resources with tips for label reading are available at the Food Allergy Research and Education (FARE) website (https://www.foodallergy.org/resources/how-read-food-label).

Cross-contact refers to the inadvertent transfer of a food allergen into a food that is not intended to contain the allergen. This may occur during food preparation or packaging and has been implicated in up to 15.1% of reactions in children under age 5 years [70]. The most commonly implicated packaged foods for cross-contact include cookies, ice cream, doughnuts/snack cakes, and snack mixes. The likelihood of cross-contact triggering a reaction depends on the amount of allergenic protein and an individual's threshold of reactivity. Baumert et al. have suggested that raising the threshold of reactivity from under 100 mg to 300 mg would likely reduce the risk of reaction due to peanut in these common snack foods by over 95% [71]. However, threshold dose varies widely among individuals and even over time for a given individual, so experts generally recommend avoidance of products with precautionary allergen labeling.

Traveling and/or eating outside the home often leads to increased anxiety about accidental ingestion, but steps can be taken to reduce the risk. Informing servers or flight attendants of allergies, provision of a "chef card", ordering simple foods with few ingredients, and avoiding fried foods (re-use of oil may increase risk of cross-contact) are some simple steps that are commonly recommended [57]. It is important to advise individuals and caregivers that allergens such as peanut are highly unlikely to aerosolize, so vigilance should be focused on avoiding ingestion of the allergen.

Recognition and Treatment of Anaphylaxis

Food-induced anaphylaxis is a severe, potentially life-threatening allergic reaction, sudden in onset, that occurs upon exposure to an allergenic food. It is the most feared outcome of food allergy and rarely may result in fatality. The most commonly implicated foods in fatal reactions are peanut, tree nuts, and—in young children—milk, but severe reactions are possible with any food allergen [72]. Case series of food-induced anaphylaxis fatalities consistently identify delay in administration or failure to administer epinephrine as a major risk factor [73–77]. In light of this, prompt recognition and treatment of anaphylaxis with auto-injectable intramuscular epinephrine is considered essential for the appropriate management of food-induced anaphylaxis. [3] The dose may be repeated if symptoms progress or fail to improve adequately. Self-injectable epinephrine and education on its use is considered mandatory for food-allergic patients. To facilitate recognition and proper management, written food allergy anaphylaxis action plans are recommended, with clear instructions on symptoms for which antihistamine treatment alone may be appropriate (e.g., scattered urticaria with no other symptoms) and situations in which epinephrine should be promptly administered (any reaction including respiratory signs/symptoms or meeting criteria for anaphylaxis). Such action plans are available from the website of FARE and that of the American Academy of Allergy, Asthma and Immunology (AAAAI) as well as most other allergy societies worldwide. Medical alert jewelry may alert first responders of a food allergy and facilitate prompt emergency care including epinephrine administration.

Therapeutic Interventions

While allergen avoidance and emergency preparedness are often quite effective for the management of food allergy, significant research efforts seek safe, effective interventional therapies for food allergy. Most research has focused on immunotherapies, which attempt to desensitize individuals to food allergens through exposure over time. Biologic therapies use monoclonal antibodies as an adjunct with immunotherapy or as monotherapy.

Immunotherapy has been used for over a century for the treatment of environmental allergies causing allergic rhinitis and asthma, usually via subcutaneous injection. The immune mechanisms of immunotherapy appear similar regardless of administration route, with induction of allergen-specific regulatory T cells and allergen-specific "blocking" IgG antibodies [78, 79]. The subcutaneous route of immunotherapy was briefly studied for peanut allergy, but research was halted due to high rates of anaphylaxis and high drop-out rates [80, 81].

Oral immunotherapy (OIT) has emerged as an alternative route of administration, with most research focusing on peanut allergy, largely due to the tendency to persist into adulthood and the association with severe reactions and fatalities. While specific methods vary, in general OIT begins with administration of several very low doses in a single observed visit (initial dose escalation) followed by continuation of the highest tolerated dose at home daily. The dose is increased at regular intervals under supervision (build-up phase) until a target dose is reached and continued for a period of time (maintenance phase). Maintenance doses vary, but the only FDA-approved therapy (Palforzia, Aimmune Therapeutics, Inc.) uses a maintenance dose of 300 mg peanut protein, equivalent to approximately one peanut kernel. In a phase 3 study, 67.2% of participants were able to ingest a single dose of 600 mg (cumulative dose 1043 mg) without significant symptoms after about 6 months of treatment with the 300 mg maintenance dose [82]. For reference, it has been estimated that raising the threshold of reactivity to 300 mg peanut protein would reduce the incidence of accidental reactions from peanut contamination in processed foods by over 95% [71].

Adverse effects with OIT are common, including gastrointestinal symptoms that may lead to treatment discontinuation. Eosinophilic esophagitis due to OIT has been estimated to occur in 2.7% to 5.1% of subjects [83, 84]. Acute allergic reactions after ingestion of doses are most common during the build-up phase but can occur at any point in therapy, even after a prolonged period on maintenance therapy [85]. Co-factors including heat, exercise, concurrent viral illness, ingestion on an empty stomach, menses, and even pollen season may increase the risk of symptoms after doses are ingested. To mitigate reactions related to these co-factors, significant lifestyle modifications are typically implemented, including avoidance of exercise or heat exposure (e.g., hot shower) prior to and for several hours after doses, adjusting or withholding doses during acute viral illness, and avoiding dose administration immediately prior to bedtime to allow observation for symptoms after ingestion. While most OIT reactions occur during a predictable time period after dose ingestion and therefore may be more easily managed than unpredictable reactions due to accidental ingestion, a recent meta-analysis concluded that peanut oral immunotherapy may cause more anaphylaxis and subsequent epinephrine use than it prevents [86]. Furthermore, the desensitization produced by OIT rarely persists after treatment cessation, so few patients are able to transition to ad lib consumption.

Given the safety concerns of OIT, there is great interest in alternative routes of administration that may pose a more favorable adverse event risk profile. Sublingual immunotherapy (SLIT) is increasingly used as an alternative to SCIT for aeroallergens and has shown promise in the treatment of food allergy, typically using doses of around 2 mg of food protein. The largest randomized controlled trial of peanut SLIT included 40 peanut-allergic adolescents and adults and 70% in the active treatment arm (~2.5 mg daily for 44 weeks) achieved a tenfold increase in successfully consumed dose from baseline versus 15% in the placebo group [87]. In a long-term study of peanut SLIT (2 mg/day for 3–5 years) in children aged 1–11 years, 37 of 48 (67%) successfully consumed 750 mg peanut protein after 3–5 years of therapy [88]. Adverse events in both studies were rare and mostly limited oropharyngeal pruritus.

Epicutaneous immunotherapy (EPIT) uses very low doses (Viaskin peanut patch contains 250 μg peanut protein) of allergen applied to intact skin. Langerhans cells in the epidermis uptake the allergen and transport it to regional lymph nodes, where it is presented to the immune system without having entered the bloodstream [89]. This mechanism and very low dose allow for a very favorable adverse effect profile, limited mostly to superficial skin reactions. However, EPIT appears to have lower efficacy than either OIT or SLIT. A phase 3 randomized controlled trial of a 250 μg peanut patch worn daily showed only 35.3% of subjects to be responders versus 13.6% in the placebo group [90].

Adjunctive therapies have also been investigated as a means of ameliorating adverse effects and improving the tolerability of OIT. Anti-IgE monoclonal antibodies including omalizumab have been shown to raise the threshold of reactivity upon OFC when used as monotherapy [91–93]. Adjunctive use, typically before and during the build-up phase of OIT, has been shown to facilitate rapid desensitization with fewer allergic symptoms for milk, peanut, and multiple food allergies [94–100]. A large multicenter phase 3 randomized controlled trial is currently underway to better define the benefits of omalizumab monotherapy including a direct comparison with omalizumab-facilitated OIT (NCT03881696). The anti-IL4rα monoclonal antibody dupilumab, which blocks the major Th2 cytokines IL-4 and IL-13, is also under investigation as adjunctive therapy (NCT03682770). Dupilumab is FDA-approved for allergic asthma and atopic dermatitis and under investigation for eosinophilic esophagitis, all of which are common comorbidities in food-allergic individuals. A probiotic therapy combined with peanut OIT (PPOIT) showed promise in an Australian cohort study, with 89.7% of those with PPOIT achieving desensitization compared to 7.1% among those receiving placebo [101].

Conclusions

Otolaryngologists will often interact with food-allergic patients as it is commonly seen with other atopic conditions. While several types of food allergies exist, IgE-mediated reactions are the most frequently diagnosed and can have the largest impact on the patient's or caregiver's quality of life. An important subtype, pollen-food allergy syndrome, will be regularly encountered due to its association with allergic rhinitis. While the diagnostic tools are currently limited, a thorough history can often lead to the correct diagnosis with testing only indicated in specific situations. A specialist trained and knowledgeable in food allergy may be helpful for the diagnosis and ongoing management of food allergies, especially as a multitude of novel treatment options are currently being investigated.

References

1. Gupta RS, Warren CM, Smith BM, Blumenstock JA, Jiang J, Davis MM, et al. The public health impact of parent-reported childhood food allergies in the United States. Pediatrics. 2018;142(6) https://doi.org/10.1542/peds.2018-1235.
2. Gupta RS, Warren CM, Smith BM, Jiang J, Blumenstock JA, Davis MM, et al. Prevalence and severity of food allergies among US adults. JAMA Netw Open. 2019;2(1):e185630. https://doi.org/10.1001/jamanetworkopen.2018.5630.
3. Boyce JA, Assa'ad A, Burks AW, Jones SM, Sampson HA, Wood RA, et al. Guidelines for the diagnosis and management of food allergy in the United States: summary of the NIAID-sponsored expert panel report. J Allergy Clin Immunol. 2010;126(6):1105–18. https://doi.org/10.1016/j.jaci.2010.10.008.
4. Sicherer SH, Sampson HA. Food allergy: a review and update on epidemiology, pathogenesis, diagnosis, prevention, and management. J Allergy Clin Immunol. 2018;141(1):41–58. https://doi.org/10.1016/j.jaci.2017.11.003.
5. Kamdar TA, Peterson S, Lau CH, Saltoun CA, Gupta RS, Bryce PJ. Prevalence and characteristics of adult-onset food allergy. J Allergy Clin Immunol Pract. 2015;3(1):114–5 e1. https://doi.org/10.1016/j.jaip.2014.07.007.
6. Peters RL, Koplin JJ, Allen KJ, Lowe AJ, Lodge CJ, Tang MLK, et al. The prevalence of food sensitization appears not to have changed between 2 Melbourne cohorts of high-risk infants recruited 15 years apart. J Allergy Clin Immunol Pract. 2018;6(2):440–8 e2. https://doi.org/10.1016/j.jaip.2017.11.018.
7. Mahesh PA, Wong GW, Ogorodova L, Potts J, Leung TF, Fedorova O, et al. Prevalence of food sensitization and probable food allergy among adults in India: the EuroPrevall INCO study. Allergy. 2016;71(7):1010–9. https://doi.org/10.1111/all.12868.
8. Keet CA, Savage JH, Seopaul S, Peng RD, Wood RA, Matsui EC. Temporal trends and racial/ethnic disparity in self-reported pediatric food allergy in the United States. Ann Allergy Asthma Immunol. 2014;112(3):222–9 e3. https://doi.org/10.1016/j.anai.2013.12.007.
9. Vyas DA, Esenstein LG, Jones DS. Hidden in plain sight – reconsidering the use of race correction in clinical algorithms. N Engl J Med. 2020;383:874.

10. Nowak-Wegrzyn A, Szajewska H, Lack G. Food allergy and the gut. Nat Rev Gastroenterol Hepatol. 2017;14(4):241–57. https://doi.org/10.1038/nrgastro.2016.187.
11. Sicherer SH, Sampson HA. Food allergy. J Allergy Clin Immunol. 2010;125(2 Suppl 2):S116–25. https://doi.org/10.1016/j.jaci.2009.08.028.
12. Yagami A, Ebisawa M. New findings, pathophysiology, and antigen analysis in pollen-food allergy syndrome. Curr Opin Allergy Clin Immunol. 2019;19(3):218–23. https://doi.org/10.1097/ACI.0000000000000533.
13. Du Toit G, Roberts G, Sayre PH, Bahnson HT, Radulovic S, Santos AF, et al. Randomized trial of peanut consumption in infants at risk for peanut allergy. N Engl J Med. 2015;372(9):803–13. https://doi.org/10.1056/NEJMoa1414850.
14. Noti M, Kim BS, Siracusa MC, Rak GD, Kubo M, Moghaddam AE, et al. Exposure to food allergens through inflamed skin promotes intestinal food allergy through the thymic stromal lymphopoietin-basophil axis. J Allergy Clin Immunol. 2014;133(5):1390–9, 9 e1–6. https://doi.org/10.1016/j.jaci.2014.01.021.
15. Burks AW. Peanut allergy. Lancet. 2008;371(9623):1538–46. https://doi.org/10.1016/S0140-6736(08)60659-5.
16. Kubo M. Mast cells and basophils in allergic inflammation. Curr Opin Immunol. 2018;54:74–9. https://doi.org/10.1016/j.coi.2018.06.006.
17. Reber LL, Hernandez JD, Galli SJ. The pathophysiology of anaphylaxis. J Allergy Clin Immunol. 2017;140(2):335–48. https://doi.org/10.1016/j.jaci.2017.06.003.
18. American Academy of Pediatrics. Committee on nutrition. Hypoallergenic infant formulas. Pediatrics. 2000;106(2 Pt 1):346–9.
19. Du Toit G, Sampson HA, Plaut M, Burks AW, Akdis CA, Lack G. Food allergy: update on prevention and tolerance. J Allergy Clin Immunol. 2018;141(1):30–40. https://doi.org/10.1016/j.jaci.2017.11.010.
20. Du Toit G, Katz Y, Sasieni P, Mesher D, Maleki SJ, Fisher HR, et al. Early consumption of peanuts in infancy is associated with a low prevalence of peanut allergy. J Allergy Clin Immunol. 2008;122(5):984–91. https://doi.org/10.1016/j.jaci.2008.08.039.
21. Togias A, Cooper SF, Acebal ML, Assa'ad A, Baker JR Jr, Beck LA, et al. Addendum guidelines for the prevention of peanut allergy in the United States: report of the National Institute of allergy and infectious diseases-sponsored expert panel. J Allergy Clin Immunol. 2017;139(1):29–44. https://doi.org/10.1016/j.jaci.2016.10.010.
22. Bird JA, Parrish C, Patel K, Shih JA, Vickery BP. Prevention of food allergy: beyond peanut. J Allergy Clin Immunol. 2019;143(2):545–7. https://doi.org/10.1016/j.jaci.2018.12.993.
23. Perkin MR, Logan K, Marrs T, Radulovic S, Craven J, Flohr C, et al. Enquiring about tolerance (EAT) study: feasibility of an early allergenic food introduction regimen. J Allergy Clin Immunol. 2016;137(5):1477–86 e8. https://doi.org/10.1016/j.jaci.2015.12.1322.
24. Natsume O, Kabashima S, Nakazato J, Yamamoto-Hanada K, Narita M, Kondo M, et al. Two-step egg introduction for prevention of egg allergy in high-risk infants with eczema (PETIT): a randomised, double-blind, placebo-controlled trial. Lancet. 2017;389(10066):276–86. https://doi.org/10.1016/S0140-6736(16)31418-0.
25. Wei-Liang Tan J, Valerio C, Barnes EH, Turner PJ, Van Asperen PA, Kakakios AM, et al. A randomized trial of egg introduction from 4 months of age in infants at risk for egg allergy. J Allergy Clin Immunol. 2017;139(5):1621–8 e8. https://doi.org/10.1016/j.jaci.2016.08.035.
26. Palmer DJ, Sullivan TR, Gold MS, Prescott SL, Makrides M. Randomized controlled trial of early regular egg intake to prevent egg allergy. J Allergy Clin Immunol. 2017;139(5):1600–7 e2. https://doi.org/10.1016/j.jaci.2016.06.052.
27. Palmer DJ, Metcalfe J, Makrides M, Gold MS, Quinn P, West CE, et al. Early regular egg exposure in infants with eczema: a randomized controlled trial. J Allergy Clin Immunol. 2013;132(2):387–92 e1. https://doi.org/10.1016/j.jaci.2013.05.002.
28. Bellach J, Schwarz V, Ahrens B, Trendelenburg V, Aksunger O, Kalb B, et al. Randomized placebo-controlled trial of hen's egg consumption for primary prevention in infants. J Allergy Clin Immunol. 2017;139(5):1591–9 e2. https://doi.org/10.1016/j.jaci.2016.06.045.
29. Katz Y, Rajuan N, Goldberg MR, Eisenberg E, Heyman E, Cohen A, et al. Early exposure to cow's milk protein is protective against IgE-mediated cow's milk protein allergy. J Allergy Clin Immunol. 2010;126(1):77–82 e1. https://doi.org/10.1016/j.jaci.2010.04.020.
30. Bergmann MM, Caubet JC, Boguniewicz M, Eigenmann PA. Evaluation of food allergy in patients with atopic dermatitis. J Allergy Clin Immunol Pract. 2013;1(1):22–8. https://doi.org/10.1016/j.jaip.2012.11.005.
31. Irvine AD, McLean WH, Leung DY. Filaggrin mutations associated with skin and allergic diseases. N Engl J Med. 2011;365(14):1315–27. https://doi.org/10.1056/NEJMra1011040.
32. Martin PE, Eckert JK, Koplin JJ, Lowe AJ, Gurrin LC, Dharmage SC, et al. Which infants with eczema are at risk of food allergy? Results from a population-based cohort. Clin Exp Allergy. 2015;45(1):255–64. https://doi.org/10.1111/cea.12406.
33. Tham EH, Leung DY. Mechanisms by which atopic dermatitis predisposes to food allergy and the atopic march. Allergy Asthma Immunol Res. 2019;11(1):4–15. https://doi.org/10.4168/aair.2019.11.1.4.

34. Bird JA, Crain M, Varshney P. Food allergen panel testing often results in misdiagnosis of food allergy. J Pediatr. 2015;166(1):97–100. https://doi.org/10.1016/j.jpeds.2014.07.062.
35. Fleischer DM, Bock SA, Spears GC, Wilson CG, Miyazawa NK, Gleason MC, et al. Oral food challenges in children with a diagnosis of food allergy. J Pediatr. 2011;158(4):578–83 e1. https://doi.org/10.1016/j.jpeds.2010.09.027.
36. Busse PJ, Nowak-Wegrzyn AH, Noone SA, Sampson HA, Sicherer SH. Recurrent peanut allergy. N Engl J Med. 2002;347(19):1535–6. https://doi.org/10.1056/NEJM200211073471921.
37. Fleischer DM, Conover-Walker MK, Christie L, Burks AW, Wood RA. The natural progression of peanut allergy: resolution and the possibility of recurrence. J Allergy Clin Immunol. 2003;112(1):183–9.
38. Carlson G, Coop C. Pollen food allergy syndrome (PFAS): a review of current available literature. Ann Allergy Asthma Immunol. 2019;123(4):359–65. https://doi.org/10.1016/j.anai.2019.07.022.
39. James JM, Bernhisel-Broadbent J, Sampson HA. Respiratory reactions provoked by double-blind food challenges in children. Am J Respir Crit Care Med. 1994;149(1):59–64. https://doi.org/10.1164/ajrccm.149.1.8111598.
40. Bock SA, Atkins FM. Patterns of food hypersensitivity during sixteen years of double-blind, placebo-controlled food challenges. J Pediatr. 1990;117(4):561–7. https://doi.org/10.1016/s0022-3476(05)80689-4.
41. To T, Stanojevic S, Moores G, Gershon AS, Bateman ED, Cruz AA, et al. Global asthma prevalence in adults: findings from the cross-sectional world health survey. BMC Public Health. 2012;12:204. https://doi.org/10.1186/1471-2458-12-204.
42. Bird JA, Burks AW. Food allergy and asthma. Prim Care Respir J. 2009;18(4):258–65. https://doi.org/10.4104/pcrj.2009.00036.
43. Vermeulen EM, Koplin JJ, Dharmage SC, Gurrin LC, Peters RL, McWilliam V, et al. Food allergy is an important risk factor for childhood asthma, irrespective of whether it resolves. J Allergy Clin Immunol Pract. 2018;6(4):1336–41 e3. https://doi.org/10.1016/j.jaip.2017.10.019.
44. Beausoleil JL, Fiedler J, Spergel JM. Food intolerance and childhood asthma: what is the link? Paediatr Drugs. 2007;9(3):157–63. https://doi.org/10.2165/00148581-200709030-00004.
45. Lack G. Clinical practice. Food allergy. N Engl J Med. 2008;359(12):1252–60. https://doi.org/10.1056/NEJMcp0800871.
46. Lopes JP, Sicherer S. Food allergy: epidemiology, pathogenesis, diagnosis, prevention, and treatment. Curr Opin Immunol. 2020;66:57–64. https://doi.org/10.1016/j.coi.2020.03.014.
47. Nowak-Wegrzyn A, Assa'ad AH, Bahna SL, Bock SA, Sicherer SH, Teuber SS, et al. Work group report: oral food challenge testing. J Allergy Clin Immunol. 2009;123(6 Suppl):S365–83. https://doi.org/10.1016/j.jaci.2009.03.042.
48. Sampson HA. Utility of food-specific IgE concentrations in predicting symptomatic food allergy. J Allergy Clin Immunol. 2001;107(5):891–6. https://doi.org/10.1067/mai.2001.114708.
49. Perry TT, Matsui EC, Kay Conover-Walker M, Wood RA. The relationship of allergen-specific IgE levels and oral food challenge outcome. J Allergy Clin Immunol. 2004;114(1):144–9. https://doi.org/10.1016/j.jaci.2004.04.009.
50. Sporik R, Hill DJ, Hosking CS. Specificity of allergen skin testing in predicting positive open food challenges to milk, egg and peanut in children. Clin Exp Allergy. 2000;30(11):1540–6.
51. Garcia-Ara C, Boyano-Martinez T, Diaz-Pena JM, Martin-Munoz F, Reche-Frutos M, Martin-Esteban M. Specific IgE levels in the diagnosis of immediate hypersensitivity to cows' milk protein in the infant. J Allergy Clin Immunol. 2001;107(1):185–90.
52. Knight AK, Shreffler WG, Sampson HA, Sicherer SH, Noone S, Mofidi S, et al. Skin prick test to egg white provides additional diagnostic utility to serum egg white-specific IgE antibody concentration in children. J Allergy Clin Immunol. 2006;117(4):842–7. https://doi.org/10.1016/j.jaci.2005.12.1304.
53. Boyano-Martinez T, Garcia-Ara C, Diaz-Pena JM, Martin-Esteban M. Prediction of tolerance on the basis of quantification of egg white-specific IgE antibodies in children with egg allergy. J Allergy Clin Immunol. 2002;110(2):304–9.
54. Sicherer SH, Morrow EH, Sampson HA. Dose-response in double-blind, placebo-controlled oral food challenges in children with atopic dermatitis. J Allergy Clin Immunol. 2000;105(3):582–6. https://doi.org/10.1067/mai.2000.104941.
55. Roberts G, Lack G. Diagnosing peanut allergy with skin prick and specific IgE testing. J Allergy Clin Immunol. 2005;115(6):1291–6. https://doi.org/10.1016/j.jaci.2005.02.038.
56. Sicherer SH, Bock SA. An expanding evidence base provides food for thought to avoid indigestion in managing difficult dilemmas in food allergy. J Allergy Clin Immunol. 2006;117(6):1419–22. https://doi.org/10.1016/j.jaci.2006.01.051.
57. Bird JA, Lack G, Perry TT. Clinical management of food allergy. J Allergy Clin Immunol Pract. 2015;3(1):1–11.; quiz 2. https://doi.org/10.1016/j.jaip.2014.06.008.
58. Kattan JD, Sicherer SH. Optimizing the diagnosis of food allergy. Immunol Allergy Clin N Am. 2015;35(1):61–76. https://doi.org/10.1016/j.iac.2014.09.009.
59. Kattan JD, Sicherer SH, Sampson HA. Clinical reactivity to hazelnut may be better identified by component testing than traditional testing methods. J Allergy Clin Immunol Pract. 2014;2(5):633–4 e1. https://doi.org/10.1016/j.jaip.2014.03.013.
60. Sampson HA. Comparative study of commercial food antigen extracts for the diagno-

sis of food hypersensitivity. J Allergy Clin Immunol. 1988;82(5 Pt 1):718–26. https://doi.org/10.1016/0091-6749(88)90070-x.
61. Hefle SL, Helm RM, Burks AW, Bush RK. Comparison of commercial peanut skin test extracts. J Allergy Clin Immunol. 1995;95(4):837–42. https://doi.org/10.1016/s0091-6749(95)70127-3.
62. Rance F, Juchet A, Bremont F, Dutau G. Correlations between skin prick tests using commercial extracts and fresh foods, specific IgE, and food challenges. Allergy. 1997;52(10):1031–5. https://doi.org/10.1111/j.1398-9995.1997.tb02427.x.
63. Verstege A, Mehl A, Rolinck-Werninghaus C, Staden U, Nocon M, Beyer K, et al. The predictive value of the skin prick test weal size for the outcome of oral food challenges. Clin Exp Allergy. 2005;35(9):1220–6. https://doi.org/10.1111/j.1365-2222.2005.2324.x.
64. Bird JA, Leonard S, Groetch M, Assa'ad A, Cianferoni A, Clark A, et al. Conducting an Oral food challenge: an update to the 2009 adverse reactions to foods committee work group report. J Allergy Clin Immunol Pract. 2020;8(1):75–90 e17. https://doi.org/10.1016/j.jaip.2019.09.029.
65. Hammond C, Lieberman JA. Unproven diagnostic tests for food allergy. Immunol Allergy Clin N Am. 2018;38(1):153–63. https://doi.org/10.1016/j.iac.2017.09.011.
66. Ko J, Lee JI, Munoz-Furlong A, Li XM, Sicherer SH. Use of complementary and alternative medicine by food-allergic patients. Ann Allergy Asthma Immunol. 2006;97(3):365–9. https://doi.org/10.1016/S1081-1206(10)60802-2.
67. Caglayan Sozmen S, Povesi Dascola C, Gioia E, Mastrorilli C, Rizzuti L, Caffarelli C. Diagnostic accuracy of patch test in children with food allergy. Pediatr Allergy Immunol. 2015;26(5):416–22. https://doi.org/10.1111/pai.12377.
68. Siroux V, Lupinek C, Resch Y, Curin M, Just J, Keil T, et al. Specific IgE and IgG measured by the MeDALL allergen-chip depend on allergen and route of exposure: the EGEA study. J Allergy Clin Immunol. 2017;139(2):643–54 e6. https://doi.org/10.1016/j.jaci.2016.05.023.
69. Bock SA, Atkins FM. The natural history of peanut allergy. J Allergy Clin Immunol. 1989;83(5):900–4. https://doi.org/10.1016/0091-6749(89)90103-6.
70. Fleischer DM, Perry TT, Atkins D, Wood RA, Burks AW, Jones SM, et al. Allergic reactions to foods in preschool-aged children in a prospective observational food allergy study. Pediatrics. 2012;130(1):e25–32. https://doi.org/10.1542/peds.2011-1762.
71. Baumert JL, Taylor SL, Koppelman SJ. Quantitative assessment of the safety benefits associated with increasing clinical Peanut thresholds through immunotherapy. J Allergy Clin Immunol Pract. 2018;6(2):457–65 e4. https://doi.org/10.1016/j.jaip.2017.05.006.
72. Parrish CP, Kim H. Food-induced anaphylaxis: an update. Curr Allergy Asthma Rep. 2018;18(8):41. https://doi.org/10.1007/s11882-018-0795-5.
73. Xu YS, Kastner M, Harada L, Xu A, Salter J, Waserman S. Anaphylaxis-related deaths in Ontario: a retrospective review of cases from 1986 to 2011. Allergy Asthma Clin Immunol. 2014;10(1):38. https://doi.org/10.1186/1710-1492-10-38.
74. Sampson HA, Mendelson L, Rosen JP. Fatal and near-fatal anaphylactic reactions to food in children and adolescents. N Engl J Med. 1992;327(6):380–4. https://doi.org/10.1056/NEJM199208063270603.
75. Pumphrey RS, Gowland MH. Further fatal allergic reactions to food in the United Kingdom, 1999-2006. J Allergy Clin Immunol. 2007;119(4):1018–9. https://doi.org/10.1016/j.jaci.2007.01.021.
76. Mullins RJ, Wainstein BK, Barnes EH, Liew WK, Campbell DE. Increases in anaphylaxis fatalities in Australia from 1997 to 2013. Clin Exp Allergy. 2016;46(8):1099–110. https://doi.org/10.1111/cea.12748.
77. Bock SA, Munoz-Furlong A, Sampson HA. Further fatalities caused by anaphylactic reactions to food, 2001-2006. J Allergy Clin Immunol. 2007;119(4):1016–8. https://doi.org/10.1016/j.jaci.2006.12.622.
78. Kulis MD, Patil SU, Wambre E, Vickery BP. Immune mechanisms of oral immunotherapy. J Allergy Clin Immunol. 2018;141(2):491–8. https://doi.org/10.1016/j.jaci.2017.12.979.
79. Feuille E, Nowak-Wegrzyn A. Allergen-specific immunotherapies for food allergy. Allergy Asthma Immunol Res. 2018;10(3):189–206. https://doi.org/10.4168/aair.2018.10.3.189.
80. Nelson HS, Lahr J, Rule R, Bock A, Leung D. Treatment of anaphylactic sensitivity to peanuts by immunotherapy with injections of aqueous peanut extract. J Allergy Clin Immunol. 1997;99(6 Pt 1):744–51. https://doi.org/10.1016/s0091-6749(97)80006-1.
81. Oppenheimer JJ, Nelson HS, Bock SA, Christensen F, Leung DY. Treatment of peanut allergy with rush immunotherapy. J Allergy Clin Immunol. 1992;90(2):256–62. https://doi.org/10.1016/0091-6749(92)90080-l.
82. Investigators PGC, Vickery BP, Vereda A, Casale TB, Beyer K, du Toit G, et al. AR101 Oral immunotherapy for Peanut allergy. N Engl J Med. 2018;379(21):1991–2001. https://doi.org/10.1056/NEJMoa1812856.
83. Petroni D, Spergel JM. Eosinophilic esophagitis and symptoms possibly related to eosinophilic esophagitis in oral immunotherapy. Ann Allergy Asthma Immunol. 2018;120(3):237–40 e4. https://doi.org/10.1016/j.anai.2017.11.016.
84. Lucendo AJ, Arias A, Tenias JM. Relation between eosinophilic esophagitis and oral immunotherapy for food allergy: a systematic review with meta-analysis. Ann Allergy Asthma Immunol. 2014;113(6):624–9. https://doi.org/10.1016/j.anai.2014.08.004.

85. Virkud YV, Burks AW, Steele PH, Edwards LJ, Berglund JP, Jones SM, et al. Novel baseline predictors of adverse events during oral immunotherapy in children with peanut allergy. J Allergy Clin Immunol. 2017;139(3):882–8 e5. https://doi.org/10.1016/j.jaci.2016.07.030.
86. Chu DK, Wood RA, French S, Fiocchi A, Jordana M, Waserman S, et al. Oral immunotherapy for peanut allergy (PACE): a systematic review and meta-analysis of efficacy and safety. Lancet. 2019;393(10187):2222–32. https://doi.org/10.1016/S0140-6736(19)30420-9.
87. Fleischer DM, Burks AW, Vickery BP, Scurlock AM, Wood RA, Jones SM, et al. Sublingual immunotherapy for peanut allergy: a randomized, double-blind, placebo-controlled multicenter trial. J Allergy Clin Immunol. 2013;131(1):119–27 e1–7. https://doi.org/10.1016/j.jaci.2012.11.011.
88. Kim EH, Yang L, Ye P, Guo R, Li Q, Kulis MD, et al. Long-term sublingual immunotherapy for peanut allergy in children: clinical and immunologic evidence of desensitization. J Allergy Clin Immunol. 2019;144(5):1320–6 e1. https://doi.org/10.1016/j.jaci.2019.07.030.
89. Bird JA, Sanchez-Borges M, Ansotegui IJ, Ebisawa M, Ortega Martell JA. Skin as an immune organ and clinical applications of skin-based immunotherapy. World Allergy Organ J. 2018;11(1):38. https://doi.org/10.1186/s40413-018-0215-2.
90. Fleischer DM, Greenhawt M, Sussman G, Begin P, Nowak-Wegrzyn A, Petroni D, et al. Effect of epicutaneous immunotherapy vs placebo on reaction to Peanut protein ingestion among children with Peanut allergy: the PEPITES randomized clinical trial. JAMA. 2019;321(10):946–55. https://doi.org/10.1001/jama.2019.1113.
91. Leung DY, Sampson HA, Yunginger JW, Burks AW Jr, Schneider LC, Wortel CH, et al. Effect of anti-IgE therapy in patients with peanut allergy. N Engl J Med. 2003;348(11):986–93. https://doi.org/10.1056/NEJMoa022613.
92. Savage JH, Courneya JP, Sterba PM, Macglashan DW, Saini SS, Wood RA. Kinetics of mast cell, basophil, and oral food challenge responses in omalizumab-treated adults with peanut allergy. J Allergy Clin Immunol. 2012;130(5):1123–9 e2. https://doi.org/10.1016/j.jaci.2012.05.039.
93. Fiocchi A, Artesani MC, Riccardi C, Mennini M, Pecora V, Fierro V, et al. Impact of omalizumab on food allergy in patients treated for asthma: a real-life study. J Allergy Clin Immunol Pract. 2019;7(6):1901–9 e5. https://doi.org/10.1016/j.jaip.2019.01.023.
94. Wood RA, Kim JS, Lindblad R, Nadeau K, Henning AK, Dawson P, et al. A randomized, double-blind, placebo-controlled study of omalizumab combined with oral immunotherapy for the treatment of cow's milk allergy. J Allergy Clin Immunol. 2016;137(4):1103–10 e11. https://doi.org/10.1016/j.jaci.2015.10.005.
95. Schneider LC, Rachid R, LeBovidge J, Blood E, Mittal M, Umetsu DT. A pilot study of omalizumab to facilitate rapid oral desensitization in high-risk peanut-allergic patients. J Allergy Clin Immunol. 2013;132(6):1368–74. https://doi.org/10.1016/j.jaci.2013.09.046.
96. Nadeau KC, Schneider LC, Hoyte L, Borras I, Umetsu DT. Rapid oral desensitization in combination with omalizumab therapy in patients with cow's milk allergy. J Allergy Clin Immunol. 2011;127(6):1622–4. https://doi.org/10.1016/j.jaci.2011.04.009.
97. MacGinnitie AJ, Rachid R, Gragg H, Little SV, Lakin P, Cianferoni A, et al. Omalizumab facilitates rapid oral desensitization for peanut allergy. J Allergy Clin Immunol. 2017;139(3):873–81 e8. https://doi.org/10.1016/j.jaci.2016.08.010.
98. Begin P, Dominguez T, Wilson SP, Bacal L, Mehrotra A, Kausch B, et al. Phase 1 results of safety and tolerability in a rush oral immunotherapy protocol to multiple foods using omalizumab. Allergy Asthma Clin Immunol. 2014;10(1):7. https://doi.org/10.1186/1710-1492-10-7.
99. Andorf S, Purington N, Kumar D, Long A, O'Laughlin KL, Sicherer S, et al. A phase 2 randomized controlled multisite study using omalizumab-facilitated rapid desensitization to test continued vs discontinued dosing in multifood allergic individuals. EClinicalMedicine. 2019;7:27–38. https://doi.org/10.1016/j.eclinm.2018.12.006.
100. Andorf S, Manohar M, Dominguez T, Block W, Tupa D, Kshirsagar RA, et al. Observational long-term follow-up study of rapid food oral immunotherapy with omalizumab. Allergy Asthma Clin Immunol. 2017;13:51. https://doi.org/10.1186/s13223-017-0223-8.
101. Tang ML, Ponsonby AL, Orsini F, Tey D, Robinson M, Su EL, et al. Administration of a probiotic with peanut oral immunotherapy: a randomized trial. J Allergy Clin Immunol. 2015;135(3):737–44 e8. https://doi.org/10.1016/j.jaci.2014.11.034.

Allergic Skin Conditions

34

Natalie M. Villa and Jennifer L. Hsiao

Introduction

Basic Structure of Skin

The skin is composed of two distinct layers on top of the underlying subcutaneous tissue. The outermost layer, the epidermis, is composed of multiple layers of keratinocytes that mature and migrate upwards towards the skin surface, where they are shed. Keratinocytes originate from stem cells in the basal layer. As they mature, they migrate upward through the stratum spinosum into the stratum granulosa where lamellar granules containing lipids and keratohyaline granules containing pro-filaggrin and keratin intermediate filaments are visible [1, 2].

Under normal conditions, keratinocytes lose their nuclei to form the stratum corneum. In addition, the cell membrane is replaced with the cornified envelope, consisting of keratin intermediate filaments cross-linked with filaggrin and coated with lipids to produce a water-tight skin barrier [1, 2]. Tight junctions between cells in the granular layer also play a role in the permeability of the skin barrier [3]. Melanocytes, which provide skin with pigment, and antigen-presenting Langerhans cells also reside in the epidermis.

The dermis is connected to the overlying epidermis via hemidesmosomes, specialized junctional complexes. It is a thick layer composed of collagen, elastin, blood vessels, glands, and nerves. Type 1 collagen is the predominant type of collagen found in the dermis, but Type III and Type V collagen may also be found [1].

Manifestations of skin pathology vary tremendously from inflammatory to autoimmune to neoplastic conditions. This chapter will focus on allergic skin conditions that can affect the head and neck region and also provide clinical pearls for each section.

Urticaria and Angioedema

Urticaria

Urticaria consists of the rapid onset of erythematous pruritic wheals, each of which resolves within 24 hours. The overall lifetime prevalence of any type of urticaria is around 8–11%, with a slight female predominance [4–8]. Chronic urticaria has been reported to have a lifetime prevalence of 1.8% [6].

Acute urticaria lasts for less than 6 weeks, while patients who experience symptoms for longer than 6 weeks are diagnosed with chronic

N. M. Villa
Department of Dermatology, Dartmouth Hitchcock Medical Center, Lebanon, NH, USA

J. L. Hsiao (✉)
Department of Dermatology, University of Southern California, Los Angeles, CA, USA

C. Damask et al. (eds.), *Allergy in Otolaryngology Practice*,
https://doi.org/10.1007/978-3-031-93455-1_34

urticaria. Acute urticaria may be triggered by foods and additives, medications, parasitic infections, upper respiratory tract infections, and insect bites [5, 8]. Physical urticaria may be diagnosed as acute urticaria until symptoms surpass the 6-week mark.

Chronic urticaria can be subdivided into chronic inducible urticaria (CIU), which occurs secondary to an identifiable trigger, or chronic spontaneous urticaria (CSU), which may be associated with different factors, but can occur at any time (see Table 34.1). CIU, also known as physical urticaria (with the exception of cholinergic urticaria), comprises about 20–48% of patients with chronic urticaria (Fig. 34.1a, b), while CSU comprises up to 80% of chronic urticaria [4, 5, 9]. In children, the lifetime prevalence of chronic urticaria is believed to be <1%, with no male or female predominance [10].

First-line treatment for any type of urticaria is a non-sedating (second generation) antihistamine or a sedating (first generation) antihistamine if tolerated [19]. No significant differences between non-sedating antihistamines available in the United States have been demonstrated [10, 19]. Oral prednisone is effective for the rapid resolution of wheals in acute urticaria if necessary but is not indicated as a long-term treatment [8, 18]. If the typical daily dose of non-sedating antihistamine does not induce symptom remission in patients with chronic urticaria, increasing the dose by up to four-fold is the next step.

Table 34.1 Types of chronic urticaria

Chronic inducible urticaria (CIU)			
Subtype	Description	Prevalence	Comments
Dermatographism [4, 9, 11–13]	Linear wheals in response to friction or trauma to the skin	46.2% of CIU (most common type). 1–5% of the general population	1.4 times more common in women than in men. Divided into simple (lacks pruritus) and symptomatic subtypes
Pressure urticaria [9, 11–13]	Occurs in areas where pressure has been applied, such as under shoulder straps or tight shoes. May be associated with chronic spontaneous urticaria (CSU)	7.7% of CIU	Wheals may last up to 72 hours after stimulus. Onset may be delayed up to 12 hours after exposure (delayed pressure urticaria)
Cholinergic urticaria [11–15]	Due to increase in body temperature from physical activity, exposure to heat, or emotional stress Classically presents as small wheals on trunk and extremities, known as pinpoint wheals	15.7–22.4% of CIU 4–11.2% of the general population	Not a true physical urticaria due to lack of a physical trigger
Solar urticaria [9, 12, 14]	Due to exposure to ultraviolet light	3.8% of CIU; 0.08% of all urticaria patients	Most commonly triggered by UVA spectrum
Aquagenic urticaria [12–14]	Due to exposure to water of any temperature	Rare	Presents with folliculocentric wheals within 20–30 minutes of water contact
Cold urticaria [9, 12–14, 16]	Due to exposure to cold temperatures or liquids	7.7–33% of CIU (second most common type)	May be inherited in an autosomal dominant fashion. Patients should avoid swimming due to the risk of anaphylaxis

(continued)

Table 34.1 (continued)

Chronic inducible urticaria (CIU)			
Subtype	Description	Prevalence	Comments
Heat urticaria [12, 13]	Due to contact with heat sources, such as hot water or sunlight, but not with increase in body temperature, as seen with cholinergic urticaria (see above)	Rare	
Vibratory angioedema [9, 11, 12, 14]	Due to exposure to vibration, such as with use of a lawnmower or jackhammer, or after dental procedures	Rare, but reported up to 23.1% of CIU in some populations	
Contact urticaria [17]	Wheals and pruritus occur in the area of skin that comes into contact with a particular trigger.	<0.4% of the general population	Most common triggers include latex, cosmetics, topical medications, and foods including eggs, seafood, mango, and melon. May be occupational. Non-immunologic form is commonly due to balsam of Peru, fragrance mix, sorbic acid, benzoic acid, or cinnamic aldehyde. Up to 42% of patients may also have atopic symptoms
Chronic spontaneous Urticaria [7, 9, 18]			
Chronic continuous urticaria	Symptoms occur almost daily	Associations: Food allergy (13.9%) Medications (5.8%) (NSAIDs and antibiotics most common) [18] Thyroid disease (4.7%) Other autoimmune diseases (4.7%)	May co-occur with angioedema in 40–50%
Chronic recurrent urticaria	Patients may experience symptom-free intervals of days to weeks before symptoms recur		

Abbreviations: *CIU* chronic inducible urticaria, *CSU* chronic spontaneous urticaria, *NSAID* nonsteroidal anti-inflammatory drug, *UVA* ultraviolet A

Third-line treatment is the anti-IgE monoclonal antibody omalizumab, administered 300 mg subcutaneously every 4 weeks [19, 20]. Prospective trials of omalizumab for treatment of urticaria have shown complete resolution of symptoms in 34–44% of patients, with responses of up to 83% in retrospective reports [19]. Omalizumab may be up-titrated up to every 2 weeks if necessary. Other treatment options include leukotriene receptor antagonists or cyclosporine, alone or in combination with antihistamines [19].

For children with urticaria, second-generation antihistamines dosed up to 4 times the normal dose are the preferred treatment, same as for adults; levocetirizine is approved by the U.S. Food and Drug Administration (FDA) to treat children older than 6 months of age with chronic urticaria [10]. First-generation antihistamines are not recommended in children due to their sedating side effects. Omalizumab is FDA-approved for the treatment of CIU in children 12 years and older. It may be added to oral antihistamines as a second-line combination therapy,

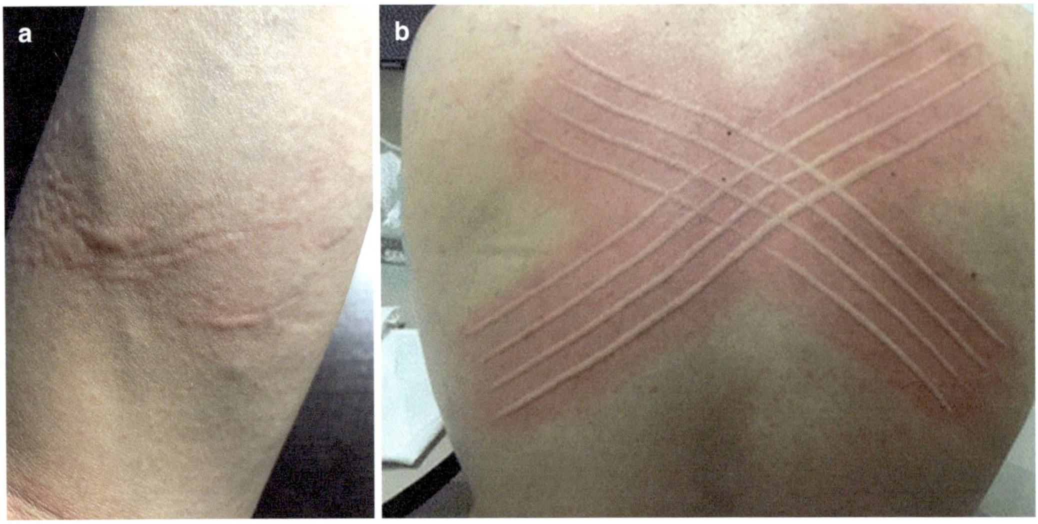

Fig. 34.1 Physical urticaria. (**a**) Pressure urticaria: Linear urticarial wheals induced after carrying grocery bags on the forearm. (Photo credit: Paul Blackcloud, MD); (**b**) Dermatographism. (Photo credit: Radonjic-Hoesli S, Hofmeier KS, Micaletto S, Schmid-Grendelmeier P, Bircher A, Simon D. Urticaria and angioedema: an update on classification and pathogenesis. Clin Rev. Allergy Immunol. 2018;54(1):88–101)

with cyclosporine and montelukast recommended as options in patients who cannot tolerate or do not have access to omalizumab [10]. Further, it is recommended to screen for thyroid disease and celiac disease in pediatric patients with chronic urticaria [10].

Urticarial Vasculitis

Urticarial vasculitis (UV) presents as wheals that are often painful or have a burning sensation and are sometimes pruritic, which persist longer than 24 hours [21]. A median duration of 10.7 days has been reported [22]. Other dermatologic manifestations of vasculitis may be present, such as palpable purpura [22]. Patients, particularly those with low complement levels, may have systemic symptoms such as arthralgias, uveitis, neuropathy, abdominal pain, proteinuria, or hematuria [22, 23]. Hypocomplementemic urticarial vasculitis syndrome (HUVS) is associated with angioedema, chronic obstructive pulmonary disease (COPD), and ocular symptoms, although the majority of UV patients with low complement levels have no systemic involvement [24, 25].

UV is a rare condition, but reports of its prevalence have ranged from 3 to 20%. It is up to 2–5 times more common in women compared to men [21, 22]. Immune complexes deposit in vessel walls, triggering complement activation. C3a and C5a trigger mast cell degranulation [23]. Triggers of immune complex formation include anti-C1q antibodies, infections (including upper respiratory tract infections, HIV, syphilis, hepatitis C, and hepatitis B), medications (including penicillin, NSAIDs, and interferon); however, a trigger may not be identified in up to 70% of patients [21–23]. Other associations with UV include systemic lupus erythematosus and malignancy (including breast, ovary, thyroid, colon, and pituitary) [22, 23].

Antihistamines may be used to treat mild disease without systemic symptoms [23]. Systemic corticosteroids are effective for patients with more severe disease, and short courses are preferred. Colchicine, dapsone, azathioprine, hydroxychloroquine, and NSAIDs have also been reported to be effective as steroid-sparing alternatives [23, 25, 26]. Hydroxychloroquine and colchicine may have similar efficacy to corticosteroids [25]. Long-term therapy may be necessary due to the chance of recurrence [22, 26]. Patients with severe necrotizing or ulcerative cutaneous disease or with systemic symptoms may require high-dose corticosteroids and/or other immunosuppressive therapies such as cyclophosphamide, cyclosporine (especially for patients with pulmonary symptoms or HUVS), or mycophenolate [19, 21, 23, 24]. There is mixed evidence on the use of methotrexate [27, 28]. More recently, omalizumab has been used to treat UV. Its use in UV is less well-studied than in chronic urticaria, but it has been reported to achieve complete remission in multiple cases; it may be less effective in patients with low complement levels [29, 30].

Angioedema

The prevalence of angioedema has been reported in a South Korean study to be 0.027% over 5 years [4] and in a Polish study to be 3.2% over lifetime [7]. A retrospective analysis of approximately 135,000 patients on an angiotensin-converting enzyme (ACE) inhibitor in the United States reported an incidence of angioedema of 0.23% within the first year after initiation and 0.1–0.12% over the subsequent four years after initiation [31]. Angioedema is more common in women [4]. It presents as swelling of the submucosal tissue of mucous membranes due to release of vasoactive mediators leading to increased vascular permeability and can involve subcutaneous tissue elsewhere on the body [7, 14]. Sites of involvement include lips, tongue, uvula, larynx, abdominal tract, and extremities [32, 33]. Symptoms develop over several hours and can take up to 7 days to resolve [32, 34, 35]. Angioedema may co-occur in around 40% of patients with chronic urticaria (see above) [9]. Angioedema related to urticaria is due to histamine release. Angioedema associated with ingestion of ACE inhibitors or inherited or acquired C1 esterase inhibitor deficiency is due to bradykinin release. Some types of idiopathic angioedema may respond to antihistamines; the exact pathogenesis of this interaction is not understood. There are two main types of angioedema without wheals: hereditary and acquired. See Table 34.2 for more details, including information on pathogenesis and treatment.

Table 34.2 Types of angioedema

Hereditary angioedema (HAE)				
Subtype	Pathogenesis	Clinical features	Treatment	Comments
Type 1 (85%) [32, 34]	Autosomal dominant or spontaneous (25%) mutation in *SERPING1* gene causes decreased levels of C1-INH and overactivation of complement and increased production of bradykinin	May be life-threatening. GI involvement presents as recurrent abdominal pain due to mucosal edema and bowel obstruction. Abdominal pain may be the presenting symptom in children; oral symptoms tend to be less severe than in adults	Acute: Replacement C1-INH (derived from human plasma or recombinant are preferred over FFP infusions); icatibant (blocks bradykinin receptor) or ecallantide (inhibits kallikrein). Patients should have access to abortive treatment at home. Prophylaxis: Androgens (stanozolol, danazol, and oxandrolone—not recommended in children); antifibrinolytics (tranexamic acid, aminocaproic acid); may also give prophylactic replacement C1-INH up to 24 hours before surgery or dental procedures. Avoid ACE inhibitors and estrogen-containing medications. Consider maintenance treatment in patients with more than 1 episode per year	Prevalence of type 1 and 2 HAE: 1.09–1.51 out of 100,000. 15–33% mortality rate Diagnose with low C4 and C2. Type 1: Low C1-INH level. Type 2: Normal or elevated C1-INH level, reduced C1-INH activity. Test children with a family history as 75% have their first episode before age 15
Type 2 (15%) [32, 34]	Autosomal dominant mutation causing normal or high levels of dysfunctional C1-INH			
Type 3 [33, 34, 36]	Autosomal dominant factor XII mutation (25%); other unknown mutations	Similar to types 1 and 2, with more frequent GI and laryngeal involvement. More common in women (83.8%), in whom attacks may be linked to oral contraceptives or pregnancy	Similar to above. Danazol favored for prophylaxis over tranexamic acid	Diagnose with genetic screening. Patients will have normal complement levels and normal C1-INH level and activity

(continued)

Table 34.2 (continued)

Hereditary angioedema (HAE)				
Subtype	Pathogenesis	Clinical features	Treatment	Comments
Acquired angioedema (AAE)				
Drug-induced [32, 34, 37–39]	Inhibition of kininase II with increased bradykinin effect	Classic angioedema with only rare reports of GI angioedema. May be life-threatening. Reported in 0.07–0.3% of patients taking ACE inhibitors. 3–4.5x more common in black patients; more common in female patients	Medication cessation; however, patients may still rarely experience relapses. Treat acute attacks with icatibant or replacement C1-INH. Icatibant may be effective for persistent symptoms. Ecallantide not effective	Tends to occur early in the course of treatment (14x higher risk in the first week of treatment) but may have a latency period of 1 year or longer. Normal complement levels
Acquired C1 esterase inhibitor deficiency [32, 34, 35]	Type 1: Patients with increased consumption of C1-INH; associated with lymphoproliferative diseases. May also have autoantibodies. Type 2: Patients with autoantibodies to C1-INH; no association with lymphoproliferative disease	Usually presents after 40 years old. Predominantly facial angioedema, although may occur anywhere on the body. GI involvement less common than with HAE	Treat the underlying disorder. May use rituximab or C1-INH replacement therapy. Antifibrinolytic agents such as tranexamic acid are more effective than steroids (danazol)	Prevalence of 1 in 500,000. Diagnose with low C4, low C1q, and decreased C1-INH levels and activity (although up to 20% of patients may have normal C1-INH level). 70% will have anti-C1-INH antibodies. Screen for lymphoproliferative disorders
Idiopathic Histaminergic [32]	Unknown	Angioedema without urticaria. Usually facial involvement with GI sparing	Antihistamines for treatment and prophylaxis	No family history or identified triggers
Idiopathic nonhistaminergic [32, 39, 40]		GI symptoms in up to one-third	Does not respond to antihistamines. Acute: Tranexamic acid, C1-INH, icatibant, and ecallantide. Prophylaxis: Tranexamic acid, omalizumab, C1-INH, progestin, methotrexate	

Abbreviations: *AAE* acquired angioedema, *ACE* angiotensin converting enzyme, *C1* complement component 1, *C1-INH* C1 inhibitor, *C1q*, complement component 1q, *C2* complement factor 2, *C4* complement factor 4, *FFP* fresh frozen plasma, *GI* gastrointestinal, *HAE* hereditary angioedema

Urticaria and Angioedema Pearls

- Urticaria presents as the rapid onset of erythematous, pruritic wheals, with many potential triggers, and should be managed with antihistamines as first-line therapy.
- Angioedema presents as swelling typically of mucosal tissues and may require emergent intervention.

Atopic Dermatitis

Atopic dermatitis (AD), or eczema, is a common recurrent inflammatory skin condition manifesting as pruritic, erythematous plaques, often with overlying serous exudate, crust, and excoriations [41, 42]. Over time, the lesions may demonstrate lichenification, or thickening of the involved skin with accentuated skin marking lines [42].

The overall global lifetime prevalence of AD has been increasing since 1960, with current reports ranging from 6 to 18%; there are geographic variations in reports of prevalence ranging from 1 to 4% in Southeast Asia and the Middle East to 8–18% in Nigeria, North America, Europe, and Australia [41, 43–46]. Historically, AD was more prevalent in more developed countries; however, recent trends show an increase in AD prevalence in developing regions as well [47]. Even within the United States, there are regional variations, with a higher risk of AD in the Northeastern states and the intermountain region states of Idaho, Nevada, and Utah [43]. However, it is difficult to separate out the effect of geographic region from other disease risk factors including urban residence, African-American race, and household education level greater than high school level [43, 45]. AD is more common in female than in male patients, with female predominance reported to range from 1.3 to 1.6:1 [44, 46]. Furthermore, in one Australian retrospective study comprising 519 adult patients, 65% of cases of adult-onset AD were found to occur in women [48].

A majority (85–90%) of patients will develop the disease within the first 5 years of life, with one Nigerian study including 774 patients under age 20 reporting 12.7% of patients had AD onset within the first 6 weeks of life [42, 44, 49]. AD tends to resolve by adulthood, but around 1–3% will have disease persistent into adulthood [41, 49]. The risk of persistence is higher with onset of symptoms after age 2; for adult patients who had onset of symptoms in childhood, the average age of disease onset was 5.8 years old [50, 51]. Patients with more severe AD are also more likely to have persistence into adulthood [52].

The physical distribution of AD lesions varies by the age of the affected patient. In infants, the face (sparing the nose), scalp, and extensor surfaces of the extremities are the most common sites of involvement, with the neck also involved less frequently [42, 50] (Fig. 34.2). In children, involvement shifts to flexural surfaces such as the neck and antecubital fossa. Adults tend to have involvement on the trunk and flexural surfaces, with up to 34% having a generalized distribution [48, 51] (Fig. 34.3a, b). Hand and foot eczema is also common in the adult AD population [48, 50].

There are several subtypes of AD. Nummular AD is a subtype of eczema that is more commonly seen in adults and consists of round or oval plaques on the extremities [50]. In addition, papular eczema may be seen in both pediatric and adult patients and presents as multiple grouped follicular papules on extensor surfaces [44].

AD patients may become superinfected with bacteria or viruses; 60–100% of AD patients have been found to be colonized with *Staphylococcus*

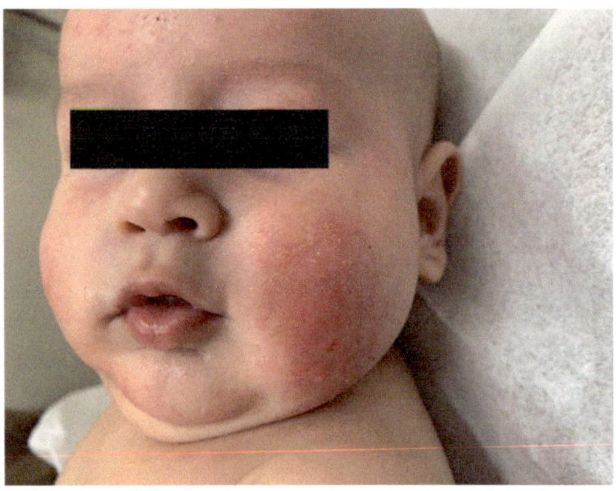

Fig. 34.2 Atopic dermatitis on the cheeks of an infant. (Photo credit: Vivian Shi, MD)

Fig. 34.3 Atopic dermatitis on the flexural wrists (**a**) and shin (**b**) of an adult patient. (Photo credits: Vivian Shi, MD)

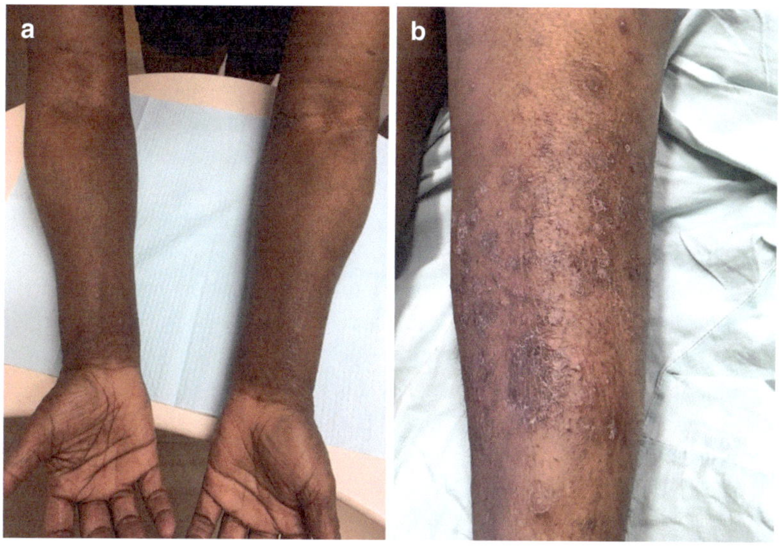

species on the skin or in the nares [41, 42, 53]. Superimposed infections with herpes-simplex virus (HSV), molluscum virus, or coxsackievirus are common in children [42, 50, 53]. Eczema herpeticum presents as monomorphic vesicles on AD-affected skin that erode to form "punched-out" appearing ulcers (Fig. 34.4). Most cases are due to HSV-1, and the condition may rarely be complicated by keratoconjunctivitis, gingivostomatitis, or meningitis [54].

Concomitant irritant or allergic contact dermatitis may also be seen in patients with AD. In one study of 34 children and 14 adults in the UK, 75% had one positive patch test result, and 39% had two, with common antigens including metals, fragrances, surfactants found in cosmetic and personal care products, and wool alcohols [55]. The presence of a sensitizing allergen should be considered in patients with refractory atopic dermatitis, as allergen avoidance may help control symptoms. Cutaneous irritants such as wool, harsh soaps, and detergents may also worsen symptoms of AD [53].

Psychological comorbidities may also occur. Pediatric AD patients have been noted to have an increased risk of depression and anxiety compared to patients without AD [50, 51]. In one series of 47 pediatric AD patients, 91.5% experienced sleep disturbances and over one-quarter were referred to psychology [56].

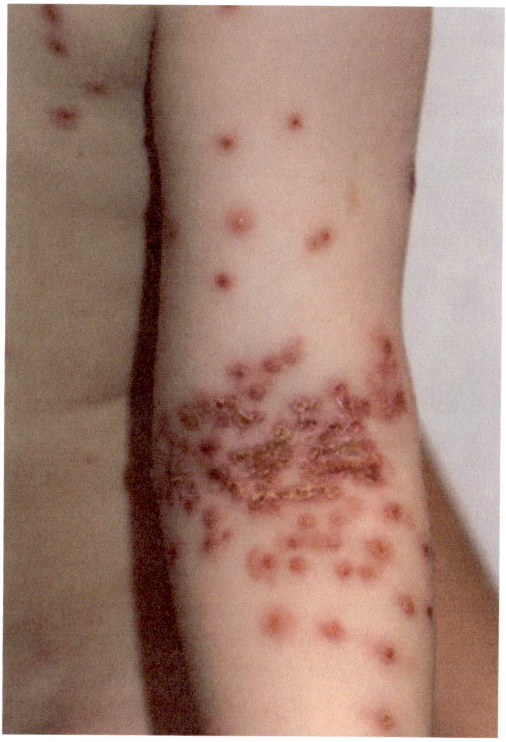

Fig. 34.4 Eczema herpeticum. (Photo credit: Damour A, Garcia M, Seneschal J, Lévêque N, Bodet C. Eczema herpeticum: clinical and pathophysiological aspects. Clin Rev Allergy Immunol. 2019)

Environmental factors may be involved in the development of AD. Increased use of indoor heating, decreased environmental humidity, and lower environmental temperature are associated with increased AD prevalence [45, 52]. Environmental allergens including air pollution and cigarette smoke (both active smoking and passive cigarette smoke exposure) have also been associated with AD [57].

The atopic march is a controversial and poorly understood pattern of development of multiple atopic conditions that has been noted in up to 80% of children with eczema [41, 58–60]. AD usually manifests first, followed by the later development of food allergies, asthma, and allergic rhinitis [50]. Treatment of AD was not found to prevent progression of the atopic march in a prospective, double-blinded study of topical pimecrolimus cream [58]. Additionally, while food allergen avoidance may improve cutaneous symptoms of AD in patients with a known food allergy, routine testing for food allergies is not recommended in the absence of symptoms, and elimination diets are not recommended in the absence of a diagnosed food allergy [42, 61]. Overall, in children with AD in the United States, asthma has been noted in 10.7–22.8%, allergic rhinitis in 22.4–30.7%, and food allergy in 15.9% [43, 58]. One study of 224 teenage and adult AD patients in the Czech Republic found that allergic rhinitis occurred in 74.1%, asthma in 40.6%, and food allergy in 29% of study patients [62]. Common food allergies include peanuts, eggs, wheat, milk, and soy, which together comprise up to 90% of the food allergies of affected patients [53, 61, 62].

Diet may be tied to the development of AD in other ways as well. Breastfeeding exclusively, or breastfeeding supplemented with hydrolyzed formula (avoiding intact milk proteins), for the first 3–4 months of an infant's life may be associated with a lower risk of AD, particularly in infants who are at high risk such as those with affected parents [63–65]. Several studies have demonstrated a protective effect against the development of atopic dermatitis in mothers who ate fish more than once per week during pregnancy and in infants who consumed fish before nine months of age [66–69]. Probiotic and prebiotic supplementation may be associated with lower rate of AD when used during pregnancy and infancy [70, 71]. Of note, a 2014 Cochrane review found that maternal dietary antigen avoidance during pregnancy does not prevent AD [72]. Further study is required before these findings can be more generally applied.

While there have been many recent developments in the study of the pathogenesis of AD, it is a complicated topic that is still incompletely understood. Two major processes appear to be intricately inter-related; however, the degree to which one causes the other remains murky [73]. On one hand, deficiencies in the skin barrier may allow for increased permeability to inciting factors (the "outside-in" hypothesis). On the other hand, underlying systemic inflammation may also impact the integrity of the skin barrier, leading to cutaneous symptoms (the "inside-out" hypothesis). It is uncertain at this time which of these factors plays the predominant role; however, both are clearly involved [73].

The skin barrier has many important roles, including hydration maintenance, pH regulation, and defense against microbes [3]. Factors such as age (e.g., increased transepidermal water loss in infants due to a thinner stratum corneum), UVB radiation, humidity, and hypoxia may affect its development [3, 50, 74, 75].

Mutations in the skin barrier have been demonstrated in patients with AD. Those with homozygous null mutations in the gene encoding the structural protein filaggrin (*FLG*) are more likely to have early onset, severe, and persistent AD [41, 76]. Up to 42% of heterozygous carriers of *FLG* mutations may also develop AD [77]. Deficiencies in filaggrin are associated with higher pH of the stratum corneum and decreased hydration of the stratum corneum through increased transepidermal water loss and decreased production of natural moisturizing factor (NMF) [3, 75, 78]. Further, byproducts of filaggrin metabolism have inhibitory effects on *S. aureus*, leading to increased risk of infection in those with a *FLG* mutation [79].

FLG mutations are also implicated in the development of asthma in atopic patients and of peanut allergies even in the absence of AD [61, 78]. Alterations in other skin barrier proteins, such as serine proteases, claudins, desmoglein-1, and desmocollin-1, may also play a role in the pathogenesis of AD [78, 80, 81]. The important role that genetics plays in AD is supported by the high (up to 82%) concordance rate in monozygotic twins and 25% concordance rate in dizygotic twins [82, 83]. Augmentation of the skin barrier with exogenous emollient use has been demonstrated to be protective; in a prospective trial, unaffected infants who received daily emollient use from age 3 weeks through 6 months had a 50% decrease in the rate of development of AD compared to infants who did not receive emollients daily [84].

The inflammation in AD is predominantly mediated by T helper cell-type 2 (Th2) and Th22 responses, with elevated levels of IL-4, IL-13, IL-22, and IL-31 in the acute phase [85]. Increased levels of these cytokines, particularly IL-4 and IL-13, suppress filaggrin levels by reducing epidermal differentiation and lead to the stimulation of Th2 cells, which propagates the above pathway [41, 73, 85]. In addition, *FLG* mutations and decreased levels of NMF are associated with increased levels of interleukin(IL)-1, which in turn amplifies additional downstream pro-inflammatory cytokine cascades [86]. There is a complex interplay between these two proposed mechanisms of the pathogenesis of AD, which will require additional study to fully elucidate.

Treatment of AD requires extreme diligence on the part of the patient and (if the patient is a child) his or her parents; daily application of thick emollients must be the cornerstone of any therapeutic regimen. It is important for parents to understand the cyclical nature of AD and for physicians to empower parents to recognize and treat the early signs of a flare. Parents should have two regimens to follow: one for flares and one for quiescent disease [42, 87]. After a daily soak in a lukewarm bath, skin should be patted dry and emollient should be applied immediately afterward to retain as much hydration as possible. During flares, wet wraps with emollients and topical steroids can be applied after bathing [42]. Emollients are preferred in ointment or cream form, which are more occlusive and therefore maintain hydration better than lotions. Ointments should be used whenever possible, but creams may be substituted during the day to avoid interfering with daily activities. When patients have moderate to severe eczema, referral to a dermatologist is indicated for discussion of additional treatment options (Table 34.3).

Dupilumab has revolutionized AD treatment as the first medication to be developed specifically for AD. It is currently FDA-approved for moderate to severe AD that is refractory to topicals in adults and children 12 years and older. Dupilumab is not yet approved for children under age 12, but it has been demonstrated to be effective and safe in off-label use [93]. Clinical trials in adults have demonstrated 39% of patients achieved complete or almost complete remission (Investigator Global Assessment (IGA) of 0 or 1) after 16 weeks compared to 12% receiving placebo [92]. Patients on dupilumab were found to have a 4-times decreased risk of infection compared to patients on placebo [91].

Atopic Dermatitis Pearls

- The majority of patients will have onset before age 2, and most will resolve during infancy or childhood, although up to 3% will persist into adulthood.
- Classic AD locations include the scalp, face, extensor surfaces (infants), and flexural surfaces including the neck in children and adults.
- Atopic skin may become superinfected with bacterial and/or viral infections, which may distort morphology and make diagnosis more challenging.
- Emollients and topical corticosteroids are the mainstay of treatment; however, for moderate to severe cases, referral to a dermatologist for management is appropriate for consideration of systemic treatment agents.

Table 34.3 Atopic dermatitis treatments

Therapy name	Mechanism of action	Dosing/Use	Adverse effects	Comments
Topical mupirocin [42, 87]	Inhibits bacterial protein synthesis	Two to three times daily to impetiginized skin or open areas of skin to prevent infection	Nausea, pain, or burning sensation upon application	Oral antibiotics may be required for refractory cases. Dilute bleach baths may also be used several times per week
Topical corticosteroids (hydrocortisone, desonide, triamcinolone, fluocinonide, halobetasol, betamethasone) [53]	Exact mechanism of action unknown; inhibit inflammatory cytokines	Twice daily for 2–3 weeks or until skin is clear, and then once or twice weekly as maintenance	Skin atrophy, rarely HPA axis suppression with prolonged use	First-line topical therapy in children under age 2. Lower-strength formulations preferred in areas with thinner skin (face, groin, axillae, skin folds) to prevent atrophy, but medium- to high-strength topical steroids appropriate for trunk and extremities depending on severity
Topical calcineurin inhibitors (tacrolimus, pimecrolimus) [42, 53]	Inhibit T cell activation by inhibiting calcineurin	Twice daily for primary treatment or as needed for maintenance treatment. Preferred over topical corticosteroids for long-term treatment or on the face and in skin folds due to lack of skin atrophy side effect	Burning and stinging sensation, which may be lessened with refrigeration of medication and/or initiation with topical corticosteroids	Pimecrolimus 1% cream and tacrolimus 0.03% ointment are FDA-approved for children older than 2 years. Tacrolimus 0.1% ointment approved and preferred for children older than 16 years and adults
Phototherapy [53, 87, 88]	Exact mechanism of action unknown; induces anti-inflammatory cytokine production	Three to five times weekly for 6–12 weeks before tapering [88]. May be considered in patients over 6 years old who fail to improve with topicals alone	Skin burning and erythema	Narrow-band (NB) ultraviolet-B (UVB) light preferred over broad-band (BB) UVB or psoralen with ultraviolet-A (PUVA) light treatment due to decreased risk of skin malignancy and erythema
Systemic anti-histamines (diphenhydramine, hydroxyzine) [53]	Block H1 receptors	Diphenhydramine: 25-50 mg orally every six hours as needed (adults), 0.5-1 mg/kg orally at bedtime (pediatric). Hydroxyzine: 25 mg orally every six to eight hours (adult), 2 mg/kg orally per day divided every six to eight hours as needed (pediatric)	Sedation, paradoxical excitation in pediatric patients	Non-sedating antihistamines (cetirizine, fexofenadine) may also be used for pruritus. Sedating antihistamines should be avoided in elderly patients. May be used to treat pruritus and help with sleep in children

(continued)

Table 34.3 (continued)

Therapy name	Mechanism of action	Dosing/Use	Adverse effects	Comments
Systemic corticosteroids [42, 59]	Exact mechanism of action unknown; inhibits inflammatory cytokines	0.5-1 mg/kg orally daily, tapering over several weeks	Adrenal suppression, steroid psychosis, hyperglycemia, hypertension, osteoporosis, glaucoma, increased risk of infections	Not preferred due to the high risk of rebound flares upon discontinuation and high risk of systemic side effects. Less effective in achieving stable remission compared to cyclosporine
Cyclosporine [53, 56, 59]	Inhibits T cells	3-5 mg/kg orally divided into twice daily dosing for at least 6 weeks (adults)	Hypertension, immunosuppression, nephrotoxicity, hepatotoxicity, leukopenia	Use for longer than 1 year not recommended due to risk of hypertension and renal failure. Up to 45% of patients may relapse within 8 weeks of discontinuation. More effective than systemic prednisolone
Methotrexate [60, 89]	Inhibits DHFR to block folate metabolism	10-25 mg orally weekly (adults); 0.2–0.7 mg/kg weekly (pediatric)	Nausea, GI discomfort, mucositis, leukopenia, anemia, skin infection	Effective in up to 76% of patients with atopic dermatitis, including children
Mycophenolate mofetil [90]	Inhibits inosine monophosphate dehydrogenase to prevent DNA synthesis	500-1500 mg orally twice daily	Headaches, GI discomfort, increased risk of infections, LFT abnormalities, nausea, constipation, myelosuppression	Can induce partial or full remission in 77.6% of adult patients, with relapse in only 8.2% of cases
Dupilumab [73, 91, 92]	Inhibits the alpha-subunit of the IL-4 and IL-13 shared receptor	300 mg subcutaneously every 2 weeks after loading dose of 600 mg subcutaneously (adults and children 12 years and older >60 kg); 200 mg subcutaneously every 2 weeks after loading dose of 400 mg subcutaneously (children 12 years and older <60 kg)	Injection site reactions, conjunctivitis, nasopharyngitis, headache, increased risk of localized herpesvirus infections	See chapter text

Abbreviations: *BBW* black box warning, *DHFR* dihydrofolate reductase, *DNA* deoxyribonucleic acid, *GI* gastrointestinal, *H1* histamine type 1, *HPA* hypothalamus-pituitary-adrenal axis, *IL* interleukin, *LFT* liver function test, *MRSA* methicillin-resistant *Staphylococcus aureus*, *NSAID* non-steroidal anti-inflammatory drug

Contact Dermatitis

Contact dermatitis presents with a well-demarcated erythematous, pruritic eruption, often with vesiculation, initially limited to the area in direct contact with the allergen [94]. If the reaction persists chronically, it may spread to involve surrounding skin, and patients can develop pruritic, lichenified plaques in the affected areas [95]. The reaction develops within 24–72 hours in previously sensitized individuals and improves within days after the exposure ceases [94]. Allergic contact dermatitis is due to a delayed (Type IV) hypersensitivity reaction with activation of CD4+ T-cells when in contact with the allergen [94, 96]. Patients must have been sensitized to the allergen prior to developing the eruption [97]. This is in contrast to irritant contact dermatitis, where prior exposure is not necessary to develop a reaction.

Several distinctive clinical patterns exist.

- Airborne contact dermatitis: Airborne contact dermatitis occurs due to exposure to an airborne allergen and affects the eyelids, neck, upper chest, and hands, including areas (such as the submandibular region) which are classically spared in photo-distributed eruptions [97–99]. Common triggers of airborne contact dermatitis include plant pollen, fragrances such as perfume or cologne, or aerosolized particles from house dust mites or pet dander [97, 98, 100].
- Eyelid dermatitis: In addition to being a common site of involvement for airborne contact dermatitis, the thin skin of the eyelids predisposes them to react with chemicals, such as toluenes and acrylates found in nail polishes and fake nails [101, 102].
- Systemic contact dermatitis: Rarely, a contact reaction may become generalized due to a systemic exposure (including inhalation, oral or parenteral ingestion) to a previously sensitized allergen causing a massive immune response [95, 101].
- Autosensitization, also known as the id reaction, describes a secondary process wherein the eruption can occur beyond the initial area of contact [103]. It is distinguished from systemic contact dermatitis due to the lack of a systemic exposure to the antigen.
- Photoallergic reactions occur only when a culprit antigen is ingested or applied to the skin and then the skin is exposed to ultraviolet light, for example, 5-methoxypsoralen found in bergamot oil and perfumes [94, 104].

The prevalence of all forms of contact dermatitis is 13.6 per 1000 per year, including allergic and irritant contact dermatitis [97]. The most common allergens include nickel and fragrances (seen in up to 1% of the general population and 10% of all patients undergoing patch testing) [103–105]. Topical corticosteroid allergies have a frequency of 2.6% in Europe [106].

Contact dermatitis has been seen in association with AD; it should be considered in atopic patients or any patients with a persistent or refractory dermatitis, as they may be continually exposed to an allergen that is perpetuating the rash [95–97, 107]. See Table 34.4 for a summary of common contact allergens, with emphasis on those that affect the head and neck.

Diagnosis begins with eliciting an accurate history of product exposure from the patient, including all personal products used, any occupational exposures, and a timeline of their use as it relates to the rash. If the patient has a partner, the partner's relevant personal care products should also be investigated, as the patient could have a consort contact dermatitis (e.g., a patient's lip dermatitis may be caused by his/her partner's lip balm).

Patch testing is the gold standard for eliciting the cause of allergic contact dermatitis. For patients presenting with a highly suspect potential trigger, avoidance of that product may be sufficient to clinically confirm the diagnosis. However, in cases where there are no, or multiple, suspected allergens, patch testing should be recommended. It is important to keep in mind that patients may have negative or false negative results with patch testing, so there are times when the patch test may ultimately not prove to be helpful in determining the cause of the patient's rash. Any positive results must be interpreted in the context of the patient's known exposures as some allergens may have a positive reaction but not be relevant to the patient's clinical disease [114].

The process of patch testing involves applying a series of potential allergens to the skin, usually on the back, for an extended period of time to test whether a reaction will develop (Fig. 34.5a). A number of standardized panels including the most common contact allergens overall and pan-

Table 34.4 Common contact allergens

Allergen category		Source	Comments
Metals [96, 101, 103, 107, 108]	Nickel	Jewelry, watches, stainless steel, implants, cell phones	May induce autosensitization. Ear piercing leads to higher rates of nickel allergies. May be seen in up to 12% of pediatric patients with atopic dermatitis who undergo patch testing. May cross-react with cobalt
	Chromate	Cement, leather, green pool table felt, paints, tattoo inks, implants	May present with hand dermatitis
Topical medications [95, 106, 107, 109–111]	Corticosteroids	Class A: Tixocortol-21-pivalate, class B: Budesonide and triamcinolone acetonide, class D1: Clobetasol-17-propionate, class D2: Hydrocortisone-17-butyrate	Patients may cross-react between and within classes. Consider use of desoximetasone in patients with topical corticosteroid allergies. May have a delayed patch reaction Preparations may also contain allergens such as propylene glycol or parabens
	Antibiotics	Neomycin, bacitracin	Bacitracin may have a delayed patch reaction. Can rarely result in anaphylaxis. Consider use of mupirocin in patients with allergies to neomycin or bacitracin. Common allergen in pediatric patients with atopic dermatitis
Fragrances (fragrance mixes I and II, and balsam of Peru) [104, 105]		Perfumes, colognes, cosmetics, toiletries, toothpaste, gum	Fragrance mixes are used to screen for reactions to commonly used fragrances including linalool, phenylethyl alcohol, linalyl alcohol, geraniol, citronellol. The use of both standard fragrance mixes captures an additional 28% compared to use of fragrance mix I alone. May present with an airborne contact dermatitis in either the user or his or her partner (consort dermatitis)
Formaldehydes and formaldehyde releasers (i.e., quaternium-15) [101]		Cutting oils, industrial products, preservatives in cosmetic products and shampoos, clothing	Consider allergy to formaldehyde in clothing when rash spares skin folds, especially the axillae
Plants [97]	Sesquiterpene lactone	Asteraceae/Compositae family: Ragweed, dandelion, chrysanthemum, sunflower, daisy	May cause an airborne contact dermatitis
	Urushiol (specifically pentadecylcatechol)	*Toxicodendron* plants of the Anacardiaceae family: Poison ivy, poison oak, poison sumac	Classic well-demarcated erythema, vesicles, and edema in area of contact but may cause an airborne contact dermatitis. May cross-react with mango skin, cashews, gingko biloba

(continued)

Table 34.4 (continued)

Allergen category	Source	Comments
Paraphenylenediamine [96, 101]	Hair dyes, temporary henna tattoos	Affects scalp, neck, ears with home use; affects hands in salon workers. May have a delayed patch reaction
Methylchloroisothiazolinone (MCI)/ methylisothiazolinone (MI) [112, 113]	Preservative in baby wipes, water-based wall paint, cosmetics, personal care products, cleaning products	May cause eyelid dermatitis if exposed to make-up remover wipes, diaper dermatitis if exposed to baby wipes, or airborne contact dermatitis if exposed to paints
Cocamidopropyl betaine [107, 110]	Surfactant found in baby shampoo, contact lens solutions, and other personal care products	May have a delayed patch reaction. Common allergen in pediatric patients with atopic dermatitis

Abbreviations: *MCI* methylchloroisothiazolinone, *MI* methylisothiazolinone

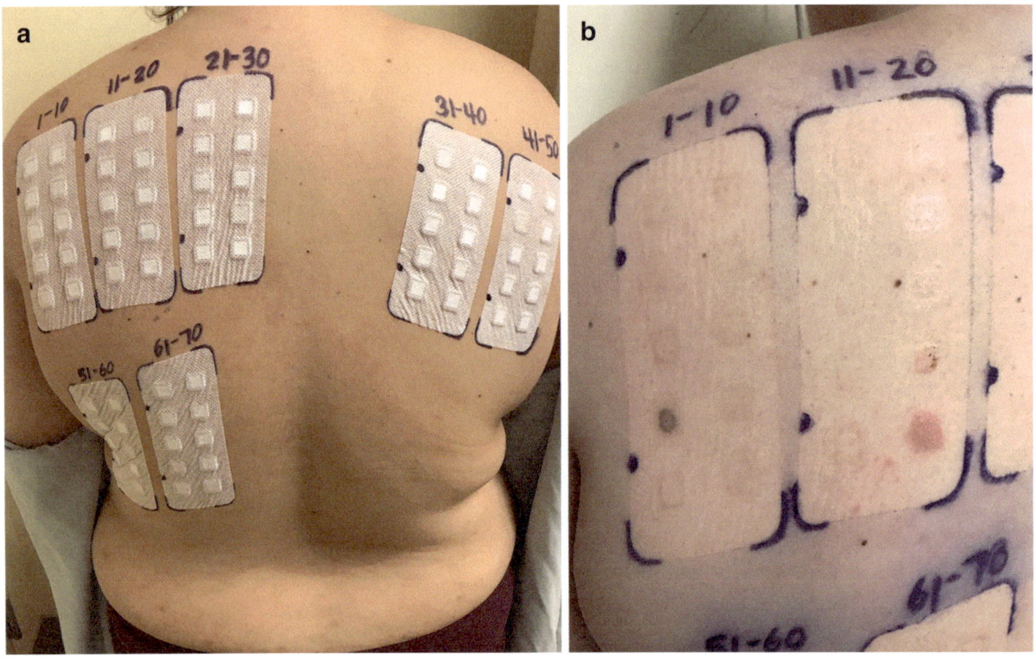

Fig. 34.5 Standardized panels applied to a patient's back for patch testing (**a**) and a positive patch test reaction (**b**)

els tailored to common exposures of specific occupations (such as dentistry) are available [110, 114]. On day 1, patches are applied; on day 3, patches are removed and an early read performed; on day 5–7, a final read is done and results discussed with patients [110] (Fig. 34.5b). Patches must be applied to an area without skin lesions so they can be accurately interpreted [101]. During this whole time, the patient must keep the back dry so as not to interfere with the possible reactions [110]. Oral corticosteroids should be stopped at least 1–2 weeks prior to the test to avoid blunting the response [115]. If this is not possible, testing at a dose of less than 10 mg per day is preferred [110]. Patients may take oral antihistamines during their patch test.

Avoidance of the allergen is the cornerstone of treatment of allergic contact dermatitis. However, sometimes not all allergens can be identified. In addition, sometimes culprit allergens cannot easily be avoided, such with patients who are exposed in the course of their occupation. Topical corticosteroids are useful for treating flares, with low-potency formulations, such as hydrocortisone 2.5% or desonide 0.5% cream or ointment, or the use of topical calcineurin inhibitors, such as tacrolimus 0.1% ointment, preferred for use on the face and skin folds.

Systemic antihistamines help with pruritus, and sedating anti-histamines may help promote sleep, but as allergic contact dermatitis is not histamine-mediated, they will not treat or prevent the rash [101]. Systemic corticosteroids may be required in rare cases [98].

Contact Dermatitis Pearls:

- In patients with suspected facial contact dermatitis, including involvement of eyelids, consider referral for patch test.
- Common allergens include metals (nickel, chromate), topical medications (corticosteroids, antibiotics), preservatives in personal care products (formaldehyde, methylchloroisothiazolinone), and fragrances in perfumes or colognes.
- Consider consort dermatitis if a positive allergen not found in any of the patient's own personal care products.

Allergic Drug Eruptions

See Table 34.5 for a summary of relevant allergic drug eruptions. See Chap. 41 for more information about drug allergies.

Allergic Drug Eruptions Pearls

- Stevens-Johnson syndrome (SJS)/toxic epidermal necrolysis (TEN) is the most severe allergic drug eruption. It should be suspected in patients with any degree of blistering on the skin or mucosal surface involvement with a possible drug exposure.
- SJS/TEN treatment consists of immediate cessation of the suspected medication along with supportive care. Dermatology and other appropriate consultant services should be involved immediately for more directed therapy.
- Other drug eruptions may be diagnosed based on clinical appearance, laboratory abnormalities, and presence or lack of systemic involvement.

Eosinophil-Associated Dermatoses on the Head and Neck

Eosinophil Biology

Eosinophils develop from myeloid progenitor cells in the bone marrow under regulation of three major cytokines including IL-3, IL-5, and granulocyte macrophage-colony stimulation factor (GM-CSF) [125]. Of these, IL-5 is the most specific and is also responsible for release of eosinophils from the bone marrow into circulation [125, 126]. Eosinophils migrate through the

Table 34.5 Selected allergic drug eruptions

Drug eruption	Clinical characteristics	Common culprit drugs	Onset	Treatment	Comments
Morbilliform drug eruption [116–118]	Erythematous macules and papules which coalesce into plaques on trunk, spreading to extremities	Antibiotics (penicillins, sulfonamides), antiepileptics (especially phenytoin), uric acid metabolism drugs, proton pump inhibitors	1–2 weeks after starting treatment, may recur within 2–3 days if previously sensitized	Prompt discontinuation of culprit medication. Topical corticosteroids	Monitor for progression to DRESS (see below). Resolves within 1–2 weeks of discontinuation of medication

(continued)

Table 34.5 (continued)

Drug eruption	Clinical characteristics	Common culprit drugs	Onset	Treatment	Comments
Stevens-Johnson syndrome (SJS)/toxic epidermal necrolysis (TEN) [119–121]	Prodrome: Fever, flu-like symptoms, skin pain precede rash by 1–3 days. Erythematous, dusky atypical targetoid macules (only 2 zones) progressing to patches and desquamation. Mucosal (oral, ocular, urogenital, esophageal) desquamation: May be substantial. Mortality: around 35% (sepsis, respiratory failure). SJS: <10% of BSA desquamated. TEN: >30% of BSA desquamated. Severe complications: Bronchiolitis obliterans, corneal scarring, symblepharon, esophageal strictures	Antibiotics (cephalosporins, beta-lactams, quinolone, sulfas), antiepileptics (carbamazepine, phenytoin, phenobarbital), NSAIDs, allopurinol, rarely infections (mycoplasma, HSV)	1–3 weeks, although may be <1 week on repeat challenge	Prompt discontinuation of culprit medication. Supportive care: Fluid replacement, wound care (consider transfer to burn center). Consult to dermatology and to ophthalmology, urology, gynecology where appropriate. No consensus on the use of immunomodulatory therapies including TNF-alpha inhibitors (etanercept, infliximab), IVIG, systemic corticosteroids, and cyclosporine in adults or children	Mortality benefits have been reported with IVIG (dose >2 g/kg), corticosteroids, combination of IVIG and corticosteroids, cyclosporine, and early transfer to burn centers, although studies on the mortality benefit of systemic therapies conflict
Drug reaction with eosinophilia and systemic symptoms (DRESS) [122–124]	Diffuse symmetric eruption of erythematous macules and papules coalescing into plaques (morbilliform) on trunk and extremities, facial edema, lymphadenopathy, fever. Mucosal desquamation: Mild, if any. Systemic findings: Peripheral eosinophilia, atypical lymphocytosis, elevations in liver function tests and creatinine, rarely myocarditis	Antiepileptics (carbamazepine, lamotrigine, phenytoin), antibiotics (beta-lactams, sulfonamides), allopurinol, dapsone, minocycline, abacavir, nevirapine	1–4 weeks, but classically 2–3 weeks, and rarely up to 8 weeks	Prompt discontinuation of culprit medication. Systemic corticosteroids (40-60 mg/day of prednisolone equivalent) with long taper usually necessary (>8 weeks). Topical corticosteroids. Supportive care	Associated with HHV-6 reactivation

Abbreviations: *BSA* body surface area, *CMV* cytomegalovirus, *HHV* human herpesvirus, *HSV* herpes simplex virus, *IVIG* intravenous immunoglobulin, *NSAID* non-steroidal anti-inflammatory drug, *SJS* Stevens-Johnson syndrome, *TEN* toxic epidermal necrolysis, *TNF* tumor necrosis factor endothelium via interactions between P-selectins and β1- and β2-integrins and then move through tissues based on the presence of eotaxins (chemoattractants) [125]. Eotaxins 1–3 have been found to be powerful attractants for eosinophils, but eosinophils respond to various other chemoattractants including leukotriene-B4 and IL-16 through interactions with the eosinophil receptor CCR3 [125, 127, 128]. Once in the target tissue, eosinophils are triggered to degranulate (through incompletely understood mechanisms), releasing pre-formed granules of cytotoxic proteins including major basic protein (MBP), eosinophil-derived neurotoxin (EDN), eosinophil cationic protein (ECP), and eosinophil peroxidase (EPX) in a piecemeal process [127, 129]. Pro-inflammatory and pro-fibrotic cytokines as well as reactive oxygen species (ROS) are also released, producing a multitude of tissue-damaging effects [126, 127, 129]. Additionally, eosinophil degranulation promotes a Th2 profile, which leads to further production of IL-4 and IL-5 and propagation of eosinophil stimulation in a feed-forward loop [126–129]. Novel treatments aimed at targeting this pathway to treat eosinophilic diseases, such as anti-IL-5 and anti-IL-5 receptor antibodies (e.g., mepolizumab), are under development and have been shown to decrease serum eosinophilia [130].

Granuloma Faciale

Granuloma faciale (GF) is a rare inflammatory condition that presents as single or multiple red to brown plaques with a rubbery or "peau d'orange" appearance on the face [126, 131] (Fig. 34.6). It is rarely seen extra-facially [132]. Patients may experience pruritus or a burning sensation and some may have a mild peripheral eosinophilia [126]. Given the rarity of GF, little is known about its epidemiology. It is believed to be more common in middle-aged men; one series of 66 patients was 62% male [126]. Sun exposure may be associated as well [132].

The pathogenesis of GF is also not well-understood. Interferon-gamma produced by CD4+ T helper cells may play a role [133, 134]. In addition, it has been seen in association with eosinophilic angiocentric fibrosis [126] and IgG4-related diseases [134]. Diagnosis is made by a skin biopsy that shows a dermal infiltrate of lymphocytes and eosinophils, which spares the area immediately inferior to the epidermis (known as the Grenz zone) [126]. Granulomas are notably absent.

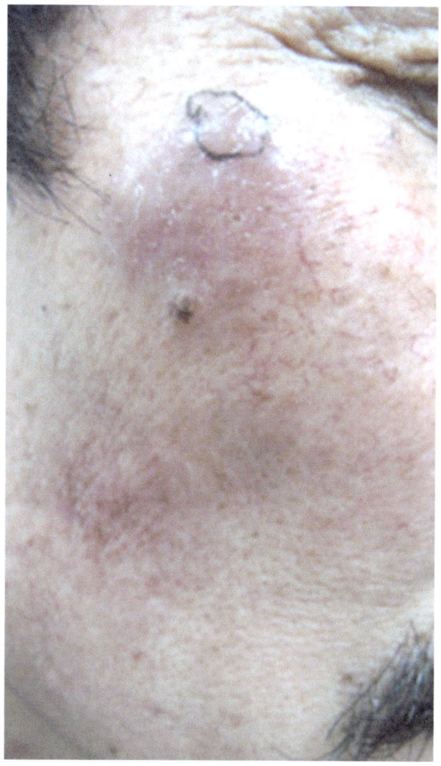

Fig. 34.6 Granuloma faciale. (Photo credit: Long H, Zhang G, Wang L, Lu Q. Eosinophilic skin diseases: a comprehensive review. Clin Rev Allergy Immunol. 2016;50(2):189–213)

GF is difficult to treat, as evidenced by the numerous modalities that have been tried, and recurrences are common [126]. Pulse-dye laser (PDL) is considered to be a first-line treatment, where available [126]. Carbon dioxide laser was also used in a patient who had recurrence after PDL [135]. Topical tacrolimus is preferred over the use of topical corticosteroids due to reports of its increased efficacy and decreased side effects [131, 133]. Tacrolimus decreases the level of interleukin (IL)-2 by inhibiting calcineurin, which leads to decreased T-cell activation and decreased interferon-gamma production, which may account for its efficacy in this condition [133]. The use of oral dapsone and antimalarials has been reported in the literature with varying success; use of adalimumab has been reported to be unsuccessful [126, 133].

Eosinophilic Angiocentric Fibrosis

Eosinophilic angiocentric fibrosis (EAF) is a rare, benign inflammatory condition that typically presents in adults as a localized submucosal or soft tissue swelling, commonly in the nose. Involvement of the nasal septum, nasal sidewalls, maxillary sinus, subglottis, orbit, and paranasal sinus has been described [136, 137]. Patients commonly present with pain, epistaxis, and slowly progressive upper airway obstruction, which may continue for years after onset of symptoms [137, 138]. Patients have rarely required tracheostomy or other procedures to maintain airway patency [136]. Diagnosis is made by skin biopsy, which shows an infiltrate of lymphocytes, plasma cells, and eosinophils, with progressive fibrosis surrounding vessels as the disease develops [138].

Around 20% of patients with EAF also have GF, although GF onset varies and has been reported before, after, and concomitantly with EAF [136, 137]. Approximately one-third may have a prior history of trauma to the area, including intubation [137]. In addition, immunoglobulin G (IgG)4-positive cells have been identified in pathologic specimens of EAF, leading some to posit that it is in the family of IgG4-related disease (IgG4-RD), which consists of infiltrates of IgG4+ cells in multiple tissues including the pancreas, salivary glands, lymph nodes, and skin [138].

EAF should be treated surgically to relieve airway obstruction. It is refractory to nasal steroids and may recur after excision as well, with some patients requiring multiple excisions [136].

Kimura Disease (Eosinophilic Hyperplastic Lymphogranuloma)

Kimura disease (KD) presents with soft tissue masses on the head or neck, usually in conjunction with regional lymphadenopathy [139]. Sites include the retroauricular region, ears, epiglottis, and salivary glands, particularly the parotid gland [140–142] (Fig. 34.7). The classic triad of KD includes slowly enlarging, painless masses on the head or neck, peripheral eosinophilia, and elevated serum IgE levels [139]. Generalized lymphadenopathy has rarely been reported [143]. Lesions are usually larger than 2 centimeters in diameter (which may be used to help distinguish this disease from angiolymphoid hyperplasia with eosinophilia) and may be pruritic [140, 144]. Malignant transformation is not expected. It has been associated with IgG4-related disease, and renal involvement, such as nephrotic syndrome, has been reported in 12–27% of patients [140, 145].

KD is most commonly reported in young Asian adult men [140]. However, it has also been reported in children and patients of other racial backgrounds [143, 145]. Trauma or persistent antigenic stimulation associated with parasitic or viral infections is hypothesized to be pathogenic in KD [139]. Work-up for Kimura disease involves skin biopsy demonstrating an infiltrate of lymphocytes forming germinal centers, eosinophils, and plasma cells with surrounding fibrosis and increased production of postcapillary venules [140].

Surgical excision is the preferred treatment modality for KD. Unfortunately, recurrence rates of up to 73% have been reported after excision [140]. Radiotherapy may have a similar recur-

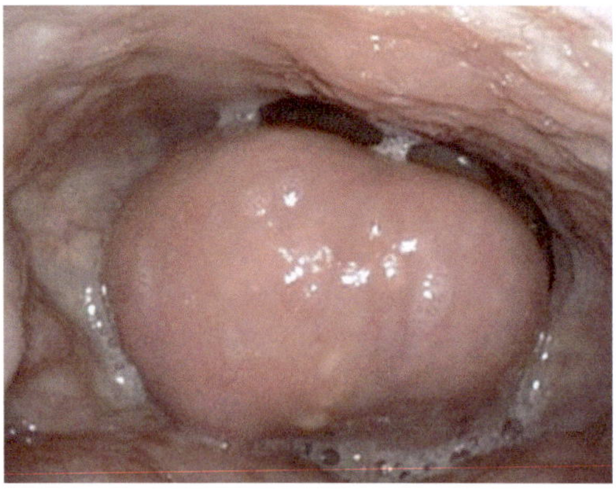

Fig. 34.7 Kimura disease. (Photo credit: Yamamoto T, Minamiguchi S, Watanabe Y, et al. Kimura disease of the epiglottis: a case report and review of literature. Head Neck Pathol. 2014;8(2):198–203)

rence rate, although its use is not reported commonly [145]. The combination of surgery and postoperative radiotherapy has been shown to be more effective compared to either modality used alone [146]. Other therapies such as cyclosporine, interferon-alpha, and cytotoxic regimens including etoposide, vincristine, and azathioprine have been reported to be successful in small numbers [140, 145].

Angiolymphoid Hyperplasia with Eosinophilia (ALHE)

Angiolymphoid hyperplasia with eosinophilia (ALHE), also referred to as epithelioid hemangioma, is a benign condition that presents as solitary or multiple pink to red dome-shaped papules or nodules. About one-third of cases occur on the ear, with other involved sites including the neck, face, and scalp; extrafacial involvement is rare [147, 148] (Fig. 34.8). Symptoms may include pruritus, pain, and bleeding [147, 148]. Peripheral eosinophilia is seen in only 20% of patients [148]. Most cases have been reported in the northern hemisphere in patients who are in their 30s and 40s [147].

There have been several reports and hypotheses regarding the pathogenesis of ALHE. It has been reported to occur or worsen in the setting of trauma including ear piercing, frostbite, incision and drainage, otitis externa, and lacerations; or in states of increased estrogen such as pregnancy and oral contraceptive use [147–149]. Diagnosis is made by skin biopsy showing vascular proliferation with inflammatory infiltrates of eosinophils, lymphocytes, and mast cells [148].

Fewer than 3% of ALHE cases resolve spontaneously [147]. Surgical excision is the preferred method of treatment with the lowest reported recurrence rate, although around 40% will recur after surgery [147]. In one case, excision margins of 4 millimeters (mm) resulted in no recurrence after a year of follow-up [150]. Lasers such as the pulse-dye laser (PDL) and CO2 laser have recurrence rates of around 50% [147]. Other treatments including topical, intralesional, and systemic corticosteroids and cryotherapy have been reported to have recurrence rates of 80–100% [147, 151]. Successful treatment has been reported with brachytherapy and propranolol [144, 152].

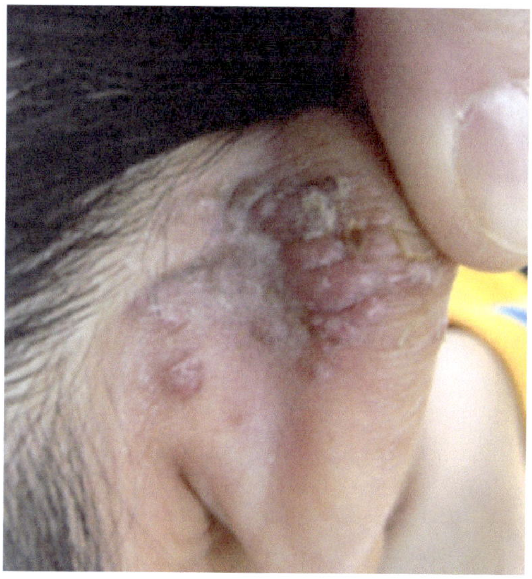

Fig. 34.8 Angiolymphoid hyperplasia with eosinophilia (Photo credit: Long H, Zhang G, Wang L, Lu Q. Eosinophilic skin diseases: a comprehensive review. Clin Rev Allergy Immunol. 2016;50(2):189–213)

Eosinophil-Associated Dermatoses Pearls

- Eosinophil-associated dermatoses that commonly occur on the head and neck require a biopsy to establish diagnosis.
- Kimura disease (KD) should be on the differential diagnosis for patients (especially young Asian men) who present with soft tissue masses on the head or neck; a biopsy should be performed and complete blood count with differential and serum IgE level checked.
- Eosinophilic angiocentric fibrosis (EAF) and KD can cause airway or nasal obstruction, respectively, and thus should be followed closely and treated surgically.

Conclusion

- In conclusion, allergic skin diseases may manifest in a myriad of forms. Their timely recognition may lead to improved patient care and decrease morbidity and, in cases of life-threatening disease, mortality.

References

1. Losquadro WD. Anatomy of the skin and the pathogenesis of nonmelanoma skin cancer. In: Facial plastic surgery clinics of North America, vol. 25. W.B. Saunders; 2017. p. 283–9.
2. Egawa G, Kabashima K. Barrier dysfunction in the skin allergy. Allergol Int [Internet]. 2018 [cited 2020 Jan 1];67(1).3–11. Available from: https://www.sciencedirect.com/science/article/pii/S1323893017301557
3. Zaniboni MC, Samorano LP, Orfali RL, Aoki V. Skin barrier in atopic dermatitis: beyond filaggrin, vol. 91. Anais Brasileiros de Dermatologia. Sociedade Brasileira de Dermatologia; 2016. p. 472–8.
4. Seo JH, Kwon JW. Epidemiology of urticaria including physical urticaria and angioedema in Korea. Korean J Intern Med. 2019;34(2):418–25.
5. Ferrer M. Epidemiology, healthcare, resources, use and clinical features of different types of urticaria. Alergológica 2005. J Investig Allergol Clin Immunol. 2009;19(SUPPL. 2):21–6.
6. Zuberbier T, Balke M, Worm M, Edenharter G, Maurer M. Epidemiology of urticaria: a representative cross-sectional population survey. Clin Exp Dermatol. 2010;35(8):869–73.
7. Raciborski F, Kłak A, Czarnecka-Operacz M, Jenerowicz D, Sybilski A, Kuna P, et al. Epidemiology of urticaria in Poland – nationally representative survey results. Postep Dermatologii i Alergol. 2018;35(1):67–73.
8. Zuberbier T, Iffländer J, Semmler C, Henz BM. Acute urticaria: clinical aspects and therapeutic responsiveness. Acta Derm Venereol. 1996;76(4):295–7.
9. Cherrez Ojeda I, Vanegas E, Felix M, Mata V, Cherrez S, Simancas-Racines D, et al. Etiology of chronic urticaria: the Ecuadorian experience. World Allergy Organ J. 2018;11(1):1.
10. Caffarelli C, Paravati F, El Hachem M, Duse M, Bergamini M, Simeone G, et al. Management of chronic urticaria in children: a clinical guideline. Italian J Pediat BioMed Central Ltd. 2019;45.
11. Kanani A, Betschel SD, Warrington R. Urticaria and angioedema. Allergy, Asthma Clin Immunol 2018;14.
12. Magerl M, Borzova E, Giménez-Arnau A, Grattan CEH, Lawlor F, Mathelier-Fusade P, et al. The definition and diagnostic testing of physical and cholinergic urticarias – EAACI/GA 2 LEN/EDF/UNEV consensus panel recommendations. Allergy [Internet] 2009 [cited 2020 Feb 16];64(12):1715–21. Available from: http://doi.wiley.com/10.1111/j.1398-9995.2009.02177.x.
13. Magerl M, Altrichter S, Borzova E, Giménez-Arnau A, Grattan CEH, Lawlor F, et al. The definition, diagnostic testing, and management of chronic inducible urticarias - the EAACI/GA2LEN/EDF/UNEV consensus recommendations 2016 update and revision. Allergy Eur J Allergy Clin Immunol. 2016;71(6):780–802.
14. Radonjic-Hoesli S, Hofmeier KS, Micaletto S, Schmid-Grendelmeier P, Bircher A, Simon D. Urticaria and angioedema: an update on classification and pathogenesis. In: Clinical reviews in allergy and immunology, vol. 54. Humana Press Inc; 2018. p. 88–101.
15. Zuberbier T, Althaus C, Chantraine-Hess S, Czarnetzki BM. Prevalence of cholinergic urticaria in young adults. J Am Acad Dermatol. 1994;31(6):978–81.
16. Singleton R, Halverstam CP. Diagnosis and management of cold urticaria. Cutis [Internet]. 2016 [cited 2020 Feb 17];97(1):59–62. Available from: https://www.mdedge.com/dermatology/article/105720/urticaria/diagnosis-and-management-cold-urticaria
17. Süß H, Dölle-Bierke S, Geier J, Kreft B, Oppel E, Pföhler C, et al. Contact urticaria: frequency, elicitors and cofactors in three cohorts (information network of departments of dermatology; network of anaphylaxis; and Department of Dermatology, university hospital Erlangen, Germany). Contact Derm. 2019;81(5):341–53.
18. Ferrer M, Bartra J, Giménez-Arnau A, Jauregui I, Labrador-Horrillo M, Ortiz de Frutos J, et al. Management of urticaria: not too complicated, not too simple. In: Clinical and experimental allergy, vol. 45. Blackwell Publishing Ltd; 2015. p. 731–43.
19. Vestergaard C, Deleuran M. Chronic spontaneous urticaria: latest developments in aetiology, diagnosis and therapy. In: Therapeutic advances in chronic disease, vol. 6. SAGE Publications; 2015. p. 304–13.
20. Kasperska-Zajac A, Jarząb J, Zerdzińska A, Bak K, Grzanka A. Effective treatment of different phenotypes of chronic urticaria with omalizumab: case reports and review of literature. Int J Immunopathol Pharmacol. 2016;29(2):320–8.
21. Kulthanan K, Cheepsomsong M, Jiamton S. Urticarial vasculitis: etiologies and clinical course. Asian Pacific J Allergy Immunol. 2009;27(2–3):95–102.
22. Loricera J, Calvo-Río V, Mata C, Ortiz-Sanjuán F, González-López MA, Alvarez L, et al. Urticarial vasculitis in northern Spain: clinical study of 21 cases. Med (United States). 2014;93(1):53–60.
23. Venzor J, Lee WL, Huston DP. Urticarial vasculitis. Clin Rev Allergy Immunol. 2002;23(2):201–16.

24. Wisnieski JJ. Urticarial vasculitis. Vol. 12, Current Opinion in Rheumatology. Curr Opin Rheumatol; 2000. p. 24–31.
25. Jachiet M, Flageul B, Deroux A, Le Quellec A, Maurier F, Cordoliani F, et al. The clinical spectrum and therapeutic management of hypocomplementemic urticarial vasculitis: data from a french nationwide study of fifty-seven patients. Arthritis Rheumatol. 2015;67(2):527–34.
26. Lopez LR, Davis KC, Kohler PF, Schocket AL. The hypocomplementemic urticarial-vasculitis syndrome: therapeutic response to hydroxychloroquine. J Allergy Clin Immunol. 1984;73(5 PART 1):600–3.
27. Morgan M, Khan DA. Therapeutic alternatives for chronic urticaria: an evidence-based review, part 2. Vol. 100, Annals of Allergy, Asthma and Immunology. In: American college of allergy, asthma and immunology; 2008. p. 517–26.
28. Borcea A, Greaves MW. Methotrexate-induced exacerbation of urticarial vasculitis: an unusual adverse reaction [8]. Br J Dermatol. 2000;143:203–4.
29. De Brito M, Huebner G, Murrell D, Bullpitt P, Hartmann K. Normocomplementaemic urticarial vasculitis: effective treatment with omalizumab. Clin Transl. Allergy. 2018;8(1)
30. Cherrez-Ojeda I, Vanegas E, Felix M, Mata VL, Cherrez A. Patient-reported outcomes in urticarial vasculitis treated with omalizumab: case report. BMC Dermatol. 2018;18(1):8.
31. Banerji A, Blumenthal KG, Lai KH, Zhou L. Epidemiology of ACE inhibitor angioedema utilizing a large electronic health record. J Allergy Clin Immunol Pract. 2017;5(3):744–9.
32. Cicardi M, Aberer W, Banerji A, Bas M, Bernstein JA, Bork K, et al. Classification, diagnosis, and approach to treatment for angioedema: consensus report from the hereditary angioedema international working group. Allergy Eur J Allergy Clin Immunol. 2014;69(5):602–16.
33. Henao MP, Kraschnewski JL, Kelbel T, Craig TJ. Diagnosis and screening of patients with hereditary angioedema in primary care. In: Therapeutics and clinical risk management, vol. 12. Dove Medical Press Ltd.; 2016. p. 701–11.
34. Gompels MM, Lock RJ, Abinun M, Bethune CA, Davies G, Grattan C, et al. C1 inhibitor deficiency: Consensus document. Clin Exp Immunol. 2005;139:379–94.
35. Bork K. Acquired and hereditary forms of recurrent angioedema: update of treatment. Allergol Sel [Internet] 2018 [cited 2020 Jan 2];2(01):121–131. Available from: https://www.dustri.com/article_response_page.html?artId=16034&doi=10.5414/ALX1561E&L=0
36. Bouillet L, Boccon-Gibod I, Launay D, Gompel A, Kanny G, Fabien V, et al. Hereditary angioedema with normal C1 inhibitor in a French cohort: clinical characteristics and response to treatment with icatibant: clinical. Immunity Inflamm Dis. 2017;5(1):29–36.
37. Kostis JB, Kim HJ, Rusnak J, Casale T, Kaplan A, Corren J, et al. Incidence and characteristics of angioedema associated with enalapril. Arch Intern Med. 2005;165(14):1637–42.
38. Javaud N, Achamlal J, Reuter PG, Lapostolle F, Lekouara A, Youssef M, et al. Angioedema related to angiotensin-converting enzyme inhibitors. Med (United States). 2015;94(45):e1939.
39. van den Elzen M, Go MFCL, Knulst AC, Blankestijn MA, van Os-Medendorp H, Otten HG. Efficacy of Treatment of Non-hereditary Angioedema. In: Clinical reviews in allergy and immunology, vol. 54. Humana Press Inc; 2018. p. 412–31.
40. Zingale L, Beltrami L, Zanichelli A, Cmaj LM. Angioedema without urticaria: a large clinical survey. Can Med Assoc [Internet]. 2006 undefined [cited 2020 Feb 18]; Available from: https://www.cmaj.ca/content/175/9/1065.short
41. Leung DYM. New insights into atopic dermatitis: role of skin barrier and immune dysregulation. Allergol Int [Internet] 2013 [cited 2020 Jan 1];62(2):151–161. Available from: https://www.sciencedirect.com/science/article/pii/S1323893015301234
42. Lyons JJ, Milner JD, Stone KD. Atopic dermatitis in children: clinical features, pathophysiology, and treatment. In: Immunology and allergy clinics of North America, vol. 35. W.B. Saunders; 2015. p. 161–83.
43. Shaw TE, Currie GP, Koudelka CW, Simpson EL. Eczema prevalence in the United States: data from the 2003 national survey of children's health. J Invest Dermatol. 2011;131(1):67–73.
44. Nnoruka EN. Current epidemiology of atopic dermatitis in south-eastern Nigeria. Int J Dermatol [Internet]. 2004 Oct 1 [cited 2020 Mar 8];43(10):739–44. Available from: http://doi.wiley.com/10.1111/j.1365-4632.2004.02360.x
45. Silverberg JI, Hanifin J, Simpson EL. Climatic factors are associated with childhood eczema prevalence in the United States. J Invest Dermatol. 2013;133(7):1752–9.
46. Williams H, Robertson C, Stewart A, Aït-Khaled N, Anabwani G, Anderson R, et al. Worldwide variations in the prevalence of symptoms of atopic eczema in the international study of asthma and allergies in childhood. J Allergy Clin Immunol. 1999;103(1 I):125–38.
47. Williams H, Stewart A, von Mutius E, Cookson W, Anderson HR. Is eczema really on the increase worldwide? J Allergy Clin Immunol. 2008;121(4):947–954.e15.
48. Bannister MJ, Freeman S. Adult-onset atopic dermatitis. Australas J Dermatol. 2000;41(4):225–8.
49. Ohtsuki M, Morimoto H, Nakagawa H. Tacrolimus ointment for the treatment of adult and pediatric atopic dermatitis: review on safety and benefits. J Dermatol. Blackwell Publishing Ltd. 2018;45:936–42.

50. Silverberg NB. Typical and atypical clinical appearance of atopic dermatitis. Clin Dermatol. 2017;35(4):354–9.
51. Son JH, Chung BY, Kim HO, Park CW. Clinical features of atopic dermatitis in adults are different according to onset. J Korean Med Sci. 2017;32(8):1360–6.
52. Sacotte R, Silverberg JI. Epidemiology of adult atopic dermatitis. Clin Dermatol. 2018;36(5):595–605.
53. Galli E, Neri I, Ricci G, Baldo E, Barone M, Belloni Fortina A, et al. Consensus conference on clinical management of pediatric atopic dermatitis. In: Italian J Pediatrics. BioMed Central Ltd; 2016.
54. Damour A, Garcia M, Seneschal J, Lévêque N, Bodet C. Eczema Herpeticum: clinical and pathophysiological aspects. In: Clinical Reviews in allergy and immunology. Springer; 2019.
55. Boonstra M, Rustemeyer T, Middelkamp-Hup MA. Both children and adult patients with difficult-to-treat atopic dermatitis have high prevalences of concomitant allergic contact dermatitis and are frequently polysensitized. J Eur Acad Dermatol Venereol. 2018;32(9):1554–61.
56. Dvorakova V, O'Regan GM, Irvine AD. Methotrexate for severe childhood atopic dermatitis: clinical experience in a tertiary center. Pediatr Dermatol. 2017;34(5):528–34.
57. Kim SY, Sim S, Choi HG. Atopic dermatitis is associated with active and passive cigarette smoking in adolescents. PLoS One. 2017;12(11)
58. Schneider L, Hanifin J, Boguniewicz M, Eichenfield LF, Spergel JM, Dakovic R, et al. Study of the atopic march: development of atopic comorbidities. Pediatr Dermatol. 2016;33(4):388–98.
59. Schmitt J, Schäkel K, Fölster-Holst R, Bauer A, Oertel R, Augustin M, et al. Prednisolone vs. ciclosporin for severe adult eczema. An investigator-initiated double-blind placebo-controlled multicentre trial. Br J Dermatol [Internet]. 2010 Mar 1 [cited 2020 Mar 2];162(3):661–8. Available from: http://doi.wiley.com/10.1111/j.1365-2133.2009.09561.x.
60. Taieb Y, Baum S, Ben Amitai D, Barzilai A, Greenberger S. The use of methotrexate for treating childhood atopic dermatitis: a multicenter retrospective study. J Dermatolog Treat. 2019;30(3):240–4.
61. Nguyen TA, Leonard SA, Eichenfield LF. An update on pediatric atopic dermatitis and food allergies. J Pediatr. 2015;167(3):752–6.
62. Celakovská J, Bukac J. Analysis of food allergy in atopic dermatitis patients-association with concomitant allergic diseases. Indian J Dermatol. 2014;59(5):445–50.
63. Saarinen UM, Kajosaari M. Breastfeeding as prophylaxis against atopic disease: prospective follow-up study until 17 years old. Lancet. 1995;346(8982):1065–9.
64. Greer FR, Sicherer SH, Burks AW, Baker RD, Bhatia JJS, Daniels SR, et al. Effects of early nutritional interventions on the development of atopic disease in infants and children: the role of maternal dietary restriction, breastfeeding, timing of introduction of complementary foods, and hydrolyzed formulas. Pediatrics. 2008;121(1):183–91.
65. Yang YW, Tsai CL, Lu CY. Exclusive breastfeeding and incident atopic dermatitis in childhood: a systematic review and meta-analysis of prospective cohort studies. Br J Dermatol. 2009;161(2):373–83.
66. Kantor R, Silverberg JI. Environmental risk factors and their role in the management of atopic dermatitis. In: Expert review of clinical immunology, vol. 13. Taylor and Francis Ltd; 2017. p. 15–26.
67. Alm B, Åberg N, Erdes L, Möllborg P, Pettersson R, Norvenius SG, et al. Early introduction of fish decreases the risk of eczema in infants. Arch Dis Child. 2009;94(1):11–5.
68. Øien T, Storrø O, Johnsen R. Do early intake of fish and fish oil protect against eczema and doctor-diagnosed asthma at 2 years of age? A cohort study. J Epidemiol Community Health. 2010;64(2):124–9.
69. Willers SM, Devereux G, Craig LCA, McNeill G, Wijga AH, Abou El-Magd W, et al. Maternal food consumption during pregnancy and asthma, respiratory and atopic symptoms in 5-year-old children. Thorax. 2007;62(9):772–8.
70. Moro G, Arslanoglu S, Stahl B, Jelinek J, Wahn U, Boehm G. A mixture of prebiotic oligosaccharides reduces the incidence of atopic dermatitis during the first six months of age. Arch Dis Child. 2006;91(10):814–9.
71. Pelucchi C, Chatenoud L, Turati F, Galeone C, Moja L, Bach JF, et al. Probiotics supplementation during pregnancy or infancy for the prevention of atopic dermatitis: a meta-analysis. Epidemiol Epidemiol. 2012;23:402–14.
72. Kramer MS, Kakuma R. Maternal dietary antigen avoidance during pregnancy or lactation, or both, for preventing or treating atopic disease in the child. Evidence-Based Child Heal. 2014;9(2):447–83.
73. Ariëns LFM, Bakker DS, van der Schaft J, Garritsen FM, Thijs JL, de Bruin-Weller MS. Dupilumab in atopic dermatitis: rationale, latest evidence and place in therapy. In: Therapeutic advances in chronic disease, vol. 9. SAGE Publications Ltd; 2018. p. 159–70.
74. Kelleher MM, Dunn-Galvin A, Gray C, Murray DM, Kiely M, Kenny L, et al. Skin barrier impairment at birth predicts food allergy at 2 years of age. J Allergy Clin Immunol. 2016;137(4):1111–1116.e8.
75. Rawlings AV, Harding CR. Moisturization and skin barrier function. Dermatol Ther. 2004;17(s1):43–8.
76. Barker JNWN, Palmer CNA, Zhao Y, Liao H, Hull PR, Lee SP, et al. Null mutations in the filaggrin gene (FLG) determine major susceptibility to early-onset atopic dermatitis that persists into adulthood. J Invest Dermatol. 2007;127(3):564–7.
77. Danby SG, Chittock J, Brown K, Albenali LH, Cork MJ. The effect of tacrolimus compared with betamethasone valerate on the skin barrier in volunteers with quiescent atopic dermatitis. Br J Dermatol. 2014;170(4):914–21.

78. Wolf R, Wolf D. Abnormal epidermal barrier in the pathogenesis of atopic dermatitis. In: Clinics in dermatology, vol. 30; 2012. p. 329–34.
79. Miajlovic H, Fallon PG, Irvine AD, Foster TJ. Effect of filaggrin breakdown products on growth of and protein expression by Staphylococcus aureus. J Allergy Clin Immunol. 2010;126(6):1184.
80. Broccardo CJ, Mahaffey S, Schwarz J, Wruck L, David G, Schlievert PM, et al. Comparative proteomic profiling of patients with atopic dermatitis based on history of eczema herpeticum infection and Staphylococcus aureus colonization. J Allergy Clin Immunol. 2011;127(1):186–193.e11.
81. Batista DIS, Perez L, Orfali RL, Zaniboni MC, Samorano LP, Pereira NV, et al. Profile of skin barrier proteins (filaggrin, claudins 1 and 4) and Th1/Th2/Th17 cytokines in adults with atopic dermatitis. J Eur Acad Dermatol Venereol. 2015;29(6):1091–5.
82. Thomsen SF, Ulrik CS, Kyvik KO, Hjelmborg JVB, Skadhauge LR, Steffensen I, et al. Importance of genetic factors in the etiology of atopic dermatitis: a twin study. Allergy Asthma Proc. 2007;28(5):535–9.
83. Larsen FS. Atopic dermatitis: a genetic-epidemiologic study in a population-based twin sample. J Am Acad Dermatol. 1993;28(5):719–23.
84. Simpson EL, Chalmers JR, Hanifin JM, Thomas KS, Cork MJ, McLean WHI, et al. Emollient enhancement of the skin barrier from birth offers effective atopic dermatitis prevention. J Allergy Clin Immunol. 2014;134(4):818–23.
85. Gittler JK, Shemer A, Suárez-Fariñas M, Fuentes-Duculan J, Gulewicz KJ, Wang CQF, et al. Progressive activation of TH2/TH22 cytokines and selective epidermal proteins characterizes acute and chronic atopic dermatitis. J Allergy Clin Immunol. 2012;130(6):1344–54.
86. Kezic S, O'Regan GM, Lutter R, Jakasa I, Koster ES, Saunders S, et al. Filaggrin loss-of-function mutations are associated with enhanced expression of IL-1 cytokines in the stratum corneum of patients with atopic dermatitis and in a murine model of filaggrin deficiency. J Allergy Clin Immunol. 2012;129(4):1031.
87. Silverberg NB, Durán-McKinster C. Special considerations for therapy of pediatric atopic dermatitis. In: Dermatologic clinics, vol. 35. W.B. Saunders; 2017. p. 351–63.
88. Wollenberg A, Barbarot S, Bieber T, Christen-Zaech S, Deleuran M, Fink-Wagner A, et al. Consensus-based European guidelines for treatment of atopic eczema (atopic dermatitis) in adults and children: part I. J Eur Acad Dermatol Venereol. 2018;32(5):657–82.
89. Anderson K, Putterman E, Rogers RS, Patel D, Treat JR, Castelo-Soccio L. Treatment of severe pediatric atopic dermatitis with methotrexate: a retrospective review. Pediatr Dermatol. 2019;36(3):298–302.
90. Phan K, Smith SD. Mycophenolate mofetil and atopic dermatitis: systematic review and meta-analysis. J Dermatolog Treat. 2019:1–5.
91. Beck LA, Thaçi D, Hamilton JD, Graham NM, Bieber T, Rocklin R, et al. Dupilumab treatment in adults with moderate-to-severe atopic dermatitis. N Engl J Med. 2014;371(2):130–9.
92. Blauvelt A, de Bruin-Weller M, Gooderham M, Cather JC, Weisman J, Pariser D, et al. Long-term management of moderate-to-severe atopic dermatitis with dupilumab and concomitant topical corticosteroids (LIBERTY AD CHRONOS): a 1-year, randomised, double-blinded, placebo-controlled, phase 3 trial. Lancet. 2017;389(10086):2287–303.
93. Treister AD, Lio PA. Long-term off-label dupilumab in pediatric atopic dermatitis: a case series. Pediatr Dermatol. 2019;36(1):85–8.
94. Belsito DV. Occupational contact dermatitis: etiology, prevalence, and resultant impairment/disability. J Am Acad Dermatol Mosby. 2005;53:303–13.
95. Cashman MW, Reutemann PA, Ehrlich A. Contact dermatitis in the United States: epidemiology, economic impact, and workplace prevention. In: Dermatologic Clinics, vol. 30; 2012. p. 87–98.
96. Mowad CM, Anderson B, Scheinman P, Pootongkam S, Nedorost S, Brod B. Allergic contact dermatitis Patient diagnosis and evaluation. In: J Am Acad Dermatol, vol. 74. Mosby Inc; 2016. p. 1029–40.
97. Schloemer JA, Zirwas MJ, Burkhart CG. Airborne contact dermatitis: Common causes in the USA. Vol. 54, Int J Dermatol. Blackwell Publishing Ltd; 2015. p. 271–274.
98. Handa S, De D, Mahajan R. Airborne contact dermatitis-current perspectives in etiopathogenesis and management. Indian J Dermatol. 2011;56:700–6.
99. Ghosh S. Airborne-contact dermatitis of non-plant origin: an overview. Indian J Dermatol. Wolters Kluwer — Medknow Publications. 2011;56:711–4.
100. Hostetler SG, Kaffenberger B, Hostetler T, Zirwas MJ. The role of airborne proteins in atopic dermatitis. J Clin Aesthet Dermatol [Internet] 2010 Jan [cited 2020 Mar 13];3(1):22–31. Available from: http://www.ncbi.nlm.nih.gov/pubmed/20725535.
101. Krasteva M, Kehren J, Ducluzeau, MS, Dupuis M, Kanitakis JFN. Contact dermatitis: II. Clinical aspects and diagnosis [internet]. European J Dermatol. 1999 [cited 2020 Mar 13]. p. 144–60. Available from: https://scholar.google.com/scholar_lookup?title=Contact dermatitis II. Clinical aspects and diagnosis&publication_year=1999&author=M. Krasteva&author=M.T. Kehren&author=M. Duclu zeau.
102. Liden C, Berg M, Farm G, Wrangsjo K. Nail varnish allergy with far-reaching consequences. Br J Dermatol. 1993;128(1):57–62.
103. Silverberg NB, Licht J, Friedler S, Sethi S, Laude TA. Nickel contact hypersensitivity in children. Pediatr Dermatol. 2002;19(2):110–3.
104. De Groot AC, Frosch PJ. Adverse reactions to fragrances. A clinical review. Contact Derm. 1997;36:57–86.
105. Krautheim A, Uter W, Frosch P, Schnuch A, Geier J. Patch testing with fragrance mix II:

Results of the IVDK 2005–2008. Contact Dermatitis [Internet]. 2010 [cited 2020 Mar 14];63(5):262–9. Available from: http://doi.wiley.com/10.1111/j.1600-0536.2010.01753.x
106. Dooms-Goossens A, Andersen KE, Brandão FM, Bruynzeel D, Burrows D, Camarasa J, et al. Corticosteroid contact allergy: an EECDRG multicentre study. Contact Derm. 1996;35(1):40–4.
107. Jacob SE, McGowan M, Silverberg NB, Pelletier JL, Fonacier L, Mousdicas N, et al. Pediatric contact dermatitis registry data on contact allergy in children with atopic dermatitis. JAMA Dermatol. 2017;153(8):765–70.
108. Larsson-Stymne B, Widström L. Ear piercing—a cause of nickel allergy in schoolgirls? Contact Dermatitis [Internet] 1985 [cited 2020 Mar 12];13(5):289–293. Available from: http://doi.wiley.com/10.1111/j.1600-0536.1985.tb02580.x.
109. Nguyen HL, Yiannias JA. Contact dermatitis to medications and skin products. In: Clinical reviews in allergy and immunology, vol. 56. Humana Press Inc; 2019. p. 41–59.
110. Mowad CM. Contact dermatitis: practice gaps and challenges. In: Dermatologic clinics, vol. 34. W.B. Saunders; 2016. p. 263–7.
111. Tran JM, Reeder MJ. When the treatment is the culprit: prevalence of allergens in prescription topical steroids and immunomodulators. J Am Acad Dermatol [Internet]. 2019 Nov [cited 2020 Jan 13]; Available from: https://linkinghub.elsevier.com/retrieve/pii/S019096221933110X.
112. Bohn S, Niederer M, Brehm K, Bircher AJ. Airborne contact dermatitis from methylchloroisothiazolinone in wall paint. Abolition of symptoms by chemical allergen inactivation. Contact Derm. 2000;42(4):196–201.
113. Leiva-Salinas M, Francés L, Silvestre JF. Update on allergic contact dermatitis due to Methylchloroisothiazolinone/Methylisothiazolinone and Methylisothiazolinone. Actas Dermosifiliogr. 2014 Nov;105(9):840–6.
114. Cohen DE, Brancaccio R, Andersen D, Belsito DV. Utility of a standard allergen series alone in the evaluation of allergic contact dermatitis: a retrospective study of 732 patients. J Am Acad Dermatol. 1997;36(6 I):914–8.
115. Condie MW, Adams RM. Influence of Oral prednisone on patch-test reactions to Rhus antigen. Arch Dermatol. 1973;107(4):540–3.
116. Yawalkar N. Drug-induced exanthems. In: Toxicology. Elsevier Ireland Ltd; 2005. p. 131–4.
117. Gerson D, Sriganeshan V, Alexis JB. Cutaneous drug eruptions: a 5-year experience. J Am Acad Dermatol. 2008;59(6):995–9.
118. Teo Y, Walsh S, Creamer D. Cutaneous adverse drug reaction referrals to a liaison dermatology service. British J Dermatol. Blackwell Publishing Ltd. 2017;177:e141–2.
119. Schwartz RA, McDonough PH, Lee BW. Toxic epidermal necrolysis: Part II. Prognosis, sequelae, diagnosis, differential diagnosis, prevention, and treatment. J Amer Acad Dermatol. Mosby Inc. 2013;69:187.e1–187.e16.
120. Micheletti RG, Chiesa-Fuxench Z, Noe MH, Stephen S, Aleshin M, Agarwal A, et al. Stevens-Johnson syndrome/toxic epidermal necrolysis: a multicenter retrospective study of 377 adult patients from the United States. J Invest Dermatol. 2018;138(11):2315–21.
121. McPherson T, Exton LS, Biswas S, Creamer D, Dziewulski P, Newell L, et al. British Association of Dermatologists' guidelines for the management of Stevens–Johnson syndrome/toxic epidermal necrolysis in children and young people, 2018. Br J Dermatol [Internet] 2019 [cited 2020 Mar 10];181(1):37–54. Available from: https://onlinelibrary.wiley.com/doi/abs/10.1111/bjd.17841
122. Shiohara T, Mizukawa Y. Drug-induced hypersensitivity syndrome (DiHS)/drug reaction with eosinophilia and systemic symptoms (DRESS): an update in 2019. Allergol Int Japanese Soc Allergol. 2019;68:301–8.
123. Chiou CC, Yang LC, Hung SI, Chang YC, Kuo TT, Ho HC, et al. Clinicopathlogical features and prognosis of drug rash with eosinophilia and systemic symptoms: a study of 30 cases in Taiwan. J Eur Acad Dermatol Venereol. 2008;22(9):1044–9.
124. Chu CY, Chen YC, Chiu HC. Drug reaction with eosinophilia and systemic symptoms: a retrospective study of 60 cases. Arch Dermatol. 2010;146(12):1373–9.
125. Rothenberg ME. Epstein FH. Eosinophilia. N Engl J Med [Internet]. 1998 [cited 2020 Feb 4];338(22):1592–600. Available from: http://www.nejm.org/doi/10.1056/NEJM199805283382206.
126. Long H, Zhang G, Wang L, Lu Q. Eosinophilic skin diseases: a comprehensive review. In: Clinical reviews in allergy and immunology, vol. 50. Humana Press Inc; 2016. p. 189–213.
127. Rothenberg ME, Hogan SP. The Eosinophil. Annu Rev Immunol [Internet]. 2006 [cited 2020 Feb 9];24(1):147–74. Available from: http://www.annualreviews.org/doi/10.1146/annurev.immunol.24.021605.090720.
128. Ahmadi Z, Hassanshahi G, Khorramdelazad H, Zainodini N, Koochakzadeh L. An overlook to the characteristics and roles played by Eotaxin network in the pathophysiology of food allergies: allergic asthma and atopic dermatitis. In: Inflammation, vol. 39. New York. LLC: Springer; 2016. p. 1253–67.
129. Diny NL, Rose NR, Čiháková D. Eosinophils in autoimmune diseases. In: Frontiers in immunology, vol. 8. Frontiers Media S.A.; 2017.
130. Sriaroon P, Ballow M. Biological modulators in eosinophilic diseases. In: Clinical reviews in allergy and immunology, vol. 50. Humana Press Inc; 2016. p. 252–72.
131. Peckruhn M, Elsner P, Tittelbach J. Eosinophilic dermatoses. JDDG J Ger Soc Dermatol. 2019;17(10):1039–51.

132. Ortonne N, Wechsler J, Bagot M, Grosshans E, Cribier B. Granuloma faciale: a clinicopathologic study of 66 patients. J Am Acad Dermatol. 2005 Dec;53(6):1002–9.
133. Lindhaus C, Elsner P. Granuloma faciale treatment: a systematic review. Acta Derm Venereol. 2018;98(1):14–8.
134. Cesinaro AM, Lonardi S, Facchetti F. Granuloma faciale: a cutaneous lesion sharing features with IgG4-associated sclerosing diseases. Am J Surg Pathol. 2013;37(1):66–73.
135. Madan V. Recurrent granuloma faciale successfully treated with the carbon dioxide laser. J Cutan Aesthet Surg. 2011;4(2):156.
136. Narayan J, Douglas-Jones AG. Eosinophilic angiocentric fibrosis and granuloma faciale: analysis of cellular infiltrate and review of literature. In: Annals of otology, rhinology and laryngology, vol. 114. Annals Publishing Company; 2005. p. 35–42.
137. Fang CH, Mady LJ, Mirani NM, Baredes S, Eloy JA. Sinonasal eosinophilic angiocentric fibrosis: a systematic review. Int Forum Allergy Rhinol [Internet]. 2014 [cited 2020 Feb 4];4(9):745–52. Available from: http://doi.wiley.com/10.1002/alr.21347
138. Ahn J, Flanagan M. Eosinophilic angiocentric fibrosis: a review and update of its association with immunoglobulin G4–related disease. Arch Pathol Lab Med. 2018;142(12):1560–3.
139. Karaman E, Isildak H, Ozdilek A, Sekercioglu N. Kimura disease. J Craniofac Surg. 2008;19(6):1702–5.
140. Kottler D, Barète S, Quéreux G, Ingen-Housz-Oro S, Fraitag S, Ortonne N, et al. Retrospective multicentric study of 25 Kimura disease patients: emphasis on therapeutics and shared features with cutaneous IgG4-related disease. Dermatology. 2015;231(4):367–77.
141. Zhang L, Yao L, Zhou WW, Ma JN, Zhang CQ. Computerized tomography features and clinicopathological analysis of Kimura disease in head and neck. Exp Ther Med. 2018;16(3):2087–93.
142. Yamamoto T, Minamiguchi S, Watanabe Y, Tsuji J, Asato R, Manabe T, et al. Kimura disease of the epiglottis: a case report and review of literature. Head Neck Pathol. 2014;8(2):198–203.
143. Fujiwara M, Fujiwara S, Kodera A, Kitada K, Araki T. Kimura disease in a 2-year-old boy with generalized lymphadenopathy. Pediatr Int. 2019;61(12):1276–7.
144. Zhang J, Li Y, Wen G, Deng Y, Yao H. Novel application of 32 P brachytherapy: treatment of Angiolymphoid hyperplasia with eosinophilia in the right auricle with 8-year follow-up. Cancer Biother Radiopharm. 2018;33(7):282–4.
145. Xu X, Fu J, Fang Y, Liang L. Kimura disease in children: a case report and a summary of the literature in Chinese. J Pediatr Hematol Oncol. 2011;33(4):306–11.
146. Ye P, Wei T, Yu GY, Wu LL, Peng X. Comparison of local recurrence rate of three treatment modalities for Kimura disease. J Craniofac Surg. 2016;27(1):170–4.
147. Adler BL, Krausz AE, Minuti A, Silverberg JI, Lev-Tov H. Epidemiology and treatment of angiolymphoid hyperplasia with eosinophilia (ALHE): a systematic review. J Am Acad Dermatol. 2016;74(3):506–512.e11.
148. Olsen TG, Helwig EB. Angiolymphoid hyperplasia with eosinophilia: a clinicopathologic study of 116 patients. J Am Acad Dermatol. 1985;12(5):781–96.
149. Okman JS, Bhatti TR, Jackson OA, Rubin AI. Angiolymphoid hyperplasia with eosinophilia: a previously unreported complication of ear piercing. Pediatr Dermatol. 2014;31(6):738–41.
150. Labib A, Estawrow M. Angiolymphoid hyperplasia with eosinophilia: new concept to lower recurrence. J Craniofac Surg. 2019;30(5):E386–8.
151. Caca-Biljanovska N, Arsovska-Bezhoska I. Angiolymphoid hyperplasia with eosinophilia successfully treated with cryotherapy. Open Access Maced J Med Sci. 2019;7(5):794–6.
152. Horst C, Kapur N. Propranolol: a novel treatment for angiolymphoid hyperplasia with eosinophilia. Clin Exp Dermatol. 2014;39(7):810–2.

Pediatric Allergic Rhinitis

35

Sofia Ellen Edwards-Salmon

Introduction

Allergic rhinitis (AR) is a common inflammatory condition characterized by symptoms of nasal congestion, rhinorrhea, sneezing, or itching in response to inhaled allergens. The majority of patients develop AR during childhood and often have other comorbid atopic conditions, including atopic dermatitis (AD) and asthma. Patients with AR report multiple negative impacts on health and development including physical activity, sleep, and school performance. Therefore, timely and accurate diagnosis and management will help ensure that children with AR achieve their full potential. This chapter will review the epidemiology, pathogenesis, diagnosis, and optimal management of pediatric AR.

Epidemiology

Allergic rhinitis (AR) is present in approximately 15% of children in the United States, although some surveys report frequencies as high as 40% [1, 2]. The typical age of onset of AR is around 18 to 24 months of age; the prevalence increases in frequency throughout childhood with a peak in adolescence [3]. Approximately 40% of patients with AR develop symptoms before the age of six and 80% will have symptoms by age 20 [4]. Therefore, determining the age of onset is often helpful in the evaluation of the rhinitis patient because onset in the first year of life or after age 35 is more suggestive of a nonallergic etiology [5].

Pathogenesis

AR results from an immunoglobulin E (IgE)-mediated inflammatory response at the nasal mucosa after exposure to environmental allergens. Both genetic factors and environmental exposures have been associated with the development of AR. Parental history of allergic disease is associated with AR, with heritability estimates as high as 90%. Genome-wide association studies have demonstrated that AR has common susceptibility with other atopic diseases such as AD and asthma [6]. Patients clinically manifest this association by following the "allergic march," which describes a natural history where AD is an initial manifestation that is followed by the development of food allergy, AR, and/or asthma.

However, studies examining the increase in allergic diseases in the last century have shown that environmental causes interact with genetics

S. E. Edwards-Salmon (✉)
Allergy & Immunology Fellow, PGY-5, Emory University School of Medicine, Atlanta, GA, USA
e-mail: sofia.ellen.edwards-salmon@emory.edu

C. Damask et al. (eds.), *Allergy in Otolaryngology Practice*,
https://doi.org/10.1007/978-3-031-93455-1_35

to lead to the development of AR. One of the earliest identified protective factors for the development of AR was a number of older siblings, which were thought to increase microbial exposure in the home environment. Children raised in farming environments were also found to have a lower frequency of atopy, and corresponding changes in the skin and nasal microbiome suggest that microbial exposure may explain this protective effect. Since reduced microbial exposure may potentially increase the risk of AR, this association has been labeled the "hygiene hypothesis." Indoor mold exposure has also been associated with AR, but other exposures such as cat or dog ownership have had variable results. Exposure to pollutants such as environmental tobacco smoke and traffic pollution such as diesel particulate matter also increase the risk of AR. These pollutants have been demonstrated to alter immune function and co-exposure of diesel particles with allergens enhances the allergic immune response [7] (Table 35.1).

The consequence of these risk factors is the production of IgE against specific airborne allergens, which is called sensitization. This allergen-specific IgE binds to mast cells which line the respiratory mucosa. Re-exposure to inhaled allergen cross-links IgE molecules on the surface of mast cells resulting in activation and release of inflammatory mediators including histamine, leukotrienes, prostaglandins, bradykinin, and platelet-activating factor. This immediate phase produces the clinical symptoms associated with AR that peak within 15–30 min after allergen exposure. A late phase which peaks 6–12 h after exposure corresponds to infiltration of nasal mucosa with inflammatory cells such as eosinophils, T lymphocytes, and basophils.

Repeated allergen exposure has been demonstrated to increase the sensitivity to subsequent allergen exposure, a phenomenon which is called "priming." Intranasal corticosteroids counteract this priming effect, suggesting an immunologic mechanism. Priming is hypothesized to be secondary to inflammation-induced barrier dysfunction and increased allergen entry, increased mast cell number, and hyper-responsiveness of nasal organs. Therefore, the management of perennial AR has been emphasized to attenuate the impact of seasonal exacerbations [8].

Table 35.1 Risk factors for development of allergic rhinitis

Parental history of atopy
Atopic dermatitis
Indoor mold exposure
Lack of microbial exposure ("hygiene hypothesis")
Exposure to pollutants

Clinical Features

AR is characterized by nasal congestion, anterior and posterior nasal drainage, sneezing, and/or nasal itching. Other common symptoms include itchy eyes and throat, repeated sniffing, snorting, throat clearing, and cough. Noisy breathing may be reported as "wheezing," although it is important to clarify whether this is a lower-pitched coarse noise from the upper airway rather than high-pitched wheeze associated with lower airway bronchospasm. Nasal obstruction can cause chronic mouth breathing and sleep-disordered breathing leading to snoring, fatigue, and irritability. Conductive hearing loss has also been reported due to eustachian tube dysfunction and middle ear effusion.

The Allergic Rhinitis and its Impact on Asthma (ARIA) subdivides AR into *intermittent* (symptoms <4 days a week or <4 consecutive weeks) and *persistent* (symptoms >4 days a week and >4 consecutive weeks). ARIA also defines AR severity based on impairment of four health-related quality of life parameters: (1) sleep, (2) daily activities, leisure, and/or sports, (3) impairment of school or work, and (4) troublesome symptoms. The disease is considered *mild* if there is no impairment in any of these areas and *moderate/severe* if one or more items are affected [9]. The United States Food and Drug Administration has adopted a classification based on the temporal pattern of exposure to the triggering allergen, which includes *seasonal* AR, typically secondary to pollens, and *perennial* AR, which are typically secondary to indoor exposures. The 2020 update to the Rhinitis Practice

Parameter also defines *episodic* AR, which refers to symptoms due to allergens not normally in the patient's home such as pets in other residences [10].

In children, the most common comorbid conditions include atopic dermatitis, allergic conjunctivitis, and asthma. Atopic dermatitis typically starts in the first year of life with xerosis and pruritus which progresses acutely to pruritic erythematous papules and patches. As the rash becomes more chronic, they develop a thick, lichenified, and potentially hyperpigmented appearance. Infants develop erythematous patches on the cheeks and extensor surfaces, but older children will demonstrate patches on the flexural surfaces of the elbows, knees, and skin folds of the neck, wrists, and ankles. Allergic conjunctivitis can be present in up to 60% of AR patients. Allergic conjunctivitis usually presents with bilateral ocular pruritus, tearing, hyperemia, chemosis, and eyelid or conjunctival edema. Finally, asthma can occur in approximately 50% of AR patients. Both entities are thought to represent a spectrum of the same condition; this is referred to as the "unified airway hypothesis." Asthma is suspected when a patient reports episodic respiratory symptoms of cough (especially nocturnal), wheezing, chest tightness, exercise intolerance, and dyspnea [10].

Allergic reactions to food mediated by IgE are not thought to be a cause of chronic rhinitis symptoms. However, up to 25% of patients with AR can develop "pollen-food syndrome" or "oral allergy syndrome." This manifests as mouth and throat pruritus and swelling secondary to cross reactive proteins contained in both pollen and foods such as raw fruits, vegetables, and nuts. However, these patients can tolerate the consumption of the same fruits and vegetables in cooked form, presumably due to the denaturation of the allergenic proteins.

Diagnosis

A thorough history is important to accurately diagnose and manage pediatric AR. The provider should determine the age of onset, type, frequency, duration and severity of symptoms, suspected triggers, indoor exposures, and response to previous medications. Risk factors such as family history of atopy and concurrent atopic diseases such as atopic dermatitis, asthma, and food allergy should be assessed. The diagnosis of *seasonal, intermittent,* or *episodic* AR can made clinically if there is a clear, reproducible association between a suspected exposure and rhinitis symptoms. For example, rhinitis symptoms reported only during the spring months in North America suggest seasonal AR due to tree pollen. Episodic AR is suggested when there is a consistent association between exposure and symptom onset, such as visiting a house with a furry animal. Conversely, *perennial* AR is more difficult to diagnose based solely on history since indoor exposures such as dust mite are ubiquitous and induce symptoms difficult to distinguish from nonallergic rhinitis.

The physical exam for pediatric AR focuses on the head, eyes, ears, nose, and throat while also assessing for pulmonary and cutaneous comorbidities. Uncontrolled active AR typically manifests as bilateral clear anterior rhinorrhea with associated inferior turbinate hypertrophy. Evidence of posterior nasal drainage manifests as "cobblestoning," which refers to hypertrophy of the lymphoid tissue lining the posterior pharynx that can be associated with upper airway causes of cough. Eustachian tube dysfunction can result in a dull, non-erythematous appearance of the tympanic membrane caused by a serous middle ear effusion. Facial findings associated with pediatric AR include the "allergic salute," which is a transverse nasal crease created by persistent rubbing of the nose, and "allergic shiners," which is a dark, violaceous discoloration and edema below the eyes caused by venous stasis. Dennie-Morgan lines are accentuated skin folds beneath the lower eyelids that are associated with allergic conjunctivitis. The "adenoid facies" refers a long, thin facial shape with malar hypoplasia, high-arched palate, and dental malocclusion associated with chronic mouth breathing [11]. Finally, a pulmonary examination for wheezing and an assessment for atopic dermatitis increase the likelihood that the rhinitis has an allergic component.

Aeroallergen testing can confirm the diagnosis of AR and is helpful in management by identifying which environmental avoidance measures are relevant to the patient. Testing can either be performed via skin prick/puncture testing (SPT), intracutaneous (intradermal) testing, or measurement of allergen-specific IgE (sIgE) from serum. SPT is advantageous for children because relatively less traumatic than other methods and provides results within 20 min after application. Intracutaneous testing has improved sensitivity over SPT but is more painful than SPT and has the potential for false positive results due to a non-IgE-mediated irritant response. Serum sIgE testing is advantageous in situations where skin testing is not possible, such as suppression of skin test responses by antihistamine medications, significant skin rashes, or uncooperative patients [12].

Differential Diagnosis

The differential diagnosis for AR in pediatric patients is broad and it is also important to remember that both allergic and non-allergic causes can co-exist in patients (Table 35.2). Since the age of onset of AR is typically around 18 to 24 months of age, nonallergic causes of chronic rhinitis should be strongly considered in children under 2 years of age. The most common causes of nonallergic rhinitis in children are infectious rhinitis due to recurrent viral upper respiratory tract infections (URIs) and vasomotor rhinitis due to irritant exposures such as environmental tobacco smoke. Recurrent URIs are suggested by a pattern of rhinitis episodes less than 2 weeks duration. Vasomotor rhinitis is suggested by triggers that include cold air, strong odors, exercise, and irritants. Vasomotor rhinitis patients are also less likely to report pruritus and sneezing than AR patients. Children under 2 years of age also may have craniofacial abnormalities due to a genetic syndrome or choanal atresia can result in nasal obstruction and rhinitis. Finally, laryngopharyngeal reflux, especially in the context of premature birth or neuromuscular disease, has also been associated with nasal congestion [10].

Table 35.2 Differential diagnosis of pediatric allergic rhinitis

Recurrent upper respiratory tract infections
Vasomotor rhinitis
Irritants (tobacco, e-cigarette, or other smoking)
Cold air
Exercise
Adenoidal hypertrophy
Nasal septal deviation
Laryngopharyngeal reflux
Nasal polyps
Hormonal rhinitis
Rhinitis medicamentosa
Nasal foreign body
Craniofacial abnormalities
Cystic fibrosis
Vasculitis
Primary ciliary dyskinesia
Inborn error of immunity
Nasal tumor
CSF rhinorrhea

In addition to infectious and vasomotor causes, toddlers between 12 and 36 months of age can also develop anatomic nasal obstruction to due adenoidal hypertrophy and therefore a lateral X-ray of the nasopharynx and neck can identify these children. A nasal foreign body would be suggested by unilateral purulent drainage and congestion. The onset of chronic rhinosinusitis in this age range, especially with concurrent dyspnea, recurrent pneumonias, and nasal polyps may suggest an underlying genetic condition such as cystic fibrosis or primary ciliary dyskinesia. Recurrent otitis media, rhinosinusitis, and pneumonia also may indicate a possible inborn error of immunity such as an antibody immunodeficiency.

Finally, older children have a similar differential diagnosis as adults. Anatomic causes of nonallergic rhinitis in older patients may be secondary to nasal polyps, nasal septal deviation, or tumors. Medications such as overuse of topical decongestants can lead to rebound congestion, called rhinitis medicamentosa. Hormonal rhinitis can occur with the onset of puberty or pregnancy. Systemic vasculitides such as granulomatosis with polyangiitis can rarely start in childhood. Finally, unilateral rhinorrhea following a skull fracture may suggest a cerebrospinal fluid leak [10].

Management

The optimal management of pediatric AR is a multimodal approach that integrates environmental control measures, age-appropriate pharmacotherapy, and/or allergen immunotherapy (Fig. 35.1). Although environmental control interventions have not consistently demonstrated a clinical benefit, studies that have included allergen measurements that demonstrate a significant reduction of exposure have shown improvement in clinical outcomes. Effective allergen mitigation is achievable but requires significant effort by the family. For example, the only effective long-term intervention for animal dander allergen reduction is removal from the pet from the house. In addition, cat allergens can be detected in the home environment months after removal of the pet. The most successful interventions for cockroach and mouse allergen reduction have been studies implementing integrated pest management, which includes sealing cracks and entryways, prompt disposal of food, baits or traps, thorough cleaning, and pesticide/rodenticide. Indoor mold exposure can be reduced by reducing dampness in the home through leak repair, reducing water intrusion, and removal (not surface cleaning) of moldy surfaces [13]. House dust mite allergen reduction can be achieved by placing mite-proof encasements on the mattress, pillow, and box spring, weekly washing of bedding, reducing indoor relative humidity under 50%, and regular vacuuming with HEPA filtration [14]. Finally, irritant exposures such as incense, candles, and smoke exposure should be eliminated from the indoor environment.

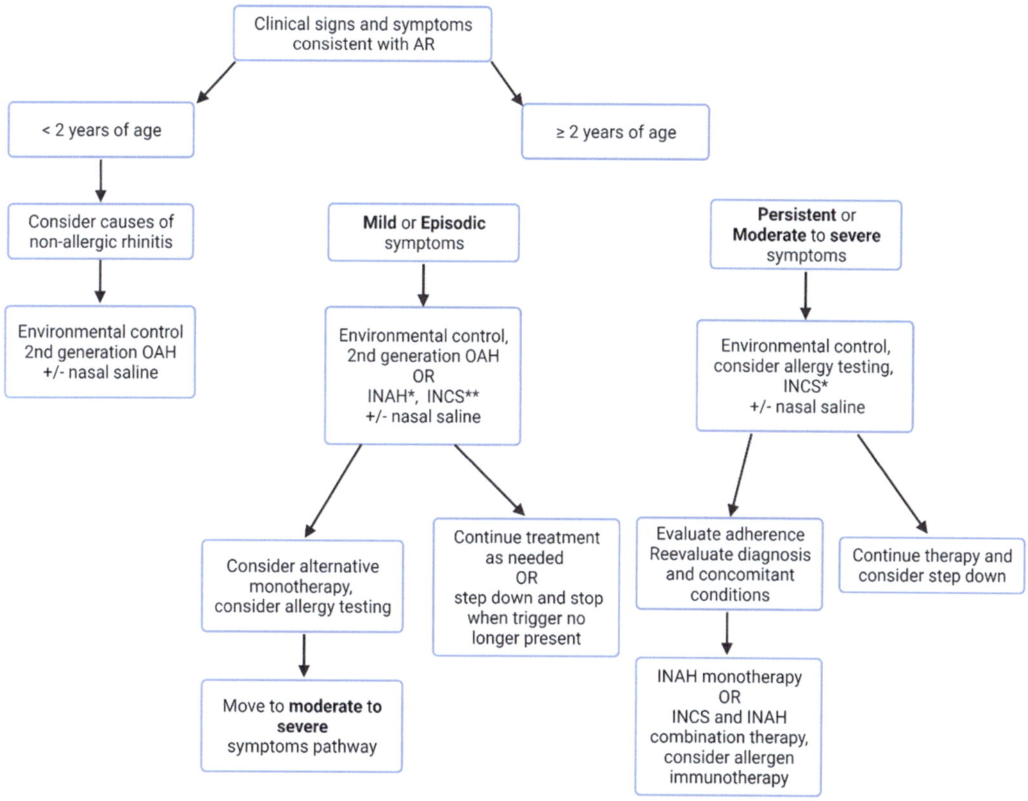

Fig. 35.1 Algorithm for the management of pediatric allergic rhinitis. *AR* allergic rhinitis, *OAH* oral antihistamine, *INAH* intranasal antihistamine, *INCS* intranasal corticosteroid, *first line, **second line, +/– consider adding adjunctive therapy. (Figure created with Biorender.com)

Intranasal corticosteroids (INCS) are recommended by multiple guidelines as first-line monotherapy for moderate to severe symptoms, especially if persistent [10, 15]. INCS are most effective with continuous use, but as-needed dosing has also been efficacious. INCS can demonstrate symptomatic improvement within 12 h of use but full benefit may not be achieved until days or weeks after starting therapy. INCS can also treat comorbid allergic conjunctivitis symptoms. The most common side effects of INCS are local dryness, irritation, and epistaxis. Nasal perforation has been reported rarely. Side effects can be minimized by spraying the medication with the head tilted slightly forward and away from the nasal septum. There is some evidence that short-term INCS use in children may decelerate short-term growth velocity, but it is not clear if long-term growth is affected.

Oral antihistamines (OAH) and intranasal antihistamines (INAH) are efficacious in the treatment for AR and either can also be used as monotherapy. First-generation OAH are associated with sedation, and therefore should not be used in children. INAH are more efficacious than OAH and have the advantage of a rapid onset of action within 15–30 min of use, and therefore has been recommended as first-line for episodic or intermittent AR [10]. However, INAH use can be challenging in children because of side effects of burning or bitter taste.

Leukotriene receptor antagonists (LTRAs) have shown similar efficacy to OAH but have not been as effective as INAH and INCS for the treatment of AR. In addition, the United States Food and Drug Administration recently added a black box warning for the LTRA montelukast due to reports of neuropsychiatric changes, mood disturbances, and suicidal ideation. Therefore, providers should consider other therapies initially in the treatment of AR, and also engage in shared decision-making with families before starting LTRAs [16].

As adjunctive therapy, nasal saline can aid in the clearing of secretions associated with AR. It can be beneficial for moisturizing dry nasal passages and clearing mucus. This can be done with simple saline solution and syringe or nasal aspiration devices recommended by the patient's pediatrician. It is associated with minimal side effects which include burning, irritation, and nausea, and has low cost. There is a risk of bacteria/parasitic infection, so if using tap water, it should be boiled for at least 5 min before use [17].

Therapies that are used less frequently in children include oral and intranasal decongestants, intranasal ipratropium, and intranasal cromolyn. Oral decongestants should be used with caution in children less than 6 years old and have been associated with agitation, hallucinations, ataxia, and death in infants and young children. Intranasal decongestants are reserved for short-term therapy due to the risk of rebound congestion with prolonged use. Intranasal ipratropium can treat rhinorrhea associated with AR, but lacks efficacy in other AR symptoms, especially congestion. Finally, intranasal cromolyn requires frequent administration to be efficacious and therefore has challenges with patient adherence [10].

AR patients may require combination therapy for severe symptoms or if symptoms are not controlled with a single agent. Combination of INCS and INAH has been proven to be effective for the treatment of moderate to severe seasonal and perennial AR that is resistant to monotherapy or for the initial treatment of moderate to severe symptoms of seasonal AR. However, studies have not demonstrated a consistent benefit of adding an OAH to INCS therapy [18]. Similarly, the addition of an LTRA to INCS therapy also does not appear to add additional efficacy [19].

Allergen immunotherapy (AIT) should be considered in patients who have moderate to severe symptoms that persist despite avoidance measures and pharmacotherapy, or for patients interested in reducing their medication requirement. In addition to alleviating symptoms, immunomodulation therapy has potential disease-modifying effects which can prevent asthma in addition to having long-term effect on rhinitis. The two major forms of AIT options are subcutaneous immunotherapy (SCIT) and sublingual immunotherapy (SLIT).

In order to start a patient on AIT, the patient should report clinical symptoms from aeroallergen exposure and demonstrate evidence of allergen-specific IgE sensitization such as skin or serum sIgE testing. After receiving the recommended time course of maintenance AIT, patients become more tolerant of aeroallergen exposure with a significant reduction of symptoms and medication use afterward. Comparative studies of SCIT and SLIT in adults suggest that SCIT leads to greater symptom reduction in AR compared with SLIT [20]. SCIT also has been demonstrated to have higher adherence rate despite in office administration [21]. However, SLIT has the convenience of administration at home and better safety profile. SLIT is associated with local symptoms such as oral pruritus, throat irritation, and local swelling with rare systemic reactions. However, SCIT has a 0.1% risk of systemic allergic reactions, and therefore it is recommended by professional societies that SCIT be administered in a medical office that can treat anaphylaxis with a 30-min wait period [22]. A shared decision-making conversation with families should include discussion of comparative efficacy, preferred location of administration, and risk of systemic side effects.

Conclusion

Pediatric AR is a common condition that can potentially lead to negative consequences on health, academic potential, and quality of life. A comprehensive assessment of clinical features, allergic and nonallergic exposures, and comorbidities are necessary to minimize these negative impacts. A management plan that integrates environmental control, pharmacotherapy, and potentially immunotherapy can help patient achieve long-term control and the best possible long-term outcomes.

References

1. National Center for Health Statistics. Health, United States, 2018. Hyattsville: NCHS; 2019.
2. Wright AL, et al. Epidemiology of physician-diagnosed allergic rhinitis in childhood. Pediatrics. 1994;94(6 Pt 1):895–901.
3. Kellberger J, et al. Prediction of the incidence and persistence of allergic rhinitis in adolescence: a prospective cohort study. J Allergy Clin Immunol. 2012;129(2):397–402.e3.
4. Meltzer EO, et al. Burden of allergic rhinitis: results from the pediatric allergies in America survey. J Allergy Clin Immunol. 2009;124(3 Suppl):S43–70.
5. Bernstein JA. Characteristics of nonallergic vasomotor rhinitis. World Allergy Organ J. 2009;2(6):102–5.
6. Portelli MA, Hodge E, Sayers I. Genetic risk factors for the development of allergic disease identified by genome-wide association. Clin Exp Allergy. 2015;45(1):21–31.
7. Murrison LB, et al. Environmental exposures and mechanisms in allergy and asthma development. J Clin Invest. 2019;129(4):1504–15.
8. Matheson MC, et al. Early-life risk factors and incidence of rhinitis: results from the European Community Respiratory Health Study—an international population-based cohort study. J Allergy Clin Immunol. 2011;128(4):816–23.e5.
9. Bousquet J, et al. Allergic rhinitis and its impact on asthma (ARIA) 2008 update (in collaboration with the World Health Organization, GA(2)LEN and AllerGen). Allergy. 2008;63(Suppl 86):8–160.
10. Dykewicz MS, et al. Rhinitis 2020: a practice parameter update. J Allergy Clin Immunol. 2020;146(4):721–67.
11. Elluru RG. Adenoid facies and nasal airway obstruction: cause and effect? Arch Otolaryngol Head Neck Surg. 2005;131(10):919–20.
12. Bernstein IL, et al. Allergy diagnostic testing: an updated practice parameter. Ann Allergy Asthma Immunol. 2008;100(3 Suppl 3):S1–148.
13. Ahluwalia SK, Matsui EC. Indoor environmental interventions for furry pet allergens, pest allergens, and mold: looking to the future. J Allergy Clin Immunol Pract. 2018;6(1):9–19.
14. Portnoy J, et al. Environmental assessment and exposure control of dust mites: a practice parameter. Ann Allergy Asthma Immunol. 2013;111(6):465–507.
15. Roberts G, et al. Paediatric rhinitis: position paper of the European Academy of Allergy and Clinical Immunology. Allergy. 2013;68(9):1102–16.
16. U.S.F.D. Administration. FDA requires boxed warning about serious mental health side effects for asthma and allergy drug montelukast (Singulair); advises restricting use for allergic rhinitis. 2020 [cited 2021 March 8, 2021]. Available from: https://www.fda.gov/drugs/drug-safety-and-availability/fda-requires-boxed-warning-about-serious-mental-health-side-effects-asthma-and-allergy-drug
17. Heatley DG, et al. Nasal irrigation for the alleviation of sinonasal symptoms. Otolaryngol Head Neck Surg. 2001;125(1):44–8.
18. Wallace DV, et al. The diagnosis and management of rhinitis: an updated practice parameter. J Allergy Clin Immunol. 2008;122(2 Suppl):S1–84.
19. Esteitie R, et al. Effect of the addition of montelukast to fluticasone propionate for the treatment of peren-

nial allergic rhinitis. Ann Allergy Asthma Immunol. 2010;105(2):155–61.
20. Lin SY, et al. AHRQ comparative effectiveness reviews. In: Allergen-specific immunotherapy for the treatment of allergic rhinoconjunctivitis and/or asthma: comparative effectiveness review. Rockville: Agency for Healthcare Research and Quality (US); 2013.
21. Nelson HS, Durham SR. Allergen immunotherapy for a teenager with seasonal allergic rhinitis due to grass pollen: subcutaneous or sublingual route? J Allergy Clin Immunol Pract. 2017;5(1):52–7.
22. Epstein TG, et al. AAAAI/ACAAI surveillance study of subcutaneous immunotherapy, years 2008-2012: an update on fatal and nonfatal systemic allergic reactions. J Allergy Clin Immunol Pract. 2014;2(2):161–7.

Pediatric Asthma

36

W. Adam Gower and Ceila E. Loughlin

Introduction

Pediatric asthma and recurrent wheeze comprise the most common chronic respiratory condition of childhood. Affected patients may initially present to a variety of pediatric providers, including allergists and otolaryngologists. Early recognition and treatment has the potential to prevent significant morbidity and improve quality of life for affected children and their caregivers. This chapter will review current epidemiology of pediatric asthma, diagnostic considerations, management approaches, and the role of comorbidities.

Childhood Asthma Prevalence and Impact

Worldwide, asthma prevalence varies across populations and geographic regions. Overall, asthma is currently more common in high-income countries, although prevalence is increasing in middle- and low-income countries, thus becoming an increasingly important cause of chronic illness and disability among children throughout the world [1]. Approximately 5.5 million children under the age of 18 years in the United States have asthma, representing about 7.5% of that population [2]. Despite improving outcomes in recent years, asthma remains a common cause for physician office visits, emergency department (ED) visits, and hospitalizations among US children [3–6]. Recent data suggest that asthma medications are used more commonly by US children than any other class of prescription drugs, including antibiotics [7]. Estimates place the annual cost for childhood asthma care around six billion USD, with substantial numbers of missed school days for patients and missed work days for parents and caregivers [8–11].

Racial and social disparities in childhood asthma are significant. Asthma is more common among children living in poverty [2]. This is likely due to several factors, including increased exposure to environmental triggers due to substandard housing conditions, poor access to care, low health literacy, and others. Both prevalence and severity of childhood asthma vary by race and ethnicity, reflecting a complex mix of social and genetic risk factors. Black children are twice as likely to have asthma as compared to white children [12]. Among Hispanic children, prevalence varies from approximately 10% in children of Mexican descent to as high as 26% among children of Puerto Rican heritage [13, 14]. Black

W. A. Gower (✉) · C. E. Loughlin
Department of Pediatrics, Division of Pulmonary Medicine, University of North Carolina School of Medicine, Chapel Hill, NC, USA
e-mail: gower@email.unc.edu; cloughli@med.unc.edu

C. Damask et al. (eds.), *Allergy in Otolaryngology Practice*,
https://doi.org/10.1007/978-3-031-93455-1_36

and Hispanic children are at higher risk of having an ED visit, hospitalization, or death due to asthma as compared to white children [12, 14].

Diagnosing Asthma in Children

Asthma presentation in children varies with age. Infants, toddlers, and preschool children typically present with episodic cough and wheeze in the setting of viral respiratory infections. Nearly half of all children have a wheezing illness at least once in the first year of life, but only about a third of those with recurrent early-life wheezing will go on to develop asthma in later childhood [15]. Nonetheless, some data suggest that even transient wheezing in the first 6 years of life may be associated with lower lung function in adolescence [16]. Because most children who experience viral-triggered lower respiratory symptoms in early life will not have persistent symptoms beyond the preschool years, many terms have been used for these episodes to reflect the uncertain future course. Often the first episode is considered acute viral bronchiolitis. If subsequent such illnesses occur, clinicians may apply a myriad of diagnoses, depending on the clinical situation, including reactive airways disease, transient wheeze, recurrent bronchiolitis, multi-trigger wheeze, preschool asthma, and many others. Clinicians may be reluctant to apply the term "asthma" until there is clear evidence for persistence beyond the first few years of life. This can be confusing and is not standardized, leading many to call for a more consistent lexicon [17]. Despite inconsistencies in terminology, the early-life episodes are often treated using asthma medications, as will be discussed later.

The modified Asthma Predictive Index (API) is a validated screening tool that uses clinical features of a young child with persistent wheezing to predict the risk of future asthma [18, 19]. In children with four or more episodes in the first 3 years, the presence of at least one major criterion (physician-diagnosed allergic dermatitis, sensitization to at least one aeroallergen, parent with asthma) or at least two minor criteria (wheezing unrelated to viral infections, blood eosinophils 4% or greater, allergic sensitization to at least one food) indicates increased risk [18]. The API can be easily applied in the clinical setting and is highly specific, with high negative predictive value. Because it lacks sensitivity, the API cannot effectively rule out later asthma development. Other predictive instruments have been published, each with its own strengths and limitations [19]. While such tools allow clinicians to identify young children at higher risk for asthma development, optimal interventions to prevent asthma and loss of lung function are less clear.

Respiratory viruses and allergic sensitization are both independent factors in the development of childhood asthma that may also work synergistically [18]. Although the role of respiratory syncytial virus (RSV) is often emphasized as a cause of acute bronchiolitis, wheezing illnesses caused by rhinovirus in the first 3 years of life seem to confer highest risk of later asthma development [20, 21]. As evidenced by its inclusion in the modified API and other predictive tools, early life sensitization to aeroallergens plays a particularly important role in asthma development [21]. This is thought to occur through skewing of the immature immune system to Th2-mediated atopy [22]. Elevated peripheral eosinophils, also included in the API, have been shown to be linearly associated with increased risk of asthma, independent of allergen sensitization [23].

The "allergic march" is a commonly observed temporal pattern of immunoglobulin E (IgE)-mediated processes in atopic children, beginning with atopic dermatitis and food allergy in early life, followed by later sensitization to aeroallergens, and culminating in allergic rhinitis and asthma [24]. Accordingly, allergic triggers are increasingly common in school-age children, especially in those with a history of atopic dermatitis or allergic rhinitis. Of course, viral respiratory infections remain an important trigger of asthma symptoms throughout life for many patients. Exercise-induced cough, dyspnea, and chest tightness may be more commonly identified as children begin to participate in organized physical activity and competitive sports in the early school years. The term "exercise-induced bronchospasm" may be used to delineate symptoms that occur only with exertion, in a patient without other identified infectious or atopic triggers. During adolescence, an important shift occurs in asthma prevalence: it is seen more frequently in boys before the age of puberty, but then more in girls and young women from puberty into adulthood [25, 26].

Differential Diagnosis and Diagnostic Evaluation of Asthma

The differential diagnosis of asthma also varies by age. Evaluation is further complicated by less reliable histories, as infants and toddlers are developmentally unable to give accurate reports of their symptoms. Parents may misperceive symptoms of asthma in young children [27, 28]. What caregivers report as wheezing may represent upper airway sounds such as stridor or stertor from fixed or dynamic airway lesions including foreign bodies, or extrinsic compression as from a vascular malformation. Dysfunctional breathing, including breathing pattern disorders and inducible laryngeal obstruction/vocal cord dysfunction (ILO/VCD), may mimic the exertional symptoms of asthma or occur as a comorbidity [29, 30].

Cough, a common presenting symptom in childhood asthma in all age groups, may be due to a myriad of other causes as well. Conditions that may present in childhood with chronic recurrent cough include but are not limited to cystic fibrosis (CF), primary ciliary dyskinesia (PCD), protracted bacterial bronchitis (PBB), recurrent croup, and chronic or recurrent sinusitis. The character of the cough may offer some clues regarding the cause. Asthmatic cough tends to be dry in character and may be worse at night or with activity. Cough associated with CF, PCD, PBB, and sinusitis is often more wet sounding. Sputum production may also point to these diagnoses, although many young children will not expectorate. With the advent of newborn screening for CF, which is conducted in all 50 US states and most parts of the world, presentation of CF beyond the newborn period has become rare [31, 32]. Poor weight gain, signs and symptoms of fat malabsorption, and other systemic symptoms should raise the concern for CF. Children with PCD often have a history of respiratory distress at birth, chronic daily productive cough, perennial thick rhinorrhea, and recurrent otitis media. Situs inversus is only seen in 50% of cases, and while examination of ciliary ultrastructure with electron microscopy and genetic testing may confirm the diagnosis, neither is sufficiently sensitive to rule it out when negative [33]. Further discussion of the diagnostic evaluations of CF or PCD is beyond the scope of this chapter. If these are being considered, referral to a pediatric pulmonologist is recommended.

Ear, nose, and throat specialists can play an important role in evaluating and managing conditions that may present with asthma-like symptoms. Endoscopic airway examination may be considered in infants with persistent wheezing despite empiric medical therapy to rule out structural lesions [34]. Recurrent croup, which may be associated with the development of asthma [35, 36], may also present to the otolaryngologist. Cough with fixed, monophonic wheeze could be suggestive of airway foreign body. Suspicion for this would necessitate bronchoscopic evaluation. Tracheomalacia, bronchomalacia, or other lower airway lesions diagnosed by direct examination can also mimic or complicate asthma in any age group.

Spirometry is less reliable in young children, especially those under 6 years of age, due to difficulty in performing the forced expiratory maneuver. It is not regularly performed in primary care asthma visits and results of such testing may be low quality [37, 38]. Having a technologist with experience in testing children is critical to obtaining accurate and useful lung function data. While presence of reversible lower airways obstruction is fairly diagnostic, children with asthma may have normal baseline spirometry. Bronchoprovocation tests, such as methacholine, cold air, or saline challenge [39] may be useful in patients with normal baseline spirometry, but they are not widely used in pediatric practice. Exercise challenge with spirometry has some utility for patients with primarily exertional symptoms if the patient is able to run on a treadmill or ride a stationary bike. Other pulmonary function tests exist for use in children, but have limited practical applications. Infant pulmonary function testing is a useful research tool, and can be used to establish obstruction with bronchodilator reversibility, but is not currently recommended for clinical use in the evaluation of wheezing infants [34]. Impulse oscillometry and multiple-breath washout require minimal patient effort and can therefore be employed in patients unable to perform spirometry [40]. These techniques, however, are not yet standardized or widely employed. Fractional exhaled nitric oxide (FeNO) may be used in patients as young as 4 years but it does not have a role in predicting future development of asthma [41–43]. The 2020 National Heart, Lung, and Blood Institute (NHLBI) asthma guidelines support the use of FeNO as an adjunct in the diagnosis and monitoring of asthma in children age five and older but recommend against using it as the only measure of control, risk, or severity [43]. Assessment of static lung volumes by plethysmography or gas washout, diffusion capacity, and the six-minute walk test may be useful in evaluating for other pulmonary disorders, but do not have a significant role in routine asthma diagnosis or management. (Table 36.1).

Table 36.1 Diagnostic evaluations to consider in children with asthma

Pulmonary function testing
Spirometry: Can assess for baseline pattern and response to bronchodilator. Child must be able to complete forced expiratory maneuver (usually age 5–6 years).
FeNO: May have a role as a surrogate marker for lower airways inflammation, as an adjunct in the diagnosis and management in asthma in children ≥5 years.
Bronchoprovocation tests: Exercise testing may be useful in patients with normal baseline spirometry and symptoms with exertion. Methacholine, saline, cold air challenge, and other forms may be useful in other cases where diagnosis is unclear, but are less commonly used in children.
Allergy testing
Skin prick testing/blood allergen panels: May be used to identify potential triggers, to limit exposure, and to predict seasonal risk of symptoms and exacerbations. Testing should include relevant local seasonal and perennial allergens. Aeroallergen sensitization may predict ICS response [56].
Other laboratory testing
Peripheral blood eosinophils: Elevation may indicate increased atopy, increased risk for asthma development in young children [18], and potentially preferential responsiveness to ICS [56].
Imaging
Plain chest films: Typically show hyperinflation, peribronchial thickening, and/or patchy atelectasis in asthma. Lateral decubitus films may be used to evaluate for airway foreign body.
Barium swallow: Compression of esophageal contrast column on standard barium swallow suggests vascular anomaly. Can evaluate for presence of severe gastroesophageal reflux.
Modified barium swallow/video fluoroscopic swallow: Evaluation of swallowing function with different consistencies may elucidate the role of aspiration in respiratory symptoms.
Chest CT: May be used to evaluate for bronchiectasis as a cause of chronic cough, or with angiography to evaluate for vascular anomalies causing airway compression.
Sinus CT: May be considered to evaluate for sinusitis.
Endoscopic airway examination
Nasopharyngoscopy: May evaluate for airway patency, and presence of adenotonsillar hypertrophy as contributing factors.
Laryngoscopy: May evaluate for anatomical or functional abnormalities.
Bronchoscopy: May be used to evaluate for lower airway compression/stenosis, malacia, clefts/fistulae, foreign bodies, and/or bronchitis. Bronchoalveolar lavage (BAL) may evaluate for lower airways infection or colonization as may be seen in CF, PCD, and PBB.

These studies may be used to evaluate for asthma and other conditions with overlapping presentation. It is important to note that normal findings on all of these are insufficient to exclude the diagnosis of asthma. Limiting exposure to ionizing radiation is a consideration in the use of imaging studies in children.

Common Triggers in Pediatric Asthma

Respiratory viruses, allergens, other environmental irritants, changes in ambient air temperature or humidity, stress, and exercise are all potential triggers of asthma exacerbations. The most common viral triggers are rhinovirus, influenza, and RSV. Lower respiratory tract infections from these viruses follow a predictable seasonal pattern, starting with bronchiolitis among infants predominantly in the fall and winter. The increase in asthma symptoms that occur in the early fall coinciding with the start of the school year, often termed the "September spike", is thought to be due in part to increased viral exposures in school-age children [44]. The most common allergen triggers are cockroaches (perennial), pet dander (perennial), dust mites (perennial), mold spores (perennial or seasonal), and pollens from trees, grasses, and weeds (seasonal). Although physical activity can also be a trigger for asthma, it should not be avoided and is considered safe, as regular exercise improves quality of life scores and asthma symptoms [45]. Children with asthma are at risk of limiting physical activity due to symptoms, which can lead to deconditioning and weight gain. It is therefore important to find ways for children with asthma to remain active. Medications may need to be adjusted for better control to allow the child to participate fully. Pre-treating with a short-acting beta agonist (SABA) 15–20 min before exercise is generally recommended.

Cigarette smoke exposure, including secondhand smoke (SHS), is a common exposure associated with both increased risk of asthma and worse asthma symptom control. Recent data suggest that more than a third of children between the ages of 3 and 17 years are exposed to SHS from tobacco, confirmed by the presence of cotinine, a metabolite of nicotine, in the blood [46]. There is increased risk of wheeze and asthma in children whose parents smoke, including infants whose mothers smoked while pregnant [47, 48]. Exposure to environmental tobacco smoke is associated with more severe asthma among children of all ages [49]. Electronic cigarettes ("e-cigarettes") and related devices represent a relatively new and increasingly popular nicotine delivery system among children and adolescents. In the 2019 Youth Tobacco Survey, over a quarter of teenagers reported use of such devices, or "vaping" [50]. There has been a significant rise in e-cigarette or vaping product use-associated lung injury (EVALI) [50]. In one study, 30% of EVALI cases reported underlying asthma, which is much higher than the rate of asthma in the general population of 8–10% [50, 51]. Even more concerning is that recent surveys revealing e-cigarettes were more popular with teenagers who had asthma than those that did not have asthma [50]. A recent survey found teens with asthma exposed to secondhand vapors of e-cigarettes reported more asthma exacerbations in the past year [52]. It is important to ask patients and their families about this potential trigger when assessing SHS exposure.

Management of Pediatric Asthma

General Principles

Asthma is considered a clinical syndrome associated with recurrent lower airways obstruction due to inflammation and bronchospasm, rather than a single discrete condition [53]. In addition to variability in presentation, substantial heterogeneity exists in disease course and response to therapy. As noted elsewhere in this book, the importance of understanding different phenotypes and endotypes of asthma in adults has been widely recognized [54]. This is an important step towards personalized medicine as many effective asthma therapies are available, but little is yet known about how to predict which patients will respond best to which ones. Table 36.2 lists many commonly used classes of asthma medications, their general indications, and major side effects. Many studies have attempted to define subgroups in childhood asthma as well [55], and clinical trials have begun to address predictive factors for differential response to therapy [56]. There are few

Table 36.2 Common asthma medications with mechanism of action with most frequent and important potential side effects [43, 69, 75]

Medications	Frequency	Indication	Mechanism of action	Side effects
Short-acting beta-agonist (SABA)	As needed	Acute symptoms "Rescue"	Relaxes airway smooth muscle Short-acting	Increased heart rate Jitteriness
Inhaled corticosteroids (ICS)	Usually BID	Persistent asthma Chronic controller	Reduces inflammation	Thrush Hoarse voice Potential slowed growth velocity
Leukotriene receptor antagonists (LTRA)	Daily	Persistent asthma Chronic controller Adjuvant therapy	Reduces inflammation and bronchoconstriction cause by LTD4	Mood or behavior changes Headaches
ICS-long-acting beta-agonist (ICS-LABA)	Usually BID SMART therapy as needed[a]	Persistent asthma Chronic controller SMART therapy—Acute symptoms "rescue"[a]	Reduces inflammation Relaxes airway smooth muscle	Same as ICS above Increased heart rate
Long-acting muscarinic antagonist (LAMA)	Daily	Persistent asthma Adjuvant therapy	Relaxes airway smooth muscle	Dry mouth Headache Sore throat Urinary retention (rare)

[a]*If LABA is formoterol*

data to guide cost-effectiveness of pediatric asthma therapies as high-quality economic evaluations are lacking [57].

In contrast to adults, children are more often treated for asthma in the outpatient setting [5]. Most outpatient asthma visits are conducted by primary care providers, especially pediatricians [6]. Referral to a pediatric asthma specialist should be considered when there is question as to the diagnosis itself, or when management has become challenging with poor control. Most guidelines endorse routine involvement of a specialist for patients with moderate to severe persistent asthma. Pediatricians and asthma specialists (including allergists and pediatric pulmonologists) report higher rates of adherence to guideline-based care than family medicine and internal medicine providers in nationwide surveys [37, 58, 59].

The optimal management of early-life wheezing episodes may be different from that of asthma exacerbations in later childhood, and like asthma in older children, optimal therapy may vary by endotype [60]. Inhaled bronchodilators may be useful in recurrent viral-induced wheezing who have shown responsiveness, but evidence does not support their use in routine acute viral bronchiolitis [61, 62]. High-quality evidence suggests that systemic steroids are not effective at reducing severity or duration of symptoms in early-life wheezing [63, 64]. Low-dose azithromycin, a macrolide antibiotic, may help prevent further episodes in children with history of severe lower respiratory tract infections [65]. The 2020 NHLBI asthma guidelines include a conditional recommendation for a short course of inhaled corticosteroids in addition to SABA at the start of viral respiratory illness for children up to 4 years old who do not wheeze between respiratory infections [43].

Allergen Identification and Control

Identification and abatement of environmental triggers is an important non-medical approach to control of allergic asthma symptoms. Most children with severe persistent asthma are sensitized to at least one aeroallergen [66]. Therefore, allergen testing may be useful to help guide reduction of exposure and inform therapy based on seasonality of the allergen. The authors of the

2020 NHLBI guidelines conditionally recommend multi-component mitigation of specific indoor inhalant allergens for asthma patients with known sensitization, symptoms, and exposure. Integrated pest management and use of pillow and mattress covers to control cockroach and dust mite allergens may be a part of this approach. While the evidence for these interventions is of low quality, they are generally regarded as low-cost and without harm, as long as they do not detract from other important aspects of therapy. Environmental interventions are considered not helpful for those without allergies [43].

Also addressed in the most recent NHLBI guidelines is allergy immunotherapy for patients 5 years and older with mild to moderate allergic asthma. Subcutaneous immunotherapy (SCIT) received a conditional recommendation as an adjunct to standard pharmaceutical therapy for those with clear allergen triggers. Immunotherapy may be designed to target specific allergen triggers that cause frequent exacerbations. Asthma must be well-controlled before the initiation, and remain so through build-up and maintenance of SCIT. Sublingual immunotherapy (SLIT) is not recommended for asthma control, although it may be used for control of allergic rhinitis in patients with asthma [43].

Food allergies in patients with asthma place them at higher risk for increased exacerbations and even fatalities [67, 68]. Education on avoidance of the food trigger and prescription of self-injectable epinephrine is critical [67].

Controller Medications

Inhaled corticosteroids (ICS) are generally regarded as the most effective form of chronic controller therapy for all ages. Thus, for persistent asthma (symptoms >2 days/week or 2 nights/month), daily ICS are the mainstay of treatment. Recommended starting dose depends upon the age of the child and the specific drug being used. Because steroid deposited in the oral cavity may cause thrush, it is recommended to rinse out the child's mouth or have them brush their teeth after administration of ICS. The main side effect of long-term concern with ICS in children is slowed height growth velocity [69].

Montelukast, a leukotriene receptor antagonist, has a role as adjuvant therapy in patients with suboptimal control on ICS but is not ideal for first-line treatment except in patients with solely exercise-induced symptoms. In children and adolescents with exercise-induced symptoms, it has been shown to improve both early and late-phase responses to exercise [70]. Behavioral changes, including suicidal ideation, have been reported as a rare side effect of montelukast that may lead to stopping therapy [71]. For children with persistent asthma or uncontrolled asthma on ICS monotherapy, switching to ICS plus long-acting beta agonist (LABA) combination inhaler can help improve symptoms and FEV_1 without increasing the cumulative ICS dose [72]. If patients remain uncontrolled on ICS-LABA therapy, tiotropium bromide, a long-acting anti-muscarinic antagonist (LAMA) bronchodilator, is an effective adjuvant approved for use down to age six, and recommended down to age 12 for uncontrolled persistent asthma in the 2020 NHLBI guidelines [43, 73, 74].

At every visit, providers should review adherence with controller therapy as well as technique of inhaled medication administration [75, 76]. Daily preventative medication adherence is a challenge in asthma as in other chronic diseases. In developed countries, 50% of patients with chronic disease do not take their medications as prescribed [77]. Studies in several different countries have shown that asthma morbidity and mortality are significantly increased by non-adherence [78]. There are multiple factors contributing to adherence issues in pediatric patients with asthma. Parental beliefs and concerns about side effects of ICS may lead to underdosing or discontinuation when the child is well [78]. Additionally, the primary responsibility for administering the medications may fall on multiple caregivers including grandparents, babysitters, and often the child at an early age [78]. Proper technique improves deposition of medication into the airways and better control of asthma with fewer exacerbations and better adherence to medication regimen [79].

Monitoring symptoms and control are also assessed at every visit to help "step up" and "step down" therapy as indicated [75, 76]. The NHLBI guidelines suggest at least 3 months of well-controlled symptoms before stepping down. Practitioners should also consider triggers when deciding to step down. As an example, for children that have spring allergies as a main trigger, it may be preferable to wait until summer to consider a trial of lower dose ICS. Similarly, providers should anticipate increased symptoms in the fall and winter for school-aged children, and plan medication adjustments accordingly.

Asthma Action Plan and Home Management

Patients should be given an asthma action plan at every visit; this is especially important when there have been changes to the medication regimen. The action plan helps patients and families organize medication use based on level of asthma control, which may change from day to day or even hour to hour. Although home peak expiratory flow monitoring was previously recommended to assess control, the NHLBI guidelines focus instead on symptoms [75], as studies have shown that peak flow measurement does not add predictive power beyond clinical symptoms [80]. Additionally, to be effective, peak flow measurements require tracking multiple daily measurements, not only when having an exacerbation. User error can occur frequently with home peak flow meters, resulting in unreliable measurements. The action plan should guide the family regarding interventions for increased symptoms. It empowers them to manage the asthma at home, but also instructs them when to seek emergency assistance [81]. The standard form of the action plan uses a "stoplight" analogy [75]. The "green zone" dictates use of daily controller medications when the patient has no symptoms. As symptoms progress, the patient transitions into the "yellow zone" which includes use of daily controllers but also increased SABA treatments, which may be given with additional doses of inhaled steroid. This may include increased use of formoterol-containing ICS-LABA if the Single Maintenance and Reliever Therapy (SMART) strategy (described further below) is being employed. If not improving, the patient can use eight puffs or an albuterol nebulizer treatment every 20 min for three treatments. An oral corticosteroid burst should be considered at this point. Typical dosing of oral prednisone for an asthma exacerbation 1–2 mg/kg/day by mouth once a day with maximum of 60–80 mg, for 3–5 days [75]. If symptoms have not responded to increased albuterol use and possibly systemic steroids, the patient is considered to be in the "red zone" and should seek medical attention without delay. Management of severe exacerbations is beyond the scope of this chapter. A newer approach to exacerbations utilizes the SMART approach, described below.

New Approaches to Exacerbations

Recent updates to both the NHLBI guidelines and Global Initiative for Asthma (GINA) Main Report emphasize use of the SMART approach [43, 82], in which ICS plus formoterol MDI is used as both controller and rescue medication, replacing SABA inhaler for acute exacerbations. The NHLBI guidelines cite moderate evidence for 4–11 years and high-level evidence for 12 years and older to support this strategy. The NHLBI guidelines suggest use of SMART for step three and four while GINA suggests it for all steps [43, 82]. It is important to note that SMART is for use with formoterol due to its quick onset of action but not to be used with salmeterol-containing products. In children older than 4 years of age, the updated NHLBI guidelines state that short-acting beta-agonists (SABA) alone for the treatment of acute symptoms is no longer recommended. In children ages 0–4 years, they recommend using a short course of daily ICS with the onset of respiratory tract infection. In children who are already on daily ICS, increasing the ICS dose during an exacerbation is not recommended. For exacerbations of mild asthma, it is recommended that low-dose ICS should be taken with every dose of SABA during an exacerbation.

Further recommendations include using ICS-formoterol as needed for mild persistent asthma. These recommendations are based on recent studies suggesting that budesonide-formoterol may have benefit over albuterol alone for an exacerbation [83]. Nonetheless, many of these recommendations represent departures from usual practice and may take time to be implemented universally.

Delivery Systems for Inhaled Medications

The delivery of inhaled medication is an especially important consideration in pediatric asthma. Very young children are often started with medication delivered by a mechanical nebulizer. With this approach, the nebulizer mask must be securely on the child's face for the full 10–15-min treatment. This often presents a challenge for families, as children may not sit still for the full duration. Caregivers may resort to using the "blow-by" method or administering nebulized medications when the child is asleep, both of which may decrease the deposition of medication into the lower airways.

Use of a MDI with spacer or valved holding chamber (VHC) has both challenges and benefits compared to use of a mechanical nebulizer. Studies examining their use in children found little over 50% of children utilized correct technique [79]. Coordination with MDI and VHC can also be difficult in children, since they may "fight" the mask and spacer, limiting its effectiveness. There are also some advantages to use of an MDI, even in the youngest patients. The MDI is more portable than a nebulizer, and can be sent to daycare, school, or taken on trips outside the home. The MDI-VHC combination provides faster delivery than nebulized treatments. Studies have shown that with proper technique MDI plus VHC with mask can achieve adequate deposition of medication in even toddlers and infants [84]. Various studies demonstrate that technique improved with education, independent of who provided the teaching (nurse, physician, pharmacist, or online tutorial), and continued to improve with each teaching session [79]. To achieve equivalent dosing of rescue medications by MDI, it often requires an increase in the number of MDI puffs to be comparable to dose delivered from nebulizer [85].

Dry-powder inhalers (DPI) do not require propellant or spacer use. These devices do, however, require the child be able to generate enough inspiratory force to release the medication [86], making them less ideal for younger children. This inhalation technique is different than that used for MDI with spacer. If prescribing both types of inhaler, it is important that the child and family understand the difference. If proper technique is used, medication delivery with nebulizer, MDI, and DPI can be considered essentially equivalent clinically [85]. Regardless the method being used, the NHLBI guidelines and GINA Main Report recommended checking device technique at every visit even when children have previously shown good technique [75, 76].

Immunotherapy and Biologic Therapy

While the recent update in NHLBI guidelines did not include recommendations regarding monoclonal antibody therapy (biologics), there is an evolving role for such drugs in pediatric asthma management. Omalizumab, an anti-IgE antibody was the first approved for children down to age 6 years and is the most studied biologic asthma therapy in children [87]. It is used in addition to maintenance therapy to reduce exacerbations and uncontrolled symptoms [87]. Mepolizumab, an IL-5 antagonist, helps to improve asthma control by reducing the circulating blood eosinophils which reduces airway inflammation [88]. It has recently been approved to down to age six as well [87]. Reslizumab (anti-IL-5) and benralizumab (anti-IL-5 receptor) are also available for use in children [89]. Dupilumab, an anti-IL4 receptor antibody used for eczema, has been shown to reduce rates of asthma exacerbations when added to adjuvant therapy in patients with uncontrolled moderate-severe persistent asthma [90]. An advantage to dupilumab is that it is approved for administration at home, which relieves the burden of regular doctor's office visits. In children, one of the downsides to these therapies is the stress and pain that may be associated with regular injections. Studies have shown that over time most children receiving repeated injections lose their fear [91].

Pediatric Asthma Comorbidities

Many children with asthma have or develop other chronic conditions, which have the potential to complicate their care [92, 93]. As described elsewhere in this book, the Unified Airway Hypothesis proposes that rhinitis, rhinosinusitis, OSA, and asthma are all expressions of the same inflammatory process, manifest at different levels throughout the airways. There is substantial evidence to support associations between these conditions in children, although the exact pathogenic mechanisms have yet to be established [94]. As has been discussed elsewhere in this chapter, atopy is common among children with asthma and control of allergen triggers as well as management of allergic symptoms may contribute to improved asthma control [92, 95]. Pediatric asthma may rarely be complicated by fungal sensitization, allergic bronchopulmonary aspergillosis (ABPA), or allergic bronchopulmonary mycosis (ABPM) [96, 97]. Eosinophilic esophagitis is an increasingly recognized comorbidity of asthma and atopy [98].

Obesity is a common comorbidity in children with asthma, although the cause-effect relationship remains poorly understood [99]. It can complicate asthma diagnosis as dyspnea on exertion and abnormal pulmonary function testing may result from obesity itself [100]. Obesity may increase risk for sleep-disordered breathing, which can contribute to nighttime awakenings and complicate asthma management [101]. Obese children with asthma may be less responsive to treatment than normal-weight children [99, 101], and frequent courses of steroids can lead to further weight gain. Children with asthma may limit exercise due to dyspnea, and this can also lead to further weight gain and deconditioning. Gastroesophageal reflux as a comorbidity of pediatric asthma has been the subject of much debate, but is thought to play a role in increased asthma symptoms among obese children [99, 101].

Breathing pattern disorders and ILO/VCD are common comorbidities of childhood asthma [29, 30]. Direct observation of paradoxical vocal fold movement can establish the diagnosis of the latter. Referral to speech-language pathologists for therapy may be useful to help the patient learn breathing techniques to mitigate symptoms.

Social, psychological, and behavioral morbidities, such as chronic stress, anxiety, and depression are common in children and adolescents with asthma [92, 102]. Stress and depression are also common among parents and caregivers of children with asthma, and these factors affect outcomes through a myriad of moderating and mediating factors [103]. Low health literacy among children with asthma and their caregivers complicates their care [104]. Attention deficient hyperactivity disorder has significant overlap with childhood asthma, but the relationship with autism spectrum disorder is less clear [105].

Conclusions and Future Considerations

Pediatric asthma is a common condition, one which nearly every practitioner who provides care to children will encounter. Understanding its presentation and management, as well as the role of common comorbid conditions, will enable the otolaryngologist to be an effective partner in diagnosis and management. Current investigations are aimed at better understanding the early life origins of chronic asthma with the goal of preventing or mitigating asthma with early intervention [106]. Defining phenotypes and endotypes of pediatric asthma is another focus of research, with the hope that this will enable more personalized/precision medicine approaches to treatment [55]. Finally, development of new and novel therapies, as well as new and more effective way of employing currently available medications, will provide a wider range of options to the pediatric asthma care provider. Ultimately, pediatric asthma is a highly treatable condition that can be managed with effective education and medical therapy to improve the quality of life of patients and their families.

References

1. Asher I, Pearce N. Global burden of asthma among children. Int J Tuberc Lung Dis. 2014;18:1269–78.
2. National Center for Health Statistics: Fast Stats – Asthma. [cited 2020 November 23]. Available from: www.cdc.gov/nchs/fastats/asthma.htm.
3. Hasegawa K, Tsugawa Y, Brown DF, Camargo CA Jr. Childhood asthma hospitalizations in the United States, 2000-2009. J Pediatr. 2013;163:1127–33.e3.
4. Akinbami LJ, Moorman JE, Garbe PL, Sondik EJ. Status of childhood asthma in the United States, 1980-2007. Pediatrics. 2009;123(Suppl 3):S131–45.
5. Akinbami LJ, Moorman JE, Bailey C, Zahran HS, King M, Johnson CA, Liu X. Trends in asthma prevalence, health care use, and mortality in the United States, 2001-2010. NCHS Data Brief. 2012;94:1–8.
6. Akinbami LJ, Santo L, Williams S, Rechtsteiner EA, Strashny A. Characteristics of asthma visits to physician offices in the United States: 2012-2015 National Ambulatory Medical Care Survey. Natl Health Stat Rep. 2019;128:1–20.
7. Hales CM, Kit BK, Gu Q, Ogden CL. Trends in prescription medication use among children and adolescents-United States, 1999-2014. JAMA. 2018;319:2009–20.
8. Sullivan PW, Ghushchyan V, Navaratnam P, Friedman HS, Kavati A, Ortiz B, Lanier B. The national cost of asthma among school-aged children in the United States. Ann Allergy Asthma Immunol. 2017;119:246–52.e1.
9. Sullivan P, Ghushchyan VG, Navaratnam P, Friedman HS, Kavati A, Ortiz B, Lanier B. School absence and productivity outcomes associated with childhood asthma in the USA. J Asthma. 2018;55:161–8.
10. Sullivan PW, Ghushchyan VH, Campbell JD, Globe G, Bender B, Magid DJ. Measuring the cost of poor asthma control and exacerbations. J Asthma. 2017;54:24–31.
11. Sullivan PW, Ghushchyan V, Navaratnam P, Friedman HS, Kavati A, Ortiz B, Lanier B. The national burden of poorly controlled asthma, school absence and parental work loss among school-aged children in the United States. J Asthma. 2018;55:659–67.
12. Akinbami LJ, Moorman JE, Simon AE, Schoendorf KC. Trends in racial disparities for asthma outcomes among children 0 to 17 years, 2001-2010. J Allergy Clin Immunol. 2014;134:547–53.e5.
13. Lara M, Akinbami L, Flores G, Morgenstern H. Heterogeneity of childhood asthma among Hispanic children: Puerto Rican children bear a disproportionate burden. Pediatrics. 2006;117:43–53.
14. Urquhart A, Clarke P. US racial/ethnic disparities in childhood asthma emergent health care use: National Health Interview Survey, 2013-2015. J Asthma. 2020;57:510–20.
15. Martinez FD, Wright AL, Taussig LM, Holberg CJ, Halonen M, Morgan WJ. Asthma and wheezing in the first six years of life. The Group Health Medical Associates. N Engl J Med. 1995;332:133–8.
16. Morgan WJ, Stern DA, Sherrill DL, Guerra S, Holberg CJ, Guilbert TW, Taussig LM, Wright AL, Martinez FD. Outcome of asthma and wheezing in the first 6 years of life: follow-up through adolescence. Am J Respir Crit Care Med. 2005;172:1253–8.
17. Douros K, Everard ML. Time to say goodbye to bronchiolitis, viral wheeze, reactive airways disease, wheeze bronchitis and all that. Front Pediatr. 2020;8:218.
18. Burbank AJ, Szefler SJ. Current and future management of the young child with early onset wheezing. Curr Opin Allergy Clin Immunol. 2017;17:146–52.
19. Castro-Rodriguez JA, Cifuentes L, Martinez FD. Predicting asthma using clinical indexes. Front Pediatr. 2019;7:320.
20. Jackson DJ, Gangnon RE, Evans MD, Roberg KA, Anderson EL, Pappas TE, Printz MC, Lee WM, Shult PA, Reisdorf E, Carlson-Dakes KT, Salazar LP, DaSilva DF, Tisler CJ, Gern JE, Lemanske RF Jr. Wheezing rhinovirus illnesses in early life predict asthma development in high-risk children. Am J Respir Crit Care Med. 2008;178:667–72.
21. Rubner FJ, Jackson DJ, Evans MD, Gangnon RE, Tisler CJ, Pappas TE, Gern JE, Lemanske RF Jr. Early life rhinovirus wheezing, allergic sensitization, and asthma risk at adolescence. J Allergy Clin Immunol. 2017;139:501–7.
22. van Tilburg Bernardes E, Arrieta MC. Hygiene hypothesis in asthma development: is hygiene to blame? Arch Med Res. 2017;48:717–26.
23. Karakoc F, Remes ST, Martinez FD, Wright AL. The association between persistent eosinophilia and asthma in childhood is independent of atopic status. Clin Exp Allergy. 2002;32:51–6.
24. Shaker M. New insights into the allergic march. Curr Opin Pediatr. 2014;26:516–20.
25. Zein JG, Denson JL, Wechsler ME. Asthma over the adult life course: gender and hormonal influences. Clin Chest Med. 2019;40:149–61.
26. Almqvist C, Worm M, Leynaert B, working group of GA2LEN WP 2.5 Gender. Impact of gender on asthma in childhood and adolescence: a GA2LEN review. Allergy. 2008;63:47–57.
27. Horak E, Grassl G, Skladal D, Ulmer H. Lung function and symptom perception in children with asthma and their parents. Pediatr Pulmonol. 2003;35:23–8.
28. Mohangoo AD, de Koning HJ, Hafkamp-de Groen E, van der Wouden JC, Jaddoe VW, Moll HA, Hofman A, Mackenbach JP, de Jongste JC, Raat H. A com-

parison of parent-reported wheezing or shortness of breath among infants as assessed by questionnaire and physician-interview: The Generation R study. Pediatr Pulmonol. 2010;45:500–7.
29. Connett GJ, Thomas M. Dysfunctional breathing in children and adults with asthma. Front Pediatr. 2018;6:406.
30. Barker N, Thevasagayam R, Ugonna K, Kirkby J. Pediatric dysfunctional breathing: proposed components, mechanisms, diagnosis, and management. Front Pediatr. 2020;8:379.
31. Naehrlich L. The changing face of cystic fibrosis and its implications for screening. Int J Neonatal Screen. 2020;6:54.
32. Scotet V, Gutierrez H, Farrell PM. Newborn screening for CF across the globe-where is it worthwhile? Int J Neonatal Screen. 2020;6:18.
33. Shapiro AJ, Davis SD, Polineni D, Manion M, Rosenfeld M, Dell SD, Chilvers MA, Ferkol TW, Zariwala MA, Sagel SD, Josephson M, Morgan L, Yilmaz O, Olivier KN, Milla C, Pittman JE, Daniels MLA, Jones MH, Janahi IA, Ware SM, Daniel SJ, Cooper ML, Nogee LM, Anton B, Eastvold T, Ehrne L, Guadagno E, Knowles MR, Leigh MW, Lavergne V. American Thoracic Society Assembly on P. Diagnosis of primary ciliary dyskinesia. An official American Thoracic Society Clinical Practice Guideline. Am J Respir Crit Care Med. 2018;197:e24–39.
34. Ren CL, Esther CR Jr, Debley JS, Sockrider M, Yilmaz O, Amin N, Bazzy-Asaad A, Davis SD, Durand M, Ewig JM, Yuksel H, Lombardi E, Noah TL, Radford P, Ranganathan S, Teper A, Weinberger M, Brozek J, Wilson KC, Wheezing ATSAHCoIwRoP. Official American Thoracic Society clinical practice guidelines: diagnostic evaluation of infants with recurrent or persistent wheezing. Am J Respir Crit Care Med. 2016;194:356–73.
35. Van Bever HP, Wieringa MH, Weyler JJ, Nelen VJ, Fortuin M, Vermeire PA. Croup and recurrent croup: their association with asthma and allergy. An epidemiological study on 5-8-year-old children. Eur J Pediatr. 1999;158:253–7.
36. Lin SC, Lin HW, Chiang BL. Association of croup with asthma in children: a cohort study. Medicine (Baltimore). 2017;96:e7667.
37. Akinbami LJ, Salo PM, Cloutier MM, Wilkerson JC, Elward KS, Mazurek JM, Williams S, Zeldin DC. Primary care clinician adherence with asthma guidelines: the National Asthma Survey of Physicians. J Asthma. 2020;57:543–55.
38. Gillette C, Loughlin CE, Sleath BL, Williams DM, Davis SD. Quality of pulmonary function testing in 3 large primary care pediatric clinics in rural North Carolina. N C Med J. 2011;72:105–10.
39. Barben JRJ. Measurement of bronchial responsiveness in children. In: Hammer JE, editor. Paediatric pulmonary function testing. Basel: Karger; 2005. p. 125–36.
40. Galant SP, Komarow HD, Shin HW, Siddiqui S, Lipworth BJ. The case for impulse oscillometry in the management of asthma in children and adults. Ann Allergy Asthma Immunol. 2017;118:664–71.
41. Heijkenskjold-Rentzhog C, Kalm-Stephens P, Nordvall L, Malinovschi A, Alving K. New method for single-breath fraction of exhaled nitric oxide measurement with improved feasibility in preschool children with asthma. Pediatr Allergy Immunol. 2015;26:662–7.
42. Lu M, Wu B, Che D, Qiao R, Gu H. FeNO and asthma treatment in children: a systematic review and meta-analysis. Medicine (Baltimore). 2015;94:e347.
43. Expert Panel Working Group of the National Heart, Lung, and Blood Institute administered and coordinated National Asthma Education and Prevention Program Coordinating Committee; Cloutier MM, Baptist AP, Blake KV, Brooks EG, Bryant-Stephens T, DiMango E, Dixon AE, Elward KS, Hartert T, Krishnan JA, Lemanske RF Jr, Ouellette DR, Pace WD, Schatz M, Skolnik NS, Stout JW, Teach SJ, Umscheid CA, Walsh CG. Focused updates to the asthma management guidelines: a report from the National Asthma Education and Prevention Program Coordinating Committee Expert Panel Working Group. J Allergy Clin Immunol. 2020;146:1217–70.
44. Pike KC, Akhbari M, Kneale D, Harris KM. Interventions for autumn exacerbations of asthma in children. Cochrane Database Syst Rev. 2018;3:CD012393.
45. Lang JE. The impact of exercise on asthma. Curr Opin Allergy Clin Immunol. 2019;19:118–25.
46. Brody DJ, Lu Z, Tsai J. Secondhand smoke exposure among nonsmoking youth: United States, 2013-2016. NCHS Data Brief. 2019;348:1–8.
47. Strzelak A, Ratajczak A, Adamiec A, Feleszko W. Tobacco smoke induces and alters immune responses in the lung triggering inflammation, allergy, asthma and other lung diseases: a mechanistic review. Int J Environ Res Public Health. 2018;15:1033.
48. Zacharasiewicz A. Maternal smoking in pregnancy and its influence on childhood asthma. ERJ Open Res. 2016;2:00042–2016.
49. Akinbami LJ, Kit BK, Simon AE. Impact of environmental tobacco smoke on children with asthma, United States, 2003-2010. Acad Pediatr. 2013;13:508–16.
50. Clapp PW, Peden DB, Jaspers I. E-cigarettes, vaping-related pulmonary illnesses, and asthma: a perspective from inhalation toxicologists. J Allergy Clin Immunol. 2020;145:97–9.
51. Adkins SH, Anderson KN, Goodman AB, Twentyman E, Danielson ML, Kimball A, Click ES, Ko JY, Evans ME, Weissman DN, Melstrom P, Kiernan E, Krishnasamy V, Rose DA, Jones CM, King BA, Ellington SR, Pollack LA, Wiltz JL, Lung Injury Clinical Task Force and the Lung Injury Epidemiology/Surveillance Task Force. Demographics, substance use behaviors, and clinical characteristics of adolescents with e-cigarette, or

vaping, product use-associated lung injury (EVALI) in the United States in 2019. JAMA Pediatr. 2020;174:e200756.
52. Bayly JE, Bernat D, Porter L, Choi K. Secondhand exposure to aerosols from electronic nicotine delivery systems and asthma exacerbations among youth with asthma. Chest. 2019;155:88–93.
53. Pavord ID, Beasley R, Agusti A, Anderson GP, Bel E, Brusselle G, Cullinan P, Custovic A, Ducharme FM, Fahy JV, Frey U, Gibson P, Heaney LG, Holt PG, Humbert M, Lloyd CM, Marks G, Martinez FD, Sly PD, von Mutius E, Wenzel S, Zar HJ, Bush A. After asthma: redefining airways diseases. Lancet. 2018;391:350–400.
54. Kaur R, Chupp G. Phenotypes and endotypes of adult asthma: moving toward precision medicine. J Allergy Clin Immunol. 2019;144:1–12.
55. Reddy MB, Covar RA. Asthma phenotypes in childhood. Curr Opin Allergy Clin Immunol. 2016;16:127–34.
56. Fitzpatrick AM, Jackson DJ, Mauger DT, Boehmer SJ, Phipatanakul W, Sheehan WJ, Moy JN, Paul IM, Bacharier LB, Cabana MD, Covar R, Holguin F, Lemanske RF Jr, Martinez FD, Pongracic JA, Beigelman A, Baxi SN, Benson M, Blake K, Chmiel JF, Daines CL, Daines MO, Gaffin JM, Gentile DA, Gower WA, Israel E, Kumar HV, Lang JE, Lazarus SC, Lima JJ, Ly N, Marbin J, Morgan W, Myers RE, Olin JT, Peters SP, Raissy HH, Robison RG, Ross K, Sorkness CA, Thyne SM, Szefler SJ, AsthmaNet NN. Individualized therapy for persistent asthma in young children. J Allergy Clin Immunol. 2016;138:1608–18.e12.
57. Halmai LA, Neilson AR, Kilonzo M. Economic evaluation of interventions for the treatment of asthma in children: a systematic review. Pediatr Allergy Immunol. 2020;31:150–7.
58. Cloutier MM, Salo PM, Akinbami LJ, Cohn RD, Wilkerson JC, Diette GB, Williams S, Elward KS, Mazurek JM, Spinner JR, Mitchell TA, Zeldin DC. Clinician agreement, self-efficacy, and adherence with the guidelines for the diagnosis and management of asthma. J Allergy Clin Immunol Pract. 2018;6:886–94.e4.
59. Cloutier MM, Akinbami LJ, Salo PM, Schatz M, Simoneau T, Wilkerson JC, Diette G, Elward KS, Fuhlbrigge A, Mazurek JM, Feinstein L, Williams S, Zeldin DC. Use of National Asthma guidelines by allergists and pulmonologists: a national survey. J Allergy Clin Immunol Pract. 2020;8:3011–20.e2.
60. Stokes JR, Bacharier LB. Prevention and treatment of recurrent viral-induced wheezing in the preschool child. Ann Allergy Asthma Immunol. 2020;125:156–62.
61. Ralston SL, Lieberthal AS, Meissner HC, Alverson BK, Baley JE, Gadomski AM, Johnson DW, Light MJ, Maraqa NF, Mendonca EA, Phelan KJ, Zorc JJ, Stanko-Lopp D, Brown MA, Nathanson I, Rosenblum E, Sayles S 3rd, Hernandez-Cancio S, American Academy of P. Clinical practice guideline: the diagnosis, management, and prevention of bronchiolitis. Pediatrics. 2014;134:e1474–502.
62. Gadomski AM, Scribani MB. Bronchodilators for bronchiolitis. Cochrane Database Syst Rev. 2014:CD001266.
63. Panickar J, Lakhanpaul M, Lambert PC, Kenia P, Stephenson T, Smyth A, Grigg J. Oral prednisolone for preschool children with acute virus-induced wheezing. N Engl J Med. 2009;360:329–38.
64. Oommen A, Lambert PC, Grigg J. Efficacy of a short course of parent-initiated oral prednisolone for viral wheeze in children aged 1-5 years: randomised controlled trial. Lancet. 2003;362:1433–8.
65. Bacharier LB, Guilbert TW, Mauger DT, Boehmer S, Beigelman A, Fitzpatrick AM, Jackson DJ, Baxi SN, Benson M, Burnham CD, Cabana M, Castro M, Chmiel JF, Covar R, Daines M, Gaffin JM, Gentile DA, Holguin F, Israel E, Kelly HW, Lazarus SC, Lemanske RF Jr, Ly N, Meade K, Morgan W, Moy J, Olin T, Peters SP, Phipatanakul W, Pongracic JA, Raissy HH, Ross K, Sheehan WJ, Sorkness C, Szefler SJ, Teague WG, Thyne S, Martinez FD. Early administration of azithromycin and prevention of severe lower respiratory tract illnesses in preschool children with a history of such illnesses: a randomized clinical trial. JAMA. 2015;314:2034–44.
66. Schatz M, Rosenwasser L. The allergic asthma phenotype. J Allergy Clin Immunol Pract. 2014;2:645–8. quiz 649.
67. Bird JA, Burks AW. Food allergy and asthma. Prim Care Respir J. 2009;18:258–65.
68. Simpson AB, Glutting J, Yousef E. Food allergy and asthma morbidity in children. Pediatr Pulmonol. 2007;42:489–95.
69. Fernandes RM, Wingert A, Vandermeer B, Featherstone R, Ali S, Plint AC, Stang AS, Rowe BH, Johnson DW, Allain D, Klassen TP, Hartling L. Safety of corticosteroids in young children with acute respiratory conditions: a systematic review and meta-analysis. BMJ Open. 2019;9:e028511.
70. Melo RE, Sole D, Naspitz CK. Exercise-induced bronchoconstriction in children: montelukast attenuates the immediate-phase and late-phase responses. J Allergy Clin Immunol. 2003;111:301–7.
71. Benard B, Bastien V, Vinet B, Yang R, Krajinovic M, Ducharme FM. Neuropsychiatric adverse drug reactions in children initiated on montelukast in real-life practice. Eur Respir J. 2017;50:170135.
72. Chauhan BF, Chartrand C, Ni Chroinin M, Milan SJ, Ducharme FM. Addition of long-acting beta2-agonists to inhaled corticosteroids for chronic asthma in children. Cochrane Database Syst Rev. 2015:CD007949.
73. Hamelmann E, Bateman ED, Vogelberg C, Szefler SJ, Vandewalker M, Moroni-Zentgraf P, Avis M, Unseld A, Engel M, Boner AL. Tiotropium add-on therapy in adolescents with moderate asthma: a 1-year randomized controlled trial. J Allergy Clin Immunol. 2016;138:441–50. e8.

74. Murphy KR, Chipps BE. Tiotropium in children and adolescents with asthma. Ann Allergy Asthma Immunol. 2020;124:267–76.e3.
75. Expert Panel Report 3: Guidelines for the diagnosis and management of asthma. National Asthma Education and Prevention Program; 2007.
76. Global strategy for asthma management and prevention. Global Initiative for Asthma; 2020.
77. Horne R. Compliance, adherence, and concordance: implications for asthma treatment. Chest. 2006;130:65S–72S.
78. Adherence to long-term therapies: evidence for action. World Health Organization; 2003.
79. Gillette C, Rockich-Winston N, Kuhn JA, Flesher S, Shepherd M. Inhaler technique in children with asthma: a systematic review. Acad Pediatr. 2016;16:605–15.
80. Mortimer KM, Redline S, Kattan M, Wright EC, Kercsmar CM. Are peak flow and symptom measures good predictors of asthma hospitalizations and unscheduled visits? Pediatr Pulmonol. 2001;31:190–7.
81. Ramratnam SK, Bacharier LB, Guilbert TW. Severe asthma in children. J Allergy Clin Immunol Pract. 2017;5:889–98.
82. Reddel HK, FitzGerald JM, Bateman ED, Bacharier LB, Becker A, Brusselle G, Buhl R, Cruz AA, Fleming L, Inoue H, Ko FW, Krishnan JA, Levy ML, Lin J, Pedersen SE, Sheikh A, Yorgancioglu A, Boulet LP. GINA 2019: a fundamental change in asthma management: treatment of asthma with short-acting bronchodilators alone is no longer recommended for adults and adolescents. Eur Respir J. 2019;53:1901046.
83. Beasley R, Holliday M, Reddel HK, Braithwaite I, Ebmeier S, Hancox RJ, Harrison T, Houghton C, Oldfield K, Papi A, Pavord ID, Williams M, Weatherall M, Novel SST. Controlled trial of budesonide-formoterol as needed for mild asthma. N Engl J Med. 2019;380:2020–30.
84. Tal A, Golan H, Grauer N, Aviram M, Albin D, Quastel MR. Deposition pattern of radiolabeled salbutamol inhaled from a metered-dose inhaler by means of a spacer with mask in young children with airway obstruction. J Pediatr. 1996;128:479–84.
85. Rau JL. The inhalation of drugs: advantages and problems. Respir Care. 2005;50:367–82.
86. Haidl P, Heindl S, Siemon K, Bernacka M, Cloes RM. Inhalation device requirements for patients' inhalation maneuvers. Respir Med. 2016;118:65–75.
87. Just J, Deschildre A, Lejeune S, Amat F. New perspectives of childhood asthma treatment with biologics. Pediatr Allergy Immunol. 2019;30:159–71.
88. Fala L. Nucala (mepolizumab): first IL-5 antagonist monoclonal antibody FDA approved for maintenance treatment of patients with severe asthma. Am Health Drug Benefits. 2016;9:106–10.
89. Ahmed H, Turner S. Severe asthma in children-a review of definitions, epidemiology, and treatment options in 2019. Pediatr Pulmonol. 2019;54:778–87.
90. Castro M, Corren J, Pavord ID, Maspero J, Wenzel S, Rabe KF, Busse WW, Ford L, Sher L, FitzGerald JM, Katelaris C, Tohda Y, Zhang B, Staudinger H, Pirozzi G, Amin N, Ruddy M, Akinlade B, Khan A, Chao J, Martincova R, Graham NMH, Hamilton JD, Swanson BN, Stahl N, Yancopoulos GD, Teper A. Dupilumab efficacy and safety in moderate-to-severe uncontrolled asthma. N Engl J Med. 2018;378:2486–96.
91. de Vos G, Shankar V, Nazari R, Kooragayalu S, Smith M, Wiznia A, Rosenstreich D. Fear of repeated injections in children younger than 4 years receiving subcutaneous allergy immunotherapy. Ann Allergy Asthma Immunol. 2012;109:465–9.
92. Mirabelli MC, Hsu J, Gower WA. Comorbidities of asthma in U.S. children. Respir Med. 2016;116:34–40.
93. Kaplan A, Szefler SJ, Halpin DMG. Impact of comorbid conditions on asthmatic adults and children. NPJ Prim Care Respir Med. 2020;30:36.
94. de Benedictis FM, Bush A. Janus looks both ways: how do the upper and lower airways interact? Paediatr Respir Rev. 2020;34:59–66.
95. Akinbami LJ, Simon AE, Schoendorf KC. Trends in allergy prevalence among children aged 0-17 years by asthma status, United States, 2001-2013. J Asthma. 2016;53:356–62.
96. Knutsen AP, Bush RK, Demain JG, Denning DW, Dixit A, Fairs A, Greenberger PA, Kariuki B, Kita H, Kurup VP, Moss RB, Niven RM, Pashley CH, Slavin RG, Vijay HM, Wardlaw AJ. Fungi and allergic lower respiratory tract diseases. J Allergy Clin Immunol. 2012;129:280–91. quiz 292–3.
97. Bush A. Kids, difficult asthma and fungus. J Fungi (Basel). 2020;6:55.
98. Durrani SR, Mukkada VA, Guilbert TW. Eosinophilic esophagitis: an important comorbid condition of asthma? Clin Rev Allergy Immunol. 2018;55:56–64.
99. Lang JE. Obesity and childhood asthma. Curr Opin Pulm Med. 2019;25:34–43.
100. Dooley AA, Pillai DK. Paediatric obesity-related asthma: disease burden and effects on pulmonary physiology. Paediatr Respir Rev. 2021;37:15–7.
101. Lang JE. Contribution of comorbidities to obesity-related asthma in children. Paediatr Respir Rev. 2021;37:22–9.
102. Landeo-Gutierrez J, Celedon JC. Chronic stress and asthma in adolescents. Ann Allergy Asthma Immunol. 2020;125:393–8.
103. Wood BL, Brown ES, Lehman HK, Khan DA, Lee MJ, Miller BD. The effects of caregiver depression on childhood asthma: pathways and mechanisms. Ann Allergy Asthma Immunol. 2018;121:421–7.
104. Morrison AK, Glick A, Yin HS. Health literacy: implications for child health. Pediatr Rev. 2019;40:263–77.
105. Kaas TH, Vinding RK, Stokholm J, Bonnelykke K, Bisgaard H, Chawes BL. Association between childhood asthma and attention deficit hyperactivity or autism spectrum disorders: a systematic review with meta-analysis. Clin Exp Allergy. 2021;51:228–52.
106. Beasley R, Semprini A, Mitchell EA. Risk factors for asthma: is prevention possible? Lancet. 2015;386:1075–85.

Index

C. Damask et al. (eds.), *Allergy in Otolaryngology Practice*,
https://doi.org/10.1007/978-3-031-93455-1

K

L

MIX
Papier aus verantwortungsvollen Quellen
Paper from responsible sources
FSC® C105338

If you have any concerns about our products,
you can contact us on
ProductSafety@springernature.com

In case Publisher is established outside the EU,
the EU authorized representative is:
Springer Nature Customer Service Center GmbH
Europaplatz 3, 69115 Heidelberg, Germany

Printed by Libri Plureos GmbH
in Hamburg, Germany